VETERINARY CLINICAL DIAGNOSIS

VETERINARY CLINICAL DIAGNOSIS

Second Edition

W. R. KELLY
M.A., M.V.M. (N.U.I.), M.R.C.V.S.

Professor of Medicine, Pharmacology and Food Hygiene,
Faculty of Veterinary Medicine, University College, Dublin

 BAILLIÈRE TINDALL · LONDON

A Baillière Tindall book published by
Cassell & Collier Macmillan Publishers Ltd, London
35 Red Lion Square, London WC1R 4SG
Sydney, Auckland, Toronto, Johannesburg

The Macmillan Publishing Company Inc.
New York

First published 1967
Second edition 1974
Reprinted 1977

ISBN 0 7020 0492 8

Printed Offset Litho in Great Britain by
Cox & Wyman Ltd
London, Fakenham and Reading

Contents

Preface

When I wrote the first edition of this book my purpose was to provide a comprehensive and well illustrated statement of the principles of clinical diagnosis as applied to domestic and farm animals with emphasis on the importance of methodical investigation and the critical evaluation of the clinical information thus obtained. Though primarily written for the student starting on a course of clinical instruction, others, such as more advanced students and general practitioners, have found the book useful and acceptable to them. A further indication of its wide acceptance is the fact that it has been translated into French, German and Spanish. I am pleased to have been able to make this contribution to the harmonization of veterinary education within the E.E.C.

In preparing the new edition, not only was the text thoroughly revised and some new material included, but it was also found necessary to re-arrange some of the material in order to render the sequence more logical, and to take account of the changes that have taken place in the interval since the first edition was published, as witness, for example, the intensification of farm animal production, which necessitates a knowledge and understanding of the disease problems arising from such farming techniques. All the experience gained from this source substantiates the view that modern animal production enterprises require the services of highly specialized and skilful veterinarians.

With the passage of time, existing laboratory-based sophisticated technology is being increasingly modified for use under field conditions, to aid the investigation and diagnosis of animal disease. It has indeed been suggested that the clinician of the future may come to have as high regard for the computer as for his stethoscope. In addition an increasing number of therapeutic agents, which in many instances possess a powerful but limited range of specificity, are now available to the veterinarian. Although rising costs are a constraint on both the over-application of laboratory procedures and excessive exuberance in prescribing therapeutic substances, both these aspects demand accuracy in diagnosis, which is best achieved by the application of clinical procedures in a careful and orderly manner. By these means all the circumstances of the individual animal or group will receive that measure of consideration necessary to the establishment of the diagnosis.

Newer concepts which must occupy the attention of the veterinarian arise in respect of the use of those chemotherapeutic agents or agricultural chemicals from which the problems of bacterial resistance and/or chemical residues in animal products arise.

Although the basic principles of veterinary clinical methodology and diagnosis do not change in any significant degree, the rapid expansion in knowledge of disease situations, and the increasing use of aids to diagnosis render it necessary to keep written texts in harmony with recent developments. This, in itself was an important motivating force in the preparation of a new edition of the book. Many other influences, however, were also at work, and acted as a stimulus providing encouragement throughout the long period given to the revision of the manuscript.

My sincere thanks are due, therefore, to a great many persons, all of whom assisted in a variety of ways. In the preface to the first edition I acknowledged the assistance of many kind friends in North America and elsewhere with regard to the provision of illustrative material and the preparation of the text. I hereby further record my indebtedness to them all, more particularly to those who supplied helpful and constructive comment relating to the substance and format of the first edition. In this context, almost all the critiques which appeared in scientific journals were also found to be helpful. I thank those persons who prepared them.

Almost all the illustrations in the previous edition have been retained. To all those concerned in supplying them I record my continuing appreciation. For new illustrative material I am indebted to the American Optical Company for the photographs for Figs 166 and 199.

For the remainder of the new illustrations I am obliged to my colleagues Mr B. A. McErlean, Mr J. D. Collins, Mr T. T. Twomey, Mr T. D. Grimes, Mr T. O'Nuallain, Dr K. Dodd and Mr J. P. O'Connor. Mr J. K. Kealy supplied the radiographs from which Figs 113, 124, 177, 204, 234 and 235 were prepared, and Dr L. N. Gleeson provided the instruments illustrated in Fig. 116. All the photographic work involved was undertaken by Mr C. J. King.

My wife has continued to give devoted assistance during the preparation and typing of the manuscript. Mr B. A. McErlean provided assistance of inestimable value by reading the finished proofs. To everyone concerned, including all the unnamed persons I consulted, who also contributed to the production of this book, I extend my sincere thanks.

In conclusion, it gives me great pleasure to record my appreciation of the forbearance shown, and kindly assistance provided by Mr R. F. West, and to express my thanks to all the other persons on the staff of Baillière Tindall who were concerned with the preparation of the book.

Dublin, November 1973   W. R. KELLY

1

General Consideration of Clinical Problems and Methods

Introduction

In the investigation of any animal disease problem, the veterinarian must, of necessity, undertake a careful and thorough clinical examination with the object of recognizing the nature of the affection, so that effective treatment and, where practicable, control measures are adopted. The situation is rendered complex by the necessity to deal with a variety of species of domestic animals and birds, with, in more recent years, the addition of a variety of exotic animal pets and fish. It is hoped that, with the passing of time, increasing specialization on the part of practising veterinarians will resolve some of the apparent problems thus presented. In general, however, the same principles may be applied in all cases to deal with the diverse difficulties that clinical diagnosis presents. It must be emphasized at the outset that performing a clinical examination involves a great deal more than directing attention to the patient; consideration must also be given to the past and the immediate circumstances of the animal, and to the environment. Not infrequently careful consideration of all these facets of a disease situation leads to the emergence of information, otherwise likely to have been overlooked, which significantly assists the diagnosis. All the relevant observations accruing from such a planned investigation should be carefully recorded for final analysis. The tyro clinician is well advised to adopt the habit of recording clinical data as the soundest basis for expanding the individual's experience and expertise.

The application of clinical methods in a systematic manner enables the veterinarian, on the basis of a sound knowledge of anatomy, physio-

logy, pathology and animal behaviour (ethology), to recognize ailing, as distinct from healthy, animals. Obviously an important requisite is complete familiarity with the state of health in all species. The presence of disease is revealed by certain changes in the structure of an organ or tissue and/or its function, as well as in the behaviour of the whole living organism. Such changes, which may be quantitative, qualitative or both, are described as the clinical signs of disease, and the process of deducing from them the nature of the disease that is present is described as 'making a diagnosis'.

It is not always possible to make an exact diagnosis, that is to establish not only the site, but also the cause and nature of the abnormality, but a special effort should be made to establish at least the aetiological diagnosis, i.e. to determine the cause of the disease, for without this knowledge treatment cannot be other than empirical. If the disease is not recognizable with certainty, the diagnosis is said to be tentative. If a particularly prominent clinical sign is present, but the site and cause of the primary abnormality are unknown, a so-called symptomatic diagnosis may have to suffice, e.g. jaundice, which is not a disease but only a clinical sign of a variety of diseased conditions, including obstruction of bile ducts, certain protozoan infections of the blood and, among others, some of those diseases which cause toxic damage to the liver. Whenever possible the diagnosis should be based on a rational consideration of all the evidence available from the three facets of any disease situation; such a reasoned conclusion will enable the most useful and worthwhile aids to diagnosis to be selected. It must be said, however, that in veterinary medicine all too many diagnoses are made on the basis of previous experience; the method breaks down when the clinical pattern of a disease changes to an unusual one or a new disease is seen for the first time.

'Giving a prognosis' means expressing an opinion as to the probable duration and outcome of the disease. The owner is interested, chiefly, in the prognosis; that is to say, he wishes to know whether an early recovery is to be expected, whether the animal will be restored to its original usefulness, and so on. For the veterinarian, however, the diagnosis is of primary importance because only this knowledge will enable him to give the required prognosis and, when necessary, to provide treatment or institute control or prophylactic measures.

There are very few individual clinical signs on the existence of which a diagnosis can be accurately based. These are known as pathognomonic signs (e.g. positive venous pulse in tricuspid insufficiency; rusty-brown watery nasal discharge in the exudative stage of infectious equine pneumonia; prolapse of the membrana nictitans in tetanus in the horse). If only pathognomonic clinical signs had to be considered, the technique of clinical diagnosis could easily be mastered. However, since the majority of clinical signs may arise from a variety of causes, diagnosis demands, in every individual case, the application of precise knowledge and intellectual effort, along with practical experience, in a rational way.

It will be clear from what has already been said that the study of clinical signs as such (clinical propaedeutics) is a necessary preliminary to the study of diagnosis. The student must therefore make himself familiar with the appearance of the various clinical signs in each species, the methods of demonstrating or eliciting them where necessary, their possible origin and their significance.

Methods used in the Detection of Clinical Signs

The clinical examination is performed by means of the senses of sight, touch, hearing and smell, and is comprised of two major parts: (a) the general and particular examination including the initial inspection and (b) the physical examination.

The preliminary general inspection, which is carried out some distance away from the animal, should never be omitted, and might best be undertaken during the period devoted to obtaining the history of the case and taking note of the environment. The outer surface of the body and the external orifices are also examined with the unaided eye at a somewhat later stage of the proceedings. The interior of hollow viscera, not otherwise visible from the exterior, can be examined (endoscopy) with the aid of instruments with built-in illumination, collectively known as endoscopes. Radiological apparatus also enables certain of the internal structures of the body to be visualized.

The techniques used in the physical examination are as follows:

Palpation

This includes direct palpation which consists of handling the tissues by means of the fingers, for which one or both hands may be employed, and indirect palpation with a probe. The object of palpation is to detect the presence of pain in a tissue by noting increased sensitivity. Other important pathological changes that may be detected in an organ or tissue by this means include variation in size, shape, consistency and temperature. The conditions identified by palpation may be defined by terms such as the following: resilient, when a structure quickly resumes its normal shape after the application of pressure has ceased; doughy, when pressure causes pitting as in oedema; firm, when the resistance to pressure is similar to that of the normal liver; hard, when the structure possesses bone-like consistency; fluctuating, when a wave-like movement is produced in a structure by the application of alternate pressure (see p. 78); or emphysematous, when the structure is swollen and yields on pressure with the production of a crepitating or crackling sound.

Percussion

This is a physical method of examination in which, by means of striking a part of the body, it is possible to obtain information about the condition of the surrounding tissues and, more particularly, the deeper lying parts. The value of the method arises from the vibrations imparted at the point of impact producing audible sounds, which vary when reflected back, because of the difference in density of the tissues. Percussion is used mainly for the examination of the thorax (lungs, heart), but it is also employed in relation to diseases of the abdominal cavity, paranasal sinuses, in subcutaneous emphysema, etc.

The traditional method of carrying out percussion in large animals is by means of a circular or oval, ivory or hardwood plate (a pleximeter) and a hammer with a firm rubber end (a percussion hammer or plexor)—hammer–pleximeter percussion. The fingers may be used instead of a pleximeter disc.

In small animals, percussion is performed by using both hands, the middle finger of one hand acting as a pleximeter and the flexed middle finger of the other hand as a hammer (finger–finger percussion). If desired the finger may be used to strike a pleximeter or a hammer to strike the finger. The use of the fingers is always preferable in animals of any size as they produce little or no additional sound. When the finger, or a pleximeter, is placed over the area being struck the procedure is termed *mediate percussion*; striking the part directly with the fingertips, which is the method most commonly employed, is termed *immediate percussion*.

The diagnostic value of percussion in large animals is rather limited because the internal organs are too large, and the overlying tissues (muscles, subcutaneous fat) in many instances too thick, to recognize the limits of the organs or abnormal areas, unless the clinician is highly experienced. The presence of subcutaneous fat in the pig, and the wool coat in the sheep, makes the application of percussion impracticable in these species.

General rules to be observed while applying percussion:

1. The pleximeter, or finger when serving the same purpose in the mediate method, must be pressed firmly against the body surface, so that no air space exists between the pleximeter and skin.

2. The hand using the hammer must be at a higher level than the hand holding the pleximeter. The handle of the hammer must not be held too firmly, but must rest loosely between the thumb and first two fingers, in order to deliver a swinging blow. The movement should come from the wrist, and not from the elbow or shoulder. When the finger acts as a striker the hands should be held in the same relative position and the movement should involve the wrist.

3. The blows should fall perpendicularly on to the pleximeter, or directly on to the part of the body being examined, because blows delivered from any other angle will evoke a response which may lead to misinterpretation.

4. The whole of the area requiring examination should be percussed in a systematic manner, and not only in isolated places, otherwise localized pathological changes in the structure of underlying tissues or organs may not be detected.

5. When the mediate method is employed the pleximeter should be struck only when it is stationary. It is then moved a distance equal to its own width, blows of equal force being delivered at each point.

6. The force of the blows should be no heavier than is necessary; the lighter they are, within reason, the easier it is to distinguish differences in resonance.

Strong percussion is used in the examination of deeply situated structures, and weak percussion for those more superficially situated. Very gentle percussion (threshold percussion), when applicable, yields particularly accurate information.

Modified forms of percussion include ballottement and fluid percussion. In the former an interrupted, firm push-stroke is applied to an appropriate part of the body with the object of evoking motion in the underlying organ and causing it to rebound on to the fingertips. Identifying the presence of the fetus in advanced pregnancy in the ox is achieved by this technique. The latter enables free fluid in a body cavity to be recognized by percussing the surface of the body on one side, and detecting the fluid wave produced by palpation of the opposite side.

These rules are intended only for general guidance. Percussion requires much practice, and its value depends on experience, and when instruments are used, familiarity with a particular one is most important. Other general factors, for which allowance must be made in the interpretation of the results of percussion, are the thickness of the body wall and the amount of air or gas in the underlying viscus; in the area of the thorax, percussion over a rib must not be compared with percussion on an intercostal space.

The quality of the sounds produced by percussion are classified as: resonant, which is characteristic of the sound emitted by air containing organs, such as the lungs; tympanic, the sound produced by striking a hollow organ containing gas under pressure, e.g. tympanitic

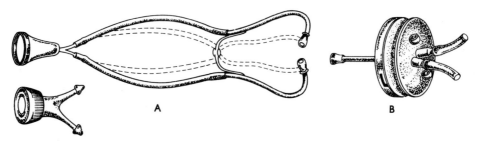

Fig. 1. *Instruments used in auscultation. A, Flexible binaural stethoscope with a diaphragm or a rubber ring on the chest-piece. B, A phonendoscope chest-piece with a diaphragm pedestal.*

rumen or caecum; dull, emitted by a solid organ like the liver or heart.

Auscultation

Auscultation means listening to the sounds produced by the functional activity of an organ located within a part of the body, in order to assess its condition. The method is used chiefly in the examination of the lungs, trachea, heart and certain parts of the alimentary tract.

Auscultation may be performed by either the direct or the indirect method. The indirect method, employing a suitable stethoscope (Fig. 1A), is the more preferable and, with adequate experience, will ensure more uniform results than the direct method. In veterinary practice, the flexible binaural stethoscope is the one most commonly employed. It consists of a chest-piece connected by fairly thick-walled, flexible rubber tubing (plastic tubing allows the entry of ex-

traneous environmental sounds, and some loss of functional sounds) to two ear-pieces. The chest-piece, which is acoustically designed, is shaped like an open bell and should have a rubber rim, the purpose of which is to eliminate friction between the chest-piece and the hair of the animal's coat. For large animals, a chest-piece about 2·5 cm or so in diameter is satisfactory, but for cats, puppies and small dogs, the size of chest-piece used for human infants is preferable. The phonendoscope (Fig. 1B) resembles the stethoscope in general appearance, but its chest-piece, which may be up to 5 cm in diameter, is surmounted by a hard plastic diaphragm which is placed in contact with the surface of the body. Since the skin is thickly covered with hair in most animals, the resultant frictional sounds seriously interfere with auscultation. There is provision, with the more elaborate phonendoscopes, for fitting on an

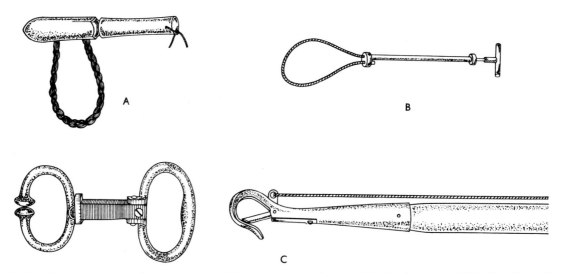

Fig. 2. *Aids to restraint.* A, *A lip or nose twitch for the horse.* B, *A loop twitch for the pig.* C, *Bull holders for cattle.*

additional diaphragm with a screw-in pedestal mount, which enables the clinician to identify functional sounds arising from restricted areas, such as the heart valves in large animals. For all general purposes, however, a stethoscope of the type described is to be preferred in veterinary clinical work. A detailed description of the normal and abnormal sounds heard during auscultation of the various organs will be given later in the appropriate parts of the text.

Direct auscultation is performed by placing the ear in contact with the body surface over the organ to be examined. The disadvantages of the method are obvious and include difficulty in maintaining contact in restless animals, friction sounds which arise from opposing movements between the clinician and the coat of the animal, difficulty in excluding extraneous sounds arising from the immediate environment of the animal, the coat of the animal may be wet, soiled with dirt, faeces or skin secretions, or the skin may harbour ectoparasites such as ticks, fleas, lice, mange mites, ringworm fungi or bacteria potentially pathogenic to man.

Methods of Restraint

Since animals often resist many of the clinical examination procedures, it may be necessary to employ some suitable means of restraint, in order to be able to carry out the examination safely and without danger to the clinician or his assistants. The methods available may be classified as physical restraint when various instruments are employed (Fig. 2) or chemical restraint when drugs inducing varying degrees of sedation or immobilization are administered.

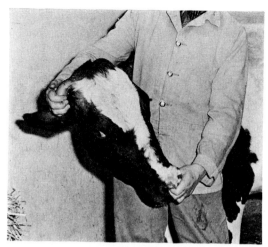

Fig. 4. *Restraining a cow by grasping the nasal septum and one horn.*

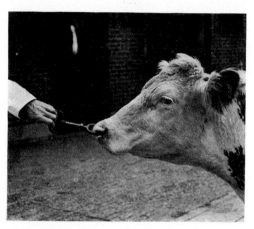

Fig. 5. *Restraining a cow by means of a bull holder.*

In the horse, a twitch is applied to the upper or lower lip or to the ear (Fig. 3); a loop of strong cord or soft rope is applied to the appropriate part and twisted up tightly enough to cause just sufficient pain to distract the animal's attention away from the part of the body being examined. It is sometimes useful to cover the eyes with the hands or to place a sack over the head as a hood or blind.

In the ox, both horns are held or tied to a strong post, or the nasal septum is gripped between the thumb and one finger (Fig. 4) or with 'bull-dogs' (Fig. 5); leg twitches are also employed. In the horse and ox, in order to obtain protection against kicks from the hindfoot, the forefoot is held up in the flexed position on the side on which the clinician is standing. In

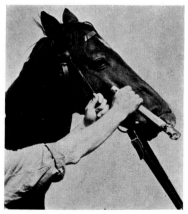

Fig. 3. *The nose twitch in use.*

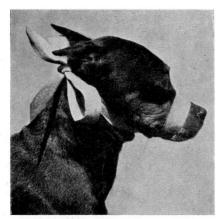

Fig. 6. *The use of the tape muzzle.*

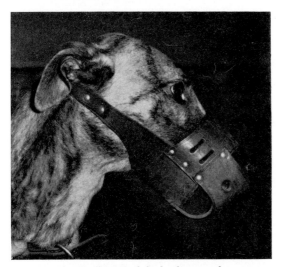

Fig. 7. *The use of the leather muzzle.*

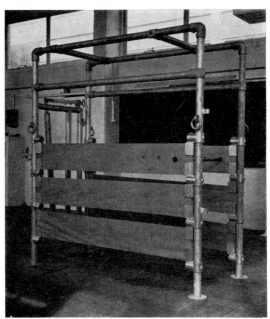

Fig. 8. *Stocks with removable wooden side boards, a yoke type gate and a retaining bar.*

the cow an udder kinch (see Fig. 181, p. 257) may be used for the same purpose. The pig is restrained by means of a wire or rope twitch (see Fig. 188, p. 264), or a pair of blunt tongs applied to the upper jaw or snout, or by confining it in a corner with a small gate or hurdle. Small animals are restrained by placing them on a table in the upright, lateral or dorsal position. In most instances the owner will assist in handling his pet animal for this purpose. In the dog a tape muzzle (Fig. 6) or a leather muzzle (Fig. 7) is used. For handling parrots or other birds, or animals apt to bite, thick leather gloves are worn.

Sometimes the animal is so refractory, because of fear or pain, that even with the aid of physical restraint examination is unsafe or impracticable. Use must then be made of special aids such as stocks or a crush (Fig. 8), hobbling and casting or the administration of sedative, tranquillizing, narcotic or immobilizing drugs (chemical restraint). Drugs that are useful for this purpose are those with ataractic or tranquillizing properties and include acepromazine, acetylpromazine, chlorpromazine, promazine and trimeprazine; members of this group can be used in most species of animals. Chloral hydrate is used mainly in large animals; its effect varies from sedation to narcosis depending upon the amount given. Morphine also induces narcosis after an initial phase of excitement, which varies in intensity according to the species; because of its excitatory action it is very rarely used for restraint purposes. Of the more recently introduced sedative drugs, azaperone is of especial value in the pig and xylazine in cattle. The morphine derivative, etorphine, is capable of producing profound narcosis and is used when immobilization is desirable. Muscle relaxants such as succinylcholine have been employed for the latter purpose.

Morphine and its derivatives pethidine and etorphine are unsuitable for cats; short-acting anaesthetics of the barbiturate group or the phenothiazine psychotherapeutic drugs are often used in this species.

Needless to say, physical or chemical restraint should, whenever possible, not be applied prior to such preliminary procedures as general observation of the patient, taking the pulse and temperature and noting the character of the respirations. It is important to perform all the physical manipulations in a quiet and gentle manner in order to avoid disturbing the patient.

2

History (Anamnesis)

Disease problems in veterinary medicine are invariably presented to the clinician through the medium of the owner's complaint, which is a request for professional assistance. This provides the opportunity to obtain all the essential information relating to the circumstances of the immediate disease problem. This procedure is termed 'taking the history' and it is a very important—if not the most important—facet of the whole procedure of clinical examination. By means of appropriate questions, phrased in the minimum of technical terms, the veterinarian must try to obtain from the owner or attendant of the animal all the information that will assist the examination and ensure the accuracy of the diagnosis. When a history is being obtained, allowance should be made for the personality, knowledge and ability of the informant to communicate. Generally speaking, the better educated the person concerned, the more likely it is that only accurate observations will be reported.

It is advisable for the clinician to check the validity of the history as related and, when possible, to evaluate and supplement it by making a detailed, systematic examination. An incomplete history can be misleading, and even stock owners themselves may attempt to excuse their neglect to obtain professional help at an earlier stage by grossly understating the length of time the animal has been ill. Whenever possible leading questions should be avoided, and an attempt should be made to establish good rapport by instilling confidence in the person concerned by exhibiting a friendly manner. The confidence of animal owners is most readily gained when the veterinarian is known by repute to provide a prompt and highly efficient service. The ability to obtain a satisfactory history depends upon a thorough knowledge of how animals react to disease, and increases with widening experience. If, at a later stage during the particular clinical examination of the animal, evidence emerges which appears to throw doubt on any aspect of the history, further enquiries should be made in order to clarify the situation. It is not possible to specify all the questions that must be asked in individual cases, but, in general, routine conformity is achieved and all aspects likely to be of significance are covered by applying them under the headings of immediate, past and general history, the latter to include consideration of the environment.

Immediate History

This relates to the sequence of events associated with the period of time that the animal has been ill. It is important to determine the chronological order in which the more important changes in behaviour and in physiological functions were observed. Specific questions should therefore be centred on such aspects as appetite for food or drink, defaecation, urination, respiration, sweating, physical activity, milk production, growth, gait, posture, voice, odour, etc. The questions should be designed to ascertain the degree and nature of any departure from normal in any of these functions.

When a proportion of a group or flock of animals is affected, a typical case should be selected as a basis for establishing the history. Significant information may be obtained, in this situation, from laboratory examination of specimens from a proportion of the living, affected animals, or autopsy investigations in a few selected cases. Information relating to any preceding surgical, therapeutic or prophylactic procedure such as docking, castration, shearing, vaccination or administration of anthelmintics, parasiticides or other chemotherapeutic substances may be important. The nature of the disease might be indicated by assessing the morbidity rate (expressed as the proportion of animals clinically affected compared with the total number at risk) and the mortality rate (the proportion of affected animals which die). It is important to realize that a proportion of animals, in a herd or flock affected by disease, may not themselves manifest overt clinical signs; in the majority of such instances productive capacity is impaired.

Particularly in those countries where therapeutic substances are freely available for treatment of animals, but also elsewhere, it is essential to determine whether any treatment has, in fact, been given and, if so, the nature and dose of the preparation used. Due allowance must be made for the effect of such treatment in modifying the clinical signs of disease. Many of the therapeutic substances now in common use are capable of producing clinical signs (iatrogenic disease) in animals when they are administered in too large doses or for too long a time. It should be remembered that unless the client is known to him, the veterinarian must satisfy himself that he has not been presented with a case that is already receiving professional attention, thus avoiding supersession.

Past History

In this respect, information should be obtained relating to the nature and timing of any previous illness which had affected the individual animal or group. Details regarding clinical features, diagnosis, treatments, morbidity and mortality rates, post mortem observations, etc., should be obtained. It is pertinent, at this juncture, to ascertain the system of animal replacement on the farm or in the home, with the object of determining whether there has been any recent introduction from outside sources. In the event that this has occurred, then further enquiries should be made concerning the health history and status of the source animals. The period for retrospective enquiry may extend to weeks, months or even years according to the information that is made available and the evidence obtained by the clinician.

General History and Consideration of the Environment

The examination of an animal must be accompanied by a consideration of its surroundings and circumstances. This is more necessary in the case of animals in groups than for individual animals, although even in the case of domestic pets the environmental aspects should not be completely overlooked. In this context consideration might be given to the epidemiological significance of the relationship between humans and animals. The consideration of the surroundings and circumstances should include an enquiry into such aspects of animal husbandry as nutrition, breeding policy, housing, etc., which might reveal information of diagnostic significance. In relation to diet, any recent change in character or constitution should be ascertained. This brings into focus the need to determine whether the ailing animal is being house-fed or grazing. Within this context, it is necessary to consider the geographical and seasonal incidence of disease for a particular region. Knowledge of the local topography is of value in relation to vector-borne diseases including louping-ill, babesiasis, anaplasmosis, trypanosomiasis, African horse sickness, Rift Valley fever and blue tongue, etc., and a number of other diseases such as fascioliasis, hypocuprosis, cobalt deficiency, etc. Nutritional diseases are, in most instances, group problems, so that a number of animals are more or less simultaneously affected. Domestic pets, however, are still occasionally found to be suffering from serious nutritional deficiency syndromes.

During the grazing season, a study of the pasture composition, along with identification of specific poisonous species, including ergotized grass or rye, or those which possess the ability selectively to absorb potentially toxic elements (selenium, copper), is advisable in certain circumstances. Stall-fed animals, in comparison with those at pasture, are in most instances fed on a nutritionally balanced diet; the quality of pasture is not easily assessed, so that, with the exception of certain recognized diseases, a nutritional deficiency may exist for quite a time before it is identified. A sudden change from stall to lush pasture feeding, during the spring season, may predispose to hypomagnesaemic tetany or rickets, even though the herbage composition is normal. Grazing animals, more particularly when adolescent, are exposed to the risk of acquiring various parasitic infestations, e.g. various forms of parasitic gastroenteritis in cattle and sheep, lungworm infestation in cattle, strongylosis in horses. By the adoption of improved fertilization programmes and the inclusion of more productive strains of plants, grazing of animals is becoming more intensive, thus increasing the incidence of parasitic diseases. The standard of grassland and grazing stock management of the particular farm should, therefore, receive appropriate consideration, with, where it is thought advisable, an examination of the pasture, grazing control and fodder conservation methods and the conserved fodder.

Housed animals are exposed to the risk of being over- or underfed or of receiving diets which are incomplete or inadequate in respect of some essential constituents. Farm compounded foods are more likely than those commercially produced to be nutritionally inadequate. The quality of the ingredients may have an undesirable effect. Grain of good quality, recognized by weighing heavier per unit volume, may cause digestive disturbance if the ration is compounded on a volume rather than a weight basis. In this context, the proportion of fibre or roughage in the diet of intensively produced animals being fed on cereal diets is a matter of some importance. A sudden change from a high- to a low-fibre, crushed barley diet causes lactic acidaemia in young cattle, unless care is taken to make the change gradually and to ensure an adequate roughage intake. The quality of the conserved fodder should be considered in relation to ragwort or sweet clover poisoning. In the case of ensiled grass, a product which has a high butyric acid content will be a cause of primary ketosis in cattle. Imported foodstuffs, particularly those of animal origin, are a possible source of entry for such conditions as foot-and-mouth disease, swine fever, anthrax and salmonellosis.

The presence of old flaking paint on woodwork, or evidence of recent painting, may be valuable knowledge in relation to lead poisoning in calves. The quality of the drinking water may be important because of possible contamination with organic or inorganic substances, or infective agents, e.g. fluorine in artesian and sub-artesian waters, nitrate in shallow water drained off soil rich in organic matter or contaminated by silage effluent, algae in stagnant pools, ponds

or shallow lakes may contain neurotoxic and hepatotoxic agents, and effluents from industrial processes may contaminate rivers. In the case of a stalled or housed animal, said to be off its food, investigation may reveal that the water supply is polluted or inadequate, or that the fodder within the animal's reach is stale or otherwise unpalatable. An adequate, and where possible continuous, water supply is a prime factor in maintaining animal health and production; in the case of pigs, water deprivation is an essential feature of salt poisoning. Faecal contamination of rivers or streams by grazing cattle is a recognized means of dissemination of salmonellae and other pathogenic bacteria.

Feeding methods should also be investigated because they may contribute to low productivity or disease. Inadequate trough space for pigs and calves and for older cattle in yards leads to overeating on the part of the vigorous animals and partial starvation in the smaller, weaker ones. The design or fittings of a box, stall, pen or kennel may suggest the possibility of certain kinds of injury, or of exposure to draughts or sudden changes in environmental temperature. The state of the bedding may reveal whether the animal has been restless, either moving about aimlessly or circling clockwise or anticlockwise.

In the context of general management there are many factors to be considered, neglect of which can contribute to the development of disease. Adequate hygienic standards are of vital importance in relation to milk production, parturition and the early postnatal period. Other factors of importance in animal health include adequate house space, satisfactory ventilation, reasonable facilities for effluent treatment and disposal and opportunity for exercise. An investigation of the breeding programmes may reveal features of significance when line breeding has led to the appearance of an inherited genetic defect. It is necessary to appreciate that selection for high productivity may result in breeds or families of animals which are more susceptible to certain diseases or which have inherited a greater than normal requirement for a specific nutrient (genototrophic disease). Consideration of the breeding management may reveal features of significance; for instance when calvings are arranged to occur early in the year the incidence of ketosis, hypomagnesaemia and calf scour may be increased. An early lambing programme, more particularly in lowland flocks, may be associated with a high incidence of pregnancy toxaemia.

Climatic conditions have an influence on many diseases. The relationship between temperature, high rainfall and clinical fascioliasis in sheep and cattle is well recognized. Similarly, warmth and humidity have an important influence on the larval stages of the internal nematode parasites which cause gastroenteritis and parasitic bronchopneumonia. Intermittent periods of warm, wet weather and cold moist conditions during the spring season may favour the appearance of hypomagnesaemic tetany in cattle and sheep. A mild, damp spring season may be responsible for the appearance of rachitogenic effects in young grazing animals in particular, because of the high carotene content in the lush pasture. Conversely a period of drought may be sufficiently prolonged to cause vitamin A deficiency in animals grazing the dried-out herbage. Hot, humid weather is associated with anhidrosis in non-indigenous horses and dairy cattle. Contamination of pastures by fumes and other effluents from brick works, ore smelters, aluminium processing plants, mines, etc., is more likely to lead to significant intoxication problems in animals grazing pasture situated in the direction of the prevailing wind or downstream.

3

General Examination of the Patient

Disease processes in the body can be divided into two main groups: those associated with inflammation and those of a non-inflammatory nature (injuries, neoplasms, obstructions, metabolic disorders, nutritional deficiencies, etc.). Inflammatory changes generally give rise to certain characteristic signs—pain, redness (only obvious when it occurs in non-pigmented skin areas), swelling, increased temperature of diseased organs, increased body temperature (fever) and impairment of function. In non-inflammatory processes, swelling and disturbance of function of the diseased organs may likewise occur but, in general erythema, heat and pain are absent. The presence of the last three signs always suggests that the disease has inflammatory characteristics. In acute processes (those running a rapid course) these signs are well marked, but in chronic processes (those running a slow course) they are much less obvious. Not every structural defect or functional change in the body will necessarily result in an obvious disturbance of health. The presence of small tumours in the liver, lung, mammary gland or other organ, although detectable by various means, may produce no overt clinical signs of disease, and the heart may function adequately in spite of minor valvular or functional defects.

Routine for Clinical Examination

Because the patient cannot communicate any verbal information as to the probable situation of the disease, the examination of the ailing animal must always be carried out in such a way that no organ or tissue is omitted from the investigation. In order that nothing is overlooked, it is advisable to carry out the examination according to a routine pattern. The order in which the various parts of the clinical examination are performed is a matter for personal choice, although it is recommended that certain procedures, such as ascertaining body temperature, taking the pulse and determining the respiratory frequency, should be performed before others which involve the risk of unduly disturbing the animal. The systematic scheme followed here can be adopted or modified to meet personal requirements; the essential point is not to omit anything and this is best accomplished by becoming so accustomed to one particular sequence that its use becomes a matter of habit. The best way to reduce errors in diagnosis is always to make a thorough and complete clinical examination. The majority of incorrect diagnoses result from the omission of one or more parts of the examination.

In all cases the history of the patient is thoroughly elucidated in the manner previously described, and a general inspection of the animal and its environment is carried out prior to the general and physical parts of the clinical examination. The general inspection of the animal is important in that it enables the behaviour of the animal to be assessed before it has been unduly disturbed by the near approach of the clinician or the need to apply any form of physical restraint. The value of the general inspection is reduced in animals brought into a strange environment, such as the veterinarian's waiting room or surgery. The following points are important in determining the identity and health status of an animal, and should always be reviewed within the preceding context.

Suggested routine for mammals. The procedure involved in making a clinical examination can usefully be classified into two phases: (a) the general examination which includes the general inspection and (b) the regional and/or systematic examination.

The general clinical examination involves detailed consideration of the following: (1) distinguishing marks; (2) physical condition; (3) general appearance and demeanour; (4) posture; (5) gait; (6) abnormal behaviour; (7) body temperature; (8) pulse; and (9) respiration.

The regional or systematic clinical examination involves the application of the various clinical methods (sensory and physical) to the various regions or systems of the body as follows: (1) coat and skin; (2) head and neck; (3) thorax; (4) abdomen; (5) urinary system; (6) reproductive system; (7) blood and blood-forming organs; (8) nervous system; and (9) musculoskeletal system.

The necessity to perform a detailed examination of any particular part of the body may have been indicated by the information obtained during the general clinical examination. If otherwise, all the component regions and systems, as indicated, may have to be thoroughly explored for evidence of disease. The details relating to the regional and systematic examination are set out in Chapters 7 to 15 of this text.

Distinguishing Marks

The distinguishing features of an animal should be carefully noted at the beginning of the examination when the general inspection is made, in order to establish its identity. This is of particular importance if legal evidence regarding the animal is likely to be required. Accurate identification of the patient is also essential for group disease records, in situations where a repeat visit may be made by a different veterinarian and for accounts purposes. The data required include: name and address of the owner, species, breed (dominant breed characteristics in crossbred animals), sex, age, height or size, colour markings, horned or polled, brands, tattoo marks and permanent blemishes or defects (large scars, blindness, overshot jaw, etc.).

In the horse, it is useful to note also the colour of the hoofs, and whether there are any unpigmented stripes, or defects, such as a false quarter, keratoma or areas of flattening, or even concavity, instead of the normal convexity. The presence of a wall eye (unpigmented iris) or the habit of showing the white (sclera) of the eye should also be noted. In some countries, e.g. the United States of America, racehorses are tattooed on the mucous membrane of the upper lip, and the size and shape of the chestnuts are recorded by means of a photograph. The whorls of hair can also be used as a means of identification; this consists in measuring the distance of the frontal whorl (situated on the upper part of the face just above the eyes) from the origin of the forelock, and of the tracheal whorl (situated on the ventral aspect of the neck) from the junction of the larynx with the first tracheal cartilage.

In cattle, ear tattoo marks, which are usually employed in conjunction with disease eradication programmes such as tuberculosis, brucellosis, etc., as well as for identification by breed societies, provide a ready means of identification. Certain distinctive breeds, such as the Friesian (Holstein), permit the use of a simple black and white colour sketch for easy and accurate identification.

In the dog, the type of coat (long, curly, smooth- or wire-haired), the form of the ears (pendulous, erect or cropped) and the state of the tail (natural or docked) are noted. In this species (and less commonly in the horse and ox) some or all of the coat may have been dyed. This can often be detected by a close examination of individual hairs near the roots; plucking out some of the hairs is usually helpful. For very accurate identification in the dog (e.g. racing greyhounds, foxhounds), and also in the ox, a coloured impression can be taken of the skin of the muzzle, on the same principle as that employed in the identification of persons by means of fingerprints. Note may also be made of the colour of the dog's claws. The written description of an animal may often be made much clearer by means of a simple sketch or photograph.

Observation of the identifying characteristics of the animal is not only necessary for purposes of recognition, but may be of assistance in diagnosis. There are, for example, diseases that occur only in the intact male or female animal (inguinal and scrotal hernia, seen most frequently in young hog pigs and colts, or diseases of the reproductive organs). There are also those which occur chiefly in the young animal (joint-ill, white scour, strangles, blackleg, canine distemper); those related to size (laryngeal paralysis in big horses); those associated with colour of

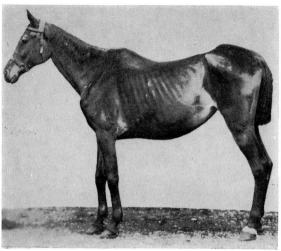

Fig. 9. *Emaciation (cachexia) in a horse after dilatation of the oesophagus.*

the coat, which may be a breed characteristic (melanomas in grey horses or photosensitization which, in cattle, occurs most frequently in the Hereford and Ayrshire breeds); those affecting only certain breeds (progressive retinal atrophy in Irish setters and miniature poodles); and many others. Determination of the age of the patient may be pertinent in relation to the economics of continued treatment, more particularly so in chronic affections.

Physical Condition

It is usually easy to assess the bodily condition of the animal by simple inspection. The method is unsatisfactory only in long-haired or long-wooled animals, in which it is necessary to run the hand over certain parts of the body (ribs, spine, shoulder, pelvis, root of tail). Physical condition may be classified as being normal, obese, thin or emaciated. In normal, well-conditioned animals, all parts of the skeleton are covered with flesh, giving the body a rounded appearance (see Figs 121, 122, p. 117). In those in poor (thin) condition, various parts of the skeleton are prominent (e.g. ribs and pelvis) and the supra-orbital fossae are deepened. The difference between thinness and emaciation is one of degree; in addition, however, the coat is lustreless, staring and dry, the elasticity of the skin is reduced (hidebound) and the mucous membranes are pale and watery. Emaciation (cachexia) is a sign of disease (Fig. 9). Fluctuation in bodily

condition can be most accurately determined by weighing the animal at regular intervals. Changes in bodyweight can occur gradually or with great rapidity. Severe wasting is a common accompaniment of old age (Fig. 10), severe intestinal parasitism and extensive or diffuse neoplasia.

Loss of bodily condition can be caused in various ways. It occurs when too little food is provided or eaten, when too much nutrient material is being metabolized or when the ingested food is inadequately digested or inefficiently utilized following absorption. The following possibilities should be considered: dietary errors; loss of power to prehend food or unwillingness to do so because of pain; chronic wasting diseases, as for example, Johne's disease, cobalt deficiency, parasitic gastroenteritis, fascioliasis, tuberculosis, pyelonephritis, internal neoplasia, etc.; diseases arising from disturbance of metabolism, such as diabetes mellitus; or excessive fluid loss from the body. A tendency towards leanness may be constitutional, hereditary (the influence of high productive capacity, which usually is the cause of leanness in the dairy cow, may originate in this way) or the result of endocrine disease or enzyme deficiency. An animal may be emaciated in spite of a good, even an excessive, appetite, e.g. in chronic nephritis, certain types of pancreatic disease and cerebral disease.

The opposite of emaciation is the excessive

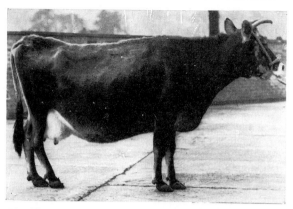

Fig. 10. *Emaciation in a cow as the result of old age. Note also the dropped back, pendulous abdomen and senile alopecia affecting the face.*

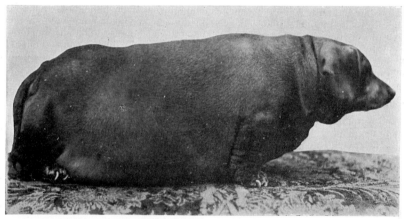

Fig. 11. *Adiposity accompanying thyroid abnormality in a dachshund. Note the gross size of the body, with the abdomen and thorax touching the ground.*

deposition of fat in the body. If this is sufficient to cause systemic disturbances (dyspnoea, etc.), it is described as obesity or adiposity (Fig. 11). In many species, excessive deposition of fat is produced by deliberate overfeeding, as in the case of cattle being fattened prior to slaughter. Even without an excessive intake of food, however, certain diseases, particularly of the endocrine glands (thyroid, pituitary), cause an excess laying down of fat because of reduced basal metabolism. Castration of male and female animals increases deposition of fat. Fat may be laid down over the whole body, or only in certain parts (e.g. in the crest in the stallion, at the base of the tail in the 'fat-tailed sheep).

Gross obesity usually indicates that the cause

has been present for a considerable length of time. Extreme emaciation may also be the result of a chronic process but, as in subacute grass sickness in the horse, it may develop within a week.

The assessment of conformation may be made when physical condition is under consideration. The evaluation is based on the symmetry, shape and relative size of the different body regions. Disproportionate enlargement of the abdomen is the more usual abnormality of conformation seen in animals. Changes in conformation occur in dropsy of the foetal membranes, ascites, chronic exudative peritonitis, rickets and nymphomania. Conformation will be given more detailed consideration in the description of the body regions.

General Demeanour

Both at the beginning and during the course of the clinical examination the general demeanour of the animal should be noted, due allowance being made for age and temperament. In the case of animals in a herd or flock, separation of an individual may be an indication of disease. When, on being approached, an animal makes a normal response to external stimuli, such as movement and sound, the demeanour is said to be bright. Normal reaction under these circumstances may consist of elevating the head and ears, turning towards and directing the attention at the source of the stimuli, walking away and evincing signs of attack or flight.

Various abnormalities of behaviour may be exhibited, including dullness or apathy, which state is appreciated by the reactions to normal stimuli being sluggish or retarded, or even somewhat suppressed. The so-called 'dummy' state is an advanced degree of failure to respond to external stimuli although the animal remains standing and is capable of movement. It occurs in liver fibrosis and encephalomyelitis in the horse, and in listeriosis and occasional cases of lead poisoning and ketosis in cattle. The most advanced degree of apathy is coma, in which the animal is unconscious and fails to respond to painful stimuli, as in the cow in the advanced stages of parturient hypocalcaemia. Increased responsiveness to external and other stimuli varies in degree from mild to frenzied. When mildly anxious, or apprehensive, the animal appears alert, looks about constantly, but exhibits normal movements. Behaviour of this type is an expression of slight constant pain, or of anxiety, as in serious defects of vision or the early stages of parturient hypocalcaemia. Restlessness is a more severe state in which movement is almost constant, consisting of lying down, rolling, getting up again, looking at the flanks, kicking at the belly and groaning or bellowing. This form of behaviour is usually caused by sharp intermittent or constant pain, as in the colic syndrome in the horse. The more extreme forms of abnormal behaviour include mania and frenzy. In mania the behaviour aberrations appear to be compulsive and include vigorous licking of some specific part of the body surface (ketosis, pseudorabies), pressing forwards with the head (meningitis) or licking or chewing inanimate objects. When frenzied, the animal's actions are uncontrolled as in acute lead poisoning, hypomagnesaemic tetany and rabies. When death is imminent, animals may show anxiety with a fixed, haggard expression.

Posture

When approached in the lying position, most normal animals will get up. Various abnormalities of posture may be shown by animals, some of which do not indicate disease, but if they occur in association with other clinical signs then a disease process should be suspected. Changes in posture take the form of curvature of the spine, high or oblique carriage of the head and neck, unusual position of the limbs, etc. Most of these postural aberrations may arise from a variety of abnormalities; their origin can, therefore, be determined only by appropriate further examination of the organs and systems concerned. Diseases of the following structures have to be considered: bones,

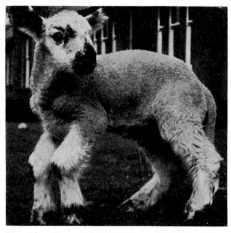

Fig. 12. *Abnormal posture caused by inability to extend the knees. Note the swelling of the carpal joints. Streptococcal arthritis.*

joints (Fig. 12), ligaments, tendons (Fig. 13), tendon sheaths, bursae, muscles, nervous system, ears, skin, hoofs and claws. Change of posture which does not indicate disease is seen in debilitated or tired horses, when they rest the limbs alternately, placing one foot on its toe, with the heel elevated and the fetlock joint flexed, a little in front of the corresponding one. When affected with laminitis, or during the early stages of osteodystrophia fibrosa, the horse continually shifts its weight from limb to limb. The presence of abdominal pain may be

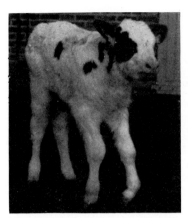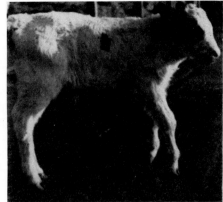

Fig. 13. *Abnormal posture caused by inability to extend the fetlock joints. Congenital contracture of the flexor tendons.*

indicated by the animal arching its back (Fig. 14), placing the feet more closely together when standing still, depressing the back and moving the feet more widely apart. The postural behavioural signs associated with abdominal pain in animals are not very characteristic in most species, except in the horse in which various changes in posture are part of the abnormal behaviour patterns giving rise to the clinical syndrome termed colic.

In acute gastric distension in the horse, pain and pressure on the diaphragm cause the animal to adopt the 'dog sitting' posture in association with periodic rolling and vigorous kicking at its belly. Pain in the chest, or difficulty in breathing, gives rise to obvious abduction of the elbows. As the result of increased muscle tone, animals affected with tetanus show erection and rigidity of the ears, restricted limb movements, immobilization of the eyelids and partial elevation and rigidity of the tail. Sheep, during the early stages of pregnancy toxaemia and scrapie, adopt a characteristic posture with the head in an elevated position and the ears pricked (listening attitude). In painful, unilateral conditions of the pharyngeal region, the head and neck are extended (see Fig. 108, p. 103) or held to one side. Abnormal posture may arise from a developmental defect (Fig. 15).

The recumbent animal may also manifest postural abnormality. Cattle affected with parturient hypocalcaemia often lie in sternal recumbency with the head deviated towards the flank. Sheep, similarly affected, assume the same posture but the hindlegs are extended posteriorly

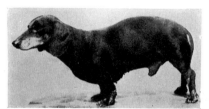

Fig. 14. *Arching of the back (kyphosis). Acute nephritis.*

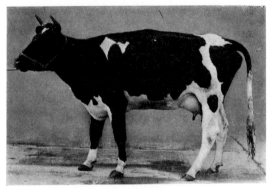

Fig. 15. *Congenital curvature of the spine (roach back) in a Friesian (Holstein) cow. Health is usually otherwise undisturbed.*

in a frog-like attitude; in cattle this latter position is indicative of bilateral hip dislocation. In cattle affected by unilateral sciatic nerve paralysis or dislocation of the hip the affected limb sticks out in an awkward position.

Gait

Locomotor disturbances are seen when the animal moves about voluntarily, or is led or driven at various paces past, towards or away from the clinician. Limb movements can be assessed by reference to their rate, range, force and direction. Abnormal movements include lameness, stiffness, shortened stride, stilted gait, exaggerated flexion (Fig. 16), abduction of one

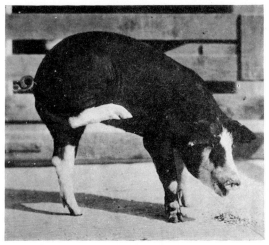

Fig. 16. *Goose-stepping gait. Moderate pantothenic acid deficiency.* (Nutritional Deficiencies in Livestock. FAO Agricultural Studies No 5)

or more limbs, stumbling, staggering, swaying of the hindquarters, forced movements, and so on. The locomotor disturbance may be constantly or only intermittently present, and may gradually disappear or become more pronounced with exercise.

As might be expected, locomotion is affected in many developmental diseases of the nervous system, including the following: swayback; enzootic ataxia; cerebellar hypoplasia, an hereditary disease occurring in calves of the Hereford, shorthorn, Guernsey and Holstein breeds; cerebellar atrophy of lambs; inherited ataxia of calves and in poisoning with *Claviceps paspali*, in all of which all qualities of limb movements are abnormal. In louping ill, affected sheep manifest a high-stepping hackney-like gait with occasional jumping movements in which all four feet are off the ground simultaneously. Walking in circles is a characteristic feature of gid and listeriosis in sheep (it also occurs periodically in ketosis and pregnancy toxaemia); it is usually associated with rotation or lateral deviation of the head. Changes in gait also occur in diseases primarily affecting muscles (blackleg, muscular

dystrophy, azoturia), bones (rickets, osteomalacia, neoplasia), joints (bacterial arthritides, osteo-arthritis) and feet (foot-and-mouth disease, 'fouls', footrot). Abnormalities of gait due to muscle dysfunction may be inherited as in inherited spastic paresis of cattle, a condition affecting calves of the Holstein, Aberdeen Angus, Red Danish and a number of German breeds. The calves are normal at birth, the signs appearing when they are several weeks to six months of age. Due to hypertonicity of the gastrocnemius muscle the hock is straightened and the affected limb is thrust backwards when the calf is walking and then advanced with a swinging motion. Compulsive movement in a forwards direction occurs in the 'dummy' syndrome characteristic of liver disease and encephalomyelitis in the horse.

It should be remembered, however, that the origin of a locomotor disturbance may lie outside the nervous or musculoskeletal system, as in laminitis in the horse, which is basically an allergic reaction to certain proteins present in cereal foods, or derived from the placenta, if retained; in cattle the disease occurs occasionally as a sequel to metritis, mastitis, retained placenta and mammary oedema. When animals are inspected indoors, the nature of the flooring should be taken into consideration. Very young pigs, for example, may have difficulty in keeping their feet on the smooth bare concrete floor sometimes seen in heated creeps.

Abnormal Behaviour

Departure from normal behaviour on the part of the animal should be considered of clinical significance, and warranting further investigation. In many cases, unusual behaviour arises from a pain stimulus. Abdominal pain is indicated by grunting, groaning, grinding the teeth, whining, looking round at the flank, etc. The signs are not very characteristic in most species except in the horse, which has a distinctive way of indicating the presence of abdominal pain. This is spoken of as colicky pain or an attack of colic. From an appreciation of the nature of the abnormal behaviour, certain diagnostic information can be deduced. In an attack of colic, its severity, duration and the assumption of abnormal postures are noted. In a mild attack, the horse looks round at the flank (Fig. 17), kicks at the abdomen, swishes the tail and lies down for short periods (mild intestinal spasm, catarrhal

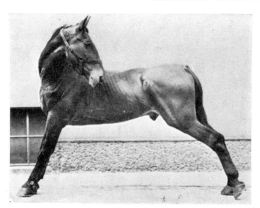

Fig. 17. *Extension of the fore- and hindlegs, and looking round at the flank. Colicky pain in severe impaction of the caecum.*

enteritis, recent obstruction of the small colon). In an attack of moderate severity, the horse is restless, frequently lies down and occasionally rolls, but usually gets up immediately (obstruction of the large colon, intestinal tympany). In a severe attack, the animal behaves recklessly, throws itself to the ground, rolls frequently, remains lying on its back for variable periods, runs against the wall, walks aimlessly, frequently injures itself and is dangerous to approach (intestinal volvulus, strangulated hernia, severe spasm of the intestine). The whole attack may be short, lasting for about 15 minutes, or prolonged, lasting for several hours or a day or more. It may be continuous (volvulus, strangulated hernia, intussusception) or there may be short or long remissions, sometimes for as long as a day (impaction of the large colon). Shortly before death, however, when a state of collapse is present, although pain is very severe, the animal stands quietly and is rigid and unmoving.

In certain types of equine colic, characteristic postures may be assumed, for example standing with both fore- and hindlimbs extended, which is a behavioural sign in severe impaction of the large colon and of the caecum (Fig. 17) and in large tumours in the abdomen (when this is accompanied by protrusion of the penis, it may be an indication of urethral obstruction); the dog may occasionally adopt this posture for brief periods when there is partial obstruction of the colon caused by volvulus or intussusception. Sitting on the haunches, like a dog, is seen in horses affected with gastric distension, and kneeling, particularly in volvulus.

Care must be exercised, in the horse, to differentiate between the pain manifestations arising from alimentary disorders (true colic) and those associated with other diseases such as pleurisy, certain genitourinary diseases, etc. (false colic).

Heavily pregnant stalled cattle, particularly after a full meal, may stand with their hindlegs extended backwards into the dung channel, in order to reduce the pressure of the abdominal viscera on the diaphragm. When recumbent, such animals may grunt slightly at each expiration for considerable periods. Neither of these manifestations, which are indicative of slight discomfort only, should be mistaken for a sign of abdominal pain.

Involuntary movements are responsible for more or less obvious changes in normal behavioural patterns; they include tremor and convulsions. Tremor is a persistent, repetitive twitching of the skeletal muscles; it may be localized or generalized and is often visible, but is always detectable by palpation. As a rule active movement by the affected animal intensifies the tremor. Convulsions may involve the whole or only a part of the body, and consist of violent muscular contractions which usually continue for short periods with intermissions of variable duration, or they may appear to be continuous, as in late stages of many acute encephalitides. Clonic convulsions, in which repeated muscle spasms are interspersed with periods of relaxation, occur much more frequently than tonic convulsions, which occur chiefly in strychnine poisoning and tetanus, and consist of continuous muscle spasm which may be intensified periodically to become clonic.

Bad habits or vices are often expressed in distinctive behaviour. Vices include persistent refractoriness while being led, ridden or worked; jibbing (balking); restiveness during saddling; undue sensitivity of the head, shying at apparently imaginary objects; jealousy with food; viciousness; weaving (swaying from one forefoot to the other); urinary incontinence in the dog. Although such behaviour is usually regarded as being habitual, it may sometimes be pathological. Viciousness and balking in the mare may be associated with ovarian cysts; urinary incontinence in the dog with disease of the bladder, kidneys or spinal cord, and in the bitch with hormonal imbalance following ovaro-hysterectomy; resentment of saddling in the horse with disease of the withers or saddle area; shying with defective vision, and so on. Certain vices may have an hereditary basis.

Other forms of abnormal behaviour originate from the acts of eating, defaecation and urination. Such conduct will be considered in detail in the appropriate section of the text. In order to extend the information available in the context of the immediate history, it is pertinent at this juncture, however, to ascertain the state of the appetite for food and water. If the animal has retained its appetite, variation in the quantity of food consumed may have been observed, along with abnormality of prehension, mastication or swallowing; in cattle, the frequency and character of rumination may be abnormal. The frequency of defaecation and the character of the faeces may have been observed to be abnormal; the faeces, if available, should always be exa-

mined. Similar consideration should be given to the act of urination. Cattle and sheep affected with foot-and-mouth disease salivate excessively and, as the result of jaw movements during attempts to swallow the saliva, produce a smacking noise in the case of cattle, and an abrupt snapping sound in the case of sheep. The act of defaecation may be difficult, and accompanied by straining with groaning (tenesmus) (see Fig. 151, p. 189) in conditions giving rise to constipation, and in paralysis of the rectum or colon, or stenosis of the rectum. In painful abdominal diseases, e.g. peritonitis, acute nephritis, etc., and inflammatory conditions of the anal region, defaecation is difficult and painful. Straining movements may also be caused by abnormalities in the urinary tract, e.g. partial obstruction of the urethra, and in the genital tract, e.g. infectious pustular vulvovaginitis of cattle.

4

Temperature

Higher animals (birds and mammals) are homeothermal, i.e. they maintain their internal or deep body temperature independently of that of the environment, within relatively narrow limits, by means of the central thermoregulating mechanism in the anterior hypothalamic area of the brain. Maximal temperature regulation against heat or cold is achieved by the combined action of peripheral thermoreceptors, situated in the skin and certain mucous membranes, and central thermodetectors in the anterior hypothalamus. The thermoregulatory mechanisms consist of neural and hormonal components. A subnormal body temperature causes a considerable increase in the secretion of adrenaline and of thyroxine, the latter being mediated by release of thyrotropic hormone from the anterior pituitary gland. An elevated body temperature has the reverse effect.

Heat production in the body results from intracellular oxidative and other processes, but is added to from the exterior by radiation, conduction and convection. The liver and heart produce heat constantly at a fairly uniform rate, but the muscles, when active, are the site of greatest heat production, contributing some 80% of the total. Insurance against overheating is provided by the physical phenomena of radiation, conduction and convection, as well as by vaporization of water from the skin and respiratory system, and the excretion of faeces and urine.

Internal Temperature

The temperature of the body, as measured by the clinical thermometer, is not indicative of the total amount of heat being produced; it only reflects the balance (steady state) existing between heat production and heat loss. The temperature of the surface of the body is usually lower than that of the deeper parts. This temperature gradient is important in relation to heat loss.

Although rectal temperature does not invariably indicate the body temperature in animals, it is the most convenient site at which to obtain this measurement. The determination is made by means of a short blunt-bulb clinical thermometer (see Fig. 190, p. 266) which records the highest temperature reached. Its range should be from about 36°C (97°F) to 42·5°C (108°F). The temperature is taken by first shaking the mercury in the column of the thermometer down below the lowest point likely to be recorded. This is achieved by means of a wrist flicking action with the thermometer held between the thumb and first two fingers. The bulb end of the thermometer should then be lubricated with soap or petroleum jelly prior to being gently inserted, with a rotary action, through the anal sphincter into the rectum. Care should be taken to ensure that the bulb of the thermometer is inserted to a constant depth in each particular species of animal and that it makes contact with the mucous membrane of the rectum; in order to obtain an accurate determination of the body temperature the instrument should be left in place for about 2 minutes. If there is any doubt about the validity of the reading obtained the temperature should be retaken. In circumstances where it is considered unlikely that an accurate temperature reading can be obtained from the rectum, e.g. because of atony of the anal sphincter or the presence of large masses of faeces (rectal paralysis), it can be taken, in the case of female animals, in the vagina, where it is

TABLE 1. NORMAL RECTAL TEMPERATURES

Animal	Temperature (°C)		Temperature (°F)	
	Range	Average	Range	Average
Horse, adult draught	37·2–38·0	37·6	99·0–100·5	99·7
Foal	37·5–38·6	38·0	99·5–101·5	100·5
Ox, over 1 year	37·8–39·2	38·5	100·0–102·5	101·3
Calf, up to 1 year	38·6–39·8	39·2	101·5–103·5	102·5
Sheep	38·9–40·0	39·5	102·0–104·0	103·1
Goat	38·6–40·2	39·4	101·5–104·5	102·9
Pig, adult	37·8–38·9	38·3	100·0–102·0	100·9
Piglet	38·9–40·0	39·4	102·0–104·0	102·9
Dog, small breeds	38·6–39·2	38·9	101·5–102·5	102·0
Dog, large breeds	37·5–38·6	38·0	99·5–101·5	100·4
Cat	37·8–39·2	38·5	100·0–102·5	101·3
Silver fox	38·9–41·0	39·9	102·0–106·0	103·8
Chinchilla	37·0–38·4	37·6	98·4–101·0	99·7
Rabbit	38·9–40·5	39·8	102·0–105·0	103·6
Guinea pig	37·5–39·4	38·4	99·5–103·0	101·1

approximately 0·5°C (1°F) higher than in the rectum.

The temperature values given in Table 1 are applicable only when the animal is at rest, the environmental temperature and humidity moderate and the ventilation satisfactory. The smaller the species the higher the normal temperature of the body. Female, pregnant and young animals have a higher normal temperature than male, non-pregnant and old animals. Some animals appear to possess a protective tolerance to low environmental temperatures, consisting of a mechanism which permits their body temperature to fall, thereby reducing the temperature gradient. Neonatal lambs, when subjected to cold, have been shown to survive low body temperatures for 48–72 hours, probably by a readjustment of the hypothalamic thermoregulator. Young piglets affected with neonatal hypoglycaemia characteristically have subnormal body temperatures. In this case the hypothermia is probably the direct result of inadequate energy supplies.

In all healthy animals the temperature varies during the day, being at its lowest in the early morning, somewhat higher in the middle of the day, and at its peak at about 6 P.M. (up to 0·8°C or 1·5°F higher than in the morning). This diurnal variation, which appears to have no seasonal trends and the phases of which complement the hours of daylight and darkness throughout the year, is most marked in healthy cattle. In certain diseases, notably tuberculosis in the horse, the temperature is higher in the morning than in the evening.

In animals under clinical observation, the temperature is usually taken twice daily (morning and evening). In a healthy animal the difference between the two readings is the daily variation. The readings are recorded on a graph chart and comprise the temperature curve. Physiological rises in temperature, varying up to 1·5°C (3°F), occur after feeding, particularly if excessive, and frequently in dairy cattle, after forced exercise, on the day of parturition (except in the bitch in which case it is usually subnormal), on exposure to very high atmospheric temperature and when the animal is excited. It must not be forgotten that the procedures associated with the clinical examination itself may cause a rise in body temperature (in sheep, nervous dogs and fur-bearing animals).

Strenuous or prolonged exercise raises the temperature of a healthy animal beyond normal limits, but when the animal is rested the temperature should quickly (within 10–20 minutes) return to normal. In a sick animal, even if the disease is non-febrile, exercise causes a greater and more rapid rise and a slower return to the original temperature (within 30–120 minutes). Diagnostic use may be made of this in examining doubtful cases of chronic pulmonary emphysema in horses.

If there is local inflammation of the rectum (proctitis), the thermometer will give a higher reading than the true temperature of the body. This is also the situation when the faeces, as a result of prolonged retention in the rectum, e.g. in paralysis of the rectum, occasionally

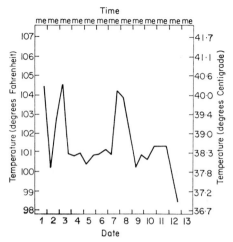

Fig. 18. *Recurrent rise in rectal temperature as a result of bacterial action in faeces impacted in the rectum of a horse. Afebrile paralysis of the rectum.*

noted in sows and mares shortly prior to parturition, undergo a spontaneous rise in temperature as a result of bacterial activity (Fig. 18). In acute enteritis with diarrhoea, immediately following normal defaecation, or the administration of a cold fluid enema, and when the anal sphincter is flaccid, the thermometer indicates a lower rectal temperature than is representative of the true body temperature. A subnormal temperature (hypothermia) is not uncommon in very old animals and in those that are emaciated because of malnutrition. It also occurs in young lambs and piglets under the circumstances referred to earlier, and in such conditions as shock, parturient hypocalcaemia, acute ruminal impaction in cattle, mulberry heart disease, hypothyroidism and just prior to death in most diseases, with some notable exceptions such as tetanus.

Hyperthermia

This is the elevation of body temperature brought about by physical factors such as excessive heat absorption or production or deficient heat loss. Excessive heat absorption occurs during exposure to high environmental temperature. The effect of such exposure in animals is likely to be exaggerated by a concomitant high humidity, muscular exertion, large amounts of body fat, a heavy hair coat or fleece and confinement, particularly when ventilation is inadequate. Animals in a state of dehydration are slightly more prone to hyperthermia because heat loss by evaporation of tissue fluids is correspondingly reduced.

The camel possesses a well-known remarkable tolerance to high environmental temperatures mainly by reason of vaporization of sweat at the skin surface rather than on the hair coat itself.

In Friesian type cattle the rectal temperature will begin to rise when the environmental temperature reaches 21°C. Other effects that are likely to follow include reduction in food intake and in milk production, with little alteration in respiratory rate until the rectal temperature reaches 40°C, when polypnoea often occurs. Sweat gland activity increases relative to the rise in temperature. Jersey cows have been observed to have rises in rectal temperature from 38·3°C at an environmental temperature of 10°C to 39·6°C at an environmental temperature of 35°C. The concomitant respiratory rates were 20 and 90/minute.

The rectal temperature in sheep starts to rise above the normal range when the environmental temperature reaches 32°C. When the body temperature rises to 41°C panting respiration begins and this, together with sweating, enables the sheep to survive for hours, even if the environmental temperature should rise to 43°C, provided the relative humidity remains below 65%.

In the pig the rectal temperature is affected when the environmental temperature reaches 30°C or so, and at a temperature of 35°C the pig cannot tolerate prolonged exposure to a relative humidity of 65% or more. Collapse from heat stroke is likely if the rectal temperature reaches 41°C in the pig.

A room temperature of 27°C, or just above, will cause the rectal temperature of the dog to rise above normal. If the environmental temperature is much above this point panting type breathing will appear. In the dog thermal equilibrium becomes unstable at a rectal temperature of 41°C, and collapse is likely if this should rise to 42·5°C.

The critical air temperature for the cat is 32°C, and collapse is likely if it is subjected to an environmental temperature of 40°C and a relative humidity above 65% for a prolonged period. The cat increases the rate of heat loss by polypnoea and by spreading saliva on its coat.

In the majority of circumstances hyperthermia is an undesirable state because the metabolic rate may be increased up to 50% with a rapid depletion of liver glycogen stores and increased metabolism of endogenous protein as a source of energy. The severity of the metabolic disturbance is indicated by the degree of hypoglycaemia and rise in blood non-protein nitrogen which occurs. Dehydration will lead to dryness of the mouth and this, together with the respiratory embarrassment, will cause anorexia with considerable loss of bodyweight.

The dry state of the mouth causes increased thirst. The peripheral vasodilatation which results from the rise in blood temperature, altering the activity of the thermoregulating centres in the anterior hypothalamus, leads to a fall in blood pressure which itself indirectly increases the heart rate by direct action and the respiratory rate by directly influencing the respiratory centres.

When the body temperature exceeds 41°C there is depression of the nervous system which, when marked, presages circulatory failure due to myocardial weakness, the pulse becoming fast and irregular, or respiratory failure preceded by laboured respirations.

Fever

An elevated temperature is one aspect of the clinical syndrome termed fever. Fever is a symptom-complex which causes, among other changes, a disturbance of the heat regulating mechanism of the body leading to a state of positive heat balance, and which is not due solely to food, exercise or environment.

Fevers may be caused by specific or nonspecific agents, the former group being most common. Specific causal agents include viruses, bacteria, fungi or protozoa. The infective process may be a localized one, in the form of an abscess or an empyema involving a body cavity, or occur in a generalized form, as in a bacteraemia or septicaemia. Non-specific agents causing fever include foreign proteins, substances which cause tissue damage, protein degradation products, necrotic tissue and damaged blood as in surgical fever.

The mechanisms associated with fever are probably better understood in the case of infective bacteria than for some of the other causal agents. Bacteria are known to produce endotoxins or exogenous pyrogens, which are capable of inducing a febrile response within one hour after being injected into an animal. This reactivity is lost following repetitive injections of the pyrogen, probably because of developing tolerance. It is considered that the pyrogenic substances do not elicit a febrile response by direct action on the thermoregulatory centres of the brain, but that they influence these centres by causing the release of endopyrogen from the neutrophil leucocytes. Other specific and nonspecific agents capable of giving rise to fever are also considered to be capable of producing an exogenous pyrogen-like substance which induces the release of endopyrogen from the granulocytes.

The significance of fever in relation to the efficiency of the defence mechanisms is uncertain, although it has been suggested that antibody production is increased when the body temperature is elevated. Artificially elevating body temperature in animals infected with certain micro-organisms has been shown to reduce the severity of the disease.

Clinical Signs of Fever

In addition to a rise in body temperature the other clinical signs of fever are shivering (rigors), increased pulse and respiratory rates, malaise, irregular external temperature, firm faeces, concentrated urine, etc., the most constant feature being the elevated temperature. An elevated body temperature alone (hyperthermia) is not indicative of fever.

Fever is usually divided into three main stages. (a) The *increment* or onset: although the internal temperature is rising the skin capillaries are constricted with the result that the animal feels cold and shivers (*rigors*). (b) The *fastigium*, acme or period of maximum temperature during which the body temperature remains more or less constant and shivering ceases. (c) The *decrement* or defervescence during which the temperature falls.

A rapid reduction of fever, with the temperature returning to the normal level within a few hours, is known as a *crisis* (Fig. 19A) and a slow subsidence as a *lysis*. In both cases the fall in temperature is roughly paralleled by that of the pulse rate. This reduction in frequency, coupled with improvement in quality of the pulse, is an additional indication that the ailing animal has commenced to recover. When the fall in temperature is accompanied by signs indicating that death is imminent, the condition is termed collapse; here, although the temperature falls, the

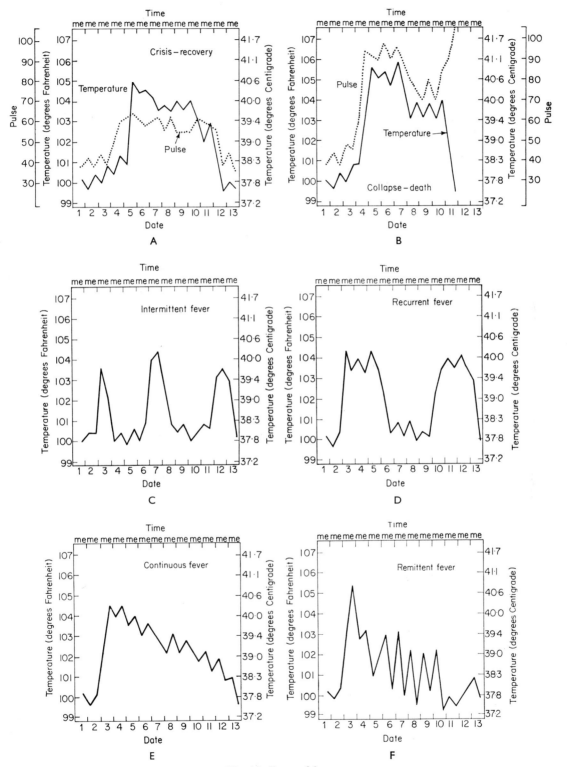

Fig. 19. *Types of fever.*

pulse rate increases and the quality of the pulse deteriorates, indicating incipient cardiac failure. Clearly there has been clinical deterioration, and the animal's life is endangered (Fig. 19B).

In a mild (low) fever the temperature is about 1°C (2°F) above normal, in a moderately severe fever (pyrexia) 1·7°–2·2°C (3°–4°F) and in severe fever (hyperpyrexia) 2·8°–3·3°C (5°–6°F) above normal.

Types of Fever (Fig. 19)

Simple fever. The temperature rises, remains high with variations of less than 1°C (2°F) for several days, and then falls as the animal recovers or collapses prior to death. When the fever subsides within about 24–48 hours after its development it is described as transient (ephemeral), as in bovine ephemeral fever.

Continuous fever. The temperature remains high (plateau temperature) for a longer period than in a simple fever. This form of fever is characteristic of tick-borne fever.

Remittent fever. The temperature rises and falls by more than 1°C (2°F) at short and irregular intervals.

Intermittent fever. There are short attacks of fever lasting for 2–3 days, interspersed with non-febrile intervals, usually forming a regular pattern.

Recurrent fever. This takes the form of relatively prolonged attacks of fever with non-febrile periods of about similar duration.

Atypical fever runs an irregular course. This is by far the commonest type of fever seen in animals, and it occurs in a great variety of febrile diseases. The form of the fever takes a biphasic pattern in some diseases, e.g. canine distemper, louping ill, strangles and swine erysipelas.

The possibility of inducing a rise in body temperature was formerly of diagnostic value in certain clinically latent diseases (allergic temperature reactions). The value of such tests depended upon whether the parenteral introduction of prepared products of bacterial origin (mallein, tuberculin) evoked a characteristic febrile and systemic response in subclinically infected animals.

Temperature of the Skin and its Appendages

The external temperature of the skin is best judged by palpation, passing the palmar surface of the hand from the ears over the horns (in cattle), neck and trunk to the extremities of the fore- and hindlimbs. Skin temperature is dependent partly upon the degree of dilatation of the cutaneous capillaries. The environmental temperature and functional activity of the heat-regulating areas in the anterior hypothalamus have a significant effect on skin temperature, by influencing the internal temperature. Normally the skin temperature shows regular gradations, the ears, muzzle, feet and root of the tail being cooler, on account of the poorer blood supply, than the neck and trunk. In disease, the external temperature may be variably irregular, and may be generally, or locally, raised or lowered.

Irregular variation of skin temperature occurs in hyperpyrexia, severe illness generally, cardiac insufficiency, collapse, etc. In these conditions, the extremities of the body (ears, feet, horns, vulva) are either cold or abnormally warm. A generalized rise in the temperature of the skin occurs during exertion, after unaccustomed exposure to sunlight (heatstroke in pigs), or high environmental temperature, also in the early stages of hyperpyrexia. The temperature over the whole body surface is lowered shortly before death, in extreme emaciation, and following severe haemorrhage, and other forms of vascular shock. A local rise in temperature occurs in the vicinity of localized inflammation of the skin and superficial tissues. A local fall in skin temperature occurs where there is a local deficiency in the blood supply (ischaemia). This occurs where there is localized death of tissue (necrosis, gangrene), and also where there is interference with the arterial blood supply on account of a thrombus, or embolus, in the related artery (iliac thrombosis, mesenteric arteritis), or localized spasm of the vessel (ergotism).

5

Pulse

The importance of examining the pulse in domestic animals is that this procedure, in conjunction with examination of the heart and the superficial veins, and when advisable the circulating blood, enables the clinician to formulate an opinion as to the condition of the circulatory system. By this means prognostication is not infrequently assisted.

In the horse, the pulse is taken at the external maxillary artery, on the medial aspect of the ventral border of the mandible where the vessel is associated with the corresponding vein and the parotid duct, and itself continues as the facial artery (Fig. 20). In certain circumstances it may

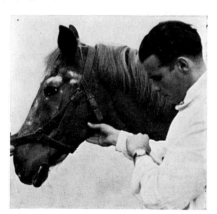

Fig. 20. *Examination of the pulse in a horse at the external maxillary (mandibular) artery.*

be taken in other positions: at the transverse facial artery, at a point posterior to the zygomatic process of the frontal bone about midway between the base of the ear and the eye; at the median artery beneath the posterior superficial pectoral muscle, at the upper extremity of the

foreleg on its medial aspect, as the artery passes downwards in company with the corresponding vein and median nerve; or at the great metatarsal artery on the lateral aspect of the large metatarsal bone in the groove formed by the latter and the lateral small metatarsal bone. In restless horses, the median artery will prove most satisfactory.

In the ox, if the animal is quiet, the pulse may be taken at the facial artery on the lateral aspect of the mandible (Fig. 21) or at the transverse facial artery. The median artery is also commonly used (Fig. 22). An alternative site is

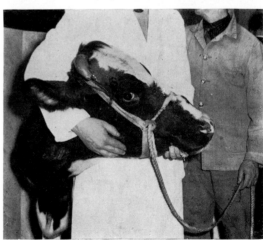

Fig. 21. *Examination of the pulse at the facial artery in an ox.*

the middle coccygeal artery, which is palpated on the under aspect of the tail about 10 cm below the level of the anus (Fig. 23). The pulse is readily detected at this site in dairy cattle, and with a little practice can be obtained here in any type of bovine animal, including fat

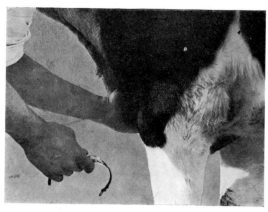

Fig. 22. *Examination of the pulse at the median artery in an ox.*

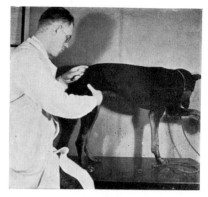

Fig. 24. *Examination of the pulse at the femoral artery in a dog.*

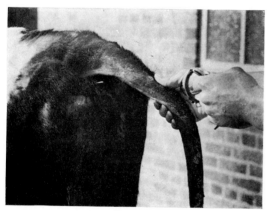

Fig. 23. *Examination of the pulse at the middle coccygeal artery in an ox. Note that the ball of the finger, not the tip, is used. The temperature is being taken at the same time.*

bullocks and very young calves. The advantages claimed for taking the pulse at this site are that the temperature can be taken, and the character and rate of the respiration noted at the same time. Important disadvantages are the small size of the artery, which precludes a proper appreciation of pulse quality as distinct from pulse rate, and the great frequency of faecal contamination of this part.

In the dog, cat, sheep, goat, small pig and young calf, the pulse is taken at the femoral artery, high up in the inguinal region, on the medial aspect of the thigh (Fig. 24). In large pigs, pulse frequency can sometimes be determined at the middle coccygeal artery.

If the pulse cannot be detected because of restiveness, generalized muscle tremors, obesity or

any other reason, the heart beats are counted, with the aid of a stethoscope if necessary. This is a somewhat unsatisfactory substitute and it is important to realize that the heart rate may not always accurately reflect the pulse rate; in conditions such as extrasystolic arrythmia some heart beats do not produce a pulse wave.

When determining the pulse frequency, a watch with a second hand should be used, and the waves counted for a minimum of 30 seconds, when the number obtained should be multiplied by 2. In many cases it is advisable to continue counting the pulse waves for 1 minute, during which time note may be taken of other features such as rhythm and quality. It is advisable to avoid counting for periods less than the minimum recommended, otherwise, unless great accuracy is achieved, significant over- or undercounting may result, more particularly in animals with a high pulse frequency.

The technique of taking the pulse consists of placing the ball part of one or more fingers on the skin over the selected artery, and applying gentle pressure until the pulse wave can be detected. Where the artery is large and tends to roll away from beneath the transversely placed fingertips, as does the external maxillary artery of the horse and the facial artery in cattle, it may be found of value to place the tips of 2, or even 3, adjacent fingers on the artery parallel to its long axis, so that the vessel is held in the groove between the fingertips; this is readily achieved by advancing the second finger beyond the first and third. Smaller arteries are palpated with the tip or ball of the second or third finger. It is better to avoid the use of the index finger because the skin of the tip of this finger is generally somewhat thicker, and therefore less sensitive, than that of the others. Pressure must be just sufficient to tense the skin and the underlying artery to make the pulse wave detectable and, in the case of a small artery, gentle pressure only is used, in order to avoid obliteration of the pressure wave. Before concluding the examination of the pulse, it is legitimate gradually to increase the pressure applied to the artery to the point at which the pulse wave disappears, and then reduce the pressure again in the same manner. With experience this procedure will prove useful in assessing certain pulse qualities.

The student is advised to practise pulse taking in the various animal species until detection of the pulse is readily achieved, the variations in frequency and character of the normal pulse are fully appreciated and the influence of physiological factors readily recognized, and their significance correctly interpreted. Only when this stage is reached will it become possible to recognize significant variations from the normal pulse in individual cases. In an examination of the pulse the following properties should always be considered: (a) rate, (b) rhythm, and (c) quality.

Physiological Factors Affecting the Pulse Rate in Normal Animals

Species. Table 2 indicates the species range and variation. The rates given are for healthy animals accustomed to being handled; in comparable animals not accustomed to the interference associated with taking the pulse the rates would be up to 25% higher. In general, the smaller the species the more frequent the pulse rate, but size is not the only factor responsible for the difference; for example, a pony stallion has a lower pulse rate than a bull of the same age, which might be more than three times the weight of the pony.

TABLE 2. NORMAL PULSE RATE (BEATS/MINUTE)

Animal	Range
Horse	28–40
Colt (yearling)	70–80
Cattle	55–80
Calf (young)	100–120
Sheep, goat	70–90
Pig (adult)	60–90
Pig (young)	100–130
Dog (large)	65–90
Dog (small)	90–120
Cat	110–130
Rabbit	120–250
Mink	115–200

Size. Within a species the pulse rate is usually, but by no means invariably, higher in small than in large individuals. A healthy working pony at rest, for example, usually has a pulse rate in the region of 40/minute, whereas a heavy draught horse under similar circumstances has a pulse rate of around 30/minute. The effect of size is not so marked in cattle.

Age. The pulse rate in very young animals is much higher than in adolescent and adult individuals of the same species. The neonatal calf, for example, has a pulse rate in the region of 120/minute compared with the rate of over 80 for yearling cattle and 50–80 for adult animals. It should be noted, however, that the comparatively high pulse rate usually accepted as being normal for the young (as compared with that of the newly born) animal is not attributable solely to immaturity; the excitement and exertion invariably associated with the examination of the healthy foal or calf by a strange person produce a much greater physiological effect on the pulse rate than does equivalent handling of the adult horse or dairy cow. Thus, although the pulse frequency of young calves is as quoted 100–120/minute and that of yearling cattle as being in the vicinity of 80/minute, the resting pulse of calves accustomed to being handled may be as low as 80/minute by the fourth, and 60/minute by the eighth week of life.

Physical condition. Athletic animals, particularly if in training, have a less frequent pulse than non-athletic animals of the same species and type. This situation is common in race horses, trotting horses, hunter ponies and certain breeds of dogs, more especially greyhounds. In the types of horses mentioned the dropping of a pulse wave when at rest, due to hypertension, partial atrioventricular block or other cause, is not invariably indicative of serious abnormality.

Sex. In most species the male animal has a slightly lower pulse rate than the female.

Pregnancy. In the later stages of pregnancy, the pulse is more frequent than it is in the same animal when in the non-pregnant state. This is probably an indication of a mild degree of hypertension. In cattle during the last 3 months of pregnancy the proportional increase in pulse rate may amount to 15–40%.

Parturition. As parturition becomes imminent, there is a further increase in the pulse frequency.

Lactation. Lactating animals have a higher pulse rate than comparable ones not lactating.

Moreover, the heavier the milk yield the greater the increase in pulse frequency. In high-yielding dairy cattle the pulse rate may be 10% more frequent than in those producing only moderate quantities of milk.

Excitement. This may cause a considerable increase in the pulse frequency, particularly in animals unaccustomed to being handled. Even in dairy cattle the approach of a strange person usually causes an immediate increase of up to 10% in the rate of the pulse. In this type of animal, when healthy, the pulse rate usually returns to the normal range within a few minutes if no further cause of excitement should occur. In readily excited subjects the increased pulse frequency persists throughout the period the animal is exposed to a fright-inducing stimulus, e.g. clinical examination procedures, restraint. This situation is the result of a coordinated, increased output of adrenal medullary secretion, and of increased activity of the sympathetic component of the autonomic nervous system bringing about redistribution of the blood supply, with an associated increase in heart rate.

Exercise. Physical exertion increases the pulse rate to an extent which varies according to the severity of the exercise and fitness of the animal. In thoroughbred and standardbred horses, electronic monitoring has shown that pulse rates of up to 200/minute may occur during severe exercise such as racing. In dairy cattle, 10 minutes of forced exercise may produce an increase of over 60% in the frequency. After 30 minutes rest the pulse rate, in such animals, may still be 10% above normal, and may not return to its original resting rate for as long as 90 minutes after the exercise has terminated. In athletic animals such as racehorses, riding horses or greyhound dogs, following exercise, the pulse rate usually returns to normal within 10–15 minutes.

Posture. Except in the horse, which can rest in the standing position, the pulse rate is appreciably less frequent when the animal is lying down than when it is on its feet. In cattle the rate of the pulse may be reduced by as much as 10% during a period of recumbency.

Ingestion of food. Eating a large quantity of food will cause a very considerable increase in the frequency of the pulse. In dairy cattle the increase in rate may be as great as 66%; a pulse rate of over 100/minute is not unusual towards the end of a large meal. When ingestion of the food is completed, the pulse rate decreases fairly rapidly, but does not return to its preprandial frequency for some time; an hour after eating it may still be up to 10% higher than it was immediately prior to the meal.

Rumination. This action is recognized to cause an increase of up to 3% in the pulse rate.

Environmental temperature. Exposure to either very high or very low temperatures produces an increase in the rate of the pulse. In the former situation, the increase is due to the rise in blood temperature acting directly on the heart, which is also affected indirectly by the fall in blood pressure resulting from peripheral vasodilatation. In the latter case increased amounts of adrenaline and noradrenaline are secreted, for calorigenic purposes, and which along with other endocrine secretions cause an increase in heart rate.

An increase in the rate of the pulse occurs in all painful conditions, in many diseases not primarily involving the cardiovascular system, and is one of the characteristic features of the fever syndrome.

Pulse Rhythm

The rhythm of the pulse is assessed by appreciation of the time intervals between the peaks of a series of successive pulse waves, and the temporal sequence may be regular or irregular. With the exception of sinus arrhythmia, which is a characteristic feature of pulse rhythm in healthy dogs and more rarely in other animals, and is related to the respiratory cycle, rhythmic irregularities may be regular or irregular in their time relationships. Regular intermittence in the pulse (Fig. 25B) is occasionally observed in animals customarily subjected to severe physical exertion; the intermittence occurs with constant periodicity and it indicates a mild degree of heart block. In such cases the pulse irregularity often disappears with exercise. Irregular intermittence occurs without any cyclical pattern being obvious, and is usually associated with irregularities in pulse amplitude due to variations in the stroke volume of the heart. The commonest causes of irregular intermittence of the pulse are second degree heart block, ventricular extrasystoles and auricular fibrillation. With exercise, pulse irregularities of this type usually become accentuated.

Pulse Quality

The quality of the pulse depends mainly upon

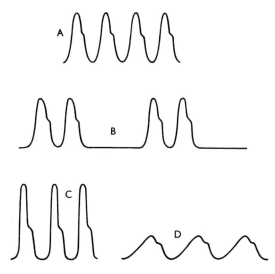

Fig. 25. *Diagrams of pulse waves.* A, *Normal pulse.*
B, *Dropped pulse.* C, *Large bounding pulse (water-*
hammer pulse). D, *Slow pulse; note that it is also small,*
a point of distinction from the infrequent pulse.

method readily available to the veterinary clinician whereby blood pressure variations and
cardiac output can be assessed.

Changes in the normal qualities of the pulse
may be caused by structural or functional disease
of the heart or by abnormalities of the blood
vessels (arterial thrombosis and embolism, vasomotor disturbance, certain types of passive
venous congestion) which only have a local or
indirect influence on the pulse. Such changes
may affect any one or all of the three properties
mentioned.

The normal pulse wave (Fig. 25A) is regular
in sequence, amplitude and strength, and the
artery is well filled, the wall being distended and
exhibiting a degree of tone which is readily
appreciated by digital palpation. In the wake of
the pressure wave it should still be possible to
detect residual tone in the wall of the artery. It
should be noted that in some species, particularly horses and dogs, the degree of distension
of the artery at the acme of the pulse wave is
proportionately greater than in other species,
such as cattle and sheep. This interspecies difference is attributable to variations in the activity
of the vasomotor mechanism, and in the amount
of elastic tissue in the walls of the arteries, influencing the distensibility and tone of the
vessels. It is important to appreciate too that
irregularities in the rhythm of the pulse, in the
absence of clinically demonstrable disease, are
by no means uncommon in the dog, goat, sheep
and horse.

the amplitude of the pressure waves which may
vary because changes in the rate of diastolic
filling influence the stroke volume of the heart.
Rhythmic irregularities in the pulse are invariably
associated with some degree of fluctuation in
pulse amplitude. The amplitude or quality of
the pulse is assessed by noting the degree of
digital pressure required to obliterate the pulse
wave in the artery. This is the only practical

6

Respiration

Those physical actions by means of which air is brought into and is expelled from the lungs are not infrequently termed *respiration*. They should, more properly, be called ventilation because, in physiological terms, respiration includes both the chemical and physical processes which enable an organism to exchange gases with its environment. In the case of higher organisms, including animals and man, survival is dependent upon the efficient functioning of a series of specialized structures which regulate the exchange between oxygen from the atmosphere and carbon dioxide in the tissues.

The physical features of respiration involve the diaphragm and intercostal muscles, which are in action during breathing. The volume and frequency of the respiratory movements are controlled by 'centres' in the brain stem which maintain inspiration and expiration. During inspiration, air enters the nose and mouth and, passing through the larynx, enters the trachea and makes its way to the pulmonary alveoli via the bronchi, bronchioles and alveolar ducts. The structure of the pulmonary alveoli is such, and the relationship with the numerous pulmonary capillaries so intimate, that exchange of oxygen and carbon dioxide occurs freely in normal conditions.

The exchange of these gases takes place by simple diffusion and is dependent on the pressure gradient (partial pressure) of the gas across the membrane separating the alveolar air and the blood in the alveolar capillaries. Although blood takes only about a second, at most, to pass through the capillaries, gaseous exchange is complete because of the enormous diffusing area.

Breathing is regulated by the respiratory centres consisting of an inspiratory centre and an expiratory centre in the medulla and a pneumotaxic centre in the upper pons. The inspiratory and expiratory centres are reflexly influenced by afferent vagal stimuli from stretch receptors in the lungs, by afferent impulses from the carotid and aortic chemoreceptors, and from the higher levels of the brain. In addition the inspiratory centre is extremely sensitive to changes in the partial pressure of carbon dioxide and in hydrogen ion concentration, less so to changes in oxygen tension, in the blood.

It is not possible to diagnose any given disease, with certainty, by observations on the physical aspects of respiration alone, but it is sometimes possible tentatively to recognize specific entities by noting the character of the respiratory movements. Respiratory activity is assessed by noting the movements of the ribs and sternum, and flanks (in response to the expansion and contraction of the lungs and the movement of the diaphragm), preferably when the animal is in the standing position, as recumbency will have a modifying effect on respiration, more particularly in ailing animals.

This part of the clinical examination is best performed in conjunction with the general inspection, prior to the physical procedures, or the application of restraint. In selected cases exposing the animal to physical effort may be a necessary part of the examination, as a means for determining respiratory efficiency. The clinician should stand behind and to one side of the animal, so that both the thoracic and abdominal areas of the body are in view. It is advisable to observe the animal from both sides, in order to determine whether the respiratory movements are bilaterally similar. In quiet animals, determining the frequency and rhythm of the respirations is facilitated by placing one hand on the lower part of the flank. The respiratory rate may

TABLE 3. NORMAL RESPIRATORY RATES

Animal	Range
Horse	10–14
Ox (adult)	10–30
Ox (yearling)	15–40
Sheep, goat	20–30
Pig	8–18
Dog	15–30
Cat	20–30
Rabbit	30–45
Rat	90–110

also be determined by observing nostril movements, or more efficiently by auscultation over the thorax or trachea. The following points are noted: (a) rate or frequency (number/minute) (see Table 3); (b) type; (c) rhythm (regularity); and (d) quality (amplitude or depth of the respiratory movements). Counting the frequency of the respirations is performed on the same basis as for the pulse. Physiological or abnormal variation may occur in any one or more of the four stated features.

The act of respiration is controlled voluntarily and reflexly through the monitoring function of the respiratory centres in the medulla oblongata. Particularly in the dog, excitement, fear or high environmental temperature and humidity may cause the animal to take sudden short breaths with great rapidity; this panting respiration (polypnoea) must not be confused with dyspnoea.

Clinical Assessment of Respiration

Respiratory Rate

The state of normal quiet breathing is called *eupnoea*. The rate of external respiration decreases directly with the bodyweight in domestic animals, with the exception of cattle. Sheep and pigs have the fastest rate and horses the slowest.

Increased respiratory frequency occurs whereever there is an increased demand for oxygen by the tissues. As a consequence it is seen when the animal is excited, after exercise or exposure to high environmental temperature or humidity and in obesity. It is a regular concomitant of fever and is observed in various pulmonary diseases, severe cardiac disease, obstruction of the upper respiratory passages, in conditions making respiration painful (pleurisy, peritonitis) and in

anaemia (deficiency of erythrocytes producing hypoxia). Increased respiratory rate, with or without an increase in the amplitude of the movements, is termed *hyperpnoea*. When there is increased respiratory frequency with reduction in depth of the associated movements the term *polypnoea* is applied.

Decreased or retarded respiratory frequency (*oligopnoea*) is rare; it occasionally occurs in animals with space-occupying lesions of the brain (chronic acquired and congenital hydrocephalus), in stenosis of the upper respiratory tract and in uraemia.

Type of Respiration

This is assessed by noting the way in which the observable respiratory movements are shared between the thoracic and abdominal walls (Fig. 26). The mechanics of respiration result from the opposing forces presented by the lungs which, because of their elastic tissue, tend to collapse, and the chest wall with its tendency to expand outwards. From the commencement of inspiration when the respiratory muscles contract, the intrapleural pressure becomes more subatmospheric. The contraction lowers the diaphragm and elevates the rib cage. In normal respiration, movement of the abdominal wall is a secondary effect; it varies in degree between species.

If the movements of both component parts are of equal extent, the respiration is said to be costo-abdominal in type. As a rule, normal respiration in horses is costo-abdominal, in dogs and cats it is mainly costal and in cattle, sheep and goats the movement of the abdominal component is greater. Predominantly costal or thoracic type of respiration occurs as an abnormal manifestation when the action of the diaphragm —the principal muscle of respiration—is impaired, e.g. by paralysis, rupture, abscessation, pressure by a neoplasm or accumulation of gas or fluid in an abdominal viscus or in the peritoneal cavity; in diseases of the lungs, particularly those, such as pneumonia and acute pulmonary oedema, in which the entry of air into the lungs is impeded; and in peritonitis, in which movement of the abdominal wall and diaphragm is suppressed on account of pain.

A wholly abdominal type of respiration occurs in acute pleurisy because of the pain caused by movement of the thoracic wall; in tuberculous pleurisy, or thoracic nocardiosis with effusion

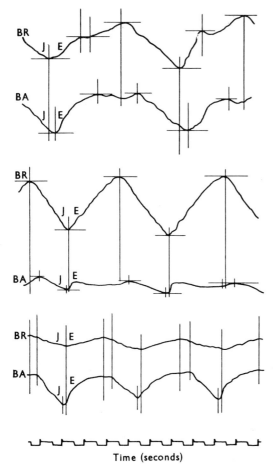

Fig. 26. *Respiratory waves.* Top, *Costo-abdominal type.*
Centre, *Costal type.* Bottom, *Abdominal type.* BR,
*movement of thoracic wall; BA, movement of abdominal
wall; I, inspiration; E, expiration.* (After Forster)

period of expiration is slightly longer than that
of inspiration; the duration of the pause in
healthy animals depends upon whether the animal is relaxed and resting, or has recently been
excited or exercised. During inspiration, contraction of the intercostal muscles causes the
costal arch to move outwards, and during inspiration it moves inwards. Inspiration is the
result of an active movement of the respiratory
muscles (diaphragm, intercostal and abdominal
muscles), initiated by the respiratory centres,
whereas expiration is almost entirely passive,
the elastic lungs contracting with the collapse
of the thorax. In equine species, expiration has a
biphasic character in that two peaks of expiratory airflow occur. This is not associated with a
double movement of the respiratory muscles, so
that confusion with chronic alveolar emphysema
does not arise.

Irregular respiration is not uncommon in
normal animals, particularly the dog and pig
(interrupted breathing or sniffing). Prolongation
of inspiration is observed when there is partial
obstruction of the upper respiratory tract and
prolongation of expiration in pulmonary emphysema (chronic alveolar emphysema in horses,
atypical pneumonia, parasitic pneumonia and
anaphylaxis in cattle), when a double movement
of the abdominal wall may be noted. In normal
animals, any increase in the respiratory rate
occurs at the expense of the pause period, which
becomes correspondingly shorter. While in the
majority of respiratory diseases involving the
lungs, the cycle of respiration consists of two
phases and the pause does not occur.

Dropped respirations (Fig. 27) cause the most
marked change in respiratory rhythm. Characteristic forms of dropped respirations are recognizable. *Cheyne–Stokes* respiration is an abnormal type of breathing in which a period of
respiratory arrest (*apnoea*) occurs for 15–30
seconds, followed by a gradual increase and then
a gradual decrease in the amplitude of the movements which are regularly succeeded by a further
respiratory hiatus. It is characteristic of advanced
renal and cardiac diseases, and severe toxaemia.
Biot's respiration is characterized by recurring
series of relatively shallow, rapid breaths (*polypnoea*), alternating with periods of *apnoea*; the
intervals of respiratory arrest, and periods of
activity, vary in length. It occurs in meningitis
affecting particularly the region of the medulla
oblongata. In syncoptic respiration, a pause is

in the dog and cat; in chronic alveolar emphysema (heaves) as a result of the decrease in the
elastic collapse of the lungs which necessitates
the voluntary use of the abdominal muscles to
bring about the forcible expulsion of air during
expiration; in paralysis of the intercostal
muscles; and in those conditions in which the
outward flow of air is impeded. In the initial
stages of acute pleurisy, the fixation of the costal
arch, resulting from the limitation of costal
movement, produces the so-called pleuritic
ridge, noted particularly in the horse.

Respiratory Rhythm

The three phases in each normal respiratory
cycle are inspiration, expiration and pause. The

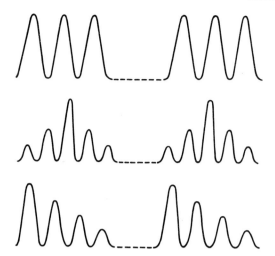

Fig. 27. *Dropped respirations*. Top, *Biot's respiration*. Centre, *Cheyne–Stokes respiration*. Bottom, *Syncoptic respiration. Note that the top diagram is drawn at a larger scale than the other two.*

followed by deep breathing (*hyperpnoea*) that gradually becomes shallow until *apnoea* prevails. These three types of abnormal respiration should be regarded as indicating an unfavourable prognosis; they reflect decreased sensitivity of the respiratory centres in the medulla oblongata to carbon dioxide in the circulating blood.

Respiratory Depth

Normally there is great variation in the amplitude of the respiratory movements. Any form of exercise increases the depth of respiration because of temporary hypoxia; at rest, amplitude is reduced. In deep breathing (*hyperpnoea*) the considerable movements of both the thoracic and abdominal walls are clearly visible. In shallow breathing the movements of these components is very slight. Very deep respiration is said to be 'laboured', it occurs in *dyspnoea*. Irregularity in depth, and in the intervals between successive respirations, is commonly seen in dyspnoea. Asymmetrical respiration occurs when there is unilateral deficiency or absence of movement; it is sometimes recognizable in severe disease in one lung, the amplitude of movement on the healthy side being normal or increased in extent, while that on the affected side is reduced to a variable degree, e.g. collapse or consolidation of one lung, unilateral pleural exudation, hydrothorax or pneumothorax and rupture of the diaphragm with unilateral herniation of abdominal viscera.

Dyspnoea

Any subjectively assessed difficulty in respiration, causing apparent distress to an animal, is known as dyspnoea. It may be a physiological occurrence following strenuous exercise but it more usually arises out of disease and is caused by hypoxia in association with hypercapnia. Dyspnoea may take the form of a change in the rate, type, rhythm or depth of respiration. According to whether the difficulty arises at inspiration, at expiration or during both phases, dyspnoea is referred to as inspiratory, expiratory or indeterminate. In order to determine the degree of dyspnoea (slight, moderate or severe) it may be necessary to have the animal exercised. The more severe the dyspnoea, the correspondingly longer the recovery period after exertion (30–60 minutes or longer, instead of the usual 5–10 minutes in healthy animals). Obviously severe cases of dyspnoea can be recognized without recourse to exercise.

Inspiratory dyspnoea is a feature of all those diseases in which entry of air into the lungs or transfer of oxygen to the blood or tissues is inhibited, e.g. in stenosis of the air passages, bronchopneumonia, pulmonary oedema, pulmonary congestion, ruptured diaphragm, pleurisy and hydrocyanic acid poisoning. When there is inflammation or congestion of the lungs or pleura, increased sensitivity of the Hering–Breuer reflex is a contributory cause of dyspnoea. In this form of dyspnoea the accessory respiratory movements become activated; dilatation of the nostrils; in cattle, dogs and cats, extension of the head and neck (Fig. 28) and opening of the

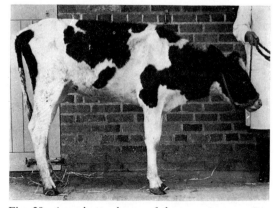

Fig. 28. *A moderate degree of dyspnoea in a yearling heifer suffering from parasitic bronchitis. Note the 'tucked-up' appearance, the low carriage of the head and the position of the ears. The animal is lean and stunted.*

mouth; costal type of respiration; depression of the intercostal spaces; forward movement of the body during each inspiration; outward rotation of the elbows; prolongation of inspiration. In the dog, the cheeks may be sucked inwards during inspiration (seen particularly in breeds with loose, mobile cheeks, when the mouth is closed or partially opened).

Expiratory dyspnoea occurs when the escape of air from the lungs is impeded, e.g. in pulmonary emphysema, as the result of the reduced elasticity of the lungs causing reduction in the volume of tidal air expelled and so leading to hypoxia, and in pleural adhesions. In these situations the dyspnoea is caused by ambient hypoxia and by the forced expiration which is an attempt to restore the tidal volume to near normal. The clinical signs of this form of dyspnoea are: development of a groove in the anterior part of the flank, along the line of the costal arch—the so-called 'heaves line' (N.B. This is observed in transient form also, in lean, healthy horses following vigorous exercise); protracted expiration; double expiratory lift involving the abdominal muscles; 'pumping' of the anus (see below). In the dog, the lips and cheeks may be blown outwards.

Indeterminate dyspnoea is the commonest type. It is seen to occur in pneumonia, bronchitis, cardiac diseases such as failure of the left ventricle leading to congestion and oedema of the lungs, severe anaemia, acidosis, occasionally in meningitis, encephalitis or space-occupying lesions of the brain, stenosis of the nasal passages, etc.—diseases in which there is a fairly severe disturbance of tissue respiration (hypoxia) or difficulty in both inspiration and expiration. Other factors which contribute to development of this form of dyspnoea include increased sensitivity of the Hering–Breuer reflex, and the influence of increased venous pressure on the respiratory centres.

'Pumping of the anus' is a sign which appears in severe dyspnoea, usually in association with dilatation of the nostrils, particularly in established chronic pulmonary emphysema in the horse. During inspiration, when the circumference of the abdomen is increased, the anus retracts into the plevic cavity, and at expiration, when the size of the abdominal cavity is reduced, more particularly during the second expiratory movement, the anus is protruded.

A double lifting movement involving the abdominal wall is observed during expiration when the elasticity of the lung is impaired. Passive contraction of the lung, which is only partial, produces the first part of the double phased expiratory movement; the remainder of the tidal air has then to be actively expressed with the aid of the abdominal muscles, this being the second phase of the expiratory movement. A double expiratory lift of the abdominal muscles in the horse is usually indicative of chronic alveolar emphysema (broken wind). In calves, it is often seen in parasitic bronchopneumonia.

Abnormal Respiratory Noises

A *hiccough* (singultus) is a short, jerky inspiration, caused by stimulation of the phrenic nerve producing sudden contraction of the diaphragm. It causes an abrupt sound which varies in volume according to the size of the animal, but in most cases it is much less obvious than in man. In the horse of intermediate or large size, a severe attack is associated with an inspiratory 'grunt', which is somewhat similar to the sound produced during attempted regurgitation in gastric tympany. The spasmodic contraction of the diaphragm is readily identified by placing the hand on the thoracic wall, or near the costal arch in the region of the attachment of the diaphragm. In hiccough, the abdominal wall is jerked outwards (in spasm of abdominal muscles, the movement is inwards) because of the sudden increase in intra-abdominal pressure produced by the sharp contraction of the diaphragm. When the horse is severely affected indoors, the sudden contractions may cause the stall and surrounding fittings to vibrate.

Other abnormal respiratory noises include *sneezing* due to nasal irritation; *snoring* caused by pharyngeal occlusion as in tuberculous lymphadenitis of the retropharyngeal lymph nodes; *roaring* and *whistling* in paralysis of the intrinsic muscles of the larynx; *grunting*, which is a forced expiration against a closed glottis, and is associated with many painful conditions, particularly those involving the respiratory tract; *coughing* (see p. 110) due to irritation of the pharynx, larynx, trachea and bronchi; and *yawning*, which is a prolonged inspiration, with the mouth opened widely and the soft palate raised, followed by an inspiration. In the dog it is accompanied by a fairly loud sound. The purpose of yawning is uncertain but when it occurs only occasionally it is not regarded as a sign indicating disease. Frequent yawning is observed in association with catarrhal gastritis, chronic 'hepatitis' and in some diseases of the brain, e.g. equine encephalomyelitis, dumb rabies. The yawning movements in rabies are suggested to be voiceless attempts to bellow or bark.

Respiratory Insufficiency

When it is functioning efficiently the respiratory system oxygenates and removes carbon dioxide from the blood in the pulmonary circulation (ventilation or external respiration). Interference with the gaseous exchange at this point, leading to reduced supply of oxygen for tissue (internal) respiration, can occur in a variety of respiratory diseases, e.g. pulmonary diseases (pneumonia, atelectasis, pleurisy, pneumothorax, pulmonary oedema and congestion, emphysema, neoplasia), partial occlusion of the respiratory passages as in bronchitis, rhinitis, tracheitis and neoplasia, etc. As a result the blood oxygen level decreases and the carbon dioxide concentration increases (hypercapnia), leading to greater respiratory activity through the overriding mediation of the respiration centres. In mild affections, in which internal respiration is only slightly disturbed, these functional changes alone may be effective in restoring tissue oxygenation to a normal state. When the interference is serious, because the extreme range of respiratory compensatory activity fails, respiratory insufficiency will develop and lead to hypoxia. Many of the important clinical signs of respiratory disease, therefore, arise from hypoxia due to respiratory insufficiency, which may become severe enough to cause death from respiratory failure. The signs include changes in the character of the respirations which may be manifest as hyperpnoea or dyspnoea, cyanosis which is recognized as a bluish discoloration of the skin and visible mucous membranes and, depending upon the nature of the particular respiratory disease, coughing and nasal discharge.

Hypoxia

It is necessary in the consideration of the clinical aspects to remember that failure of tissue oxygenation can occur in other ways than by means of primary respiratory disease which produces *ambient hypoxia*. In this type of hypoxia the oxygen tension in the arterial blood is lower than normal so that haemoglobin is not saturated with oxygen to the normal extent. In *anaemic hypoxia* which occurs when there is a significant reduction in the blood haemoglobin concentration the total transporting capacity of the blood is inadequate to meet essential demands even although the percentage saturation and oxygen tension of the available haemoglobin are normal. This type of hypoxia occurs with anaemia due to any cause; a similar effect is produced when haemoglobin is converted to non-oxygen carrying pigments. In nitrite or chlorate poisoning haemoglobin is converted into methaemoglobin and in carbon monoxide poisoning conversion to carboxyhaemoglobin occurs; both these haemoglobin derivatives are stable products and are completely inactive in relation to oxygen transportation or release. In *stagnant hypoxia* the blood flow rate through the capillaries is reduced so that a tissue oxygen deficit occurs even although the oxygen saturation and tension of arterial blood and the total oxygen load are normal. This form of hypoxia occurs generally in congestive heart failure and in peripheral circulatory failure (arterial thrombosis and embolism) and locally in venous obstruction. In *histotoxic hypoxia* which occurs in cyanide poisoning tissue oxidation is inhibited by paralysis of cytochrome oxidase even although the blood is fully oxygenated. Narcotics also depress tissue oxidation to a variable degree by inhibiting dehydrogenase systems.

The common causes of ambient hypoxia in animals are those diseases associated with lesions or dysfunctions of the respiratory tract and which reduce alveolar oxygen tension. These various diseases all cause a reduction in the vital capacity; they include pneumonia, in which the alveolar epithelium is altered, pulmonary atelectasis, pneumothorax, pulmonary oedema and congestion, and painful conditions such as pleurisy which decrease the amplitude of chest movements (tetanus, strychnine poisoning, botulism and tick paralysis also cause impairment of chest movements). A similar effect is produced in those diseases in which accumulation of exudate causes partial obstruction of the air passages. Depression of the respiratory centre by drugs, or in toxaemia, also causes this type of hypoxia. Other non-respiratory conditions which cause this state include low atmospheric oxygen tension (altitude disease) and congenital cardiac and vascular defects in which serious arterio-venous shunts occur.

The degree to which compensatory mechanisms come into operation in the various hypoxic states depends upon their rate of development. Almost immediately (except in anaemic hypoxia) the chemoreceptors situated in the carotid and aortic bodies mediate an increase in amplitude of the respiratory movements (hyperpnoea). A compensatory increase in the heart rate and stroke volume leads to an increase in the minute volume of the heart; this degree of improvement is unlikely in cases of hypoxia caused by major congenital cardiac and vascular defects and in congestive heart failure. An increase in the erythrocyte population of the blood (polycythaemia) may follow almost at once as the result of contraction of the spleen (most likely to be marked in the horse) or at a later stage following increased erythropoiesis in the bone marrow. When in spite of these compensatory mechanisms tissue oxygen lack becomes severe the function of certain organs becomes impaired. Because of its high oxygen demands, dysfunction of the central nervous system appears as an early sign followed by cardiac decompensation, hepatic and renal dysfunction and reduction of motility and secretory activity of the digestive tract.

Respiratory Failure

This, which is the terminal stage of respiratory insufficiency, is recognized clinically by cessation of movement of the respiratory muscles following a period of diminishing activity of the respiratory centres. The character of the respiratory failure, which can be asphyxial, paralytic or tachypnoeic, depending on the primary disease, may be suggested by the clinical signs. Asphyxial (dyspnoeic) failure gives rise to hypercapnia and hypoxia of varying severity, so that the respiratory movements are dyspnoeic, with alternating periods of apnoea, and gasping, in the terminal phase. It occurs when tidal volume is seriously reduced in upper respiratory tract obstruction, in pneumonia and in pulmonary oedema. Depression of the respiratory centres by anaesthetic agents, other toxic chemicals, nervous shock, acute heart failure and severe haemorrhage precedes paralytic respiratory failure in which the respirations rapidly decrease in frequency and amplitude, and finally cease, without dyspnoea supervening. In all forms of hypothermia, hyperventilation of the lungs produces hypoxia and acapnia and because of the reduced carbon dioxide tension in the blood the respiratory movements become rapid and shallow—tachypnoeic respiratory failure. This is the least common form of the condition.

7

The Skin, Coat and Associated Structures

The skin is a heterogeneous organ which serves as the principal medium of communication between the animal and its environment. The main functions of the skin include maintenance of water and electrolyte balance of the body, participation in temperature regulation, mechanical protection and limitation of penetration of noxious physical and chemical agents, sensory perceptivity and elaboration of vitamin D.

The skin is a stratified tissue consisting of two major layers: the outer epithelial layer called *epidermis* and the inner *corium* or *dermis*. The associated structures, including hairs, quills, horns, claws, nails, hoofs and sebaceous and sweat glands, all develop from the epidermis. Smooth muscle fibres comprising the *arrectores pilorum*, which are attached to the hair follicles, are distributed at intervals throughout the dermis.

The epidermis which extends over the whole surface of the body in mammals is comprised of two main layers: the *stratum Malpighii* and *stratum corneum*. The deeper stratum Malpighii is subdivided into a basal layer *stratum germinativum*, one cell thick overlying the dermis, and the *stratum spinosum* (prickle cell layer) of varying thickness. The upper prickle cells comprise the *stratum granulosum*, superimposed on which is a hyaline layer, the *stratum lucidum*, seen only on the digital pads and muzzle of the dog, cat and other animals. The outer stratum corneum is composed of dead keratinized cells which are continuously shed from the skin surface.

The dermis consists of a fibrous connective tissue layer, the bulk of which comprises collagen along with elastic and reticular fibres, capillary loops and nerve endings. Cutaneous appendages including hairs and sebaceous and sweat glands extend from the epidermis into and even beyond the dermis itself.

As well as being directly involved in a variety of disease processes, the skin and coat are indirectly influenced by the general health status of the individual animal. It is worthwhile, therefore, at this stage in the clinical examination, to perform the simple procedures of inspecting and palpating the body surface, and in selected cases to apply other methods of examination in order to assist the diagnosis.

The incidence of skin disease in domestic animals is high. It may be primary or secondary in origin. In primary skin diseases, initially at least, the lesions are restricted to the skin and its associated structures; spread to other tissues may occur as a complication. Secondary skin disease occurs as the result of extension of a disease process from elsewhere in the body. Elucidation, through the medium of the history, of the chronological order and character of the changes that have been observed to occur in the skin, in association with a complete clinical examination of the patient, may assist in establishing whether or not the disease is primary. When the evidence revealed by the clinical examination indicates that only the skin is involved in the disease process, the condition can be assumed to be primary in origin. Involvement of other organs presents the need to determine whether such involvement was followed by the development of skin lesions or whether the reverse course of events occurred. In a considerable proportion of cases of skin disease in animals, the condition is a reaction to an irritant, so that it is inflammatory in character. Other cases are attributable to malfunction on the part of an associated skin structure. In either event, the application of available knowledge in respect of the specific diseases of the skin, and their pathology, occurring in animals of differing species, should enable the various entities to be recognized.

Skin diseases may also be classified into parasitic and non-parasitic categories, according to their aetiology. Skin parasites in animals include certain members of the dermatophyte and metazoan groups, many of which will be referred to later in this section. It is important to remember that some skin diseases are contagious, so that prompt recognition is essential in order to prevent further dissemination of infection and to assist control. In this context there are several parasitic skin diseases, including sheep scab and parasitic mange in equine species, which are subject to statutory control* in many countries.

The risk to persons handling animals affected with certain parasitic skin diseases is an important public health responsibility for the veterinary clinician. Sarcoptic mange and certain forms of ringworm are a problem in this respect. Temporary personal embarrassment can arise from acquisition, through contact with animals, of certain of the larger arthropod parasites such as ticks and fleas.

* It is essential that all veterinarians should be aware of those diseases which are included in the notifiable list in their own countries.

Clinical Examination

In the general examination of the patient, visual inspection would reveal when obvious skin disease was present. At all events the history of the case, as vouchsafed by the owner or attendant, would, in many instances, have drawn attention to the situation of the trouble. In such circumstances, the general clinical examination would be followed by a special examination of the skin, consisting of more detailed inspection and also palpation, coupled with other procedures, such as the taking of skin scrapings for examination for parasites, skin swabs for bacteriological examination and skin biopsy for histological examination in selected areas.

In the text which follows the various skin structures will be considered in sequence, and changes from normal structure or function, along with any other associated clinical signs, will be discussed. Reference will also be made to the application of any of the special methods of examination where they are considered to be appropriate.

Condition of the Coat

In any persistent disturbance of nutrition the coat is affected and becomes lustreless, dry and staring; conversely, a smooth, shiny coat usually implies that the animal is not suffering from significant nutritional deficiency. In the examination of the coat it is necessary to take into con-

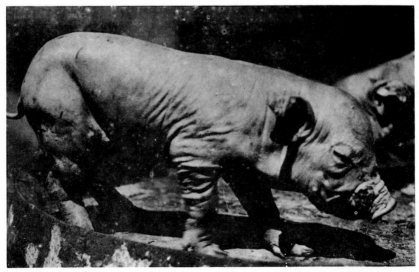

Fig. 29. *Hairlessness and thickening of the skin in a newborn pig. Iodine deficiency. Note the swelling caused by enlargement of the thyroid gland.* (Diseases of Swine. USA Department of Agriculture Bulletin No. 1914.)

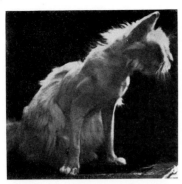

Fig. 30. *Loss of hair over the anterior part of the body, extending to the anterior lumbar region. Alopecia in an Angora cat.*

sideration the species, breed, grooming and housing of the animal. In healthy cattle, even when running outdoors during winter, lick marks can be seen over the body. Certain breeds of animals are naturally rough-coated or shaggy, e.g. Scottish highland cattle, old English sheep dog. Horses and cattle that are allowed to run at grass for a long period, particularly during the winter, grow a rough coat of long hair (see Fig. 121, p. 117). Lack of grooming leads, even in housed animals, to a dirty, rough, lustreless coat. In such neglected animals, long hair may become matted into locks or balls. The hair is greasy in seborrhoeic eczema.

Transient bristling of the hair (produced by contraction of the *arrectores pilorum* muscles) is a nervous reaction occurring in emotional states associated with the release of adrenaline (excitement, fear, anger). It is also present during the shivering (rigor) stage of fever, i.e. when there is a feeling of coldness in spite of a normal or even an elevated body or skin temperature, sometimes even accompanied by sweating. Erection of hair occurs locally over areas of serous infiltration into the skin, e.g. in urticaria.

In the spring and autumn it is normal, in most species for the coat to be changed (moulting). Occasionally at moulting the hair, for some unknown reason, may be shed so suddenly and rapidly that the whole body of the animal is denuded. Loss of hair occurs mainly, however, in demonstrable diseases of the skin itself, such as eczema, dermatitis, mange, ringworm (see Figs 71–73, pp. 69, 70) etc., and in generalized diseases, which also involve the skin, such as iodine deficiency (Fig. 29), hyperkeratosis (see Fig. 56, p. 57) etc., when it is known as symptomatic hair loss. Sometimes, however, the skin itself shows no structural lesions, in which case the condition is known as alopecia (Fig. 30); it is due to follicle dysfunction, the cause of which is sometimes difficult to ascertain. It may occur in certain forms of poisoning (Fig. 31) (mercury, selenium, thallium, potato poisoning in the horse); in copper deficiency; in hormonal imbalance; in hypothyroidism; in dystrophia

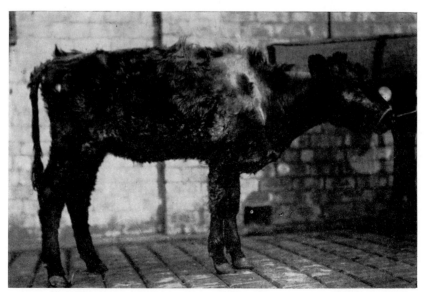

Fig. 31. *Loss of hair in a yearling bullock suffering from advanced molybdenosis. Note also the emaciated condition.*

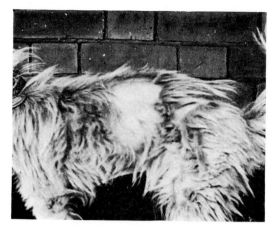

Fig. 32. *Alopecia of the abdomen in a dog, caused by a Sertoli cell tumour. Other effects observed in this case include softening of the skin, some degree of gynaecomastia and enlargement of the prepuce.*

adiposogenitalis (Fröhlich's syndrome); and in Sertoli cell tumour of the testicle in the dog (Fig. 32). It may be hereditary (inherited symmetrical alopecia, inherited congenital hypotrichosis and baldy calves in cattle); it may be a senile change (Fig. 33).

In inherited symmetrical alopecia, which has been observed in Friesian cattle, animals are born with a normal coat, but progressive hair loss commences on the head at 6 weeks to 6 months of age, and extends in a symmetrical manner to involve the neck, back and hindquarters, progressing to the root of the tail and hindlegs as well as the forelimbs. Hair follicles in the affected area appear normal. The condition is inherited through transfer of a single autosomal recessive character. Inherited congenital hypotrichosis is similar in its general aspects, except that it is present at birth or develops soon afterwards, and there may be other developmental defects. Six known forms of the condition have been recognized. In one form occurring in Guernsey and Jersey cattle, inherited as a single recessive character, hair follicles fail to develop. Affected calves survive provided they are protected from cold weather or exposure to the warm sun. Guernsey and Jersey calves with adrenohypophyseal hypoplasia invariably manifest hypotrichosis. A lethal form of the condition, associated with hypoplasia of the thyroid gland, has occurred in Friesian cattle. Another form of hypotrichosis, occurring together with adontia in calves, is transmitted as a conditioned

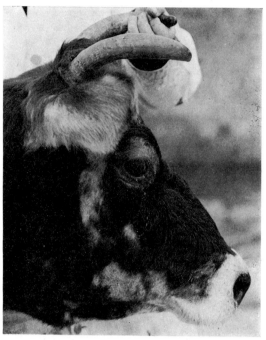

Fig. 33. *Senile alopecia in an aged dairy cow. Note the absence of changes in the skin and the irregular shape of the denuded areas. (Differentiation from mange and ringworm.) Depigmentation and greying of the hair may occur as a preceding change.*

sex-linked recessive gene. A sex-linked semi-dominant gene is responsible for the condition in female Friesian calves, in which the hairlessness occurs in narrow streaks. Partial hypotrichosis, associated with fine curly hair and later coarse hair, and transmitted as a simple recessive, has been observed in Hereford calves. Baldy calves, occurring in the Friesian breed, makes its appearance at one to two months of age and is characterized by loss of condition, alopecia, skin lesion and lack of horn growth. The skin lesions, which take the form of thickened, scaly and folded patches on the neck and shoulders, and raw areas in the axillae and flanks, are inherited by means of an autosomal recessive gene.

In a temporary form, alopecia may be a sequel to severe generalized disease or disturbance of nutrition. The feeding of excessive amounts of animal (whale) or vegetable (palm or soya) oil in milk replacer foods to calves has been found to cause the development of a zone weakness in the growing hair, followed by loss of the abnormal fibres. Primary or secondary zinc deficiency in young calves gives rise to sudden hair loss around the muzzle, vulva, anus, base of the tail, hindlegs, flank and neck. The skin in the denuded areas is usually infiltrated and hyperaemic in appearance. In nervous alopecia, which is the result of peripheral nerve injury, it is local in extent. Partial or complete hairlessness with thick, horny scales separated by fissures occurs in inherited congenital ichthyosis, which has occasionally been observed in calves of the Holstein, Norwegian red poll and brown Swiss breeds.

Excess development of hair (hypertrichosis, trichauxis) is usually an inherited condition, but sometimes an abundant growth of hair occurs where the skin has been subjected to some form of irritation (inflammation, pressure). The hair of so-called harness marks (white patches in areas subjected to prolonged or repeated pres-

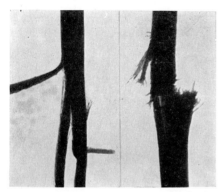

Fig. 34. *Hairs showing nodulation and splitting. Trichorrhexis nodosa.*

sure, particularly from the harness in the horse) is often longer than that of the surrounding area.

Individual hairs may show signs of disease such as abnormal brittleness (trichorrhexis) or irregular swellings resembling nodes, at which the hair tends to break off (trichorrhexis nodosa; Fig. 34). The cause of these conditions is often obscure, some cases may be of hereditary origin, while others may be the result of metabolic or toxic disturbance. Sheep on copper-deficient diets produce wool which has lost its crimp and the fibres become straight and steely. Regular constrictions along the length of the hair shaft are a result of interruptions during development and may arise from periodic disturbances of nutrition. Sometimes a number of hairs may unite to form a single horny, structure, which

might be mistaken for a neoplasm arising from the epidermis.

Changes in pigmentation of the coat include a decrease or an increase. Decreased pigmentation causing greying of the hair occurs physiologically in old age, particularly on the head of the horse, dog and ox. Sometimes, it occurs prematurely in the young animal, when it is usually difficult, or impossible, to identify the cause. Harness marks are composed of white hairs, or hairs with an alternately white and pigmented shaft. The position of these depigmented areas indicates that they are due to the effects of pressure caused by various kinds of harness, bandages, cribbing straps (Fig. 35), surgical

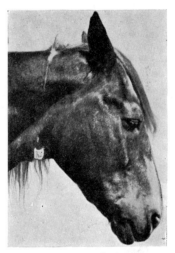

Fig. 35. *Depigmented areas (harness marks) on the neck, caused by wearing a cribbing strap.*

dressings, etc. In most other cases of changes in the pigmentation of the hair, the same considerations apply as for the skin. Normally pigmented hairs rarely grow again in places where irritation has been intense. Reduced pigmentation of the coat occurs in certain chronic debilitating diseases (Johne's disease, molybdenosis, hypocuprosis). In cattle on diets containing inadequate copper or excess molybdenum, the characteristic depigmentation produces speckling of the coat, which is most obvious around the eyes; otherwise cattle with dark-coloured coats develop light brown areas over the abdomen and chest. An increase in pigmentation is usually a very local event and occurs following irritation of rather short duration.

In the examination of the keratogenous

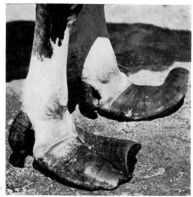

Fig. 36. *Deformity of the feet in an ox, caused by over-growth of horn. Note that the toe of the medial digit on the near foot has been cut back.* (After Habacher)

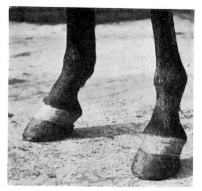

Fig. 37. *Change in texture of the hoof wall below the coronet in a horse which had been suffering for 3 months from chronic enteritis. All four feet were equally affected. The abnormal horn is pale, rough and dry.*

appendages (horns, hoofs, claws and chestnuts of mammals), the shape, size, colour, surface character, brightness and texture are noted. The examination of the interdigital cleft and the interdigital folds is conveniently carried out at this stage. Changes in size and shape of the horny structures (Fig. 36) result from malformations, lack of exercise (keeping in stalls or boxes on a deep layer of decomposing straw and faeces) and from diseases of or injury to the peripheral tissues from which the various keratogenous appendages develop. In foot-and-mouth disease, bovine malignant catarrh and virus diarrhoea the coronary band is deep pink or red (unpigmented skin), swollen and painful. A similar state, along with a thickened, brittle, uneven hoof wall, occurs in inherited dermatitis vegetans of pigs, which is apparent at birth. In animals convalescent from foot-and-mouth disease, and in generalized nutritional disorders of long standing, the hoofs become dull and dry, with loss of colour in the affected areas (Fig. 37), and may become fissured, or the entire horny structure of the hoof may be shed (more usual in pigs), thus interfering with locomotion. When nutrition is temporarily disturbed, e.g. in severe systemic disease of some duration, transverse grooves are formed in the developing keratinized tissue. The presence of these, months after recovery, indicates that a disturbance of nutrition, causing a deficiency in horn production, has previously occurred. In cows with horns, the presence of grooves at this part reflects the fluctuating nutritional status of the animals relative to pregnancy; the number of grooves is said to indicate the number of pregnancies.

Structures consisting of typical keratogenous tissue sometimes arise from the skin of various parts of the body (Fig. 38).

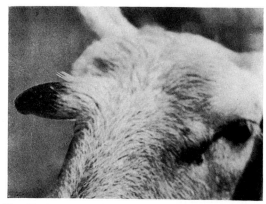

Fig. 38. *Horn growing from the skin below the right eye of a Cheviot wether. Sheep of this breed are normally polled in both sexes.*

Elasticity of the Skin

The elasticity of the skin is tested by lifting up, and then releasing, a fold of skin in the region of the neck, back or ribs. In a healthy animal, the fold of skin is easily grasped at these sites and on release immediately flattens out again. This is particularly well demonstrated in the dog, in which species a proportionately large fold of skin may be raised readily from the region of the back.

When its elasticity is reduced, the skin is less easily picked up and the fold tends to remain

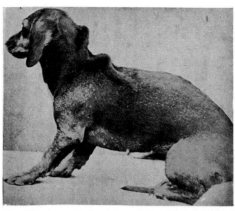

Fig. 39. *Loss of elasticity of the skin. A fold of skin picked up over the neck and shoulders has not resumed its normal position.*

after the grip has been released (Fig. 39). When the elasticity of the skin is completely lacking it is impossible to pick up even a small fold. The animal is then said to be hidebound. Loss of elasticity arises when there is reduction in the semifluid ground substance of the dermis and subcutaneous tissue, as well as of the elastic fibres. The elasticity of the skin is reduced when it itself is affected with disease, particularly in those diseases which are extensive and of long standing (eczema, mange), and in various systemic disorders associated with marked loss of condition (malnutrition, tuberculosis, leptospirosis, etc.) and/or severe dehydration (salmonellosis, white scour, enteric colibacillosis of pigs, transmissible gastroenteritis of pigs, vomiting and wasting disease of suckling pigs, Johne's disease, subacute grass sickness, diabetes insipidus).

Surface of the Skin

Absence of skin over various parts of the body surface has been observed as an inherited congenital defect (epitheliogenesis imperfecta) occurring at birth in pigs, calves and foals. There is complete absence of all skin layers in the affected areas, which vary in size and distribution. In piglets, the defect is located on the flanks, sides, back and other parts of the body. In the calf the lower parts of the limbs and occasionally the muzzle are affected.

Changes in the colour and/or structure of the skin not only occur in primary diseases of the integument, but may also be secondary to many systemic diseases, e.g. a vesicular and pustular exanthema may occur in canine distemper, an urticarial eruption in association with feeding high-protein diets and in swine erysipelas, and subcutaneous inflammatory oedema in anthrax in pigs and horses, and in pasteurellosis in cattle.

In the horse suffering from chronic alveolar emphysema, callosities and abrasions are often present on the elbows, because in order to reduce the pressure of the upper part of the forelimb on the chest the animal, when recumbent, lies with its hoofs turned inwards and so injures the skin over the elbows with the heels of the shoes.

The colour of the skin (as opposed to that of the hair) plays only a small part in veterinary diagnosis, because the skin is naturally pigmented in most animals, and usually the coat is so dense that it reduces the effectiveness of the examination, which is practicable, at best, only in the relatively hairless areas, e.g., on the ventral part of the abdomen.

Absence of pigment may occur in a general or a local form and is inherited or acquired. Albinism (white skin) is a developmental or hereditary absence of melanin in the skin; it is seen as a breed characteristic, particularly in rabbits. Vitiligo means an induced deficiency of pigment, e.g. white patches permanently affecting a pigmented skin; it is sometimes seen as a sequel to a disease of the skin, e.g. ringworm and glanders. When a discharge, e.g. from the nose, has been present for a long time, the skin over which the excretion flows tends to lose its pigment. Loss of skin pigment may occur in alopecia (the reverse is more generally the rule), and in the vicinity of the external genital organs in occasional cases of dourine.

Excessive pigmentation, causing the affected part to become much darker or even black, occurs in certain chronic skin diseases, e.g.

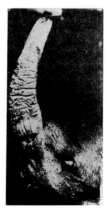

Fig. 40. *Rough and black skin on the tail and perianal region of a dog; the corrugation of the skin is clearly shown. Acanthosis nigricans.*

acanthosis nigricans (Fig. 40), in some cases of ovarian (hyperoestrogenism) and testicular disorders (hypoandrogenism) causing alopecia in dogs, sometimes in alopecia due to other causes and in chronic dermatitis. Acanthosis nigricans is characterized by pigmentation, thickening and lichenification of the skin in the axillae, with areas such as the forearms, groin, ventral neck, pinnae and tail and perianal region becoming involved later. Excessive pigmentation may also occur in thyroid hypoplasia in the dog, if coat loss is marked, and in Sertoli cell tumours of the testicle, when the skin of the abdomen and scrotum, particularly, is affected.

The colour of unpigmented skin depends upon the number of capillary blood vessels in the dermal layers; in addition the diameter of the capillaries, and the state and volume of the blood passing through them, have an influence on skin colour. Pallidness of the skin due to reduced blood supply occurs in anaemia caused by defective nutrition (cobalt, iron and certain vitamin deficiencies), intestinal parasites (haemonchosis, hookworm infestation, chronic fascioliasis), leukaemia, etc. Sudden generalized pallor of the skin occurs in acute cardiac insufficiency, syncope, shock and severe internal and external haemorrhage (as a result of contraction of the capillaries, or blood loss). Regional pallor is caused by spasm of local blood vessels or constriction of the related arteries. Both conditions occur in the blood vessels of the extremities in ergotism.

Increased redness, or hyperaemia, of the skin may be circumscribed or diffuse; it occurs in inflammatory diseases of the skin (acute dermatitis), and underlying structures in photosensitivity reactions, and also as a result of extreme dilatation of the cutaneous capillaries in certain systemic diseases of the pig, e.g. swine erysipelas, swine fever, salmonellosis and pasteurellosis, and in sunburn and heatstroke. When only individual small blood vessels stand out clearly, they are said to be injected.

Cutaneous haemorrhage is caused by rupture or increased permeability of the walls of the dermal and subcutaneous blood vessels (warfarin and sweet clover poisoning). Haemorrhages into (bruising) or under the skin appear as red areas. With the passage of time, changes occur in the colour of these patches (blue, green, yellow). Haemorrhages into the skin do not disappear on application of light pressure,

whereas hyperaemic areas are temporarily blanched. Punctiform (pinhead or larger) haemorrhages are known as petechiae, larger macular (0·5 cm in diameter) haemorrhages as ecchymoses and diffuse haemorrhages as sugillations or suffusions (extravasations of blood). Haemorrhage onto the surface of the skin is recognized by the fact that it can be washed off.

Apart from recently inflicted wounds, haemorrhage from the skin in horses is associated with local lesions produced by the filarial nematode *Parafilaria multipapillosa* (Fig. 41). The lesions, in the form of circular, raised areas of

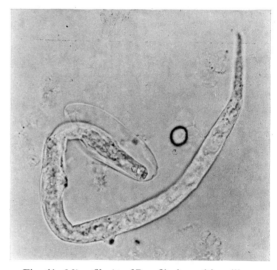

Fig. 41. *Microfilaria of* Parafilaria multipapillosa.

skin 2–5 cm in diameter (Fig. 42), are usually located in the saddle area, less frequently on the shoulders, posterior neck or upper arm regions. In cattle, non-traumatic haemorrhage occurs in conjunction with 'cutaneous angiomatosis', the lesions of which, varying in size from 0·5 to 2·5 cm in diameter and only slightly raised above the surface of the skin, are sited along the dorsum of the back, on or near the midline, or elsewhere, including the outer surface of the ear.

Bluish discoloration of the skin, or cyanosis, occurs when the capillaries contain venous blood; it disappears if the blood is squeezed out from an area of skin. It occurs to a variable degree, in a generalized form, in all diseases associated with respiratory distress (chronic pulmonary congestion, pneumonia, respiratory paralysis, airway obstruction, hydrothorax, pneumothorax,

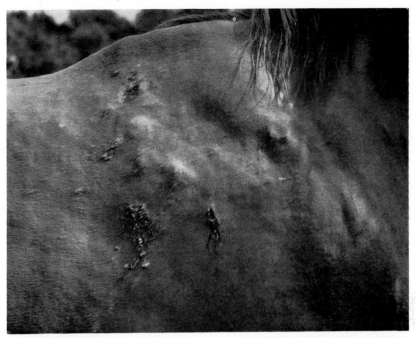

Fig. 42. *Parafilariasis in the horse, associated with cutaneous haemorrhage.* (Figs 41 and 42 from T. E. Gibson, G. A. Pepin & P. J. N. Pinsent (1964) Vet. Rec., *76*, 774; Crown Copyright)

lung collapse), also when there is undue admixture of oxygenated with unaerated blood in right-to-left congenital shunt through a significantly patent interventricular septum, in uncompensated cardiac insufficiency, when haemoglobin is altered (methaemoglobinaemia which may be caused by ingestion of nitrate, chlorate or certain sulphonamides) and when the partial oxygen pressure is too low to oxygenate the circulating haemoglobin adequately. Locally, cyanosis occurs as a result of venous stasis, caused by compression or obstruction of a blood vessel. In most cases the presence of cyanosis is more readily appreciated by examination of the visible mucous membranes. In the early stages of local gangrene the bluish area of affected skin is cold and lacking in elasticity. These changes occur in the skin of the mammary gland and teat of cows and sheep, in the relatively early stages of acute mastitis caused by *Staphylococcus aureus*.

Yellow discoloration of the skin (jaundice, icterus), which can only be identified in non-pigmented areas, occurs when an excessive quantity of free bile pigment, or conjugated bilirubin, passes into the blood and is deposited in the tissues. In all cases, more particularly those in which the skin is naturally pigmented and/or covered with hair, jaundice is more readily detected in the mucous membranes of the lips, tongue, gums, conjunctiva and membrana nictitans.

Pruritis (Itchiness)

This is a characteristic sensation, having much in common with pain, but it creates the desire to scratch, which pain does not. Pruritis can be differentiated from hyperalgesia by observing the absence of scratching and the increased reactivity to normal stimuli when the latter state exists. Itchiness is associated with a variety of skin diseases in animals, and is indicated clinically by scratching, biting and rubbing against any convenient object (Figs 43, 44). The stimulus for itching may originate peripherally or centrally. Damage to the epidermal or deeper cells, by stimulating the pain-recording endorgans situated immediately beneath the epidermis and in the epidermis itself, produces itching of peripheral origin. This type of itching is characteristically present in many forms of ectoparasitism, such as mange and many other verminous infestations. Itching does not occur when the epidermis has been completely destroyed, as in moderately deeply ulcerated areas, nor when skin

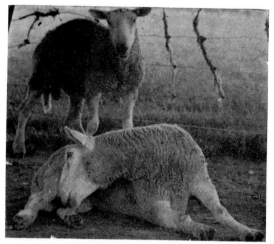

Fig. 43. *Itchiness on the leg and hindquarters. Note the wool caught up on the wire fence. Scrapie.*

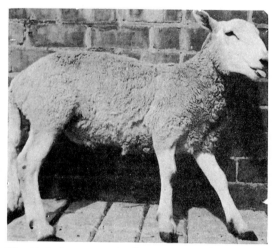

Fig. 44. *Itchiness in the hindquarters. Note the protrusion of the tongue, indicating nibbling movements of the mouth. Scrapie.*

damage is only superficial, as in most cases of ringworm. The sensation of itching, and its expression by scratching, is usually most marked when the lesions of skin disease involve the mucocutaneous junctions rather than other areas because of the greater number of pain-recording endorgans at these sites.

Itching of central origin occurs in scrapie and Aujeszky's disease (pseudorabies), in certain forms of hepatitis, obstructive jaundice, chronic nephritis, diabetes mellitus and the nervous form of acetonaemia. Apparent itchiness, indicated by licking and biting one of the extremities,

is a feature, associated with other neurological signs, in occasional cases of canine distemper. In scrapie and pseudorabies, the itching sensation may have a structural basis, the sensory stimuli being conveyed to the medulla via the spinothalamic tracts in the dorsal horns of the spinal cord; otherwise it is probably functional in its derivation, being motivated from the scratch centre below the acoustic nucleus in the medulla.

Local histamine release, as in urticaria, is a known chemical mediator of itching. It is doubtful whether mnemodermia or 'skin memory', a well known form of pruritis in man, in which skin hypersensitivity evinced by scratching persists after relatively mild lesions have disappeared, occurs in animals.

Although the animal may not be observed in the act of scratching, the existence of denuded or rough, sometimes moist, patches on the coat may serve to indicate that self-inflicted damage has occurred; in more severe cases superficial injuries (excoriations, abrasions) may be found. The presence of itchiness in the horse or ox can be demonstrated by gently scratching the animal with the fingernails or a small piece of wood; if itchiness is present the animal makes nibbling movements of the lips, salivates (particularly the ox), stretches out and partially rotates the head and neck and presses the body towards the examiner. If, on the other hand, the condition is painful, the animal draws the body away and may even strike out, or bite. It should be remembered, however, that the existence of itchiness, as expressed in this manner, does not necessarily indicate the presence of disease. Many healthy cattle respond very strongly to light. scratching of the dorsal surface of the base of the tail and surrounding parts of the rump. Most horses show signs of pleasure on being rubbed, or gently pinched, on the crest just anterior to the withers. Pigs that are accustomed to being handled usually appear to derive enjoyment from being scratched or rubbed on almost any part of the body surface, and even timid pigs, as is well known, usually respond to being lightly scratched on the back with a stick. The so-called scratch reflex in the dog appears to be completely mechanical in its reaction.

Itchiness in the ear of the dog and cat (otodectic mange, other forms of otitis externa caused by allergens, bacteria and fungi, and trauma including foreign bodies and overtreatment) is shown by shaking the head, rotating the head so that the affected ear is dependent and scratching at the ear with the hindfoot. A dog suffering from anal irritation (tapeworm segments, impaction of the anal glands) usually adopts a sitting posture and drags its hindquarters over the ground ('scooting'). Itchiness in the legs of the horse (chorioptic mange, seborrhoea or greasy heels), is indicated by stamping the feet and rubbing one limb against the other. In the horse irritation of the anus caused by *Oxyuris equi* is shown by persistently rubbing the hindquarters against solid objects, often resulting in a 'rat-tail'. (In the gelding an accumulation of smegma in the prepuce may also cause tail-rubbing.) Similar rubbing of the hindquarters occurs in mild dermatitis of the tail, while more generalized itching is a feature of 'summer itch'.

Acral lick dermatitis (lick granuloma) which occurs primarily in adult dogs of the large breeds (great Danes, Labrador retrievers, Doberman pinschers, etc.), is associated with an apparent localized pruritus manifested by licking and even biting. The lesions in the form of initial alopecia, followed by erosion and ulceration with epithelial hyperplasia leading to nodular plaque formation, are usually located in the anterior carpal or metacarpal area (Fig. 45), followed in order of frequency by the anterior radial, metatarsal, tarsal or tibial regions. Lack of exercise and boredom are considered to be of major aetiological significance. In a similar con-

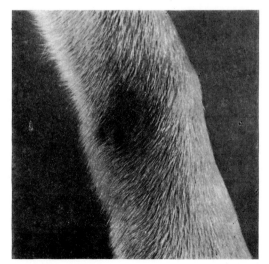

Fig. 45. *Acral pruritic nodule on the medial aspect of the metacarpus in a dog. Note the loss of hair and the ulceration of the skin.*

dition in the cat (feline neurodermatitis) the lesion is most commonly located on the inside of the thigh region, although it may be found on other parts of the cat's body.

Sweat Gland Activity

There are two types of sweat glands: (*a*) eccrine glands which are innervated by cholinergic fibres present in the sympathetic nerves and (*b*) apocrine glands which develop from hair follicles and are susceptible to adrenaline in the blood stream. In the sheep and goat, evidence suggests that the apocrine sweat glands are under direct nervous control. Most mammals have eccrine sweat glands somewhere on the body surface, particularly on frictional surfaces; those in the paw of the dog and cat are similar to the eccrine glands of man. Apocrine glands occur in most mammals. They are disseminated over the body surface of the dog and cat, except on the footpads and muzzle in the dog. The glands are especially large in the perianal region and in the lower eyelid (glands of Moll). Horses, sheep and cattle also have a general distribution of apocrine glands. The function of apocrine sweat glands, which is influenced by emotional stimuli, is of minor significance in central temperature control, although it may serve to control local skin temperature. The rabbit and bird do not possess sweat glands.

True sweating as in man, in which liquid sweat is copiously secreted over the whole body, is seen only in the horse and to a lesser degree in heat-tolerant breeds of cattle. The other breeds of cattle, which are mainly of temperate origin, possess sweat glands which are much less active, so that while beads of moisture appear on the coat in warm weather, and in certain conditions of stress, such as painful affections, the significance of these glands in heat dispersal is much less important than that of capillary dilatation leading to increased heat conduction and vaporization of moisture from the respiratory tract. The sheep and pig sweat to a limited degree and extent (in the pig the mechanism is not physiologically effective), and only at the base of the ears, on the flank and in the region of the mammary glands. The cat sweats only on the pads, and occasionally sweating is obvious at this site in the dog.

In the species possessing sudoriferous glands, the ability to sweat varies with the individual, and the degree of sweating has a considerable physiological range, determined largely by the need to lose heat produced either by exertion or exposure to high environmental temperature or humidity, or both. As a means of controlling the internal temperature, heat loss by evaporation of moisture from the body surface is much less important in animals than in man; other more important mechanisms, in some species, are panting respirations with evaporation from the respiratory tract, salivation and in the sheep insulation from the fleece, which prevents body temperature from rising under environmental influences.

Heat loss from the body occurs most rapidly when the atmospheric temperature and humidity are low. Heat conservation and heat loss by the body are controlled by the heat-regulating functions of the thermoregulating centre in the anterior hypothalamus. The afferent impulses originate from peripheral sensory receptors and the temperature of the blood flowing through the hypothalamus. The efferent impulses are conveyed via the sympathetic nervous system to the eccrine sudoriferous glands, respiratory centre, adrenal medulla, peripheral blood vessels and muscles.

Pathological sweating takes the form of an increase or decrease in volume or a change in chemical composition. Sweating does not play a significant role in excretion of waste matter from the body, because sweat itself is very dilute, the solute and solid matter being small in amount.

Increased secretion of sweat (hyperhidrosis) may be generalized, i.e. occurring over the whole body, or localized, i.e. restricted to a small area of the body. Generalized sweating to an obvious degree occurs in painful diseases ('equine colic'), and as the result of excitement (in some cases sweating may occur before the body temperature is significantly elevated), in certain diseases involving the nervous system, in muscular spasm (tetanus, transit tetany in mares) and also in severe dyspnoea when there is danger of asphyxiation. The sweating that occurs just prior to and during the decremental stages of fever is described as being 'critical', i.e. accompanying the crisis. Very severe disease of the urinary system (acute renal insufficiency) may be accompanied by uraemic sweating, i.e. the sweat has a uraemic odour due to increased urea content. In acute febrile diseases associated with jaundice, the sweat may be slightly yellowish.

The well known 'bloody' sweat (haemathidrosis) is a feature of the hippopotamus, being the normal reddish coloured product of its apocrine sweat glands when the animal is angry or excited. Apparent sweating of blood occasionally occurs in the group of diseases known as the haemorrhagic syndrome (haemophilia, sweet clover poisoning, warfarin poisoning) and is caused by haemorrhage into the hair follicles, sebaceous and sudoriferous glands.

Localized sweating usually results from disorders of the peripheral nervous system (paralysis, bruising, local inflammation involving nerves, particularly of the sympathetic nervous system), or obstruction of sweat gland ducts. In such cases it should be noted, for example, whether the sweating occurs over only half of the body (fore- or hindquarters, right or left side) or on only one side of the face. Subcutaneous injection of adrenaline may, in the horse, produce intense sweating at the site of injection only.

Reduced secretion of sweat (anhidrosis) is difficult to detect clinically; it is most readily identified by feeling the skin under the mane which, in a normal horse, is almost always damp. As a generalized condition anhidrosis occurs in various systemic diseases, more particularly those in which excessive fluid loss occurs from the body by routes other than the skin and/or the respiratory tract (enteritis, diabetes insipidus, diabetes mellitus), and in chronic nutritional disorders. The 'non-sweating syndrome' is noted to occur mainly in horses and occasionally in cattle (high-producing dairy cattle are more susceptible) of non-indigenous origin, in countries with a hot, humid climate. The problem is most serious in racehorses imported into tropical countries from temperate areas. Affected horses and cattle have their efficiency impaired to such a degree, in some cases, that they have to be returned to a cooler climate in order to recover. The cause of the disease is not clearly established; investigations in the horse suggest that, under hot weather conditions, the sweat glands become insensitive to the action of adrenaline because they have become conditioned to the high blood levels of the catecholamine which occur under such circumstances. The hyponatraemia which occurs is a result of the initial heavy sweating which persists for a period prior to the onset of anhidrosis. Evidence from studies in cattle suggest that the ability to acclimatize to hot weather is genetically based. In a local form, decreased sweating results from reduction in the blood supply to an area of skin following arterial spasm (frost-bite, ergotism, terminal dry gangrene in calves), or thromboembolic obstruction of an artery (e.g. external iliac artery in the horse).

Sebaceous Glands

Normally the skin and hair are kept somewhat greasy (this gives the hair its lustrous, shiny appearance and slight moisture-repellent quality), by the secretion (sebum) of the sebaceous glands which is composed of the disintegrating epithelial cells of the glands themselves (holocrine secretion). Abnormally, the secretion of the sebaceous glands may be reduced or become excessive, in which case the animal gives off an unpleasant rancid odour. Reduced sebaceous gland activity occurs during the course of many nutritional deficiency diseases, parasitic infestations and other chronic debilitating diseases and most febrile states, giving the hair a dry lacklustre appearance. When excessive, sebaceous secretion may be either liquid, making the hair in the affected area appear oily (it occurs in exudative epidermitis of baby pigs and greasy heels in horses), or solid, forming crusts that feel greasy on being crushed between the fingers. This latter may occur in the horse, particularly the gelding, pig and ox in the form of smegma accumulations in the preputial cavity. The cause of sebaceous hypersecretion is not fully understood; it probably originates as a condition secondary to dermatitis or eczema; in exudative epidermitis of pigs the exciting cause is a *Staphylococcus*-like bacterium which sets up an inflammatory state involving the sebaceous glands.

External Ear

The outside and inside of the pinna are inspected, as is the external auditory meatus, which normally contains a certain amount of wax produced by the ceruminous glands present in considerable numbers in the thin lining skin. Inspection of the concave surface of the pinna and of the cutaneous pouch along its posterior border in the dog will reveal the presence of macroscopic parasites such as fleas, ticks and forage mites. Trauma to the pinna will be indicated by laceration; in some breeds of dogs, e.g. dachshund, the margins of the pinna are often found to be dried, fissured, hairless and slightly scaled. The existence of a haematoma involving the pinna (this occurs most frequently in the dog, cat and sheep and is usually situated between the cartilage and the skin of the inside of the pinna) is readily recognized.

Whenever necessary, the distal part of the external auditory meatus should be squeezed between the fingers and thumb of one hand gently applied at the base of the ear, as close to the head as possible. A crackling or squelching sound indicates the presence of a fluid exudate (otitis externa). For an examination of the interior part of the external auditory meatus, it is advantageous to use a source of light (pocket torch, head lamp) or a concave mirror; for a more thorough inspection of the deeper parts it is necessary to use an auriscope fitted with a speculum of appropriate size and a magnifying lens (Fig. 46). Care should be exercised in using

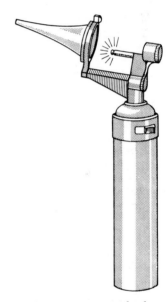

Fig. 46. *An auriscope with a large speculum in position. Smaller specula are also available.*

the auriscope in order to avoid injury to the delicate skin of the meatus, and the infliction of pain.

The necessity to perform these examinations is greatest in the dog, which usually behaves in a characteristic manner (shaking the head, which is often held to one side or rotated with the affected ear dependent, and scratching the affected ear with the hindfoot) when afflicted with irritation of the external ear canal. In many cases of prolonged otitis externa in the dog, proliferative lesions, which tend to possess corrugated characteristics, give rise to a variable degree of narrowing of the external auditory meatus.

When considered desirable, a sample of the material present in the meatus may be removed by means of a small pair of forceps and a wisp of cottonwool, or a suitable swab, for further examination. By these means, mange mites, which in the case of the dog may have been observed during the auriscopic examination (*Otodectes cynotis*; see Fig. 61, p. 62), foreign bodies, fungi or recognized pathogenic bacteria can be identified, and in the case of the last, antibiotic sensitivity tests made. Gentleness should be employed when handling the ears of animals, particularly those with obvious pain in this part; whenever necessary, in the dog and cat or in other animals, a suitable narcotic or even a general anaesthetic should be administered to aid the examination.

Odour

Bacterial and chemical decomposition of the secretion of the apocrine sweat glands and the holocrine secretion of the sebaceous glands gives animals their species odour. Otherwise, a distinctive odour, noticed during the examination of an individual animal, may have arisen from a medicinal substance that has recently been applied and is still adherent to the skin and coat. In cutaneous seborrhoea there is a rancid smell; in generalized dermatitis, advanced demodectic mange, canine distemper and also heavy infestation with ascarid worms, a strong and unpleasant smell may be detected. Necrotic disintegration of tissue, particularly of bone, gives rise to a very offensive odour. In ketosis of ruminants, and in advanced diabetes mellitus, there is an odour of acetone, and in uraemia a urinous odour.

Lesions

A distinction is made between primary lesions (eruptions) and secondary lesions. Eruptions (exanthemas) are characteristic changes in the skin and mucous membranes. As a general rule, eruptions originate with a characteristic appearance, whereas secondary lesions may develop from the primary ones, or follow some form of interference, which may be self-imposed during biting or scratching the affected part, or occur following injudicious treatment. Eruptions may be inflammatory or non-inflammatory in origin, and may occur in the skin or mucous membranes in certain diseases of the skin or internal organs. Important points in the recognition of skin eruptions are their size (discrete or diffuse), shape, number and distribution over the body. Most primary lesions are discrete and some of the secondary type tend to be diffuse.

Primary Lesions

A *macule* or spot is a circumscribed area of discoloration of the skin which is not elevated above the level of the surrounding skin, e.g. the local hyperaemia of the skin which occurs at the outset of many skin diseases, including the pox group. Lesions of this type, arising from erythema of the skin, can be temporarily obliterated by pressure, in contrast to those due to haemorrhage into the skin caused by the bite of a tick or louse. Maculae may be large or small, circular or irregular (Fig. 47).

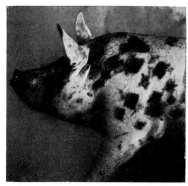

Fig. 47. *Rhomboidal red areas on the skin. Swine erysipelas.*

A *papule* or pimple is a solid elevation on the surface of the skin, varying in size from a pinhead to a pea, caused by cellular infiltration. A similar lesion of larger size is described as a *nodule* and a still larger lesion of this type is termed a *node*. The situation of a papule in an area of skin covered by hair can be recognized by the erection of the overlying hair of the coat, in the form of a tuft. Papules may involve only the superficial layers of the epidermis, in which case they are comparatively avascular and painless, or they may extend more deeply, when they

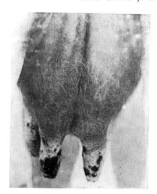

Fig. 48. *Blood-filled vesicles on the teats of a cow. Foot-and-mouth disease.*

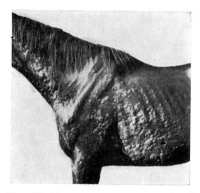

Fig. 49. *Numerous cutaneous weals of irregular size and shape in the horse. Urticaria.*

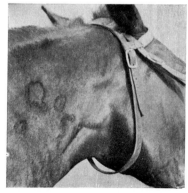

Fig. 50. *Annular weals in a horse. Dourine.* (Gratzl)

are likely to be associated with a vascular reaction in the surrounding tissues, and evidence of pain. A nodule may be firm or soft in consistency, its surface may be smooth or irregular, and it may vary in colour. Eruptions of a papular or nodular character occur in the early stages of acne, furunculosis, eczema, various forms of animal pox, contagious pustular dermatitis ('orf') of sheep, in lumpy skin disease and malignant catarrhal fever of cattle and in glanders in horses. Nodular swellings in the subcutaneous tissues, as in calcinosis in dogs and *Hypoderma* larvae in cattle, may give the appearance of primary cutaneous involvement.

A *vesicle* is a small elevation of the superficial epithelium of the skin caused by a lenticular-shaped accumulation of serous fluid or lymph between the epidermal (prickle cell) or dermal layers. A *bleb, bulla* or *blister* is a larger lesion of a similar type. The vesicular type of eruption may be unilocular and smooth on the surface (foot-and-mouth disease, vesicular exanthema), or sharply pointed (acuminated) (pseudo-cowpox), or multilocular and irregular on the surface (umbilicated) (poxes). A *pustule* is a similar lesion containing pus, which gives it a yellow colour. Vesicles containing blood are black in colour (Fig. 48).

A *weal* is a circumscribed swelling in the skin caused by local serous infiltration and erythema, as in urticaria. The lesion has a flat surface, and in unpigmented skin it is beetroot coloured. The number, size and shape are variable (Fig. 49); in dourine the weals possess annular characteristics (Fig. 50) while in pityriasis rosea they are whorl-like, with central areas of normal skin (Fig. 51). Similar whorl-like centrifugally expanding rings of erythema occur in ringworm in the pig. If the affected area is small, it is recognized visually only by the bristling of the overlying hair. Urticarial lesions usually appear and disappear rapidly.

Secondary Lesions

Scurf (scales, pityriasis) is discarded epithelial tissue retained in the coat. A certain amount of desquamation is a normal consequence of the continual proliferation of the germinative layer of the skin. Pityriasis is exaggerated in certain dietary, parasitic or fungal diseases, and in some forms of chemical intoxication. The important dietary deficiencies include avitaminosis A, nicotinic acid, riboflavine, and linolenic acid. Pityriasis

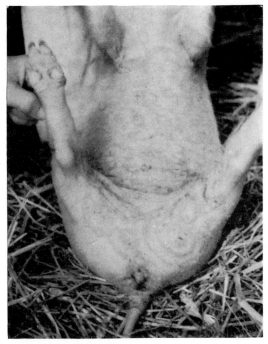

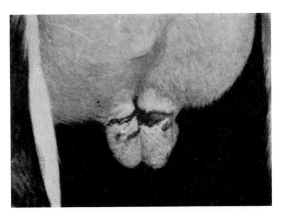

Fig. 51. *Pityriasis rosea in a pig. Note the whorl-like character of the urticarial weals. The lesions are fairly advanced, with superficial scab formation.*

Fig. 52. *Clearly demarcated ulcers on the teats of a cow. Bovine ulcerative mammilitis (herpes virus infection).*

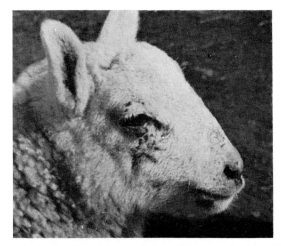

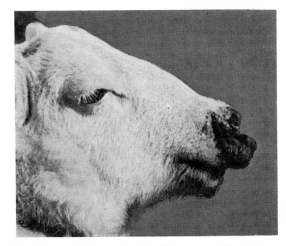

Fig. 53. *Crusts on the skin below the eye, on the lower lip and on the muzzle in two lambs. A late stage of contagious pustular dermatitis (orf).*

is often associated with infestation by fleas, lice or mange mites, and is pronounced in the early stages of ringworm. Shedding of thin bran-like scales from the skin occurs in most cases of chronic iodism, chronic arsenic or chlorinated naphthalene poisoning and pityriasis rosea in the pig.

An *erosion* is a destructive loss of the superficial layers of the skin (epidermis). Erosive lesions, which tend to develop other characteristics, occur in the interdigital cleft and on the teats, as well as the more usual sites, in cattle in foot-and-mouth disease and vesicular stomatitis, and on the muzzle in malignant catarrhal fever and mucosal disease. An *excoriation* involves also the deeper layers (corium) and is usually the result of self-inflicted trauma.

An *ulcer* (Fig. 52) is the result of localized destruction or breakdown of tissue which may occur as part of an inflammatory reaction or may result from trauma. Ulceration of the skin occurs at the site of earlier vesicular or necrotic lesions in foot-and-mouth disease, vesicular exanthema, bovine ulcerative mammillitis, malignant catarrhal fever, rinderpest, mucosal disease, lumpy skin disease, ulcerative dermatitis and certain diseases of equidae which will be referred to almost immediately. Observing the characters of an ulcer may be of diagnostic value. An ulcer may be large or small, circular, irregular or elongated, shallow or deep. Its margin may be raised above or remain level with the floor, which may be smooth or tuberculate. Characteristic ulcers occur in cutaneous glanders (clean-cut border with a depressed floor), equine ulcerative lymphangitis (rapidly granulating floor), equine epizootic lymphangitis (inverted border) and contagious pustular dermatitis (very actively proliferating and irregular).

A *chap* is a small fissure in the skin which extends to the subcutaneous tissues. Fissuring usually develops where ulceration involves a fold in the skin; it shows a tendency to increase in length and depth.

A *crust* or scab is a firm mass, consisting of dried inflammatory exudate and epithelial debris (Fig. 53), or of blood, in which case it is black, and closely attached to the underlying tissues. Scab formation is a recognized phase in the animal pox diseases and in many other conditions in which a cutaneous exanthema or ulcer occurs at an earlier stage. Characteristic crusts occur in ringworm in cattle and in certain instances also in rabbits, dogs and cats.

A *scar* is formed by the proliferation of fibrous tissue at the site of a lesion which has destroyed the corium of the skin. Causes include diseases associated with severe, extensive or deep ulceration or trauma which may have been self-inflicted, of surgical origin or result from injudicious use of irritant drugs or cauterization. Scars may be small, flat, raised or depressed, linear or stellate, and white, red or purple in colour. Scars are invariably devoid of hair but, when they are situated in haired areas, their presence may be overlooked, unless they are of moderate or large size. Small scars are readily noticed on hairless skin, and even on the haired parts when the coat is lifted and a careful search is made.

Eczema

Eczema has been defined as an inflammatory reaction of the epidermis to exogenous or endogenous substances which may act in the manner of sensitizing agents. In many instances, a predisposing factor such as nutritional deficiency, trauma, certain chemicals or ectoparasites may play a not insignificant part in its development. With increasing understanding of the pathological changes occurring in inflammatory diseases of the skin, the term 'eczema', has been largely replaced by 'dermatitis'.

In typical cases the skin reaction, which shows a tendency to extend to the dermal layers, is characterized by a variety of lesions including any combination of papules, vesicles and pustules, with a varying degree of cutaneous erythema, which results in moist, crusted or scaly, itching lesions. In the mature, long-haired dog, an acute, moist form of eczema is of fairly frequent occurrence, particularly during the spring to autumn seasons. The lesion, which is usually single, and situated on the back, loins, croup or base of the tail, is circumscribed, hyperaemic, oedematous, hot and painful. There is considerable exudation of serous fluid, which may later coagulate and form a thin crust; the hair is thoroughly soaked with the fluid, and is quickly lost (Fig. 54). This form of the condition develops rapidly, sometimes reaching an advanced degree in less than 24 hours. In the cat, the moist lesions of acute eczema are found on either, or both sides of the vertebral column from the shoulders to the croup, on the ventral

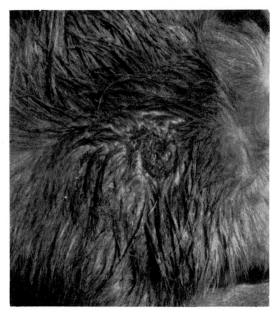

Fig. 54. *Acute moist eczema, with matting of the surrounding hair in a dog. An early stage of the condition.*

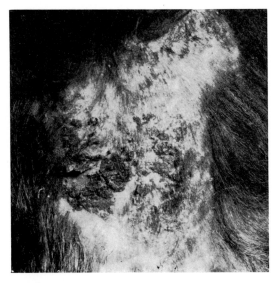

Fig. 55. *Chronic eczema in a dog with exfoliating crusts indicating an earlier and more acute phase.*

aspect of the abdomen, and also on the posterior aspect of the thighs; in this form, the condition may resolve quickly and completely, or it may be succeeded by chronic inflammation associated with proliferation of epidermal cells, extending hair loss, hypertrophy of all skin layers with resultant pachydermia, but the skin remains intact. In many such cases, dermatitis supervenes as a result of the local establishment of bacterial infection. In both the dog and cat, a mild form of eczema (Fig. 55), with limited exudation, is probably more prevalent than the acute exudative form of the disease. The lesions of this type may be found on almost any part of the body and, in the cat, are usually small and discrete, particularly in the initial stages. True eczema is rare in large animals. Occasionally it is seen in the horse, but the other farm animals are only rarely affected.

There is evidence to suggest that some animals have a marked predisposition to eczema, which in a proportion of instances appears to be genetic, viz. dogs of the long-haired breeds. In the majority of cases it is due to factors within the environment of the animal, such as external parasites, application of irritant substances such as some soaps, detergents and antiseptic substances to the skin, internal parasites and possibly certain proteins ingested with the food. External parasites (fleas, lice) and accumulation of dirt on the skin cause constant scratching, and so predispose to eczema. Frequent dampness, as in exposure during wet weather and repeated sweating, will have a similar effect.

Dermatitis

The term dermatitis includes those conditions characterized by inflammation of the deeper layers of the skin, including the blood vessels and lymphatics, with secondary involvement of the epidermis. The causes of dermatitis in animals may be classified as follows: *bacterial* (mycotic dermatitis of cattle and sheep, infectious dermatitis of pigs, ulcerative granuloma of pigs, pyoderma in puppies); *viral* (cowpox, pseudo-cowpox, swine pox, horse pox, sheep pox, bovine ulcerative mammilitis, contagious pustular dermatitis of sheep, lumpy skin disease of cattle, ulcerative dermatosis of sheep); *fungal* (ringworm, initially in all species, only involves the stratum corneum, but in some cases, more especially in horses, may spread to the dermal layers, sporotrichosis in horses); *metazoan ecto-*

parasites (mange and other mites, myiasis caused by blowflies or screw-worm fly larvae, stephano-filariasis, cutaneous habronemiasis, elaeophor-iasis); *physical agents* (sunburn, frost-bite, photosensitization, fleece rot in sheep due to excessive wettings, radiation burn); *irritant or toxic chemicals* (mercuric iodide, arsenic, sodium and potassium hydroxide applied to the skin, or arsenic taken orally); *nutritional* (deficiency of nicotinic acid or biotin in the diet is considered to produce dermatitis in pigs); or *undetermined* (excessive consumption of potatoes in cattle, 'collie nose' in dogs). Allergy to certain substances which are innocuous to most animals more usually results in the development of eczema involving the epidermis alone; when the reaction is severe, the deeper tissues are likely to be affected, as in allergic dermatitis of horses.

The inflammatory reaction associated with dermatitis varies in intensity depending, to some degree, on the character of the causal agent and whether self-inflicted trauma has taken place. It may be acute or chronic, suppurative, exudative, seborrhoeic, ulcerative or necrotic. Erythema is observed in unpigmented skin and pain or itching is evident. The temperature of the affected area is raised and cellular and fluid infiltration produces thickening of the skin. The main histological changes in acute dermatitis consist of leucocyte infiltration and cellular necrosis. When the lesions remain localized and uncomplicated, healing follows crust or scab formation. In some cases, more often in thin-skinned breeds of dogs, diffuse, spreading cellulitis results when bacterial infection extends to the subcutaneous tissues. When the area of skin so affected is extensive, shock, with peripheral circulatory failure, is likely to develop in the early stages, and toxaemia or septicaemia in the later stages.

Dermatitis is readily recognized by its clinical features; its specific nature may be indicated by the characteristic syndrome some of the aetiological agents produce. Differentiation from eczema is sometimes difficult unless contact with a known allergen can be established. Examination of skin scrapings or swabs for parasites, bacteria or fungi is always advisable. Skin biopsy is also worth serious consideration as it provides the opportunity to examine the deeper structures of the skin in a variety of ways. Some of the types of dermatitis referred to will be considered in more detail later in this chapter.

Hyperkeratosis

Hyperkeratosis (thickening of the skin, with or without loss of hair) is produced by accumulation of excessively keratinized epithelial cells on the surface of the skin. Although thickening of the skin may occur in any part of the body in all species, hyperkeratosis is recognized most often as a clinical entity in cattle (particularly calves), in which it is caused by contact with or ingestion of certain chemical substances, such as highly chlorinated naphthalene compounds, which are incorporated in wood preservatives, lubricating oils and insulating materials and creosote, arsenic, etc. In chlorinated naphthalene and creosote poisoning, the excessive keratinization is due to interference with conversion of carotene to vitamin A by the liver (hyperkeratosis is not a feature of nutritional hypovitaminosis A) and with normal cell division in the granular layer of the epidermis, leading to hypertrophy of the stratum corneum and adhesion of epithelial scales. The skin of the upper two-thirds of the trunk and the sides of the neck, is thickened and wrinkled, and that over the angle of the jaw and upper part of the neck is characteristically dry, grey, wrinkled and hairless (Fig 56). (There are also papillary proliferations on

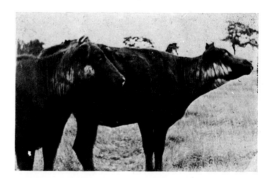

Fig. 56. *Hyperkeratosis in two heifers. Note the position of the affected areas.* (R. M. Loosmore (1953) Vet. Rec., *65*, 908)

the mucous membrane of the mouth, tongue, oesophagus and other parts of the alimentary tract.) In newborn animals, especially calves, rare cases of congenital hyperkeratosis (ichthyosis, fish-scale disease) may occur. Local areas of hyperkeratosis may result from repeated trauma at pressure points, such as the elbows, in animals lying on hard surfaces. Hyperkeratosis of the footpads and muzzle is a feature of some cases of canine distemper; the footpads are not infrequently affected in apparently normal Irish terriers, more rarely in other breeds.

Parakeratosis

This is a condition of the skin in which keratinization of the superficial epidermal cells is incomplete. The initial abnormality consists of oedema of the prickle cell layer, with lymphatic dilatation and leucocyte infiltration. The abnormal cells, which retain their nuclei, are soft and sticky and tend to remain adherent to the underlying tissues or fall off in the form of scales. The lesions may be extensive and diffuse or localized. The condition is recognized as a specific entity in pigs, in which a relative dietary deficiency of zinc, an excess of calcium and a deficiency of unsaturated fatty acids are considered to be involved as aetiological factors. It appears that, in rapidly growing pigs, when the diet is high in calcium, essential fatty acids do not meet requirements and, in addition, there is decreased digestibility of the fat in the ration. Additional dietary zinc and copper alleviate the condition, which is effectively prevented by supplements of soyabean oil or some other suitable source of linoleic acid.

Parakeratosis also occurs in a diffuse form in calves being reared on whole milk, or processed milk diets, when these are deficient in zinc (less than 40 ppm). Areas of skin affected include the legs, scrotum, neck and head, especially around the nostrils. There is swelling of the coronets, hocks and knees, with wrinkling of the skin and alopecia, which is often first noticed around the nostrils, but also appears elsewhere. If the affected areas of skin are unpigmented, marked erythema is noted when hair loss first occurs. The calves lose condition and fail to thrive unless additional zinc is provided. In sheep, parakeratosis is characterized by loss of wool with thickening and wrinkling of the skin in the exposed areas.

In a local form, parakeratosis is often confined to the flexor aspects of joints where it results from non-specific chronic inflammation. Clinical examples include mallenders and sallenders. Parakeratosis occurs along with other skin changes, including superficial desquamation and alopecia, in thallium poisoning. Differentiation of parakeratosis from hyperkeratosis is made by noting that the skin crusts in the former are soft, and when removed leave a raw surface beneath.

So-called 'Skin Tuberculosis' (Acid-fast Lymphangitis)

Particular note should be taken of this condition, which occurs only in cattle, and is important in relation to the interpretation of herd tuberculin tests, because affected animals may give a suspicious or positive reaction to the test when they are free of tuberculosis. As a consequence greater attention is paid to the condition in areas and countries in which bovine tuberculosis eradication is in progress. The disease is worldwide in distribution, the incidence being higher in housed cattle. The lesions take the form of clearly demarcated nodules (tuberculoid granuloma) or abscesses, varying in size from that of a pea to a tangerine, and containing either firm, light-brown living tissue, dry necrotic material or thick yellow caseopus. The nodules and abscesses are situated in the skin itself, and after a varying time they rupture, discharge the caseopurulent contents and heal.

The lesions occur most commonly on the legs, particularly the forelegs, where they tend to develop along a line ascending from the posterior aspect of the carpus, round the lateral aspect of

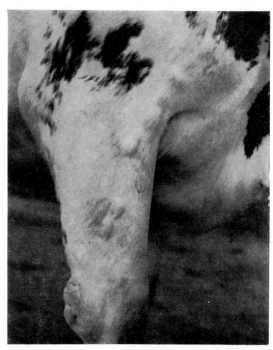

Fig. 57. *'Skin tuberculosis' (acid-fast lymphangitis) in a cow. Note the typical distribution of the lesions along a line running from the back of the knee towards the prescapular region.*

the forearm to the prescapular region (Fig. 57). In the hindleg, the lesions (commonly of the abscess type) are usually found on the posterolateral aspect of the hock, metatarsus and fetlock joint.

The situation of the lesions suggests cutaneous abrasion as the most probable portal of entry of the causative organism. There is considerable doubt as to the identity of the causal agent; the acid-fast bacterium which is often observed in small numbers in smears prepared

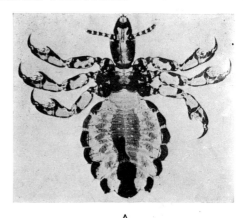

A

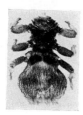

Fig. 58. Ixodes ricinus, *the common sheep or cattle tick.* ×4.

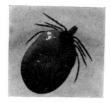

Fig. 59. Melophagus ovinus, *the sheep ked.* ×4.

from typical lesions is not considered to be a true pathogen.

Ectoparasites

A number of important ectoparasites are responsible for producing skin disease in animals. The larger species include ticks, keds, fleas and lice, which are readily seen and recognized as such with the naked eye (Figs 58–60). The sheep ked (*Melophagus ovinus*) is a bloodsucker, and heavy infestations may cause anaemia; otherwise it is a source of irritation resulting in scratching, biting and damage to the fleece; staining of the wool may depreciate the value of the fleece. Keds are suspected to be vectors of Q fever in sheep. Goats are also sometimes infested by keds.

Like the sheep ked, lice are usually host-specific and pass their whole life on the host. There are a considerable number of species of lice (Table 4) but only two types are recognized: (*a*) biting lice which have broad, blunt heads with chewing mouth parts and (*b*) sucking lice with long, narrow heads and mouth parts designed for sucking blood. For morphological descrip-

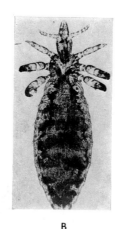

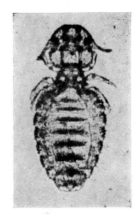

B   C

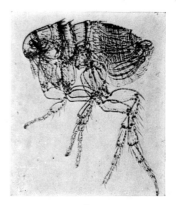

D

Fig. 60. A, Haematopinus suis, *the sucking louse of the pig.* B, *A typical sucking louse.* C, *A typical biting louse.* D, Ctenocephalides canis, *the dog flea.*

TABLE 4. COMMON LICE OF DOMESTICATED ANIMALS

Animal	Biting Lice	Sucking Lice
Horse	*Damalinia equi*	*Haematopinus asini*
Cattle	*Damalinia bovis*	*Haematopinus eurysternus*
		H. quadripertusus
		Linognathus vituli
		Solenopotes capillatus
Sheep	*Damalinia ovis*	*Linognathus pedalis*
		L. ovillus
		L. africanus
		Haematopinus quadripertusus
Goat	*Damalinia caprae*	*Linognathus stenopsis*
	D. limbata	
	D. crassipes	
Pig	—	*Haematopinus suis*
Dog	*Trichodectes canis*	*Linognathus setosus*
	Heterodoxus shiniger	
Cat	—	*Felicola subrostratus*

tions and details of life cycles see standard textbooks of parasitology.

In louse infestations (pediculosis), which show seasonal periodicity, being more prevalent in winter, there is sufficient irritation of the skin to cause scratching, licking and restlessness, leading to damage to hair, fleece and skin and to loss of weight or milk yield. Heavy infestation with sucking lice may lead to serious anaemia; this has been observed most often in cattle. *Haematopinus suis* has been incriminated as being of importance in the transmission of swine pox.

Ticks are of great importance as vectors in the transmission of many diseases in animals. In addition they may have more direct effects on animal health, e.g. *Ixodes ricinus* and *Argas* spp. as well as some others are active blood-suckers so that in heavy infestations they are capable of causing very severe anaemia. Otherwise tick infestation may interfere with food intake and cause loss of weight and depressed production. Ticks spend only part of their lives feeding on animals, and they lay eggs away from the host. The life cycles of the different species of ticks vary according to the number of hosts they parasitize. Some are single-host ticks, passing their entire life on one host, during which time they may become mature; others pass the different stages of the cycle—larval, nymphal and adult—on successive hosts, while others are parasitic at some stages and not at others. Table 5

TABLE 5. TICKS: NUMBER OF HOSTS DURING LIFE CYCLE

One-Host	Two Hosts	Three Hosts
Boophilus spp.	*Rhipicephalus evertsi*	*Ixodes* spp.
Dermacentor albipictus	*R. bursa*	*Haemaphysalis* spp.
Margaropus wintheimi	*Hyalomma* spp.	*Ambylomma* spp.
Otobius spp.	(may have three hosts)	*Rhipicephalus* spp.
		(except *R. evertsi* and *R. bursa*)
		Hyalomma spp.
		(may have two hosts)
		Dermacentor spp.
		(except *D. albipictus*)
		Ornithodorus spp.
		(many hosts)
		Argas persicus
		(many hosts)

classifies the ticks according to the number of hosts necessary for the completion of the life cycles. It must be remembered that ticks are not rigidly host specific, so that they may parasitize a considerable variety of animals.

In addition to their direct effects on animals ticks may transmit a variety of protozoal, bacterial, viral and rickettsial diseases. Adult female ticks of certain species can cause paralysis in animals by means of a toxin secreted by the salivary glands, which interferes with the synthesis or action of acetylcholine.

A number of species of fleas infest animals (Table 6); they are identified by their gross

TABLE 6. SPECIES OF FLEAS FOUND ON ANIMALS

Animal	Flea
Dog and cat	Ctenocephalides spp.
Rabbit	Spilipsyllus cuniculi

Fleas do not occur on any other species of domestic animal.

morphological characters. Fleas live for long periods away from a host and in their life cycle pass through a complete metamorphosis. Eggs are usually laid in dust and dirt in the environment of the infested host. Apart from the direct effect they produce by means of their bites being extremely irritating, thereby causing erythema and sometimes dermatitis, fleas serve as an intermediate host for certain tapeworms (*Dipylidium* spp.) and, it has been suggested, could perform a similar function for filarid worms (*Dipetalonema* spp.).

Mange Mites

Certain species of the mange mites (*Psoroptes Chorioptes* and *Otodectes*) are also visible to the unaided eye, but require the use of a microscope for their identification. Many of the other mange mites (*Sarcoptes* and *Notoedres*) however, can be found and identified only by microscopical examination of suitable material (Figs 61, 62).

Suitable material for this type of examination is obtained from the periphery of the active skin lesions. Scales are scraped off with a sharp-bladed knife held at a wide angle to the skin surface until slight bleeding occurs. (When working out of doors, the examiner may find it helpful to rub a little 5% caustic potash solution, or water, onto the selected area by means of a cottonwool swab, so that the skin scrapings adhere to the knife blade instead of being blown

away by the wind.) Some of the material is then placed on a microscope slide, triturated with a few drops of a 5–10% solution of potassium hydroxide (and may be gently heated to near boiling point over a small flame) until the crusts and scales are softened and somewhat clarified. The preparation on the slide is then gently pressed out into an even layer with a cover-slip or another slide, taking care to exclude air bubbles. Alternatively, the scrapings from the skin may be gently boiled in the potash solution in a suitable testtube, using a water bath. When the liquid becomes syrupy, centrifuge and, after discarding the supernatant fluid, place the deposit on a microscope slide and examine the preparation with minimum delay. Preliminary examination is carried out under low-power magnification (about 100 diameters); for species identification, the detailed morphology of the mites is obtained with medium magnification (about 300 diameters).

For a diagnosis of mange, recognition of mites, portions of mites or eggs is sufficient, but a negative finding may not mean that mange is absent. Further material from the same and different lesions on the skin must be examined. Care is essential to differentiate the larval stage of certain forage or harvest mites (Fig. 63), which may be found on the skin of animals, in some instances causing disease, from the pathogenic mange mites.

Adult mange mites have 8 legs, nymphs have 8 legs but no genital pore and the larvae have 6 legs. The mite ova, which are large and oval in outline, may be found empty or containing larvae at various stages of development. The recognition of the individual species of mange mites is of considerable clinical and, in certain cases, legal importance. The information given in Table 7, stating the morphological detail, will enable the species to be recognized even when only fragments of the mites are found. A knowledge of the usual hosts and predilection sites of each species of mange mite is of considerable value in diagnosis, but it must be remembered that in heavy infestations the lesions may extend considerably beyond these sites.

Sarcoptic mange affects many species, including man. It is caused by *Sarcoptes scabiei*, which is usually considered to have individual host subspecies, e.g. *S. scabiei* var. *bovis*, etc.; this host-specificity is by no means absolute, so that interspecies transmission can occur fairly readily.

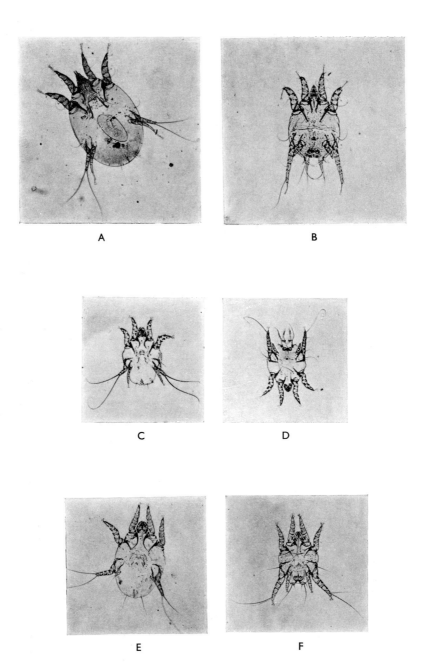

Fig. 61. *Non-burrowing mites.* A, Psoroptes, *female.* B, Psoroptes, *male.* C, Chorioptes, *female.* D, Chorioptes, *male.* E, Otodectes, *female.* F, Otodectes, *male.* *All* ×40.

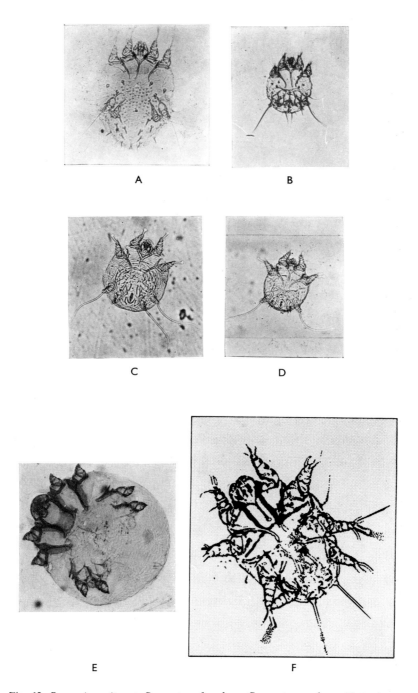

Fig. 62. *Burrowing mites*. A, Sarcoptes, *female*. B, Sarcoptes, *male*. C, Notoedres, *female*. D, Notoedres, *male*. E, Cnemidocoptes, *female*. F, Cnemidocoptes, *male*. A–D ×*100*; E, F ×*115*. (R. B. Griffiths & F. J. O'Rourke (1950) Ann. trop. Med. Parasit., *44*, 93)

TABLE 7. DIAGNOSTIC CHARACTERISTICS OF IMPORTANT ADULT MANGE MITES OF DOMESTIC MAMMALS

Genus	Body	Rostrum	Epimera of leg	Legs	Pedicles	Sucker	Sucker formula Male	Sucker formula Female	Other characteristics
Burrowing									
Sarcoptes	Round	Horseshoe-shaped	Epimera of each side joined, forming Y behind rostrum	Only two front pairs project beyond body margin	Unsegmented	Small, bell-shaped	1, 2, 4	1, 2	Anterior group of 3 peg-like cones on each side of dorsum of both sexes Posterior group of 14 stout spines on dorsum of female and 12 in male Several rows of posteriorly directed sharp-pointed scales on dorsum of female Anus terminal
Notoedres	Round	Horseshoe-shaped	Epimera of each side joined, forming Y behind rostrum	Only two front pairs project beyond body margin	Unsegmented	Small, bell-shaped	1, 2, 4	1, 2	Anterior peg-like cones absent Scales on female much reduced and obtuse Anus dorsal
Non-burrowing									
Psoroptes	Oval (visible naked eye)	Long, conical pointed	Not joined	All 4 pairs project	Long, 3 segments	Long, narrow, funnel-shaped	1, 2, 3	1, 2, 4	Posterior lobes in male rounded; 5 hairs on each
Chorioptes	Oval (visible naked eye)	Blunt, triangular	Not joined	All 4 pairs project	Very short, unsegmented	Large, bell-shaped	1, 2, 3, 4	1, 2, 4	Posterior lobes in male rectangular; 4 hairs on each, 2 being spatulate
Otodectes	Oval (visible naked eye)	Blunt, triangular	Not joined	All 4 pairs project (in female last pair very short)	Very short, unsegmented	Large, bell-shaped	1, 2, 3, 4	1, 2	Posterior lobes in male very poorly developed; 3 hairs on each

Psorergates resembles *Sarcoptes* in general outline but has a broader rostrum, longer hindleg and is slightly less than half the size of the sarcoptic mite of sheep.

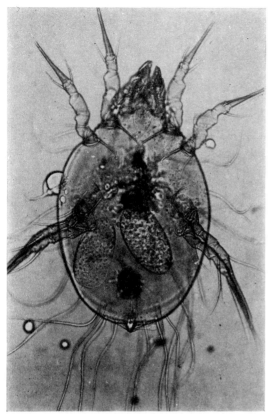

Fig. 63. *A forage mite. An ovigerous female,* Tyroglyphus sp.

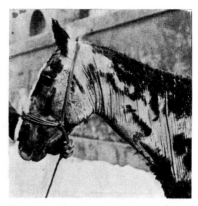

Fig. 64. *Extensive hair loss and corrugation of the skin. Advanced sarcoptic mange*

In the early stages of development the lesions are characterized by the appearance of small, red papules and general hyperaemia of the affected area, with excoriation by biting and scratching because of the intense itchiness. Later because of exudation, dry scales and crusts form which, when the disease is severe, become extensive and may be up to 1 cm thick. In the horse and ox, the head and neck are chiefly affected (Fig. 64); the medial surface of the thighs and around the root of the tail are also likely to be involved in cattle. In the pig the lesions appear on the inner aspect of the pinna of the ear and spread to the limbs and trunk; in the sheep, goat and rabbit, the head and ears are first affected, with spread to involve the whole trunk (Fig. 65), except in the sheep, where the lesions do not occur in the woolled areas. In the dog the areas involved include the face behind the muzzle, posterior border of the ear, elbow, sternal region, base of the tail and posterior aspect of the thigh.

Notoedric mange affects only the cat, rabbit and rat. The causal species, *Notoedres cati,* is occasionally isolated from dogs and rarely from man. The lesions occur on the face and ears, and occasionally on the legs and external genitalia.

Psoroptic mange is of greatest importance in the sheep, in which species it is known as 'scab', but it occurs in all species of animals. The causal parasite, *Psoroptes communis,* is much more host-specific than *S. scabiei* so that biological evidence suggests that each species of animal is affected by a distinct species of psoroptic mite, viz. horse, *P. communis equi* and *P. hippotis;* ox, *P. communis bovis* and *P. communis natalensis;* sheep, *P. communis ovis;* and goat, *P. communis caprae.* In sheep the areas chiefly affected include the dorsal part of the shoulders, along the sides and back, and at the base of the tail (Fig. 66B). Later, because the mite migrates widely to areas covered with hair or wool, the lesions may occur on any part of the body covered by the fleece. In the horse this type of mange causes lesions under the mane, in the saddle area, at the base of the tail and in some hairless areas, including the axilla, prepuce and mammary gland. *P. hippotis* infests the external auditory meatus, giving rise to severe otitis externa. In the ox this form of mange affects the neck, the region around the base of the tail and the escutcheon; spread to the rest of the body may occur in severe cases. In the goat and rabbit the lesions appear mainly on the ears (Fig. 67).

The early lesions of psoroptic mange take the form of small papules (5 mm diameter) which ooze fluid which later coagulates to form thin

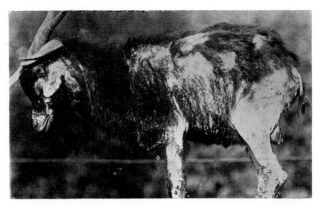

Fig. 65. *Loss of hair in a goat. Note the numerous squamous areas among the remaining hair. Sarcoptic mange.*

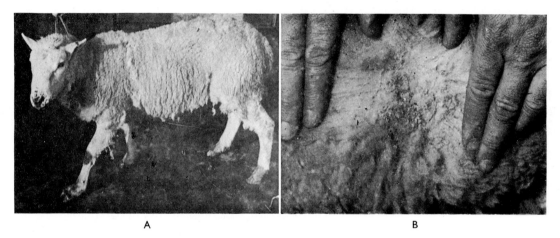

A   B

Fig. 66. *Psoroptic mange in sheep.* A, *Extensive lesions. Note the loose tufts with some shedding of wool.* B, *Dry scab formation at the base of the wool fibres on the side of the chest.*

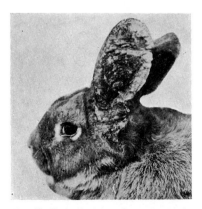

Fig. 67. *Extensive crust formation in the ear. Psoroptic mange.*

crusts and, eventually, if the parasites remain active, becomes converted into scab material. In sheep attention may be attracted to the condition by reason of the wool presenting a ragged appearance, with later shedding of wool (Fig. 66A). Itchiness is a feature in all species and is manifested by biting, rubbing and scratching the affected areas, resulting in hair or wool loss and secondary damage to the skin.

Chorioptic mange is caused by host-specific mites as follows: horse, *Chorioptes equi*; ox, *C. bovis*; sheep, *C. ovis*; and goat, *C. caprae*. This type of mange occurs most frequently in horses; the lesions affect mainly the feathered parts of the legs causing 'itchy leg'. In cattle it may affect any part of the body, but particularly the fetlock region, base of the tail and region of the groin, from where it may extend forwards along the scrotum or udder to the legs and face. Clinically obvious infestations are most prevalent during the winter season, although the mite persists in the region of the pasterns and muzzle during the summer time. In sheep the lesions are located in the non-woolled areas, chiefly the lower parts of the limbs.

In horses, attention is drawn to the existence of this type of mange because the intense irritation causes affected animals to stamp the feet in a violent manner and rub the back of the hind pasterns against fixed objects or with the front of the other leg. The affected skin areas are moist and greasy with scab formation and fissuring, the skin itself being thickened. Signs of irritation are much less obvious in cattle, and the skin lesions take the form of small scabs.

Otodectic mange affects the external auditory meatus in the dog and cat. The causal mite *Otodectes cynotis* has also been recovered from the external ear canal of foxes and ferrets. It is considered that all of these mites are biologically indistinguishable and are varieties of the one species. The mites cause irritation of the sensitive skin lining the ear canal by thrusting their long mouth parts directly through the skin and, at the same time, producing a very irritant saliva. As a result, quantities of serum exude and become mixed with the cerumen, which is produced in excessive amounts, and form a characteristic scab, often occluding the ear canal. Secondary bacterial infection often results

leading to severe inflammation and even ulceration of the epithelial tissue.

Demodectic mange occurs in all species of domestic animals. The incidence is highest in the dog, although it may be severe in the goat, and in some areas large proportions of cattle in individual herds may be affected. The causal mites, which differ from other mange mites by invading hair follicles and sebaceous glands, are host-specific, being thereby designated as *Demodex bovis* for cattle, *D. equi* for horses, *D. ovis* for sheep, *D. caprae* for goats, *D. phylloides* for pigs and *D. canis* for dogs.

As the pathogenesis of demodectic mange involves invasion of the hair follicles and sebaceous glands, i.e. the deeper parts of the skin, irritation is slight, itchiness does not occur and the inflammation is chronic in intensity. It occurs in two main types: a *squamous* (scaly) form usually found in the region of the head and neck (very often around the eyes) and a *pustular* (follicular) form resulting from secondary staphylococcal infection, which may affect almost any part of the body surface. The squamous form is most commonly seen in the dog, and is relatively uncommon in large animals. The pustular form occurs in the dog, occasionally in the ox, pig and goat, and very occasionally in the horse. A third type occurs in the dog, which in the initial stages simulates acute eczema and may be of the nature of an allergic type of reaction. The moist, painful lesions which may occur on the head and abdomen with reddening of the skin, develop rapidly and coat loss is obvious within a short time.

The initial signs of the disease take the form of small nodules and pustules which may enlarge. There is partial hair loss and thickening of the skin. If not readily seen, the lesions can be detected by palpation, when the contents of the pustules or small abscesses can be readily expressed. In cattle and goats the areas most commonly affected include the brisket, lower neck and shoulder; in horses the face and around the eyes are usually involved. Mites have been demonstrated in lymph node tissue of affected dogs, and in the skin of clinically normal dogs.

Material suitable for laboratory examination in suspected cases of demodectic mange consists, in the squamous form, of a fairly deep scraping taken with a sharp blade from the most severely affected parts of the skin and, in the pustular form, of the squeezed-out contents of a pustule. Some of the collected material is placed on a microscope slide, a drop of glycerine or liquid paraffin is added (treatment with caustic potash makes this mite too transparent to be readily observed) and a cover-slip applied. Examination is performed immediately using the low-power objective of the microscope with the iris diaphragm partially closed down. Demodectic mange mites are relatively small and elongated (about 250 μm in length), with 4 pairs of rudimentary legs in the anterior part of the body (Fig. 68). The larvae have 3 pairs of legs; the

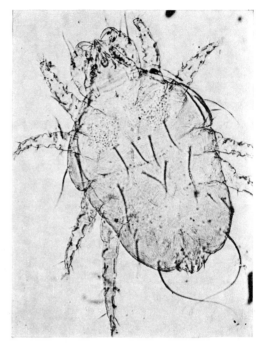

Fig. 69. *Male* Cheyletiella yasguri, *a non-burrowing mite. Note the enlarged pedipalps with prehensile claws.* × *100.*

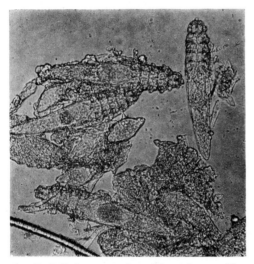

Fig. 68. *Follicle mange mites of* Demodex spp. *Note the characteristic operculate egg.* × *100.*

eggs are lemon-shaped and operculate. The mites are readily found in material from the pustules, but are sometimes difficult to demonstrate in the squamous form. In such circumstances it is recommended to make a deep incision into the skin in an affected area, fold the skin so that the cut edges of the wound are exposed and then take a scraping from both surfaces.

Trombidiform Mites

Various species of trombidiform mites infest animals, causing dermatitis. The harvest or grain mites primarily infest harvested cereals and only secondarily parasitize animals. Other species of this family include *Psorergates ovis* and *P. bos* (the latter is not considered to be of pathogenic significance), and *Cheyletiella* spp. (Fig. 69).

Psorergates ovis, the 'itch mite', has been recognized as a parasite of sheep in Australia, USA and South Africa. The mite completes its entire life cycle on the host; only the adult form is motile, spread of the infestation occurring only at this stage by means of direct contact between shorn sheep. Lesions appear first on the sides of the abdomen and later on the flanks, rump and thighs. There is an accumulation of loose dry scales with slight thickening of the skin (hyperkeratosis is apparent on histological examination). Crusts are rare—a point of difference from psoroptic mange—so that the lesions resemble those of louse infestation. The skin irritation causes affected sheep to rub and bite so that the fleece becomes ragged and may be shed. Owing to the slow progress of the disease, the worst cases are usually seen in mature animals and in the winter time.

For diagnosis, superficial skin scrapings should be taken over an extensive area after being closely clipped and smeared with an oil or liquid paraffin. For microscopic examination a portion of the scrapings are mounted in oil on a glass slide, or may be clarified as recommended for the mange mites. The mites are fragile so that the scrapings should not be overheated in the caustic solution; they are on average about half the size of a mange mite.

Cheyletiella parasitovorax (rabbit fur mite) is commonly found on the skin and in the fur of rabbits; it has been recovered from the hair of squirrels, cats and dogs and the feathers of birds. *C. yasguri* (Fig. 70) is also of importance

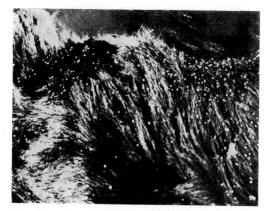

Fig. 70. *Mange-like lesions caused by* Cheyletiella yasguri *in a dog. Note the characteristic small bran-like scales in the coat hair.*

in the dog. Both species of mites can produce mange-like lesions in the dog. The lesions are variable in extent and in severe infestations may be distributed over the entire body surface. There is excessive scaling with some hair loss, and the skin becomes thickened with profuse exfoliation, fissuring and yellow scab formation. The mites are located or partially embedded in the keratin layer, and as the whole of the life cycle is spent on the host, all stages of development may be demonstrated in skin scrapings. Material for microscopic examination is most satisfactorily obtained by brushing the skin in the affected areas and collecting the scales which come off by placing the animal on a spread-out newspaper.

Harvest Mites (Chiggers)

The larvae of certain trombiculid mites, for which the natural hosts are small rodents, frequently parasitize man and many species of animals, causing dermatitis, usually in the autumn when the animals are grazing or, if confined in houses, are being fed newly-harvested cereals. The important species include *Pediculoides ventriculosus, Leptus ryleyi, Trombicula*

autumnalis, T. alfredugesi, T. splendens, T. botatasis and *Tyroglyphus farinae* (Fig. 63).

Herbivorous animals are usually affected on the face and lips, while dogs and cats are more usually affected between the toes, around the ears, the eyes, the abdomen and the base of the tail. The larvae, which may be found in clusters and are red in the unfed state, becoming straw-coloured when engorged, cause intense irritation and scaling of the skin with some loss of hair. Infestation with *Tyroglyphus* spp. in the pig causes pruritus and the development of thin scabs up to 3 cm in diameter distributed over the body; the skin beneath the scabs appears normal. The infestation is usually acquired from mite-infested ground cereal fed in the dry state. Examination of the lesions by means of a hand lens giving a magnification of some 10–30 diameters is usually sufficient to enable a diagnosis to be made. Detailed morphological examination necessitates the use of a microscope; no special preparation is required.

Ringworm

Ringworm is a disease caused by dermatophytic fungi which invade the superficial layers of the skin or its appendages, the hairs and nails. Although ringworm affects animals in all countries the incidence is highest when animals are kept in close contact, such as occurs when they are confined in houses or yards. The disease is most prevalent during the winter months and affected animals tend to recover spontaneously during spring. A number of species of two genera of fungi are recognized to cause ring worm in domestic animals. According to the specific character of the affection it can be classified as (*a*) trichophytosis (Figs 71–73), which

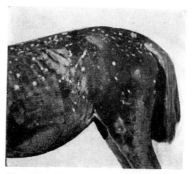

Fig. 71. *Numerous circular hairless patches distributed over the harness areas of a horse. Ringworm (trichophytosis).*

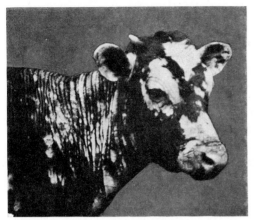

Fig. 72. *Extensive lesions of ringworm (trichophytosis) in a calf.* (C. J. La Touche (1952) Vet. Rec., 64, 841.)

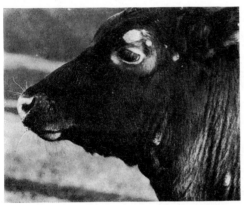

Fig. 73. *Early lesions of ringworm (trichophytosis) in a calf. Note the thick asbestos-like crust which occurs even at this early stage. The position of the lesion above the eyes is characteristic.*

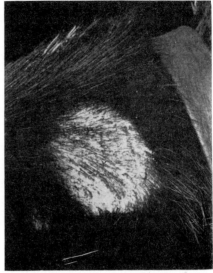

Fig. 74. *The typical asbestos-like crust formed in microsporosis.* Microsporum canis *infection in a young dog.* (C. J. La Touche (1952) Vet. Rec., 64, 398)

occurs in all species, the commonest form of ringworm being associated with *Trichophyton verrucosum* var. *discoides* infection in the calf, and (*b*) microsporosis (Fig. 74) which occurs in the horse, pig and small animals, mainly in the form of *Microsporum canis* infection in the dog and cat. Ringworm is an important zoonosis; it has been determined that in rural areas about 80% of human ringworm is acquired from animals.

The species which occur in cattle are *Trichophyton verrucosum, Tr. verrucosum* var. *album, Tr. verrucosum* var. *discoides, Tr. mentagrophytes, Tr. megnini* and *Scopulariopsis brevicaulis*; the last is a soil saprophyte. The appearance and distribution of the lesions caused by *Tr. verrucosum* var. *discoides* in the calf are typical of ring-

worm in this species, and are usually sufficiently characteristic to enable a diagnosis to be made on inspection alone. Points of significance include: age, calves being more commonly affected than adult cattle; time of year, the incidence being highest in housed cattle in late winter; situation of lesions, commonly on neck, head and perineum, although a generalized distribution may occur; the appearance of the lesions themselves, which are greyish-white, with thick crusts and roughly circular about 2·5 cm in diameter.

In the horse, the species which occur are *Trichophyton equinum, Tr. quinckaenum, Tr. mentagrophytes, Tr. verrucosum, Microsporum equinum, M. gypseum* and *Keratinomyces ajelloi*; the last two are soil saprophytes. The lesions of ringworm in the horse develop, initially, on the trunk and croup, and may later spread to the neck, head and limbs. In racehorses the saddle and girth areas are the usual sites. In the majority of cases the lesions are superficial, being more usually manifested by irregular areas of alopecia and desquamation and, in some cases, by the appearance of thick crusts. Less commonly the fungus invades the deeper structures through the hair follicles causing small areas of inflammation and suppuration. Secondary damage may arise in such cases from the trauma caused by irritation and itching.

The fungi which cause ringworm in pigs are *Trichophyton mentagrophytes, Tr. verrucosum* var. *discoides, Microsporum canis* and *M. nanum.* In the pig ringworm develops typically as a peripherally extending circular weal with a central area of alopecia covered by a relatively thin crust. The areas affected include the back and sides. The lesion produced by *M. nanum* is much less obvious because of its superficial nature. There is no pruritus or hair loss, and the crusts consist of flakes of epithelial exfoliations.

In sheep the fungi causing ringworm are: *Trichophyton verrucosum* var. *ochraceum, Tr. quinckeanum, Tr. mentagrophytes, Tr. gypseum* and *Microsporum canis.* In sheep the lesions develop on the woolless areas, particularly the head.

In the dog and cat ringworm is most commonly caused by *Microsporum canis, M. gypseum* and *Tr. mentagrophytes.* A number of other species have occurred occasionally, including *M. audouini, M. vanbreusegheni, M. distortum. Tr. schoenleini* and *Keratinomyces ajelloi.* As is the case in cattle, there is a significantly higher incidence of ringworm in younger dogs and cats. The lesions of ringworm in the dog are frequently located on the head and forequarters and appear, initially, as small incrustations, involving a few hairs, which then develop into circular areas with slight scaliness of the skin and some loss of hair. At a later stage, a moderately thick crust may form, with a few truncated hairs projecting above the surface.

In the cat the clinical picture may simulate that in the dog, or the lesions may be diffusely distributed over the body in the form of very small incrustations which present an appearance like flakes of cigarette ash when the coat is parted. In the dog, cat, rabbit and mouse *Trichophyton quinckeanum* infection may be associated with favic scutula. The appearance of the clearly demarcated orange-yellow or silvery saucer-shaped crusts is almost diagnostic. When they are broken down the lesions emit a musty odour. On microscopical examination, material from the crusts is found to contain many branching filaments (hyphae) with comparatively few, rather large spores.

Fungal infections of the superficial layers of the skin give rise to fairly characteristic lesions. In species other than cattle, however, diagnosis of ringworm depends upon microscopical examination of hairs, and to a lesser extent of scrapings, taken from the periphery of active lesions.

Evidence that an animal is affected with *Microsporum canis* or *M. audouini* is obtained by exposure, in a darkened room, to light from a Wood's lamp (Fig. 75) (i.e. ultraviolet light

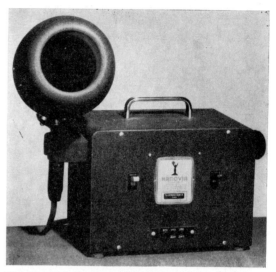

Fig. 75. *A Wood's lamp, of assistance in the diagnosis of microsporosis.* (Newton Victor)

passed through nickel oxide glass) or a purple-X bulb. Infected hairs show a bright pale-green fluorescence. Hairs infected by other *Microsporum* spp. and *Trichophyton* spp. do not fluoresce. This method of examination is often effective in detecting microsporosis in the cat, in which species macroscopic lesions may be very small and widely dispersed, or not otherwise detectable, only individual or small numbers of hairs being affected. It is also essential to remember that skin scales, nails, teeth and substances such as petroleum jelly and some other oily preparations, which may be applied to the skin and coat, also evince fluorescence when examined in this way, but usually with a bluish-white colour.

If fluorescent hairs are seen, they should be plucked out; otherwise, hairs which are dull and broken or those with a greyish-white band at their base should be selected in the same way along with skin scrapings as recommended. Some of the collected material is placed on a microscope slide with a few drops of 10% potassium hydroxide solution; a cover-slip is applied and the slide gently warmed. Although it is possible to recognize the fungus at this stage on many occasions, it is advisable to allow the preparation to stand for several hours, at the end of which time the fungus, if present in any quantity, will be more readily detectable under high-power magnification in the form of chains (*Trichophyton*) or an irregular mosaic (*Microsporum*) of highly refractile arthrospores, which may form a sheath, sometimes of considerable thickness, around the shaft of an infected hair (Figs 76–78). Mycelia may be seen in the interior of the hair.

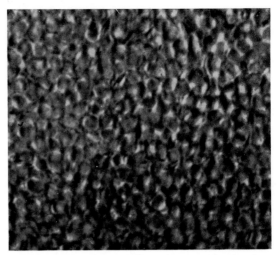

Fig. 78. Microsporum canis. *The 'mosaic' of arthrospores in the spore sheath of cat's hair. 20% KOH mount, × 1000.*

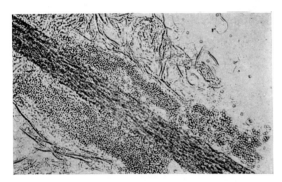

Fig. 76. Trichophyton verrucosum *var.* discoides. *An infected cattle hair showing a sheath of arthrospores. A late stage of the infection; at this stage it would be indistinguishable from infection with* Microsporum. *20% KOH mount,* ×200.

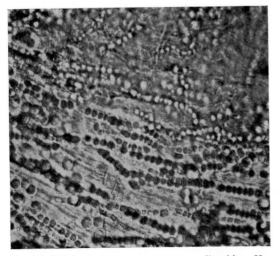

Fig. 77. Trichophyton verrucosum *var.* discoides. *Hyphae and chains of arthrospores in infected cattle hair. 20% KOH mount,* ×500.

When repeated microscopical examination of selected material from suspected ringworm lesions fails to reveal the presence of the causal fungus, specimen material may be submitted to a laboratory for cultural examination. For this, the specimen is packed in a sealed envelope, as tightly capped containers favour the growth of non-pathogenic fungi. Cultural examination enables the causal agent to be specifically identified. Sabouraud's dextrose agar containing antibiotics and cyclohexamide is usually employed because, while it inhibits the growth of both bacteria and saprophytic fungi, it does not alter the growth of pathogenic fungi. In most cases 2–3 weeks elapse before significant growths are obtained.

Bacterial Infections of the Skin

The skin may be invaded by bacteria, giving rise to a variety of diseases including impetigo, acne-like conditions, furunculosis, cutaneous pyoderma, and the various forms of bacterial dermatitis mentioned earlier. A variety of bacteria including streptococci, staphylococci (sycosis), diphtheroid species, *Dermatophilus* spp. and others are associated with these conditions.

Impetigo

This is a superficial eruption consisting of small, thin-walled vesicles which develop into pustules, followed by rupture and scab formation. In animals the main organism is usually a

Staphylococcus, sometimes in association with a *Streptococcus*. Primary impetigo occurs most commonly on the udder in cows, especially near the base of the teats. The lesions are usually less than 5 mm in diameter, but in the occasional case in which they extend to involve the deeper tissues, they develop into furuncles. The causal *Staphylococcus* may invade the udder or set up an infection of the hands of milkers. In infectious dermatitis (cutaneous pyoderma) of pigs in which pustules, caused by streptococci together with staphylococci, develop on the face and neck, spread occurs through abrasions caused by the sharp teeth of the young piglets. Clinical recognition of these diseases depends upon consideration of the site involved and the character of the lesions as well as the determination of the causative bacterium by cultural investigations.

Acne

The term acne properly relates to an infection of the hair follicles by a specific diphtheroid bacterium. More generally infection of hair follicles (non-specific acne) may be caused by pyogenic organisms such as staphylococci. In furunculosis extension to the deeper skin layers and subcutaneous tissues has occurred.

Non-specific acne occurs sporadically in the horse, affecting particularly those areas where pressure is exerted by the saddle or harness. Staphylococci can be readily isolated from the lesions. The lesions, which are somewhat painful, commence as nodules at the base of the hair and later develop into pustules. At the pustular stage the lesions rupture under pressure, and this leads to infection of other hair follicles because of local contamination. A somewhat similar condition occurs occasionally in the dog, affecting the nose, chin and ventral aspect of the neck. Inflammation of the hair follicles and sebaceous glands arises as the result of occlusion of the follicle orifices with sebum, followed by secondary infection by pyogenic bacteria.

Contagious acne of horses (Canadian horsepox) is a specific dermatitis caused by *Corynebacterium pseudotuberculosis*. The lesions, which develop in the form of nodules which are painful, occur in groups in the harness areas. Infection is transmitted by means of contaminated grooming utensils or harness, while pressure from harness causing blockage of sebaceous gland ducts predisposes to the infection. A specific diagnosis is achieved by cultural investi-

gations. The pustular form of demodectic mange is also a specific acne.

Furunculosis

This is a condition in which acne-like lesions extend to involve the deeper dermal layers and the subcutaneous tissues. It may arise as a secondary development in impetigo and acne. As a primary condition it occurs in the large, short-haired breeds of dogs such as the Great Dane. The lesions, which are characterized by the development of a painful erythematous nodule which may have fluctuant qualities like a cyst, occur most commonly on the interdigital skin, lips, ears and nose. The fluid contents of the lesions are purulent or haemorrhagic. The condition is chronic.

A form of furunculosis (juvenile pyoderma), which may often develop into a cellulitis, occurs in young puppies 4–8 weeks of age. A variable proportion of the litter may be affected. The lesions which develop in the lips, eyelids and pinnae are painful and cause thickening of the skin, which becomes ulcerated after local suppuration has occurred. The regional lymph nodes are enlarged and painful, and the affected animal loses condition quite rapidly because of difficulty in ingesting food. The majority of cases are caused by *Staphylococcus aureus* which can be isolated from the lesions.

Ulcerative Granuloma (Necrotic Ulcer)

This infectious disease affecting the skin in pigs is caused by a spirochaete, *Borrelia suis*. It occurs in Australasia, particularly when hygienic standards are low. The lesions, which develop as small, hard, fibrous swellings, occur on the face of sucking pigs and the ventral abdomen of sows. In 1–2 weeks, the nodules rupture to form a persistent ulcer, the edges of which are raised and the floor, comprised of proliferating granulation tissue is covered with a film of sticky grey pus. In the sow, the ulcer may extend to 20–30 cm in diameter while in the piglet, erosion of the cheeks and the jawbone may cause shedding of the teeth. Bacteriological investigation based on swabs from the ulcers enables a specific diagnosis to be made, thereby differentiating actinomycosis in the sow.

Mycotic Dermatitis

This disease, which occurs in cattle, sheep, goats and horses (Figs 79, 80), is most prevalent

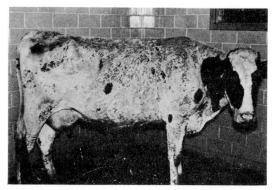

Fig. 79. *Mycotic dermatitis (streptothricosis) in a cow. Note the distribution of the lesions, which are more marked over the back.*

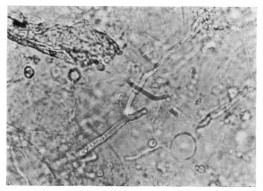

Fig. 81. *An impression smear showing branching filaments of* Dermatophilus congolensis. *Giemsa stain.*

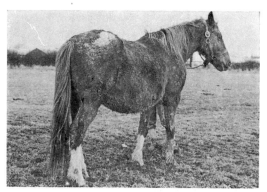

Fig. 80. *Mycotic dermatitis in a horse (streptothricosis). The lesions are most extensive in the croup region.* (Crown Copyright).

in tropical and semitropical climates, but it also occurs fairly extensively in northern temperate climates. In Africa a similar disease affecting cattle is known as cutaneous streptothricosis. The disease in horses and cattle is caused by *Dermatophilus congolensis* and in sheep by *Derm. dermatonomus.*

Infection is transmitted by contact between diseased and healthy animals. The lesions, in the form of crusts which result when the causal organism invades wool and/or hair follicles, occur on the neck, body or escutcheon in cattle (in young beef cattle more usually on the rump), and on the dorsal parts of the body, spreading laterally, and on the nose, face and ears in sheep. The initial lesions in young cattle may develop on the muzzle and spread to the head and neck; a similar development occurs in the goat, with a tendency to spread to the feet, possibly as the result of biting. In the horse, the lesions are

mainly associated with the head, beginning at the muzzle and spreading up the face to the eyes. In some cases the distribution of the lesions is more variable than indicated for the different species.

The lesions cause no itching or irritation, and the crusts are 2–5 cm in diameter, thick and cream to brown in colour. In many cases the causal bacterium is demonstrated by making an impression smear from the undersurface of a scab. Following suitable staining (Giemsa 1:10) the branching filamentous organism is recognized (Fig. 81). Cultural isolation on blood agar may be attempted from scrapings or a biopsy section.

Strawberry Footrot

This proliferative form of dermatitis has been recorded in Britain, particularly Scotland, but it has also been observed in Ireland. The causal agent, *Dermatophilus pedis*, is probably transmitted from ground contamination. It has been confirmed that, in dried crusts from the natural lesions of the disease, *Derm. pedis* can survive for long periods. All ages and types of sheep are susceptible and the majority of outbreaks of the disease occur during the summer season. The lesions, which develop on the leg from the coronet to the knee or hock take the form of heaped-up scabs which enlarge to 3–5 cm in diameter, becoming thick and wart-like. If the scab is removed the exposed bleeding mass has a strawberry-like appearance. The surrounding narrow ulcer tends to become deeper. The condition resembles contagious pustular dermatitis but can be distinguished by the absence of lesions elsewhere than on the limbs. A specific diagnosis is achieved by microscopic and cultural examinations of swabs and scrapings.

Other Bacteria

Secondary bacterial involvement of the skin may occur in glanders*, ulcerative lymphangitis*, demodectic mange, certain *Sphaerophorus* (*Fusiformis*) *necrophorus* infections ('fouls', infectious pododermatitis, footrot of cattle) and occasion-

sence of the larvae in a wound is generally easy to recognize but differentiation from blowfly larvae may be a matter of considerable importance.

Blowfly calliphorine myiasis causes considerable losses in sheep in all countries, especially in Australia, South Africa and Great Britain where heavily woolled breeds with deeply wrinkled skin are kept. Table 8 includes the flies

TABLE 8. FLIES CAUSING CUTANEOUS MYIASIS

Significance	Species	Distribution
Primary	*Lucilia sericata*	Britain and Ireland, Australia, New Zealand, North America
	L. cuprina	Australia, South Africa, North America
	Phormia terrae-novae	Britain and Ireland, North America
	P. regina	North America
	Calliphora stygia	Australia, New Zealand
	C. australis	Australia
	C. auger	Australia
Secondary	*Calliphora erythrocephala*	Britain and Ireland
	C. vomitoria	Britain and Ireland
	Sarcophaga spp.	Australia, New Zealand
	Chrysomia spp.	Australia

ally in some other diseases. Microscopic examination of a thin smear of material from a lesion, appropriately stained, is sometimes of value in diagnosis, but often the lesion, more particularly when on the extremities, is so contaminated with non-pathogenic organisms from soil, faeces, skin etc. that identification of pathogens by this method is impracticable.

Myiases

The important myiases affecting animals are screw-worm infestation and blowfly strike. In the former condition the female flies, *Callitroga americana* and *Chrysomia bezziana*, lay their eggs in fresh surgical and other wounds (the navel of newborn animals is a common site). The screw-worm flies are obligatory parasites; they can utilize any homeothermic species of animal or bird as a host. Newly hatched larvae penetrate from the wound into the deeper tissues, where they cause considerable damage as well as producing secondary effects such as bacterial infection and toxaemia. This form of myiasis occurs in the tropical parts of Africa, Asia and North and South America. The pre-

* This disease does not occur in many Western European countries, including Great Britain and Ireland.

capable of causing cutaneous myiasis, their distribution and their significance in the development of 'strike'.

The most common site for 'strike' is the breech, especially when soiled and excoriated by soft faeces or by urine in ewes. Deeply wrinkled skin over the perineum and back of the thighs, narrow perineum and crutch, and a long tail contribute to 'strike' because they permit soiling of the parts. Urine contamination around the prepuce, excessive wrinkling of the skin over the poll and fleece rot along the dorsum of the back in very wet seasons permit strike in these regions. Otherwise, wounds, especially docking and castration wounds, and wounds on the head in rams as the result of fighting are likely sites for blowflies to deposit eggs.

Sheep may be 'struck' at any time from spring to autumn depending on the weather conditions and the attractiveness of the animal. Affected sheep are restless, move around with the head lowered, wriggle the tail and tend to bite or kick at the infested area, which is moist and brownish in colour. If the maggots are in contact with the skin it becomes hyperaemic and then ulcerated; later a moist scab forms and the wool separates from the surrounding fleece and the larvae move to the periphery of the area. Blowfly myiasis is readily recognized but specific identification of the flies involved necessitates examination of larvae and fly trapping.

Nematodes

Certain species of nematodes are recognized causes of skin disease in animals in some countries. In the United States *Stephanofilaria stilesi*, a filarid worm, produces lesions clinically similar to those of sarcoptic mange on the ventral aspect of the body, near or on the midline, in cattle. The scab covered lesions vary from 2 to 15 cm in diameter. The causal parasite, both in the adult and larval forms, can be found in scrapings made from active parts of the lesions. Other *Stephanofilaria* spp. causing dermatitis include: *S. dedoesi* which causes dermatitis ('cascado') in cattle in the East Indies; *S. kaeli* and *S. assamensis* which cause 'humpsore' in cattle in India and Malaya; and *S. zaheeri*, which causes 'earsore' of buffalo in the same countries.

Parafilaria multipapillosa (see Fig. 41, p. 46) is associated with the development of subcutaneous nodules which ulcerate, bleed and heal spontaneously, in horses in Asian and eastern European countries. The disease only occurs during the summer season, so that flies are thought to be involved as vectors. *P. bovicola* causes a similar disease in cattle in eastern Europe, India and the Phillipine Islands. A similar disease affecting pigs in South Africa is caused by *Suifilaria suis*.

Filarial dermatitis (elaeophoriasis) of sheep, which occurs in North America and Italy, is caused by the microfilaria of *Elaeophoria schneideri*. The lesions, which are found on the poll of the head and extend over the face to the lips and other parts, as well as the feet and ventral abdomen, develop initially as small areas which, because of scratching, become extensive and have a bleeding, proliferative surface spotted with numerous small abscesses. The microfilariae may be detected by maceration of a skin biopsy specimen, or by histological examination.

Infestation of skin wounds in horses by the larvae of *Habronema muscae*, *H. microstoma* or *H. megastoma*, causes cutaneous habronemiasis. The larvae are deposited in wounds by the house fly (*Musca domestica*), the stable fly (*Stomoxys calcitrans*), and a variety of bush and blowflies all of which, at the larval stage, are themselves invaded by the *Habronema* larvae passed out in the faeces of horses. Habronemiasis is only of importance in countries with a warm climate. When the larvae are deposited in wounds they cause an inflammatory reaction with the production of quantities of granulation tissue ('summer sores', 'swamp cancer'). The lesions occur on the face below the eye and on the midline of the abdomen, areas where the vector flies are not readily disturbed. Larvae may only be found following biopsy, in the central part of early lesions; in later lesions a marked local eosinophilia is characteristic.

Rhabditis strongyloides, a saprophytic nematode, has been observed to invade the skin, causing dermatitis, in cattle and dogs, more especially in animals exposed to filthy conditions. The lesions occur on those parts of the body which become caked with faeces and filth. Loss of hair is usual in the affected areas and the skin becomes thickened, wrinkled and scurfy, with pustules up to 1 cm in diameter, containing thick yellow pus and both larval and adult worms.

Photosensitization

Secondary dermatitis, following damage to the superficial layers of relatively unpigmented skin by the energy released from interaction between light of certain wavelengths and certain photodynamic agents, occurs in the disease phenomenon known as photosensitization. The photodynamic agents may be ingested in an active form (hypericin in *Hypericum perforatum*, fagopyrin in *Polygonum fagopyrum*, perloline in *Lolium perenne* and miscellaneous substances including acridine dyes and rose bengal) or may arise as a product of metabolism (phenothiazine sulphoxide from phenothiazine), thus causing primary photosensitization. Aberrant pigment metabolism occurring in inherited congenital porphyria, a rare disease, is an occasional cause of photosensitization. Phylloerythrin, a product of chlorophyll metabolism normally excreted in the bile, may accumulate when biliary function is impaired. A variety of plants and some chemical substances have been especially incriminated as important sources of this so-called hepatogenous photosensitization. A variety of other plants has also been found to be associated with photosensitization syndromes in which the nature of the reaction has not been determined.

In photosensitization two factors are required

before a reaction can occur; these are the presence of a photodynamic agent in the dermal layers containing light pigmentation and sunlight.

The lesions are confined to those unpigmented parts of the body most exposed to sunlight, so that they are usually most obvious on the dorsal aspects with diminishing intensity down the sides and are virtually absent from the ventral aspect. The main sites affected are the ears, the face including the eyelids and muzzle, along the back, the lateral aspects of the teats in cattle and occasionally the vulva and perineum. The initial sign is erythema followed by oedema, both stages being associated with severe irritation which causes the animal to rub the affected parts, thereby producing lacerations. Exudation causes matting of the hair, and oedema may cause drooping of the ears, dysphagia because of swelling of the lips and dyspnoea due to nasal obstruction. The affected areas are sharply demarcated from the neighbouring areas of normal skin. Necrosis and gangrene with sloughing of peripheral structures may occur in severely affected cases. Systemic effects, involving the cardiovascular and respiratory functions, are related to the degree of shock and toxaemia in individual cases. Diagnosis depends upon appreciation of the distribution and nature of the lesions. Recognition of the type of photosensitization requires consideration of other aspects.

Cutaneous Oedema (Anasarca)

This is a swelling on the surface of the body caused by increased diffusion of serous fluid into the tissue spaces of the subcutis and secondarily of the dermis (other organs and tissues may show oedema simultaneously). The term anasarca is applied when the abdomen is affected in this manner. Cutaneous oedema is recognized by the appearance of a doughy swelling that pits on pressure; when pressed firmly with the fingertips, it retains the indentation for a considerable period of time. In the consideration of oedema involving the body surface, the following points should be noted: rate of development, site, size and shape, nature of demarcation from surrounding tissue, consistency, condition of the overlying skin, colour, temperature and pain sensitivity, inflammatory damage to capillary walls and obstruction to lymphatic drainage.

Oedema of the cutaneous tissues is caused either by increased hydrostatic pressure in the capillaries or by reduced osmotic pressure of the blood, inflammatory damage to capillary walls and obstruction to lymphatic drainage.

Capillary dilatation and damage caused by local or general liberation of histamine are associated with certain allergic states such as angioneurotic oedema (urticaria), which occurs most frequently in grazing horses and cattle, insect bites, contact with stinging plants and the local action of diagnostic agents such as tuberculin, mallein, etc. In all these cases the oedema may affect the cutaneous tissues only. It also occurs in purpura haemorrhagica, the fog-fever syndrome (acute alveolar emphysema and oedema) and drug sensitivity reactions, in which various other tissues are involved. Inflammatory oedema is due to bacterial infections (*Clostridium* spp., pasteurellosis, anthrax) causing damage to capillary walls; this form is quite common in animals.

Oedematous conditions involving the skin may therefore be classified according to their origin as follows:

1. *Non-inflammatory oedema.* The signs of inflammation are missing so that there is neither reddening nor pain and the affected areas are cool (cold oedema). It occurs: (*a*) as a sequel to increased hydrostatic pressure in the veins and capillaries, arising from congestive heart failure in old horses and dogs, severe udder engorgement in cattle (especially heifers near calving), traumatic pericarditis in cattle, fibrosis of the liver and in compression of veins by tumours (obstructive oedema) (Fig. 82); or (*b*) as a sequel to a fall in plasma protein concentration (hypoproteinaemia), such as occurs in cattle and

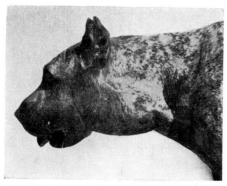

Fig. 82. *Severe infiltration of the subcutaneous tissues causing swelling of the head and neck. Obstructive oedema following enlargement of the lymph nodes in leukaemia.*

mares in late pregnancy and is partially responsible (see above) for oedema of the mammary gland and ventral abdominal wall. Oedema from this cause also occurs in chronic hameorrhage caused by heavy parasitic infestations such as strongylosis in horses, certain forms of parasitic gastroenteritis in ruminant species and hookworm infestation in dogs, in certain forms of hepatic fibrosis, e.g. chronic fascioliasis, in nutritional diseases such as avitaminosis A in beef cattle, cobalt deficiency in sheep and protracted chronic bacterial affections such as Johne's disease.

2. *Inflammatory oedema.* This is associated with inflammation resulting in damage to small blood vessels by toxins or infectious agents, e.g. abscesses, anthrax, blackquarter (*Clostridium chauvoei*, sometimes accompanied by *Cl. septicum*), malignant oedema (*Clostridium septicum, Cl. chauvoei, Cl. perfringens, Cl. sordellii, Cl. oedematiens*, 'bighead' of sheep (*Cl. oedematiens, Cl. sordellii*), septicaemic pasteurellosis of cattle (*Pasteurella multocida* Type 1); bowel oedema (*Escherichia coli*), equine infectious anaemia and equine viral arteritis (herpes virus). Inflammatory oedema is characterized, in the initial stage at least, by local increased temperature (hot oedema), redness (unpigmented skin) and pain. Obstruction of lymphatic vessels plays some part in the production of local oedema caused by neoplasms and inflammatory swellings. Sporadic lymphangitis in the horse and so-called collateral oedema affecting tissues surrounding deep-seated inflammatory conditions are examples of obstructive oedema.

Oedema is also differentiated, according to its extent, into local and generalized types. The latter is usually of systemic origin (structural or functional circulatory disorder, nutritional deficiency, generalized inflammatory disease). In local oedema, the causal factor is operating in one part of the body.

The lesions produced by cutaneous oedema may be described as being of hard or soft consistency. This depends, as a rule, upon whether the subcutaneous tissue in the affected area is loose (brisket region) or tense (head, lower part of leg). When oedema develops in a superiorly situated part of the body, the excess fluid in the tissues tends to gravitate downwards, this being known as dependent oedema. Here again, the oedematous swelling appears at a point distant from that at which the causal factor is operating

—in this case below it. Transitory oedema appears during a period of inactivity and disappears with exercise; it is seen in the lower part of the legs of otherwise healthy horses that have been deprived of exercise for a few days ('filling of the legs'), and it also occurs in certain forms of heart disease. This type of oedema may also affect the prepuce and ventral aspect of the abdomen in the horse. In heavily pregnant dairy cattle, particularly heifers, and also occasionally in mares, oedema of the abdominal wall, extending from the udder to beyond the umbilicus, is not uncommon. An oedematous swelling on the body surface may merge into the surrounding tissues or be clearly demarcated at its periphery (Fig. 83).

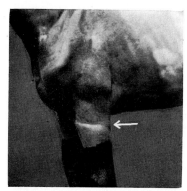

Fig. 83. *Sharply demarcated oedema of the foreleg in a horse. Purpura haemorrhagica.*

Fluctuation

This is the production of a wave-like movement in a subcutaneous fluid-filled cavity (abscess, haematoma, cyst). To demonstrate it, pressure is applied in an alternate manner with 2 fingers, of one or both hands; when one finger is pressed downwards, the other rises (the result of equal distribution of pressure in a fluid). A similar response is obtained over large relaxed muscles, this being known as pseudofluctuation.

Subcutaneous Emphysema

This occurs when air or other gases accumulate in the subcutaneous tissue spaces. (Emphysema may occur in other organs such as the lungs.) Subcutaneous emphysema is recognized by the presence of a soft yielding swelling that crepitates (makes a crackling sound) on palpation and sometimes gives an abnormally resonant or tympanic sound on percussion. Two types of subcutaneous emphysema are described:

1. *Aspiratory or exogenous emphysema.* In this type the swelling contains air, or occasionally intestinal or other gas, that has reached the subcutaneous tissues by aspiration from tissue movements following accidental, or surgical, injury to the skin, or to an air or gas containing internal organ (lung, guttural pouch, oesophagus, rumen, intestine). Lung puncture may result following fracture of a rib or penetration by a foreign body in traumatic reticulitis; rumen gas may escape through trocarization sites. This form of emphysema is also a feature of severe pulmonary interstitial emphysema in cattle.

2. *Endogenous emphysema (septic emphysema).* In this form, gas has been produced locally by gas-forming bacteria (usually *Clostridium* spp.). It occurs in blackleg of cattle, sheep and deer, and in malignant oedema of sheep, horses and pigs.

Epizootic Lymphangitis

This is a chronic disease of horses and very occasionally of cattle, occurring in Asia, Africa and the coastal areas of Mediterranean countries. The causal fungus, *Histoplasma farciminosum* is transmitted by both direct and indirect contact, and infection is established through cutaneous abrasions. The lesions occur most frequently on the limbs, involving particularly the hocks, but may also be found on the back, sides, neck, vulva and scrotum, and occasionally on the nasal mucosa just inside the nostrils. The cutaneous form of the disease develops slowly, as an ulcer, at the site of infection, with evidence of local lymphangitis and enlargement of local lymph nodes. The enlarged thickened lymphatic vessels develop nodules along their course which rupture and discharge thick, creamy pus. The skin of the affected area is usually thickened. The causal fungus is readily found in the discharges and occurs as Gram-positive, yeast-like cells with a double-walled capsule. It can be grown on selective media but special treatment is necessary because it dies in a short time. Apart from the complement fixation test, which is only specific for a short time in infected animals, serological tests are of no value.

Sporotrichosis

This is a slowly spreading contagious disease of horses, and very rarely of man, dogs, cats, camels and cattle, occurring in parts of Europe, India and the USA. The causal fungus, *Sporotrichum schencki*, forms single-walled spores which stain Gram-positive. Infection is acquired by direct, or indirect contact with discharges from infected animals. Following local invasion through wounds and abrasions on the lower parts of the legs, cutaneous nodules develop in the fetlock area. The painless nodules exude a little serum which is followed by scab formation and discharge of a little pus. Successive crops of lesions are a not unusual feature, and lymphangitis, with thickening and distension of the lymphatic vessels may be a feature in some outbreaks. The sporadic nature of the disease is a useful diagnostic feature. Cases which develop lymphangitis are diagnosed by identification of the causal fungus in the discharges. Direct microscopic examination may be sufficient, but in doubtful cases a biological test using a rat or hamster will prove of value.

Warbles

During the spring and early summer, swellings, caused by the development of the larvae of *Hypoderma* spp. in the subcutaneous tissues, are commonly found along the back in cattle in the northern hemisphere. The swellings are rather larger than a hazel nut, and are detected by inspection or palpation (depending upon their size and the length of the animal's coat). The number of larvae present in individual animals varies considerably. Of the two species of warble flies, *Hypoderma bovis* and *H. lineatum*, the larvae of which are involved, the latter favours a warmer climate and is largely located in more southerly parts of the hemisphere. Infestation with warble larvae is of importance because they cause serious damage to hides, loss of condition because of 'gadding', and sudden death or severe anaphylactic reaction if any of the larvae are ruptured *in situ*.

Cutaneous Neoplasms

Papillomas (Warts, Fibropapillomas)

These benign epithelial tumours are found on the skin of the head or neck, abdominal wall and teats (Fig. 84) of young cattle. In most cases the condition, which tends to undergo spontaneous cure, has a nuisance significance only, spoiling the appearance of the animal for sale or interfering with milking, but in occasional instances the warts are extensive, cause loss of condition and create concern because of secondary bacterial invasion. A similar condition has

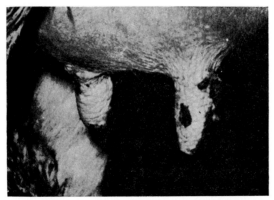

Fig. 84. *Warts on the teats of a cow. This condition is most prevalent in animals during the first lactation.*

been observed in white goats. The typical lesions vary in size from 1 cm upwards, and present a dry, horny cauliflower-like appearance; they may be sessile or pedunculated. Similar, though smaller, papillomas (up to 1 cm in diameter) occur in horses, in which species they are usually sessile and confined to the muzzle, nose and lips. A similar condition occurs on the mucous membrane of the buccal cavity in the dog, and on that of the oesophagus and rumen in cattle. In both horses and cattle cutaneous papillomas are caused by a host-specific papovavirus, which in the case of cattle also causes fibropapillomatosis of the vulva and penis. Buccal warts in the dog have a similar origin. The sarcoid-like lesion found on the skin of the legs, prepuce, abdomen and around the base of the ears in the horse is a fibrosarcoma of mild malignancy. The condition is probably caused by a virus; a similar lesion has been produced in the horse following intradermal injection of bovine papillomatosis virus.

Carcinoma

Carcinomas of the squamous cell type are occasionally seen on the eyelids and the globe of the eye in horses and cattle. The neoplasm may originate from the membrana nictitans, the cornea or the eyelid, and it is colloquially termed 'cancer eye'. The incidence appears to be highest in Hereford cattle. Once established the tumour grows rapidly, evincing its invasive properties by also metastasizing to the parotid and pharyngeal lymph nodes. A similar type of neoplasm, originating from the mucous membrane of the frontal sinus, causes the common 'cancer of the horn core' in cattle, in which species the vulva is also affected by squamous cell carcinomas.

Neoplasms of the skin and penis in the horse are not infrequently of the squamous cell type, and cancer of the ear in sheep is, in most cases, of this character also. In the latter, the neoplastic proliferation commences at the free edge of the pinna and spreads rapidly until the entire ear is converted into a large cauliflower-like mass.

Melanoma

Melanomas may be benign or malignant, although it is customary to consider that all melanomas are potentially, if not actually, malignant. This type of neoplasm is particularly frequent in old, grey horses, although it occasionally occurs in horses of other colours and also, even more rarely, in other species, e.g. dark-skinned cattle, also in sheep, goats and pigs. In horses, the initial location is the perineal or perianal region from where it tends to metastasize, via the pelvic lymphatics, to the abdominal and thoracic viscera. The rate of growth is variable, and ulceration of the skin involved in the neoplasm only occurs when growth is rapid.

8

The Head and Neck

During the preliminary stage of the clinical examination a detailed inspection of the animal, preferably on a regional basis, should be made before it is subjected to any disturbing influence, such as restraint or the near approach of a strange person, which might modify its behaviour. This inspection provides the opportunity to observe, among many other features, the general appearance and conformation of the animal, as well as to assess its behaviour and demeanour. In the case of animals normally kept in herds or flocks, separation of an individual from its group is usually indicative of illness. The significance of any change in the behavioural pattern of animals can only be correctly interpreted when the observer has a sound knowledge of the ways in which the various species are likely to react under changing circumstances and conditions. Changes in bearing are also most meaningful when the clinician appreciates the full range of reactivity that may be exhibited by animals to constantly changing environmental stimuli.

When inspecting the head, attention should be paid to the facial expression which is a good indicator of the mental state and, therefore, of the demeanour of the animal. An animal in good health has an alert appearance and reacts to external stimuli such as sound and movement in the expected manner. Abnormal positioning of the eyes or eyelids will alter the facial expression; the character and causation of these abnormalities will be discussed later in this chapter. Disturbances in mental condition, including depression or excitation, are appreciated by noting any alteration in behaviour as well as in expression (see p. 19). When an animal exhibits signs of mental disturbance it is more than likely that it is caused by primary or secondary modification of brain function.

Diseases associated with rapid loss of bodily condition, severe dehydration or exhaustion, because of pain, give rise to a haggard expression. When affected with tetanus, the horse has an anxious expression caused by muscular rigidity in conjunction with dilatation of the nostrils and wide separation of the eyelids. The somewhat maniacal expression occurring in rabies and acute lead poisoning is produced by the very intense expression, with partially opened lips and rolling of the eyes.

Evaluation of the anatomical conformation and symmetry of the bony structures and soft tissues of the head and neck region is frequently rewarding. Bulging of the frontal region occurs in calves with congenital achondroplasia, and also in some cases of congenital hydrocephalus and inherited chondroplastic dwarfism. Symmetrical enlargement of the mandibles and maxillae, causing swelling of the lower part of the head, occurs in osteodystrophia fibrosa; the maxillae are similarly enlarged in chondroplastic dwarf calves. Asymmetrical enlargement of the bones of the lower or upper jaw is a feature of actinomycosis in cattle. Changes in the contours of the soft structures, usually in the form of swellings, involve the intermaxillary space in such inflammatory states as actinobacillosis and strangles, or oedematous conditions including acute anaemia, protein starvation and congestive heart failure. Unilateral or bilateral swelling of the cheek region occurs in actinobacillosis and necrotic stomatitis (calf diphtheria). The soft tissues of the nose and face are swollen in necrotic rhinitis (bullnose) of young pigs. Tumours of the head may originate from either

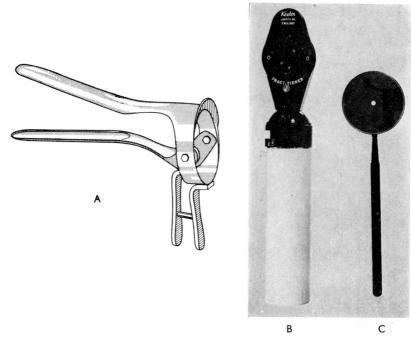

Fig. 85. *Instruments used in the examination of the mucous membranes and the eye.* A, *Metal vaginal speculum.* B, *Electric ophthalmoscope.* C, *Simple ophthalmoscope.*

bone or soft tissue. Neoplasms, involving the eye and other periorbital structures in horses and cattle, the horn core in cattle and the ear in sheep, are in most cases squamous cell carcinomas. Other changes in the soft tissues include increased muscle tone in tetanus which, more noticeably in the horse, is responsible for dilatation of the nostrils, rigidity of the ears, and protrusion of the membrana nictitans. Asymmetry of the soft structures, in the absence of swelling, is most likely to involve the positioning of the ears, the degree of eyelid closure and the position of the lower lip relative to the upper. In facial nerve paralysis there is drooping of the ear and unilateral flaccidity of the lips so that the upper lip is drawn towards the normally functioning side and the lower lip hangs down on the affected side. Drooping of the upper eyelid (ptosis) occurs when the function of the oculomotor nerve is defective.

Changes in the carriage of the head are indicative of functional or organic disease of the central nervous system. Rotation occurs when there is unilateral interference with the function of the vestibular apparatus, as in otitis media in which the affected side is turned downwards, so that the animal invariably falls towards that side.

Lateral deviation is a feature of unilateral dysfunction of the vestibular nucleus and of the medulla oblongata and cervical region of the spinal cord, as in listeriosis. Opisthotonus (elevation of the head) and orthotonus (extension of the head) occur when there is intermittent generalized increase in muscle tone during the convulsive episodes associated with tetanus, strychnine poisoning, hypomagnesaemic tetany, the encephalopathy arising from acute lead poisoning and some cases of encephalitis; extension of both the head and neck is a characteristic feature of strangles and pharyngitis in the horse (see Fig. 108, p. 103).

Examination of the Visible Mucous Membranes

Several of the clinically important visible mucous membranes are associated with the head, so that it is expedient to consider certain general aspects of the clinical examination of all mucosal structures at this point. When considering the condition of any of the visible mucous membranes, which include the conjunctival, nasal buccal, vaginal, urethral and rectal, the tissues surrounding the orifice by means of which the particular mucosa communicates with the surface of the body, should be included in the inspection.

Changes in these tissues are often closely associated with disease of the related mucous membrane or its contiguous structures.

Inspection of the mucous membrane should be carried out in daylight whenever possible, but if this is not feasible, an electric torch or suitable reflecting mirror should be employed. For examining the mucous membrane of the vagina or rectum an appropriate speculum is used (Fig. 85A; see also Figs 172–3, p. 246). The concealed mucous membranes (pharynx, larynx, trachea, stomach, bladder) may be inspected in small animals with the aid of endoscopic instruments; in large animals the mucosa of the pharynx, larynx and bladder are ordinarily examined in this way.

During the visual examination, attention is directed towards determining if any of the following conditions are present: pallor, hyperaemia, cyanosis, jaundice, eruptions, ulcerations, haemorrhages, swellings, discharges, etc.

A discharge may be the secretion of a gland (mucous, lacrimal, anal), the product of inflammation (exudate) or the result of venous congestion (transudate) or of vascular trauma (haemorrhage). It should be remembered that discharge from a mucous membrane may also contain abnormal forms of the secretions or excretions of the body, and that solid and liquid foodstuffs may be discharged from the nostrils as well as the mouth (vomition in horses), and faeces from the vulva as well as the rectum (rectovaginal fistula).

EYELIDS, CONJUNCTIVAE AND EYES

Abnormalities affecting the eyelids include swelling, position, movement, structure and other changes which may occur in the skin. Swelling of the eyelids is a feature in bowel oedema, photosensitization, allergy and traumatic injury. Except in injury the swelling is invariably bilateral. In tetanus, particularly in the horse, the normal curvature of the palpebral border of the upper eyelid may form an obtuse angle. The eyelids may be kept closed in acute conjunctivitis and other painful eye conditions, and when there is gross swelling of the eyelids, as in local oedema due to photosensitization, allergy or purpura haemorrhagica. Excessive movement is seen in painful eye conditions including acute conjunctivitis, acute keratitis, and injury, or in cases of deranged nervous function

including hypomagnesaemic tetany, lead poisoning and sometimes encephalitis. Tumours on the eyelids are readily observable.

The palpebral conjunctiva—that part of the mucous membrane comprising the conjunctival sac which covers the inner surface of the eyelids—is examined by opening and gently everting each eyelid in turn with the forefinger and thumb of one hand while, at the same time, the eyeball is pushed back into the orbital cavity by pressure on the corresponding eyelid (Fig. 86).

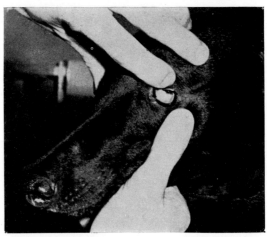

Fig. 86. *Everting the lower eyelid in the dog in order to expose the conjunctiva. The eyeball is pushed back into the orbit by pressure on the upper eyelid and the lower eyelid is pulled down.*

The membrana nictitans, which is covered with an extension of the conjunctiva, is exposed for examination, readily so in the horse and dog, by laying the forefinger and thumb along the upper eyelid and pressing it gently but firmly onto the eyeball, with, at the same time, the thumb pressing downwards on the lower eyelid (Fig. 87).

In the horse protrusion of the membrana nictitans (often noted only when the animal is tapped lightly under the jaw or walked on hard ground) is one of the early signs of tetanus (see Fig. 217, p. 312). Continuous protrusion occurs in painful eye diseases, in the later stages of tetanus and in encephalitis. In the cat, protrusion of the membrana nictitans is usually a sign of debility, but it may occur even in apparently normal animals.

The condition of the conjunctiva should be considered carefully, both eyes being included in the examination. On account of its accessibility

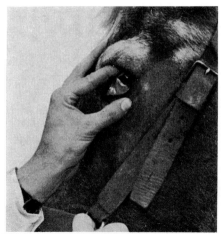

Fig. 87. *Exposing the membrana nictitans.*

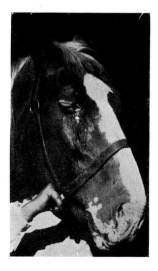

Fig. 88. *Photophobia, closed eylids and conjunctival discharge. Infectious equine arteritis.*

and freedom from soiling with foreign matter such as foodstuffs or faeces, it is of particular value in assisting in the diagnosis of diseases which produce changes in the mucosae in general, such as jaundice (yellow colour), anaemia (pallid and watery), shock (pallid and dry), arsenic poisoning (brick-red colour). Certain other diseases, including equine viral arteritis, malignant catarrhal fever, swine fever and canine distemper, affect the conjunctival mucosa with varying severity, causing it to become swollen and hyperaemic. Conjunctivitis occurs in association with inflammatory changes in other eye structures in infectious keratoconjunctivitis and contagious ophthalmia. When the swelling of the palpebral conjunctiva is so great that the mucous membrane protrudes beyond the free margin of the eyelid the condition is called chemosis.

Photophobia (Fig. 88) is a clinical sign which develops when light of normal daytime intensity causes pain in the eye, with the result that the eyelids are kept closed. It occurs in diseases of the eye itself, including all forms of acute conjunctivitis and keratitis. Blepharospasm is a feature of some cases of conjunctivitis and is usual when a foreign body irritates the cornea or conjunctiva. It is produced by reflex contraction of the orbicularis oculi muscle which then causes spasmodic closure of the eyelids. Wrinkling of the skin over the upper eyelid, which is observed in many pathological conditions of the eye, is the result of contraction of the corrugator supercilii muscle.

The detailed examination of the eye, more particularly of the deeper structures, is part of the subject of ophthalmology. Some of the general aspects relating to the more superficial structures will be given immediate consideration; those relating to examination of the deeper structures will be considered in Chapter 14. Structural abnormalities of the eyelids, including entropion (inversion of the palpebral margins), ectropion (eversion of the lower eyelid), trichiasis (abnormal deviation of eyelashes so that they impinge upon the cornea or conjunctiva), distichiasis (two rows of eyelashes), the incidence of which is probably highest in dogs and sheep, and various forms of maldevelopment including virtual absence of eyelids or eyelashes, are appreciated by direct observation.

Abnormalities of the eyeball are the result of local or systemic influences. In the former the changes may be unilateral; in the latter they are invariably bilateral, although both eyes may not be equally severely affected. Microphthalmos, which is usually associated with abnormality of various eye structures, is developmental in origin and may have a genetic or nutritional basis, as in the eye anomaly in rough collies and vitamin A deficiency in young pigs, respectively. Corneal conditions including keratitis, which varies in degree from slight haziness in mild cases and in the early stages of acute cases, to the dense white colour (leucoma) of the advanced phase, with a variable degree of vascularization (pannus) as the result of blood vessels growing in from the conjunctiva, are frequently associated with conjunctivitis. Ulceration, scarring and focal pigmentation are other changes that may be observed following keratitis. Increased convexity of the cornea occurs in a generalized form (keratoglobus) in hydrophthalmos and hypopyon, and in a localized form (keratoconus), causing a cone-shaped bulge, in a proportion of cases of keratitis. Protrusion of the eyeball (proptosis, exophthalmos) is a species or breed characteristic (it occurs to a mild degree in Jersey cattle and Pekingese dogs); it occurs as a clinical sign in cases of hyperthyroidism. In unilateral form it is due to pressure from behind the orbit; periorbital lymphoma in cattle, dislocation of the mandible and periorbital haemorrhage are the common causes. Bilateral retraction of the eyeballs, with exposure of the sclera and conjunctiva, is associated with emaciation and severe dehydration, and is due to reduction in the quantity of fat and fluid in the retro-orbital tissues. Abnormal movements of the eyeball (nystagmus), which may take place in a horizontal, vertical or rotatory direction, are periodic and involuntary, the initial movement being slow with a rapid return to the original position. Nystagmus occurs in hypoxia and when there is damage to the cerebellum or vestibular tracts. Limitation of movement of the eyeball occurs when there is paralysis of the motor nerves to the extrinsic ocular muscles with resulting malpositioning. In paralysis of the oculomotor, trigeminal and facial nerves, blinking may be restricted, infrequent or entirely absent, and the aperture between the eyelids is reduced in width (ptosis).

The deeper structures of the eye, consisting of the iris, lens and fundus, are only satisfactorily examined by means of an ophthalmoscope (Figs 85B, C, 89). Certain pathological changes in these structures can result from systemic diseases. The presence in the anterior chamber of the eye of blood (hyphaema) or pus (hypopyon) is readily recognized by direct vision when changes are moderate to severe. (In hypopyon there is a yellow to white opacity with, in the early stages, a horizontal upper border obscuring the iris.) The former condition is occasionally observed in warfarin poisoning, and the latter in most forms of severe keratitis.

Determining the size, shape and position of the pupil is important in recognizing certain diseases. Mobility of the pupil, determined by exposure to variations in light intensity, is decreased in functional disorders including severe hypoxia and botulism, in diffuse encepha-

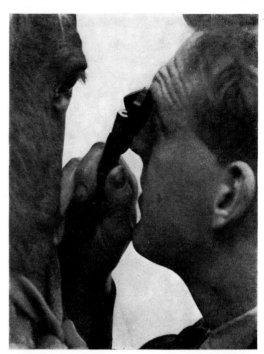

Fig. 89. *Examining the eye with an illuminated ophthalmoscope. This type of examination is best carried out in a darkened room.*

lopathies and when there are lesions affecting the oculomotor nucleus. In these circumstances the pupils are bilaterally overdilated (mydriasis). Unilateral dilatation suggests the existence of a lesion in the orbital region or in the eye itself; both pupils are dilated in peripheral blindness due to bilateral lesions of the orbits. Drugs with a parasympatholytic action, e.g. atropine, have a mydriatic effect of variable duration following systemic or local absorption. Conversely, overdosage with parasympathomimetic drugs including organophosphorus compounds produces excessive constriction of the pupil (miosis). The shape and position of the pupil are abnormal when the iris is adherent to the posterior surface of the cornea (anterior synechia), or to the lens (posterior synechia). Iritis, which produces these conditions, frequently occurs during the course of equine viral arteritis, canine distemper, some other virus infections and purpura haemorrhagica. Partial absence of the iris (coloboma) may vary in extent and in some cases does not affect the shape or size of the pupil. Opacity of the lens (cataract), most commonly observed in aged dogs, is in most cases readily visible, particularly in advanced cases when the whole of the pupil-lary area is greyish-white in colour. Retinal changes are seen in tuberculosis, progressive retinal atrophy (Irish setters, miniature poodles) and hydrophthalmos, when detachment occurs. The conjunctival, corneal and pupillary reflexes, and the various nervous disorders affecting the eye, are discussed in Chapter 14.

Diseases of the eye may cause changes in the surrounding skin, e.g. periorbital dermatitis, caused by the discharge in conjunctivitis, or the lacrimal secretion when the tear duct is obstruc-ted or the punctum lacrimalium abnormally situated (entropion).

A certain quantity of lacrimal fluid is always present in the conjunctival sac and is regularly distributed over the cornea by the normal blink-ing movements of the eyelids. An overflow of tears down the face (epiphora) may be caused by excessive secretion, obstruction of the lacrimal duct or deviation of the punctum lacrimalium. A discharge from the conjunctival sac may also consist of inflammatory exudate or blood. Cer-tain nematode parasites (*Thelazia* spp.) occa-sionally occur in the conjunctival sac; the larval stage of the worms is deposited in the conjuncti-val sac by flies (*Musca* spp.) which are the inter-mediate hosts. The worms are associated with the appearance of conjunctivitis, keratitis, oph-thalmia and abscessation of the eyelids during the summer months. Inanimate foreign bodies, such as grass seeds, cereal husks, chaff, etc., are frequently found in the conjunctival sac in cattle.

Laboratory aids may be of assistance in diag-nosing infective conditions of the eye. When normal the conjunctiva is almost free of bacteria because of the activity of lysozymes and other factors. Microscopical examination of stained smears prepared from conjunctival scrapings may be found useful in recognizing intracyto-plasmic inclusion bodies in canine distemper, or rickettsia in contagious ophthalmia. Cultural techniques are more useful for confirming the presence of *Moraxella bovis* in cattle and *Mor-axella* spp. in infectious keratoconjunctivitis and contagious ophthalmia in cattle and sheep res-pectively. As these organisms can be isolated from the eyes of normal animals, their signifi-cance in typical cases of eye disease is deter-mined by assessment of the clinical features and the numbers of organisms present. Other orga-nisms that may be recovered from conjunctival

swabs include streptococci, staphylococci, *No-cardia* spp. and fungi. In many cases these may be of secondary origin, so that a detailed clinical examination is essential in order to discover the type of primary lesion present.

The behaviour and actions of the patient may indicate that it is suffering from a defect of vision for which, as yet, there is no describable cause. Tests for visual acuity can be performed at this stage, including those for eye preservation involving the corneal and conjunctival reflexes, and an obstacle test. In peripheral and central blindness, reflex closure of the eyelids does not occur when a blow is aimed at the eye; similarly in facial nerve paralysis when, however, there may be withdrawal of the head. An obstacle test is best arranged in unfamiliar surroundings so that the animal's behaviour in relation to the obstacles can be more readily assessed. The test for night-blindness (nyctalopia), which is one of the earliest clinical signs of avitaminosis A, should be performed at dusk or in moonlight conditions. Reduced visual acuity in the absence of a demonstrable eye lesion is termed amblyopia; complete blindness in similar circumstances is called amaurosis.

NASAL REGION, NASAL MUCOSA AND NASAL SINUSES

In the examination of the nasal region the following structures and details are noted: (*a*) nostrils and the surrounding tissues; (*b*) move-ments of the nostrils; (*c*) respiratory sounds; (*d*) expired air; (*e*) nasal discharge; (*f*) mucous membrane; and (*g*) paranasal sinuses.

Tissues Surrounding the Nostrils

The changes that may occur in the skin of the nasal region include swelling of the alae nasi (purpura haemorrhagica, neoplasia, actinobacil-losis), vesicles, pustules and scabs (contagious pustular dermatitis; see Fig. 53 p. 54); abscesses, depigmented streak (chronic persistent nasal discharge), etc. Such changes may either origi-nate in the skin and then spread to involve the mucous membrane, or they may be secondary to diseases of the mucosa.

The nose of the dog, the muzzle of the ox and the snout of the pig are normally moist and cool because of continuous secretion of a watery fluid. Occasionally it may occur that the nose of a healthy dog or pig is dry and warm, e.g. in animals that have recently been digging or rooting in the ground.

Movement of the Nostrils

Distension of the external nares, involving movements of the alae nasi, is to a large extent voluntary in healthy animals. The thick rigid nostrils in the ox prohibit movement altogether. The large, flexible nostrils of the horse permit considerable movement, which is also noted in the rabbit. Inspiratory dyspnoea causes a particularly distinct, involuntary dilatation of the nostril (again most prominently in the horse) which coincides with the inspiratory phase of the cycle; during expiration the nostrils collapse to the normal position and size. This sequence of events is observed in advanced pulmonary emphysema, bronchitis, pneumonia, rupture of the diaphragm, oedema of the larynx, etc.

Respiratory Sounds

In certain diseases, respiration is accompanied by audible, abnormal sounds (stridors). When these arise from constriction of the respiratory passages they are known as stenotic sounds. They may be inspiratory or expiratory, and originate in the nasal cavities, pharynx, larynx or trachea. Stenosis of the respiratory passages may be caused by swelling of the mucous membrane, the presence of excessive mucus, inflammatory oedema, neoplasia, paralysis of the nostrils (facial nerve paralysis in the horse), enlargement of retropharyngeal lymph nodes, paralysis of the larynx, etc. Stenotic sounds are manifested by whistling, roaring or stertorous tones, and are usually louder during inspiration than at expiration. In paralysis of the larynx the abnormal sounds only occur during inspiration, whereas in paralysis of the soft palate they occur only at expiration. The sounds caused by the presence of nasal tumours, distortion of the nasal structures (atrophic rhinitis, osteomalacia), fracture of nasal bones, etc., are audible during both inspiration and expiration. Snoring (stertorous) respiratory sounds are normal in brachycephalic breeds of dogs such as the bulldog, boxer, Pekingese, etc. Some such cases are due to a congenitally elongated uvula. In other animals, sounds of this type are usually heard in lymphadenitis (actinobacillosis, tuberculosis, abscessation caused by *Corynebacterium pyogenes*) or neoplastic involvement of the pharyngeal lymph nodes, and in laryngitis, arising from vibration of the enlarged lymph nodes in the former two conditions, and of the relaxed soft palate in the latter. Snuffling, bubbling, or rattling sounds are heard when there is an accumulation of secretion, or discharge, in the nasal cavities, larynx or trachea. In many cases the stenotic sounds are audible when the animal is resting, whereas in others they develop after gentle, or in some instances only after strenuous, exercise, and disappear, sometimes very soon, after exercise is terminated (e.g. in paralysis of the larynx or of the soft plate in the horse).

The place of origin of the stenotic sounds can often be discovered by listening carefully with the unaided ear; in other cases a more thorough investigation is necessary, comprising palpation, auscultation and other methods of examination (endoscopic, radiological) of the nasal cavities, larynx or trachea. If the lesion causing the abnormal sound is unilaterally situated in a nasal cavity, the sound will disappear on occluding the nostril of that side, and will be accentuated by occluding the nostril of the normal side. Stenotic sounds originating in the larynx become temporarily softer on occluding one nostril because of the reduction in airflow volume.

A sneeze is a sudden, noisy expiration produced reflexly by irritation of the nasal mucous membrane stimulating the sensory nerve endings of the olfactory and facial nerves, e.g. by foreign bodies or parasites (*Oestrus ovis* in sheep, *Linguatula rhinaria* in the dog), irritant odours or gases or inflammation of the nasal mucosa. It is preceded by a deep inspiration, with closure of the oropharynx and contraction of the vocal cords; during the early phase of the subsequent forceful expiration movement, the glottis is closed and pressure is elevated so that when it is finally opened the expiration is explosive having as its objective the removal of foreign material from the nasal cavity (Fig. 90).

Other abnormal respiratory sounds which may be heard include coughing and grunting (see p. 36).

Expired Air

The stream of expired air is examined by holding the back of the hand in front of both nostrils. In the normal animal the flow of air from the left and right sides is equal in strength. If there is an obstruction in the nasal passage (neoplasm, fracture, exostosis), the airflow is weaker on the affected side. Variations in airflow

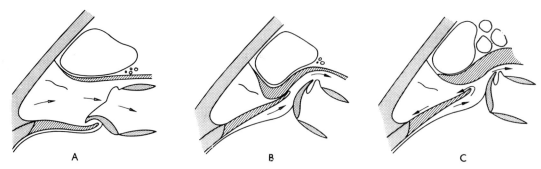

Fig. 90. *Position of the soft palate, epiglottis and posterior wall of the pharynx during respiration* (A), *swallowing* (B) *and regurgitation* (C) *in the horse.*

volume between nostrils can be further assessed by occluding the nostrils one at a time. When there is significant obstruction of one nasal cavity, severe respiratory embarrassment is produced by temporary occlusion of the other nostril. When respiration is so shallow that there is doubt as to whether the animal is breathing, holding a previously cooled hand-mirror close to the nostrils may prove of assistance; condensation on the surface of the mirror will occur as the result of expiration.

In certain diseases of the nasal cavities and neighbouring structures, or of other respiratory organs, the expired air has a very offensive odour, which can be perceived some distance away from the animal. This odour is usually produced by putrefaction of the tissues, e.g. gangrenous pneumonia, necrosis of the turbinate bones, pus in the paranasal sinus, accumulation of nasal exudate. If the origin of the odour is unilateral, it can be detected on one side only; otherwise if it originates distal to the pharynx it can be detected at both nostrils. There is usually a sweet, sickly odour from the exhaled air in cattle with ketosis. Putrefactive conditions in the mouth, arising from deposits on the teeth, decaying teeth or necrosis and ulceration of the mucous membrane may also impart an offensive odour to the air exhaled through the nostrils, but in this case the odour from the mouth is more obvious and it can also be detected in the saliva. Odours originating in the respiratory tract are usually detectable with each expiration.

Nasal Discharge

This may be unilateral or bilateral (when nasal discharge is observed both nostrils should always

be examined), continuous or intermittent, scanty or copious, and may be serous, mucoid, mucopurulent, purulent, sanious, or haemorrhagic in character. If it has been in existence for several months it may have caused an area of dermatitis, or a depigmented streak.

The nasal discharge usually originates in the nasal cavities or pharynx, but it may also arise in a paranasal sinus, the trachea, bronchi, bronchioles, lungs, mouth, oesophagus or stomach (the guttural pouch is an important source in the horse). Excretions from the conjunctival sacs may also appear in small amounts as apparent nasal discharge (via the lacrimal ducts).

A unilateral nasal discharge occurs in unilateral disease of a nasal cavity (necrosis of turbinate bone, *Oestrus ovis* infestation in sheep, *Linguatula rhinaria* infestation in the dog, neoplasia), in diseases of the paranasal sinuses (pyogenic infection, defective drainage) and in some cases of empyema of the guttural pouch in the horse. A bilateral nasal discharge occurs in inflammatory affections of the nasal cavities and in diseases involving the parts of the respiratory tract beyond the posterior nares (allergic rhinitis, atrophic rhinitis, strangles, equine viral arteritis, equine viral rhinopneumonitis, glanders, malignant catarrhal fever, mucosal disease, infectious bovine rhinotracheitis, bluetongue, feline viral rhinopneumonitis, infective pneumonias when there is an accompanying inflammation of the upper respiratory tract or the exudate in the bronchioles is copious, etc.).

A nasal discharge may be constantly present or appear only intermittently when the head is lowered (empyema of the paranasal sinuses), or spontaneously (rupture of abscesses in the nasal cavities, pharynx or lungs). The discharge may contain bubbles giving it a frothy appearance; the bubbles are usually of large size when they originate in the pharynx or nasal cavities, and are small in those cases where the origin is the lower respiratory tract.

Bleeding of varying severity from the nostrils (epistaxis) is not uncommon in young race-horses during exertion. Nasal haemorrhage some-times results from local trauma caused by passage of a stomach tube, entry of a foreign body into the nostril or accidental injury to the facial bones. The quantity of blood which escapes varies considerably, it is mainly unclotted and not ad-mixed with exudate or any other solid material. Haemorrhage from the nasal cavities, pharynx or guttural pouches (horse) may originate from lesions of the mucous membrane, e.g. ulceration (glanders), aspergillosis of the guttural pouch, neoplasia or granulomas. Small quantities of blood may escape from the nostrils in purpura haemorrhagica, warfarin or sweet clover intoxi-cation and bracken fern poisoning. In haemor-rhage from the nose or pharynx the escaping blood is dark red (venous). In acute pulmonary congestion, equine infectious pneumonia, equine infectious anaemia and congestive heart failure, small amounts of rusty-coloured serous fluid are not infrequently observed in the nostrils. In acute pulmonary oedema the discharge from the nostrils consists of greyish-white or bright-red froth which contains innumerable small bubbles; the quantity of the discharge is often considerable and its passage is often accompanied by cough-ing and severe dyspnoea.

In pharyngitis, paralysis of the pharynx, oeso-phageal obstruction or occlusion and oeso-phageal spasm, the nasal discharge may contain recognizable, masticated food particles (regurgi-tation) mixed with saliva, and which may impart a characteristic green colour (chlorophyll from fresh vegetable matter). Vomiting, particularly in the horse, is associated with discharge of food material from the nostrils. The vomitus contains partially digested food particles and has a sour odour; free hydrochloric acid is usually demon-strable.

Regurgitation

In dysphagia (difficulty in swallowing), the masticated food is returned from the pharyngeal region via the nasal cavities and mouth, and water that is drunk runs out through both nos-trils. This is regurgitation. It is observed chiefly in the horse and dog, and occurs when, as a result of inflammatory swelling of the pharyngeal mucosa, paralysis of the upper part of the pharynx, neoplasia in the pharynx, foreign body in the pharynx, etc., contact of the soft palate with Passavant's cushion in the posterior wall of the pharynx is not sufficiently intimate to shut off the cavity of the phraynx from the nasal cavities, and so food escapes through the aper-ture into the posterior nares. Regurgitation, re-sulting from dysphagia, is also associated with structural or functional obstruction of the oeso-phagus. In these circumstances repeated, vigo-rous swallowing movements may have been noted to precede regurgitation. Regurgitated material is usually slightly alkaline in reaction.

Nasal Mucous Membrane

This can be adequately inspected only in equine species, because in these animals the nostrils are wide and flexible, so that the anterior third of the nasal cavities are accessible to direct visual examination (Fig. 91); this is not the case

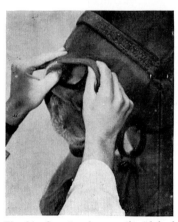

Fig. 91. *Opening the nostril with both hands to allow inspection of the mucous membrane.*

in other species of domestic animals. On the floor of the nasal fossae, at the junction between the skin and the mucous membrane, lie the openings of the lacrimal ducts, one at each side, which are fairly large and clearly visible in equine species. A nasal discharge, in whole or part only, may therefore have originated in the conjunctival sac. In equine species the nasal diverticulum ('false nostril') is readily examined by inserting the finger into the nostril at the upper commissure; if necessary an endoscopic examination can be performed. Sebaceous cysts occasionally develop at this site.

The short ducts of the mucous glands opening on to the surface give the nasal mucosa a finely punctate appearance, which is accentuated in inflammatory conditions causing hyperfunctioning of the glands. The proximal part of the nasal mucosa is somewhat pinkish in colour; the more distally situated parts of the mucous membrane have a bluish-red colour on account of the numerous venous blood vessels and spaces occurring there. When infiltrated by exudate, the nasal mucous membrane has a velvety appearance and is slightly spongy on palpation.

The more important changes affecting the nasal mucosa include pallor, injection, petechiation, erosion, ulceration or proliferation. Recognizing and correctly interpreting the significance of any change may be important. Pallidness occurs in anaemic states and in shock. Injection arises from simple hyperaemia which is noted in allergic rhinitis. Petechiation is a feature of the early stages of purpura haemorrhagica in the horse and of dicoumarol poisoning. Necrosis succeeded by erosive and ulcerative lesions of the nasal mucosa are a typical feature of rinderpest, malignant catarrhal fever and mucosal disease. The ulcerative lesions of glanders, melioidosis and epizootic lymphangitis are characteristic and have important diagnostic merit. Proliferative lesions in the form of small nodules (0·5–2·0 cm in diameter) develop on the mucosa of the anterior third of the nasal cavity in rhinosporidiosis (nasal granuloma) in cattle.

In good light the anterior part of the nasal cavity of the horse can be inspected directly, otherwise an electric torch or illuminated speculum is used to project light into the cavity. In the horse and ox, the use of a suitable rhinolaryngoscope (see Fig. 110, p. 105) permits adequate visual examination of those parts of the nasal cavities that cannot be inspected directly or by means of an illuminated speculum.

With the aid of the rhinolaryngoscope, or a suitable sound, the patency of the nasal passages and the presence of any constriction (stenosis) can be established. Care is essential when inserting the instrument into the nasal cavity in order to avoid injury to the mucosa and, in the case of restless or excitable animals, sedation is usually desirable. Further information about the state of the nasal cavities may be obtained by radiological examination.

Paranasal Sinuses

Anatomically the paranasal sinuses connect directly, or indirectly, with the nasal cavity, of which they are diverticula; there are four pairs, viz. maxillary, frontal, sphenopalatine and ethmoidal.

The maxillary sinus lies approximately in the area between the eye and the zygomatic ridge, and the frontal sinus above the level of a line joining the eyes (the position of the sphenoidal sinus and the guttural pouch in the horse will be discussed later).

The first part of the examination of the sinuses consists in observing whether there is any abnormal bony prominence (Fig. 92) or depression, and then, by palpation, determining whether

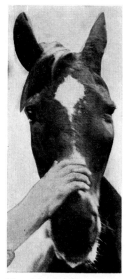

Fig. 92. *Swelling in the region of the maxillary sinus, and narrowing of the left eyelids with strabismus. Sarcoma of the maxillary sinus.*

there is rarefaction or fracture of bone, or local elevation of temperature. Percussing with the fingers (Fig. 93), or with a percussion hammer, determines the character of the sound elicited. In normal animals the sound is clear and loud, but if the sinus is filled with exudate, neoplastic tissue or a cyst, the percussion note is dull. These examinations are always carried out by comparing the findings on one side of the head with those observed on the contralateral side. Only distinctive differences in the features re-

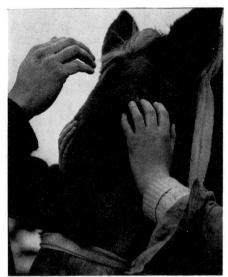

Fig. 93. *Percussion of the frontal sinus. An assistant covers the animal's eyes to prevent a reaction to the movement of the upraised hand.*

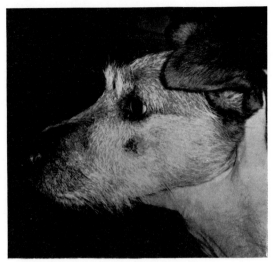

Fig. 94. *A chronic fistula in the face of a dog, arising from infection of the maxillary sinus.*

vealed are of diagnostic value. If in a completely darkened room, a very powerful, protected electric torch is introduced into the mouth, the sinuses are transilluminated and appear as clear areas (diaphanoscopy) when normal. This procedure is particularly useful in determining the condition of the maxillary sinuses in the dog. The most common cause of sinusitis in the dog is infection of the medial root of the fourth upper molar tooth (carnassial). The inflammatory exudate and pus within the sinus may, under pressure, erode the maxillary bone and break through the skin and give rise to a chronic fistula on the face below and in front of the eye (Fig. 94). Prior to the formation of a fistula, a swelling may develop on this part of the face. In cattle, apart from very occasional cases of actinomycosis or neoplasia of the maxillary sinus, it is the frontal sinus that is mainly involved in disease. Frontal sinusitis occurs as an extension of infection from the nasal cavity in malignant catarrhal fever, allergic rhinitis, injuries to horns, contusions and fractures in the area, and most commonly as a sequel of dehorning. Horn core tumours, particularly when malignant, invariably extend to involve the frontal sinus. Radiographic examination may be of diagnostic value in certain instances when the existence or nature of a sinus disease is in doubt. Exploratory puncture (trephining) of a sinus might also be undertaken when other methods fail to indicate its state.

A nasal discharge originating in a paranasal sinus is unilateral, persistent, sometimes foetid, and occurs intermittently as a result of the head being lowered. Diseases of the air sinuses may affect adjacent structures as a result of either inflammation (escape of lacrimal secretion from the corresponding conjunctival sac, erosion of the maxillary bone in the dog producing a dental fistula) or swelling (strabismus, stenotic sounds in the affected nasal cavity, bulging of the hard palate interfering with mastication).

Microscopical Examination of Nasal Discharge

Besides examination for various bacteria, including *Streptococcus equi, Strep. zooepidemicus,* other streptococci, *Actinobacillus mallei, Mycobacterium tuberculosis* and fungi, e.g. *Aspergillus* spp., etc., nasal discharges are occasionally examined microscopically for the presence of virus inclusion bodies or of parasite ova. Virus inclusion bodies occur in the cells of the nasal mucosa in inclusion body rhinitis in pigs, also in infectious bovine rhinotracheitis for a few days only, and in feline viral rhinotracheitis. Identifying the inclusion bodies in smears of nasal discharge requires specialized experience. The parasite ova may originate in the nasal cavity (*Linguatula rhinaria* which produce oval, thick-shelled, double contoured· ova), in the trachea and bronchi (*Capillaria aerophila, Crenosoma vulpis, Filaroides osleri*) or in the lungs (*Meta-strongylus* spp.; see Fig. 160B, p. 205).

If gangrene of the lung is suspected (it occurs in some cases of aspiration pneumonia and causes the expired air to have a foetid odour), the nasal discharge can be examined for the presence of elastic fibres. These are recognizable as slender, wavy, colourless, refractile threads, which are distinguished from fibrin and connective tissue by being soluble in potassium hydroxide solution. Examination of unstained preparations is satisfactory.

Parasite ova can be recognized at a low magnification; elastic fibres require higher magnification. In fungus infections of the nasal structures (epizootic lymphangitis of horses, rhinosporidiosis of cattle and chronic granulomatous rhinitis of dogs and cats caused by *Histoplasma farciminosum, Rhinosporidium seeberi* and *Histoplasma neoformans*, respectively) or lungs (aspergillosis), the causal organism can sometimes be demonstrated in the nasal discharge. Specific identification would, in most cases, require cultural techniques.

APPETITE AND THE ORAL CAVITY

Disturbances of Eating and Drinking

Appetite in animals is generally assessed by reference to food consumption in healthy individual animals in identical circumstances. Variations in appetite include increase, decrease, or abnormality (depravity). When an animal's appetite is impaired, the cause may be unsuitable food, lack of desire for food or inability to prehend or masticate the food. In all cases of reduced appetite, it is advisable to determine that the food provided is of reasonable quality.

Partial reduction in appetite (inappetence) is associated with many types of gastric disease because of reduced hunger, but all toxaemic and febrile diseases are frequently accompanied by decreased food intake (anophagia). In the more acute forms of these conditions, appetite is completely absent (anorexia). Dietary deficiencies, e.g. cobalt in ruminants and thiamine in carnivores, are other important causes of inappetence. Hunger sensations are sometimes submerged by others such as fear, excitement or severe pain; this is exemplified by lack of appetite in some dogs when put into strange kennels, or when range cattle or horses are housed.

Increased appetite (hyperorexia) manifest by increased food consumption (polyphagia) is observed in pancreatic deficiency, chronic gastritis, certain forms of intestinal parasitism, functional diarrhoea, certain metabolic diseases, such as diabetes mellitus, and as a physiological expression of hunger following a period of starvation. Because there is either a defect in absorption and/or utilization of food or excessive metabolic demand, an animal may be emaciated in spite of excessive intake of food. Increased consumption of water (polydipsia) occurs when there is excessive loss of body fluid (dehydration) which may be caused by persistent vomiting, diabetes insipidus, diabetes mellitus, chronic interstitial nephritis, and in many cases of catarrhal gastritis. Desire for water in increased amounts is manifested, as a temporary feature only, during the initial stages of many febrile diseases.

A depraved (perverted, unnatural) appetite exists when an animal ingests substances that do not normally form part of the diet of the species concerned. It is manifest by varying degrees of pica or allotriophagia. Abnormal appetite occurs in some nutritional deficiencies, more particularly of phosphorus (rickets, aphosphorosis), sodium chloride and less obviously cobalt, as well as when there is inadequate protein, bulk or fibre in the diet. Other causes include chronic peritonitis, chronic gastritis, parasitic enteritis (strongylosis) in horses and certain diseases (rabies, ketosis) which disturb the function of the nervous system. In some animals an unnatural appetite becomes habitual although the cause of its appearance has ceased to operate.

According to the preference exhibited by the affected animal an abnormal appetite can be classified: eating the faeces (seen most frequently in puppies and young horses) is coprophagia; chewing bones (occurs in cattle affected with aphosphorosis) is osteophagia; eating the young, infantophagia, is an important form of cannibalism sometimes observed in farrowing sows; eating earth is allotriophagia. Other types of pica include excessive coat-licking because of salt hunger, wool eating in sheep, eating decomposing animal carcasses, litter eating, etc.

Even when the appetite is normal, the ingestion of food may be rendered difficult, or impossible, by reason of disease in one or other of the associated mouth structures. Depending on whether the abnormality affects the lips, teeth, tongue, oral mucous membrane, soft palate, tonsils, pharynx or oesophagus, there will be difficulty in prehension, mastication or deglutition. An abnormal manner of feeding may also result from even mild disturbance of consciousness, e.g. in chronic acquired hydrocephalus in the horse. Horses and cattle recovering from chloral hydrate narcosis sometimes exhibit a compulsion to consume almost any fibrous material within reach. In order that the state of the appetite and the feeding behaviour should be correctly determined, it is necessary to undertake prolonged observation of the animal while it is eating and drinking.

Prehension and Mastication

The method of prehending solid food varies according to the species, but in all domestic animals the lips, teeth and tongue are the principal organs concerned. The sheep, goat and horse, when feeding from a manger, seize the food with the lips and incisor teeth; sheep have a cleft upper lip which permits close grazing. When grazing, the horse draws back the mobile lips and severs the grass with the incisor teeth. The tongue is the main prehensile organ in the ox, being well constructed for this purpose by reason of its length, mobility and rough surface. In the pig the food is taken into the mouth by the lower lip and teeth. The dog and cat take up solid food with the teeth, but they often use the forelimb to hold it. The horse, ox, sheep and pig draw liquid into the mouth by suction. This is accomplished by almost closing the mouth, which is submerged into the fluid, and producing negative pressure by a pumplike movement of the tongue. The dog and cat convey fluids to the mouth by using the tongue as a ladle. In very young animals sucking is achieved by creating negative pressure in the mouth by suction with the cheeks and tongue. The manner of food and water prehension is abnormal in painful conditions or malformations (Fig. 95) of the lips, tongue and incisor teeth, e.g. stomatitis, glossitis, gingivitis, penetrating or occlusive foreign bodies, fluorosis, malocclusion and broken, misaligned and deficient incisor teeth. Unilateral or bilateral paralysis of the lips, tongue or muscles of mastication, dislocation of the temporomandibular joint and fracture of the mandible or maxilla also interfere with prehension. Animals with torticollis, caused by dysfunction of the vestibular nerve or middle ear disease, have difficulty in eating and drinking

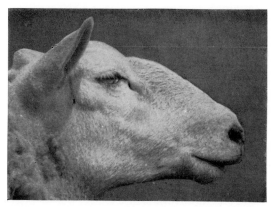

Fig. 95. *Shortness of the lower jaw (overshot jaw). A malformation of this degree is not lethal, but, owing to the reduced grazing efficiency, it may prevent the animal from thriving.*

because of their inability to orientate the mouth correctly. In these conditions the appetite for food is obviously retained.

Mastication consists of chewing with the teeth, assisted by movements of the tongue and cheeks which keep the food between the teeth. The motive power originates mainly in the masseter muscles. With sufficient trituration the food is broken down so that it can be formed into a bolus preparatory to being swallowed. Mastication usually takes place involuntarily although, basically it is a voluntary act under the control of centres in the brain. In all species, mastication consists mainly of grinding the food between the molar teeth. The degree of grinding varies between carnivorous and herbivorous species and the molar teeth are structured to meet the particular requirements. An important concomitant of mastication is the production of saliva and its admixture with the triturated food. In herbivores the upper jaw is wider than the lower and there is considerable lateral movement of the jaws so that mastication occurs only on one side at a time. In carnivores and omnivores the jaw movements, during mastication, take place in a vertical plane so producing a shearing effect on food.

Mastication is impaired, the movements of the jaw being performed slowly and with apparent caution, in painful diseases of the buccal mucous membrane (stomatitis, glossitis, gingivitis, etc.), the molar teeth, the muscles of mastication (eosinophilic myositis, actinobacillosis, paralysis), the temporomandibular joint (fracture) and the mandible (actinomycosis). In herbivorous animals, diseases causing pain during mastication are usually characterized by 'quidding', i.e. dropping of semi-masticated food from the mouth, and the presence of undigested food particles in the faeces.

Deglutition

Deglutition, or swallowing, is the action of transferring food from the mouth through the pharynx and oesophagus to the stomach. The normal act of swallowing occurs in three stages, the first of which is voluntary; the other two are reflexly controlled and are, therefore, involuntary. The deglutition centre is composed of nerve cells situated in the floor of the fourth ventricle.

Following mastication and lubrication with saliva, the food is compressed into a bolus which is initially placed in the midline between the tongue and hard palate and then thrown back between the pillars of the fauces to reach the posterior wall of the pharynx. At the commencement of the second phase, the soft palate is elevated to close off the posterior nares, and the epiglottis closes off the larynx (see Fig. 90, p. 88). Respiration is momentarily inhibited and, with approximation of the posterior pillars of the fauces, the mouth cavity is shut off. Then the pharyngeal muscles contract so that the bolus is propelled into the oesophagus which simultaneously dilates. The third phase is concerned with propelling the bolus along the oesophagus. The structures of significance in deglutition include the tongue, floor of the mouth, hard and soft palate, fauces, laryngeal muscles and oesophagus. Afferent receptors at these sites transmit impulses along the maxillary division of the trigeminal nerve, the glossophrayngeal nerve, and the superior laryngeal branch of the vagus nerve to the deglutition centre. Efferent impulses are transmitted via the trigeminal, glossopharyngeal, vagus, hypoglossal and spinal accessory nerves.

Disturbances of swallowing are attributable to structural or functional defects in any of the component structures essential for the act and include painful inflammatory swelling of the pharyngeal tissues, oesophageal dilatation and diverticulum, paralysis or cleft state of the soft palate and paralysis or dilatation of the oesophagus. In addition physical causes, such as partial or complete obstruction of the pharynx or oesophagus by a foreign body, tumour or enlarged lymph node, may interfere with swallowing, or even prevent it altogether.

In the horse, more rarely in the ox, various movements of the lips, tongue or jaws may be seen that have no immediate connection with eating or drinking, and which may be regarded as vices or bad habits. These include smacking the lips, blowing air out of the mouth between the closed lips, playfully licking objects with the tongue, crib-biting and wind-sucking.

In the dog affected with extensive pneumonia or advanced congestive heart failure, severe dyspnoea causes oral breathing with obvious movements of the lips.

Oral Cavity

All the structures comprising the mouth can be subjected to clinical examination. In order to examine the labial mucous membrane the upper and lower lips are gently grasped, lifted and turned back. In the larger species of animals, if the interior of the mouth is to be examined only briefly, the free portion of the tongue is grasped inside the mouth by inserting one hand at the interdental space, the hand is then rotated so that the thumb is uppermost (Fig. 96); alter-

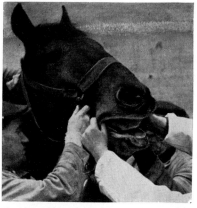

Fig. 96. *Opening the mouth. The tongue is grasped firmly inside the mouth with the right hand, the thumb of which is uppermost.*

natively the tongue is grasped in the same manner and then drawn out of one side of the mouth so that part of the attached portion is pulled between the tables of the opposing molar teeth (Fig. 97), and so prevents the animal from closing the mouth. This, in conjunction with pulling the cheek on the other side outwards with the

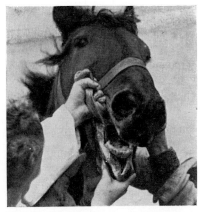

Fig. 97. *Opening the mouth. The tongue is grasped with the left hand and drawn sideways out of the mouth.*

fingers at the oral commissure, permits visual examination of a part of one side of the oral cavity; in order to complete the examination it is necessary to repeat the manoeuvre by withdrawing the tongue from the opposite side of the mouth. In the dog, the upper jaw is grasped with one hand and the lower jaw with the other, the animal's lips being pushed inwards over the crowns of the molar teeth on both sides with the thumb and middle fingers while the forefingers rest against the canine teeth (Fig. 98). If the dog is inclined to bite, the mouth is opened by means of tapes placed round both jaws just behind the canine teeth. One assistant holds the tapes, one

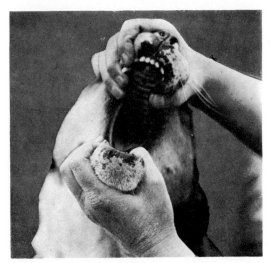

Fig. 98. *Opening the mouth of a quiet dog. The upper and lower lips are pressed inwards against the molar teeth. The forelegs are held by an assistant.*

in each hand, and by pulling them apart opens the mouth, while another assistant holds both forefeet (Fig. 99). The clinician is thus able to carry out a detailed examination of all parts of the mouth and a substantial area of the pharynx. In a quiet cat, the mouth can be opened by placing the dorsal surface of the little finger against the nape of the neck, grasping the upper jaw between the thumb and forefinger, with the eyes covered by the palm of the hand, and bending the animal's head upwards, using the little finger as a pivot (Figs 100, 101). The lower jaw is then depressed by applying downward

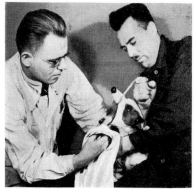

Fig. 99. *Opening the mouth of a dog inclined to bite. Loops of tape are applied to both jaws behind the canine teeth. Traction on the tapes opens the mouth, allowing the tongue to be drawn out with the aid of a towel.*

pressure with the finger of the free hand. It is essential for an assistant to hold both forefeet. When the deeper parts of the oral cavity require thorough examination, in all but the smaller species, it is advisable to use a gag (Figs 102–105). If the animal resents handling, because of painful conditions of the mouth, or fear, a suitable sedative or narcotic drug should be administered prior to undertaking the examination. This is made by means of inspection and palpation of selected tissues. In the horse and ox, and in all circumstances when the light is poor, an electric torch is required.

Abnormalities of the buccal mucous membrane include changes in colour of a focal, or more general, distribution such as jaundice, cyanosis and the pallor of anaemia and those associated with alteration in vascularity (hyperaemia, haemorrhages, etc.) which are clinical features of diseases with an inflammatory or allergic origin.

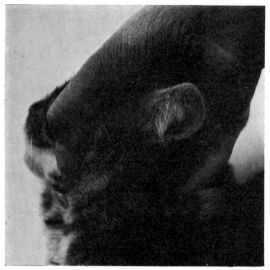

Fig. 100. *Opening the mouth of a cat (first stage). Note the position ot the little finger at the base of the cat's neck. The thumb and forefinger are grasping the cheek.*

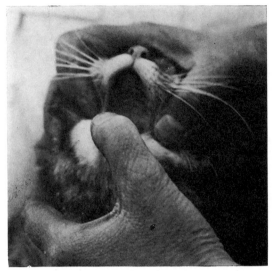

Fig. 101. *Opening the mouth of a cat (second stage). The cheeks are gripped between the forefinger and thumb and the head is bent backwards; the lower jaw is then easily pressed downwards with the other hand. The forelegs are held by an assistant.*

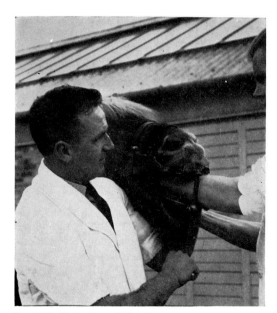

Fig. 102. *Palpation of the pharynx using a gag of the Haussman–Dunn type.*

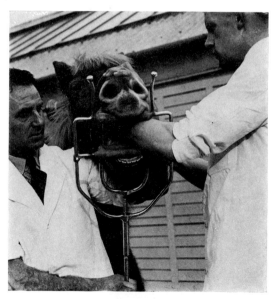

Fig. 103. *Palpation of the pharynx using the Elam gag. Note the freedom of access to the mouth.*

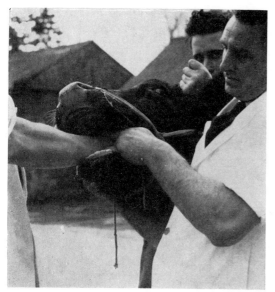

Fig. 104. *Palpation of the pharynx using Drinkwater's gag, which is wedged between the upper and lower molar teeth on each side. The cords attached to both parts of the gag (for rapid removal should the risk of their being swallowed arise) can be seen on either side.*

Inflammation of the oral mucosa may be more severe in one part than in another (stomatitis, glossitis, gingivitis) and may be caused by infectious, chemical or physical agents. The infective agents are bacterial, viral and fungal in character. Bacterial stomatitis is manifested by necrosis and ulceration as in fusospirochaetal infection in the dog caused by *Fusiformis fusiformis* and *Borrelia vincentii*; oral necrobacillosis (calf diphtheria) caused by *Sphaerophorus necrophorus*; ulcerative granuloma of pigs caused by *Borrelia suilla* which may spread from the lips and cheeks to involve the labial mucosa; actinobacillosis (*Actinobacillus lignieresi*) in the ox, which initially involves the tongue causing ulceration in many cases, may spread to the lips, and the gums may be involved in actinomycosis.

The oral lesions in viral stomatitis vary in character and may be vesicular, ulcerative or proliferative. In foot-and-mouth disease, vesicular exanthema and vesicular stomatitis the initial stage is vesicular but the lesions become ulcerative within a few days. Malignant catarrhal

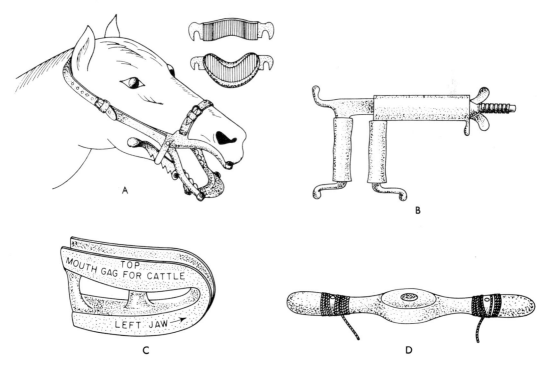

Fig. 105. *Gags for large animals.* A, *Haussman–Dunn type.* B, *Varnell's gag for horses.* C, *Drinkwater's gag (left jaw).* D, *Probang gag for cattle.*

fever, mucosal disease, rinderpest, bluetongue, infectious ulcerative stomatitis and diseases such as contagious pustular dermatitis, sheep pox and ulcerative dermatosis, when the lesions extend from the lips into the oral cavity, are manifested by erosion and secondary ulceration of the oral mucosa. Ulcerative glossitis involving the tip of the tongue is a feature of some cases of feline panleucopenia. Necrotic lesions confined to the anterior part of the tongue have been reported in feedlot steers in the USA; no specific cause has been identified. Buccal papillomatosis, seen in the dog and very occasionally in other species, and proliferative stomatitis and papular stomatitis of cattle are associated with proliferative lesions.

Vesicular, erosive or ulcerative lesions tend to be modified by secondary bacterial invasion so that they become suppurative and ulcerative, resembling the lesions of bacterial stomatitis. In a small proportion of such cases an extensive cellulitis, involving the facial tissues may develop. In certain diseases, including blacktongue and interstitial nephritis in the dog, stomatitis develops as a result of toxaemia and general debility permitting abnormal bacterial activity on the oral mucosa. Ulceration of the gingival mucosa occurs in old dogs and cats, most commonly those with dental calculus.

Mycotic stomatitis, a somewhat rare affection of the oral mucosa, is mainly caused by *Monilia* spp.; in dogs it is usually caused by *Candida albicans* which is responsible for diffuse, patchy areas covered by a whitish film. Chemical agents which may cause stomatitis are corrosive acids or alkalis, counter-irritants improperly applied so that the animal licks them off the surface of the body (mercuric iodide, cantharides) or chloral hydrate administered orally in strong concentrations. Toxic irritants contained in plants such as hemlock, buttercup, mustard, spurge, water hemlock and water dropwort may produce somewhat similar effects.

Physical agents that may be associated with the development of stomatitis include sharp awns, especially from certain cereals, thorns or spines on plants, sharp-edged or pointed pieces of bone or other foreign objects, particularly in dogs and cats, maloccluded teeth, frozen or very hot food or water and trauma during the administering of medicine.

Salivation

Saliva is the mixed secretion of the three main paired glands, the parotid, submaxillary and sublingual, together with that of numerous small glands in the oral mucosa. The glands are serous, mucous or mixed in character according to their structure and the nature of the secretion they produce. The cells of the serous glands contain zymogen granules which are thought to be the precursors of enzyme. The parotid gland in most mammals is serous. The submaxillary gland is mixed in ungulates, the dog and the cat; it is serous in rodents. The sublingual gland is serous in domestic animals.

Saliva is produced spontaneously and in response to neural or hormonal stimuli. Neural stimulation, which is of most significance in animals, is through the medium of efferent innervation from both sympathetic and parasympathetic components of the autonomic nervous system. Sympathetic preganglionic fibres originate from the spinal cord in the first few thoracic nerves and pass, via the cervical chain, to the superior cervical ganglion where they form synapses with nerve cells, the fibres of which are distributed to the blood vessels and cells of the glands. Parasympathetic preganglionic fibres traverse the glossopharyngeal and then the trigeminal nerve to the parotid gland; those to the submaxillary and sublingual glands are contained in the facial nerve and reach their destination in the chorda tympani. Afferent impulses originate in the mouth, pharynx and olfactory area and are conveyed via the trigeminal and glossopharyngeal nerves to the salivary centres in the medulla.

In normal animals the secretion of saliva is abundant, particularly in ruminant species, in which the parotid salivary gland secretes spontaneously. Reduction in the quantity of saliva secreted, resulting in a dry condition of the oral mucosa, is seen in very acute febrile conditions, in diseases accompanied by excessive loss of body fluid with severe dehydration (enteritis, nephritis, diabetes insipidus, etc.) and in poisoning with belladonna alkaloids. Dryness of the mouth occurs in animals that are breathing through the mouth, but here the dryness is caused by excessive evaporation rather than by deficient secretion.

The quantity of saliva produced is increased in painful inflammatory conditions of the mucous membrane of the mouth, tongue, pharynx or oesophagus. Foot-and-mouth disease, mucosal disease, rinderpest and actinobacillosis when the tongue is involved are some of the important causes. Foreign bodies in the mouth, more particularly when they penetrate the soft tissues, because they cause excessive chewing movements and interfere with swallowing, are a common cause of excessive salivation in the dog and cat and occasionally have a similar effect in the ox and horse. In obstruction or paralysis of the oesophagus, particularly in the ox, the flow of saliva from the mouth is an indication of the inability of the animal to swallow, not of excessive secretion. Ptyalism is a clinical feature of certain forms of mineral intoxication, e.g. chronic mercury and acute lead poisoning in young cattle. In the former it is due to a mild stomatitis and in the latter because the encephalopathy which develops involves the salivary nucleus.

Increased salivation may be revealed by observing that the animal makes frequent swallowing movements not associated with feeding (empty swallowing). With experience it is possible to recognize an increased flow of saliva by inspecting the tissues contiguous to the openings of the salivary ducts (Stensen's duct from the parotid gland opens onto the labial mucous membrane adjacent to the third upper molar tooth; Wharton's duct from the submaxillary gland opens, in association with the duct from the sublingual gland, on either side of the fraenum linguae.) Particularly abundant secretion of saliva is easily recognized: the saliva hangs from the mouth in strands and movements of the lower jaw and tongue, when they occur, are accompanied by smacking or snapping sounds (foot-and-mouth disease in cattle or sheep). Pus or blood mixed with saliva indicates purulent or haemorrhagic inflammation or injury, affecting the mucous membrane of the oral cavity or pharynx. Admixture with air causes the saliva to become frothy, as in dyspnoea, epileptiform convulsions, etc.

Owing to its exposed situation on the lateral aspect of the ramus, the duct (Stensen's) of the parotid salivary gland may suffer an injury resulting in a salivary fistula. The condition is recognized by its anatomical position, and by the fact that the escape of fluid is greatly increased when the animal is eating.

The odour of the mouth in healthy animals is not usually unpleasant, except possibly in cattle when they are fed on a diet containing silage or roots. Unpleasant odours may arise from local or remote local organs, although in many cases they are associated with general debilitation arising from acute or chronic diseases of the alimentary tract, or specific diseases causing ulceration of the mucous membrane of the mouth and pharynx. In the horse, gangrene of the lung causes the odour of the mouth and the expired air to be particularly offensive. Calves with necrotic stomatitis have a sour, rather putrid odour. In the dog, acute and advanced chronic nephritis, and deposits of tartar on the teeth, are recognized causes of unpleasant odours.

Tongue

Changes similar to those affecting the other parts of the oral mucous membrane also occur on the surface of the tongue. A covering of white, somewhat viscous, mucoid material, readily scraped off, is found on the dorsal surface of the tongue, more particularly towards the posterior part, when the intake of food has ceased, as in various febrile and alimentary diseases, etc. This 'fur' is formed when, as the result of the intake of food being diminished or absent, desquamation of the lingual epithelium is in abeyance. When the tongue is furred, the mucosa is dry, and there is an unpleasant odour. The tongue may also show changes in colour (e.g. in the dog, severe toxaemia and uraemia may cause the development of a copper-red colour), oedema, injuries, hardening with enlargement and not uncommonly ulceration (*Actinobacillus lignieresi* infection in the ox), or reduction in mobility, and sometimes size, as a result of paralysis. The underside of the tongue, close to the fraenum linguae, may be affected with a ranula (a salivary or mucous gland retention cyst).

Teeth

Tartar (dental calculus) often occurs on the teeth, more especially in dogs and cats, in the form of a hard yellowish-brown deposit, which usually commences to accumulate near the alveolar margin and causes the gingival tissues to recede, thus leading to alveolar periostitis and periodontitis. Heavy deposits of tartar are injurious to the labial mucosa as well. Note should be taken of missing, damaged, excessively worn, displaced or defective teeth, dental caries and foreign bodies wedged between the teeth. Teeth may be missing because of very old age, or delayed eruption, which in sheep signifies mineral deficiency. Missing incisor teeth may also arise from trauma or, as in sheep, from grazing on poor, stony soil, or infection of the alveoli with *Actinobacillus lignieresi*, in which case a variable number will be absent.

Chronic fluorosis in cattle and sheep causes mottling and pitting of the enamel of the incisor teeth, with excessively and unevenly worn molar teeth. These defects only appear in those permanent teeth which developed while the animal was on a diet containing excessive amounts of fluorine. In dogs which were affected with distemper prior to the eruption of the permanent teeth, it will be observed that the enamel layer is present, to a variable degree, only on the crowns of the teeth, the exposed dentine giving the teeth a dirty, yellowish-brown colour. The deciduous teeth have a bluish, translucent appearance in young animals, especially puppies, affected with rickets. Transillumination of the mouth will outline the pulp cavity of the teeth in such cases. In adolescent herbivorous animals, retention of some of the deciduous molar teeth on the crowns of the erupting permanent teeth in the lower jaw is a possible cause of impaired mastication.

In a horse that is addicted to crib-biting, the anterior edge of the teeth in both incisor arcades is worn down (Fig. 106). It is particularly impor-

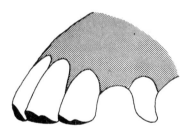

Fig. 106. *Excessive wear of the anterior edge of the upper incisor teeth in a crib biter.*

tant to examine the molar teeth for evidence of uneven wear, because sharp edges on these teeth can make mastication painful, cause ulceration of the labial and lingual mucosae, which may permit bacterial invasion of the deeper tissues, and lead to loss of condition because of impaired appetite and digestion. In the horse, it is very commonly found that both the labial edge of the tables of the upper and the lingual edge of the tables of the lower molar teeth are sharp and

pointed. A more severe form of this condition ('shear-mouth', scissors-mouth), possibly of genetic origin, occurs in horses and sheep and is caused by undue narrowing of the mandible. Other abnormalities of wear which occur in the molar teeth of the horse include step mouth (step-formed table surfaces), wave mouth (undulating table surfaces) and smooth mouth (smooth table surfaces); they are characteristically seen in aged horses.

Overgrowth of the incisor teeth in rodent species is readily recognized because the affected animal is unable to close the mouth properly, so that prehension is impaired. An important form of this condition is malocclusion in chinchilla. Anatomical defects, which cause malapposition of the incisor teeth, include prognathia (undershot jaw) in Hereford, Shorthorn, Jersey, Holstein and Ayrshire calves, and brachygnathia (parrot mouth) of Merino and Rambouillet lambs; both are congenital and hereditary in origin and are readily recognized. Displacement of the lower premolar teeth, in conjunction with shortening and narrowing of the mandible, occurs in calves as an expression of an hereditary defect. In advanced cases of actinomycosis and neoplasia of the jaw bones, tooth displacement is a usual feature.

Supernumerary teeth include wolf teeth in the horse, the more common form of excess incisors (usually a double row is present) and the more rare excess form involving the molar teeth. A dentigerous cyst, which is unique to the horse, and is thought to represent an aberrant dental follicle, is usually located in the vicinity of the mastoid process of the petrous temporal bone, at the base of the ear; the malformation may also occur on the frontal bone or in the paranasal sinuses. The condition becomes obvious, in many cases, during adolescence when normal dental changes are most active.

Tonsils

The tonsils are situated in the fauces, on either side of the root of the tongue; they show anatomical variation between species. In the horse there is a series of masses of lymphoid tissue and mucous glands which extend backwards for about 10 cm; the bovine tonsil is bean-shaped and about 1 cm long; in the pig the main mass of tonsillar tissue is situated on each side of the midline of the oral surface of the soft palate, with additional tonsillar tissue situated in the fauces lateral to the root of the tongue; the tonsils of the dog are somewhat similar to those of man. They are about 2·5 cm long, reddish in colour and almost completely concealed by folds of mucous membrane. The tonsils are most easily observed in the dog by opening the mouth and then depressing the tongue at its posterior part. Examination of the tonsils should never be omitted in the dog. The size and colour and the presence of abscesses (often pinhead in size and of varying number), haemorrhages, neoplasia, foreign bodies, etc., are noted. In other species the tonsillar tissues are difficult to inspect on account of their position, relatively small size and anatomical relationships.

Vomiting

Vomiting (emesis) is the forceful ejection of solid and liquid gastrointestinal contents through the oesophagus, mouth and/or nostrils to the exterior. It is much more common in carnivorous than herbivorous species, although it is contended that the basic mechanisms for the act are present in all species. A distinction is made between central and reflex vomiting. The former arises from direct stimulation of the vomiting centre in the medulla oblongata, and occurs in certain diseases of the brain, in uraemia resulting from nephritis and hepatitis and following the administration of apomorphine to the pig, dog and cat and, not infrequently, of morphine to the dog. The latter is caused by reflex stimulation of the vomiting centre as the result of irritation in various organs; it is observed in pharyngitis, oesophageal obstruction, foreign bodies in the stomach, gastric distension, pyloric hypertrophy, intestinal obstruction or distension, nephritis, pyometritis, peritonitis, hepatitis, etc.

The initial phenomena of vomiting consist of increased salivation, irregular, rapid and deep respiration, followed by retching, which arises from spasmodic contraction of all the muscles of respiration. The succeeding events consist of reflex mechanisms which prevent the vomitus from entering the respiratory tract. Following a deep inspiration the glottis is closed and the nasopharynx sealed off by elevation of the soft palate (see Fig. 90, p. 88). With the glottis still closed, expiration commences and is accompanied by contraction of the abdominal muscles and diaphragm. In the next sequence the pyloric area of the stomach contracts, with relaxation of the fundic and cardiac areas and of the oesopha-

gus. The increased abdominal pressure propels the stomach contents into the oesophagus, thereby creating antiperistaltic waves which carry them to the pharynx, from where they are ejected. Studies in the cat have shown the act of vomition is preceded by periods of retroperistalsis in the duodenum with reflux of duodenal contents into the flaccid stomach. This phase possibly occurs in other animals. When emesis occurs as a means of relieving an overloaded stomach, noted particularly in young puppies and kittens, retching is not observed and vomiting is projectile in character.

Except in the dog and cat, vomiting is always pathological, and in some species is of grave prognostic significance. In the horse, because of the long soft palate, vomited material is mainly regurgitated through the nostrils, and in other species through the mouth. In ruminant species, 'vomiting' in most instances is really regurgitation of rumen contents, not an emptying of the true stomach, although cattle and goats, and to a lesser extent sheep, manifest all the usual features of vomiting when they are poisoned by rhododendron or *Convallaria majalis* (lily-of-the-valley). Other causes of vomiting in cattle include spoiled foods or highly acid silage and, in individual cases, diaphragmatic hernia, foreign body or papillomas in or near the oesophageal groove, impaction of the abomasum and ulceration of the abomasum impinging on the pyloric sphincter. Dogs, cats and pigs vomit readily, and do so fairly frequently. In young pigs vomiting occurs as a feature in many systemic diseases, more consistently in vomiting and wasting disease and transmissible gastroenteritis. The bitch not uncommonly regurgitates recently ingested food in order to encourage its offspring to start eating solid food. It must be remembered, however, that persistent vomiting in the dog may indicate serious disease, e.g. pyloric obstruction or hypertrophy, intestinal obstruction or occlusion, nephritis, pyometritis, peritonitis and hepatitis, as well as less serious conditions such as pharyngitis, mild catarrhal gastritis, etc. Many of the diseases which cause persistent coughing in the dog may give rise to mild emesis. The horse vomits only rarely and then with great difficulty and distress. In this species it is always an ominous sign, indicating very serious disease, including gastric impaction or distension with gas, or rupture of the stomach. Regurgitation of considerable quantities of greenish coloured fluid, which trickles from the nostrils, is seen to occur with little discomfort in grass sickness in the horse.

Retching is frequently observed without actual expulsion of stomach contents. In all conditions which predispose to reflex vomiting, retching can be induced artificially by strong pressure along the left jugular furrow, in the depth of which the oesophagus is situated. A similar response is obtained by applying pressure on each side, above and behind the larynx.

Points to note in regard to vomiting are its frequency (occurring once only or repeatedly) and the time at which it occurs in relation to the last meal, i.e. immediately after feeding or not until later at a time when food should normally have left the stomach.

The nature of the vomitus should be noted, attention being directed to the degree of digestion, amount and presence of abnormal constituents, e.g. foreign bodies, blood, pus, parasites, faecal material, etc. Small quantities of blood, or toxic chemicals which have been ingested, can be detected by various chemical and other analytical methods, and bacteria, fungi and parasites by microscopical or cultural examination.

Proof that the vomited material has actually been derived from the stomach, and not from an oesophageal diverticulum, in the case of monogastric animals, is provided by demonstrating that the pH is acid by means of litmus or other suitable chemical indicator substance. The presence of blood is suggested by a positive reaction to the orthotolidine test; conclusive proof depends upon a positive spectroscopic examination, although intact red blood cells may be demonstrated microscopically by examining suitably stained smears. In carnivorous animals receiving raw animal flesh as food the chemical test is not suitable.

Ova of parasites may be found in the vomitus, chiefly in the dog (ascarids, *Spiroptera*) (see Fig. 161A, p. 206). If sputum has been coughed up into the pharynx and swallowed, embryonated lungworm eggs may also be found in the vomitus (see Fig. 160B, p. 205).

Eructation

Eructation is the expulsion of gas from the stomach, via the oesophagus, to the exterior. It occurs when there is excessive gas formation or accumulation of air in the stomach. In ruminant species, moderate eructation is physiological and occurs from increase of gas pressure in the rumen initiating contraction in the dorsal sacs, the motion then passing to the oesophageal cardia and, in association with relaxation of the reticulum, depressing the upper level of the fluid in that organ. The gas is expelled when the cardia relaxes. The rate of the eructation contractions (normally 1–3 per minute) depends upon the pressure of gas in the rumen, and is independent of other cycles of ruminal motility.

ANTERIOR CERVICAL REGION AND NECK

The anterior cervical region lies behind the vertical ramus of the mandible and includes the pharynx, soft palate, guttural pouch, parotid salivary gland, larynx, thyroid gland and parotid and pharyngeal lymph nodes. The clinically important structures in the neck include the oesophagus and jugular veins, which are situated in the jugular furrow, and the trachea, located on the ventral aspect. The area is examined by inspection and palpation and in the case of the larynx and trachea by auscultation; needless to say both sides are included in the examination.

External inspection reveals whether any swelling is present, e.g. parotitis, suppurative lymphadenitis of the parotid or pharyngeal lymph node, neoplasia of the lymph nodes or other tissues, empyema or tympany of the guttural pouch, etc. Direct inspection of the pharyngeal cavity is achieved by viewing it through the opened mouth or by endoscopy. The former method gives satisfactory results only in the dog and cat. Enlargement of the thyroid gland (goitre or neoplasia) causes local swelling in the anterior, ventral area of the neck. Local or general enlargement of the oesophagus (oesophageal diverticulum, foreign body obstruction, stenosis and paralysis) is associated with a swelling in the left jugular furrow.

External palpation in the larger animals is usually performed with both hands (Fig. 107), one either side, stroking lightly at first and gradually increasing the pressure, because otherwise the animal will flinch even although there is no pain in the region. Such behaviour is more usual in nervous, temperamental animals. Palpation will reveal heat, swelling and pain, indicating inflammatory conditions, and deep-seated swelling which may be caused by foreign bodies or neoplasia. In all cases an attempt should be

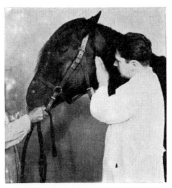

Fig. 107. *Palpation of the anterior cervical region.*

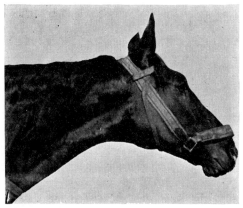

Fig. 108. *Extended carriage of the head and neck. Pharyngitis.*

made to identify the tissue which is abnormal and, if possible, the nature of the affection. Painful conditions of the anterior cervical region may result in an extended carriage of the head and neck (Fig. 108), the object of which is to relieve pressure on the structures in this area. If the pain focus is unilateral, the head is inclined towards the unaffected side.

Internal Palpation of the Pharynx

In the ox, and to a lesser extent in the horse, the whole of the pharyngeal cavity can be explored with the hand, protection against bites being afforded by the use of a suitable gag (Figs 102–105). This examination, in the horse, may require the administration of a sedative or narcotic drug in order to yield satisfactory results. The method is particularly applicable in the identification of foreign bodies, enlargement of

the pharyngeal lymph nodes, which is mainly caused by bacterial invasion or neoplasia, and diffuse cellulitis of the region (consideration should be given to anthrax in the case of the last). A large increase in the circumference of the sphenoidal sinuses can sometimes be detected by this means.

When the hand is introduced into the isthmus of the fauces in healthy horses and cattle this structure is felt to contract, and the pharyngeal reflex is initiated (constriction of the pharynx followed by a swallowing movement and then mild retching); this reaction is absent, or weak, when there is paralysis of the pharynx, as in botulism, grass sickness, peripheral nerve damage (glossopharyngeal, pharyngeal branch of vagus, spinal accessory and hypoglossal) caused by trauma and pressure by a tumour or local pyogenic focus, etc.

The parotid salivary gland is situated subcutaneously in the anterior cervical region where it impinges on the lateral aspect of the vertical ramus. Its lobulated structure makes it easily and distinctly palpable. Swelling in the area of this gland does not, however, necessarily indicate disease of the gland itself (diffuse or local parotitis); it may be caused by affections involving underlying structures (lymphadenitis of the parotid or pharyngeal lymph node, primary or metastatic neoplasia of the local lymph nodes, acute pharyngitis, etc.).

Guttural Pouch

This is a paired structure in the form of a large mucous sac which is a vertical diverticulum of the Eustachian tube; it is present only in equidae. The sacs are located between the base of the cranium and the atlas dorsally, and the pharynx ventrally; they are in apposition medially, but are separated by the ventral straight muscles of the head to some extent. The relationships of the guttural pouch with other cranial structures, particularly on its lateral aspect, are many and complex and in some instances fairly intimate, e.g. the external carotid, internal maxillary and external maxillary arteries, the internal maxillary and jugular veins. In addition the vagus, spinal accessory and sympathetic nerves, along with the internal carotid artery, are located in a fold of the dorsal part of the pouch. The guttural pouch contains air derived from the pharynx through the Eustachian tube; expansion and filling with warm air occurs during expiration, deflation and exchange with cold air takes place during inspiration. The mucous membrane lining the pouch is similar to that lining the Eustachian tube.

The guttural pouch is quite susceptible to infection which is usually introduced via the Eustachian tube. Not uncommonly infection follows strangles or other respiratory tract infections. Disease of the guttural pouch, which is invariably inflammatory and pyogenic or mycotic in character, causes, in severe cases, swelling of the anterior cervical region in the vicinity of the parotid salivary gland and, in some cases, pain. Tympanitis of the guttural pouches occurs occasionally in the newborn foal and in yearlings, as the result of inflammation or a congenital defect. In this case the unilateral or bilateral swelling is painless but tense. Severe distension of both pouches may cause dysphagia and dyspnoea (Fig. 109). The swelling, which in most

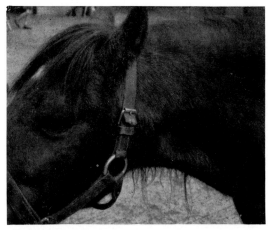

Fig. 109. *Swelling of the posterior pharyngeal region in a horse. Infection of the guttural pouch.*

cases is unilateral, is soft and cushion-like, often reducible on pressure, and sometimes it omits a splashing (succussion) sound on percussion. This sound is produced by agitation of the free surface of a fluid exudate in the cavity or pouch. If the contents of the distended pouch consist of air or gas, percussion will evoke a resonant or tympanic note. Many cases of mycotic (*Aspergillus* spp.) infection of the guttural pouch do not produce distension and lateral swelling. Pharyngeal paralysis resulting from nerve damage has been observed in some cases, while in others nasal haemorrhage of varying severity from

mild epistaxis to profuse, recurrent and fatal has occurred following ulceration of the mucous membrane and erosion of the wall of one of the major arteries.

By means of the rhinolaryngoscope, the opening of the Eustachian tube into the pharynx, on each side, can be viewed directly and, by careful manipulation, the distal end of the instrument can be inserted into the slit-like aperture and advanced into the interior of the pouch. The pouch requiring examination may be indicated by noting some discharge seeping from the Eustachian orifice into the pharynx. The rhinolaryngoscope is a rather fragile instrument; horses undergoing examination should be given a sedative or narcotic drug. Radiological examination, where practicable, may yield valuable information regarding the condition of the guttural pouches.

Larynx

In the examination of the larynx, external palpation is employed to establish its condition by noting the presence of pain, liability to coughing, any change in shape (neoplasia) and degree of rigidity (ossification). Swelling at the posterior part of the larynx may be associated with the thyroid gland. Auscultation over the larynx, in normal animals, reveals sounds which simulate those heard over the bronchial area (see p. 120). In local inflammatory states, when exudation has occurred, rattling or wheezing sounds are heard. When the glottis is constricted, the laryngeal sounds are whistling (stenotic). In such cases, a vibration or thrill (laryngeal fremitus) is recognized when the hand is placed firmly on the skin adjacent to the larynx. Constriction of the larynx occurs in oedema, originating in enlargement of the thyroid gland as the result of local venous stasis, or as part of an allergic syndrome, or following inhalation of irritant fumes or smoke, in acute inflammatory diseases with local infiltration, e.g. anthrax in the horse and pig, and in gut oedema to a mild degree only. Partial obstruction may arise from inhalation of vomitus, and in horses with unilateral paralysis of a vocal cord (roaring or whistling), during exercise.

In the clinical examination for detecting paralysis of the larynx in horses which on exercise have evinced roaring or whistling inspiratory sounds, a particular technique is employed. One side of the larynx is supported by the extended fingers and palm of one hand while the fingertips of the other hand are pressed inwards, above the larynx, from the opposite side. In this way, if laryngeal paralysis is present, an abnormal inspiratory sound is produced by the narrowing of the rima glottidis which results. The stenotic sound arising from laryngeal paralysis occurs only during inspiration because it is during this phase of respiration that the flaccid, paralysed arytenoid cartilage and vocal cord are drawn into the lumen of the larynx, thus causing stenosis. Slight stenotic sounds can be accentuated by strenuous, forced exercise, such as driving or riding at a brisk pace, walking on three legs with a foreleg tied up or extended backing. Other causes of stenotic, upper respiratory tract sounds include oedema of the pharyngeal mucosa, tumours such as lipomas, papillomas or carcinomas, or pedunculated retention cysts, when located near the epiglottis. In all these conditions the abnormal sounds are heard during both inspiration and expiration.

Laryngitis, characterized by abnormal inspiratory sounds and respiratory rhythm, and coughing, occurs as part of the syndrome in all infections of the upper respiratory tract in animals. In those of an acute nature, palpation of the larynx will induce a pain reaction and intensify the severity of the cough and the degree of respiratory embarrassment. Upper respiratory infection is a prominent feature in equine viral rhino-pneumonitis, equine viral arteritis, infectious equine bronchitis, equine influenza and strangles; infectious bovine rhinotracheitis and calf diphtheria; swine influenza; kennel cough (*Klebsiella bronchiseptica*) in dogs.

Laryngoscopy

The rhinolaryngoscope (Fig. 110) is one of the instruments used for endoscopy, i.e. the exami-

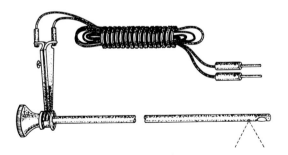

Fig. 110. *A laryngoscope for large animals, with optical system, right-angled vision, which rotates in a detachable handle. Switch and twin cables for the battery.*

nation of the interior of a body cavity that is inaccessible to direct inspection. It consists of a tube some 75 cm in length, containing a built-in optical system by means of which it is possible to project and collect light rays at varying angles. The distal end of the instrument carries a small electric bulb which is supplied with current from a portable battery. The rays of light from the illuminated interior of a hollow organ fall on a prism and are thus directed into the tube of the laryngoscope.

The rhinolaryngoscope is more regularly used in equine practice, but it can be used in cattle. It is introduced through a nasal cavity. Premedication with a suitable sedative or tranquillizer is desirable and further restraint is achieved by means of a twitch or by holding up a foreleg. Thoroughbred and excitable horses should be given a general anaesthetic in order to ensure that a satisfactory examination can be made. After initial insertion the instrument is held so that its end is placed medially against the lower border of the nasal septum. It is then carefully inserted to the desired extent. The projecting portion of the instrument should, in all circumstances, be held with the hand steadied by a simultaneous grasp of the medial wing of the nostril (to avoid injury should the animal move its head).

With the aid of the laryngoscope, it is possible to examine thoroughly the whole extent of the nasal mucosa (rhinoscopy), and in addition the ethmoturbinates, the pharyngeal mucosa, the larynx, and the entrance to and interior of the guttural pouches; even the soft palate is sometimes visible. It is possible in this way to diagnose swellings of the pharyngeal wall (oedema), haemorrhages (rhinitis, pharyngitis, purpura haemorrhagica), ulcers (glanders), exudate, neoplasms and foreign bodies.

The larynx is situated on the floor of the pharyngeal cavity, towards its posterior part. It is possible to see the epiglottis, the arytenoid cartilages, the vocal cords, the laryngeal ventricles and the upper part of the tracheal lumen. An important application of laryngoscopy consists in the demonstration of paralysis of the vocal cords (roaring or whistling). In this condition the vocal cords and larynx are seen to be asymmetrical and the mobility of one or both cords is lost. The left side alone is affected in the vast majority of cases. During forced inspiration the paralysed vocal cord is set in vibration. In catarrhal laryngitis, the mucous membrane is greyish-pink and coated with mucus. In tumours, and in oedema of the glottis, the outlines of the layrnx are indistinct or completely unrecognizable, as the result of extensive swelling.

When the distal end of the laryngoscope is above the larynx, rotation to right or left, through an angle of 45° will reveal a vertically directed fold in the wall of the pharynx—the entrance to the Eustachian tube on that side. In suppurative conditions (empyema) of the guttural pouch there is a discharge of pus from the ventral commissure of the slit-like opening. If fitted with an angled lamp-mounting, the laryngoscope can be introduced into the guttural pouch itself, where normally it is possible to see the divergence of the external carotid artery and its lingual branch, as well as the medial and lateral divisions of the pouch. In addition to accumulations of pus, blood, or concretions, diphtheritic membranes or ulcerations, it is possible to recognize abscesses in the pharyngeal lymph nodes (guttural pouch lymph nodes) which may be discharging into the pouch.

On the upper aspect of the pharyngeal cavity, opposite the larynx, the ethmoturbinates appear in the form of a pair of large smooth convexities.

In the dog, and some of the other small animals, the anterior part of the larynx can be exposed to view by opening the mouth with the aid of a suitable gag or loops of tape, drawing the tongue forward and depressing its root with a spatula or tongue depressor. An electric torch greatly facilitates the examination.

Thyroid Gland

The thyroid gland consists of two smooth ovoid structures joined by a narrow ventrally placed isthmus which is not detectable by palpation. As a rule the lobes of the normal gland are easily identified by this method. The two main lobes are situated laterally in close contact with the thyroid cartilage of the larynx and extend backwards to the proximal part of the trachea. This preliminary examination will reveal whether the thyroid gland is present; in rare cases it is absent because of a developmental defect.

Enlargement of the thyroid gland can be readily appreciated by palpation and, if it is considerable, can even be seen, as in goitre (Fig. 111). Goitre in its primary form is caused by iodine deficiency; the secondary form is attributable to interference with the absorption and utilization of iodine by factors such as

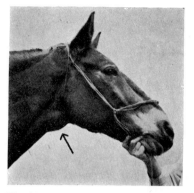

Fig. 111. *Swelling of the thyroid gland (goitre)*. (*See also Fig. 29, p. 40.*)

excessive calcium intake, diets consisting mainly of *Brassica* spp. and gross bacterial contamination of food or drinking water. The goitrogenic influence on the dam of diets containing low levels of cyanogenetic glycosides may be clinically apparent in newly born lambs (stillbirths, soft lambs). The position and nature of the thyroid swelling, which may be smooth, nodular, soft or firm, are readily determined. In well established goitre, the increased vascularity of the enlarged thyroid gland causes pronounced, local arterial pulsation and oedema of the surrounding tissues. Radiological examination, or the administration of radioactive iodine, may provide information to supplement the other findings. Alterations in the shape, size and consistency of the thyroid gland are the result of inflammation, neoplasia, injuries or endocrine dysfunction. Inflammation usually terminates in abscess formation; heat, swelling, pain and, in the later stages, fluctuation typify the condition. With tumour formation, the enlargement is irregular and eventually assumes considerable proportions. Depending upon which component tissue of the gland is primarily involved in the neoplastic state there may be other signs indicative of hyperthyroidism (increased heart and respiratory rates and, sometimes, exophthalmos).

Trachea

The trachea extends from the larynx to the hilus of the lungs. It consists of a tube-like structure which is kept patent by a series of 50–60 incomplete, cartilaginous rings. In the neck the trachea is ventrally situated, and is related dorsally to the proximal part of the oesophagus, but mainly to the longus colli muscles. Laterally it is related to the lobes of the thyroid gland, the carotid artery, the jugular vein, the vagus, sympathetic and recurrent laryngeal nerves, the oesophagus (on its left side from the third cervical vertebra backwards), the tracheal lymph ducts, and the cervical lymph nodes.

The trachea is examined by inspection of the overlying skin and coat, which will reveal changes in shape or position, scars or tracheotomy wounds; by palpation, which is valuable in the detection of pain, local swellings, and deformities; and by auscultation. Bronchial sounds (p. 120) are usually heard by auscultation over the trachea; they are usually somewhat greater in volume at this position. Moist râles indicate the presence of mucus, blood, exudate or other fluid in the trachea. Tracheal râles are detectable in tracheitis, bronchitis, parasitic bronchitis, severe pneumonia, pulmonary oedema and pulmonary haemorrhage. Sounds from this source can be detected in all the upper respiratory tract infections referred to earlier in discussing the larynx. Stenotic or whistling sounds are audible when the mucous membrane is dry (early stages of inflammation), and when there is reduction in the size of the lumen of the trachea. This last occurs in constriction from tracheotomy or other wound scars, or pressure from a neoplasm or an enlarged thyroid gland. Radiography provides conclusive evidence as to the presence of neoplasms, and the shape, position and course of the larynx and trachea. Tracheal auscultation resolves doubt as to the origin of abnormal sounds heard during auscultation of the lungs. If the sounds originate in the upper respiratory tract they will be heard only during inspiration. The methods employed to obtain a sample of fluid contents (sputum) of the trachea will be described later in this chapter.

Oesophagus

The oesophagus is a musculomembranous tube, varying in length according to the size of the animal, which extends from the pharynx to the stomach. At its origin it is medially situated, but at the fourth cervical vertebra it is located on the left side of the trachea, which relationship is continued as far as the third thoracic vertebra. In the dog the greater part of the oesophagus is located medially above the trachea.

The cervical portion of the oesophagus is examined in the depth of the jugular furrow; in rare cases it is situated on the right side of the

neck. A number of diseases cause difficulty in swallowing (dysphagia); it usually results from physical obstruction by a foreign body or neoplasm in the pharynx or oesophagus, although in occasional cases it is caused by local pain or inflammatory swelling. Oesophageal diverticulum, or segmental paralysis, invariably contributes to functional obstruction, which is manifested by dysphagia. The signs of dysphagia are forceful attempts to swallow, initially accompanied by extension and then flexion of the head, with contractions of the cervical and abdominal musculature. They can be detected by observation during and immediately after the ingestion of food or water. When deglutition occurs, the bolus can be seen passing downwards, along the left jugular furrow, as a mobile swelling in the oesophagus. When assessing the functional condition of the oesophagus, the first point to be determined, provided the animal is feeding, is whether deglutition occurs at all.

If dysphagia exists, apart from exhibiting the usual clinical signs, the animal takes an unusually long time to consume its food; slow feeding may, however, be caused by disturbances of consciousness, such as those arising from space-occupying lesions of the brain (hydrocephalus) and in the so-called 'dummy syndrome'. In herbivorous animals, finding completely masticated food in the manger indicates the occurrence of regurgitation, whereas the dropping of semi-masticated food from the mouth ('quidding') suggests a painful condition of the mouth. When the difficulty in swallowing is less severe, liquids can still be swallowed fairly readily, but not solids.

Abnormalities of the cervical portion of the oesophagus which cause changes in shape or contour are detectable by inspection or palpation, e.g. impacted foreign bodies or tumours. In dilatation of a part or the whole length of the oesophagus (diverticulum as in Fig. 112, ectasia), or in constriction (stenosis), a swelling develops at the site of or anteriorly to the lesion while the animal is feeding. This swelling is reducible on pressure and disappears spontaneously after a variable time, but recurs whenever the animal feeds. Firm pressure at almost any point along the left jugular furrow may cause eructation, regurgitation and vomiting in certain conditions (oesophagitis, dilatation, spasm). Primarily oesophagitis may follow the ingestion of chemical or physical irritants and is usually accompanied by

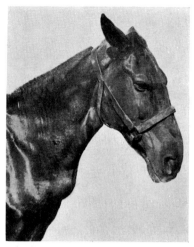

Fig. 112. *Oesophageal diverticulum, distended, at the posterior cervical portion.*

stomatitis and pharyngitis. Inflammation of the oesophagus is a concomitant, but usually unrecognized, feature of many specific diseases, particularly those causing stomatitis.

Dilatation of the oesophagus in the dog occurs in achalasia (cardiospasm, mega-oesophagus, ectasia) and in persistent right aortic arch or similar congenital vascular anomalies. Achalasia is due to abnormal innervation of the lower oesophagus and cardia because of absence of, or degenerative changes in, the neurons of the myenteric plex-

uses. A variable number of puppies in the same litter may be affected, suggesting the possibility of genetic inheritance. Adult dogs may occasionally develop the disease. The important clinical signs consist of persistent vomiting, which usually commences as soon as the puppies are weaned onto solid food. Nausea and retching do not occur. The cervical oesophagus is usually somewhat dilated and it fluctuates during breathing. The condition is diagnosed by endoscopic or radiographic examination employing a contrast medium (Fig. 113).

Vascular anomalies which cause dilatation of the oesophagus occur most frequently in the Alsatian breed. The most common abnormality of this type is persistent right aortic arch. The most obvious clinical sign is vomiting, which appears when the affected puppy begins to eat solid food, and becomes persistent by the time the animal is 3–8 months of age. Diagnosis is based upon consideration of the history and clinical signs, and radiographic examination employing contrast medium (see Fig. 132, p. 142).

By introducing a suitable sound in the form of a stomach tube or probang (Figs 114, 115), i.e. a sufficiently flexible, firm, rubber, plastic or leather covered tube, it is possible to determine whether the oesophagus is patent and whether constrictions, foreign bodies, food masses, neoplasms, etc. are present. Enlargement of the posterior mediastinal lymph nodes in the ox,

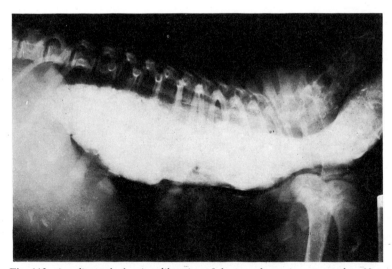

Fig. 113. *A radiograph showing dilatation of the oesophagus in a young dog. Note the pooling of the contrast medium in the precordial and lower cervical segments.*

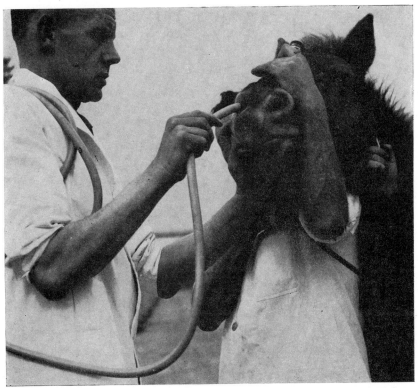

Fig. 114. *Passing an oesophageal or gastric sound in the horse. A stomach tube is being used.*

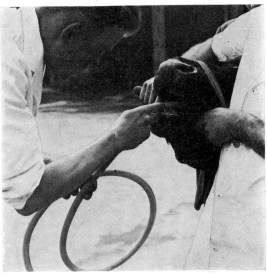

Fig. 115. *Passing an oesophageal or ruminal sound in the ox. A stomach tube is being used with the probang gag. A stomach tube is sometimes passed via the nostril, as in the horse; no gag is then required.*

which may be caused by actinobacillosis, tuberculosis or leucosis, may be detected by this method because the compression stenosis, which is produced by the enlarged node, offers some resistance to the passage of the instrument. The sound must be lubricated before use and should be introduced only when the head and neck are fully extended and the patient is adequately restrained. In the horse and in adult cattle it is introduced through the nasal cavity in the same manner as the laryngoscope and, more generally, in the ox and in other species, through the mouth, when a suitable gag (Fig. 115) is required to prevent the animal damaging the instrument with the molar teeth.

In the dog and cat, the lumen of the oesophagus can be viewed by means of a suitable illuminated oesophagoscope (Fig. 116). By this means lesions affecting the mucous membrane and foreign bodies are readily appreciated. This method of examination can only be performed under general anaesthesia. The oesophagus in the

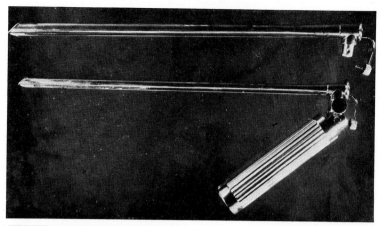

Fig. 116. *Oesophagoscopes with a source of illumination contained in a detachable handle. Suitable for use in dogs.*

dog is constricted at its origin by the existence of a prominent fold of mucous membrane at its ventral part. In addition, radiography and fluoroscopy may be employed in the examination of the whole extent of the oesophagus in small animals. For this purpose it may be necessary, in order to complete the examination, to administer a suitable contrast medium.

Coughing

A cough is initiated by reflex stimulation of the cough centre in the medulla oblongata by irritation of sensory receptors in one of various organs, particularly the respiratory mucosa. The stimulus may therefore originate in the pharynx, larynx, trachea, bronchi, pulmonary tissues or pleura. Coughing may also be initiated by irritation of the oesophagus, as in choking, or of an abdominal viscus, e.g. the stomach. The act of coughing consists of several stages; deep inspiration followed by approximation of the vocal cords; compression of the air in the lungs by vigorous forced expiration; sudden abduction of the vocal cords, which permits explosive expiration (the linear air velocity attains a speed of several hundred miles per hour). The purpose of coughing is the removal of excess mucus, inflammatory products or foreign bodies from the respiratory passages. Fluid of low viscosity may, however, be forced back into the secondary and tertiary bronchioles by the sudden variations in air pressure. Coughing indicates the existence of primary or secondary disease of the respiratory system, so that its existence should not be disregarded.

When the cough is infrequent, the animal may not exhibit it during the period of examination; it is then necessary to be able to induce the animal to cough when required. Coughing can be induced, particularly in the horse, by repeated application of light pressure to the larynx in the region of its junction with the first cartilaginous ring of the trachea (Fig. 117). Even the healthy horse, if not too restive, can usually be made to cough by this method. In inflammatory conditions of the larynx and pharynx, a cough is very easily provoked, but it is induced only with difficulty, or not at all, when the larynx is largely ossified (this state occasionally occurs in

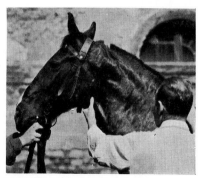

Fig. 117. *Induction of a cough by pressure on the posterior part of the larynx.*

aged horses and cattle). If, in a case of spontaneous coughing, pressure on the larynx fails to provoke a cough, its origin is probably elsewhere than in this region. Other methods of inducing coughing in large animals include applying intermittent pressure over the trachea in front of the entrance to the chest or giving a sharp blow with the hand, within the respiratory area, on the thoracic wall. Occlusion of both nostrils for 30–60 seconds—with the hands in the horse or with a folded towel in the ox (Fig. 118) —will also provoke coughing, as a result of

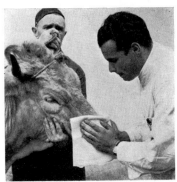

Fig. 118. *Occlusion of the nostrils of the ox with a towel in order to induce a cough.*

hypoxia causing an immediate deep inspiration following the removal of the impediment to breathing. This applies particularly to diseases of the thoracic respiratory organs. In small animals, compression of the thorax between the hands, or lifting up a large fold of skin from the back behind the shoulders, so that the weight of the animal is almost supported, will usually induce coughing. An examination of this type should always be made when there is any suspicion of pulmonary disease.

It is important to determine the frequency and periodicity of coughing. In the early stages of an inflammatory disease of the respiratory tract, coughing is infrequent, but as the condition progresses it may become relatively frequent. Numerous coughs following one after another are described as a paroxysm of coughing. As a rule, coughing is painless, but in a few diseases, e.g. those in which pleurisy, acute catarrhal laryngitis or bronchitis occurs, it is accompanied by pain, in which case it is noticeable that the animal makes an effort to suppress the cough. A simple cough may be protracted or of short duration. Protracted coughs occur when there is inflammation of the vocal cords, as a result of incomplete closure of the glottis, and in chronic

alveolar emphysema. The cough is short in acute bronchitis and in pleurisy, because of pain; in chronic tuberculous and similar forms of pleurisy, owing to adhesions restricting the elastic recoil of the lungs; and in extensive pneumonia, because of the reduced volume of the expired air.

A cough may be loud, soft, croaking, wheezing, whistling, barking or tremulous (when the soft palate vibrates). Depending upon the volume of air expelled, the cough may be distinguished as deep or shallow. If the cough causes obvious expulsion from, or upward movement of secretion in, the respiratory tract, it is said to be productive or moist; if it is unaccompanied by movement of fluid material, it is said to be unproductive or dry. Deliberate expectoration of the secretion (sputum), as seen in man, does not occur in animals. That sputum has been coughed up into the pharynx is recognized by observing that, immediately after coughing, the animal makes the movements characteristic of chewing and swallowing. Small particles of sputum may be expelled involuntarily during coughing; this occurs when respiratory dyspnoea is relatively severe. In stalled or tied animals the particles of sputum may be seen on the wall in front of the animal.

The character of the cough is not dissimilar in all the diseases with which it is associated. In a number of conditions, however, the type of cough is sufficiently characteristic to arouse suspicion that a particular disease is in evidence, e.g. the infrequent, single, prolonged, unproductive, hollow cough of a horse affected with chronic alveolar emphysema, and the dry, husky, paroxysmal cough of a calf with parasitic bronchitis. Chronic bronchitis in the dog is associated with a barking type of cough. Irritation caused by the presence of *Filaroides osleri* in small nodules, involving the submucosal tissues, usually at the bifurcation of the trachea in the dog, may cause a persistent harsh cough. In infectious equine pneumonia, the cough is infrequent, occurs singly and, in the early stages, is unproductive. In catarrhal pharyngitis or laryngitis, in all species, the cough is frequent, paroxysmal, strong and painful, and very easily induced by pressure on the larynx or pharynx. In the exudative stage of acute bronchopneumonia, it is frequent, paroxysmal, productive and explosive. A specific diagnosis, of course, cannot be made from the nature of the cough alone.

Microscopical Examination of Sputum

In certain diseases, notably bovine pulmonary tuberculosis, which because of the success of national eradication programmes is now very rarely seen, examination of the tracheal mucus by microscopic means may be diagnostic but a satisfactory sample of mucus from the respiratory tract is often difficult to obtain, and furthermore it must be remembered that excretion of the causal bacterium is variable. In the case of large animals, when tied up, it may sometimes be possible to obtain a mucus sample by affixing a large sheet of paper to the wall in front of the animal, and leaving it in position for some hours. Another method is to place the sheet of paper on the ground below the animal's head and then induce it to cough. More certain results are obtained by one of the following methods: swabbing the pharynx with a wad of sterile cottonwool attached to a suitable swab-forceps immediately after the animal has coughed and before the mucus can be swallowed (the rapid insertion of a mouth gag would be required for the method to be successful); administering a draught of cold water which will induce coughing by causing irritation of the pharynx; flushing the oesophagus free of food particles then passing the sputum cup (Fig. 119) down the oeso-

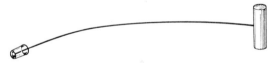

Fig. 119. *A sputum cup.*

phagus, so that the respiratory mucus, which remain adherent to the mucous membrane after being swallowed, is collected in the container (this method is used mainly in cattle); inserting the sputum cup into the trachea, via the larynx, is also practicable in cattle, but it usually requires the administration of a potent ataractic drug;

puncture of the trachea with a suitable cannula through which is then introduced a swab of cottonwool firmly attached to a short length of wire (adequate restraint and suitable sedation or local analgesia are necessary). In small animals a wire carrying a sterile cottonwool swab of appropriate size can be introduced into the trachea from the mouth. It is usually essential to induce a state of narcosis, or even anaesthesia, to enable this to be achieved.

Helminth parasites, e.g. *Dictyocaulus* or *Metastrongylus* spp., *Spirocerca* spp., *Filaroides osleri, Capillaria aerophila, Crenosoma vulpis, Aleurostrongylus abstrusus*, etc., may be seen in the mucus, or their ova identified by microscopical examination. The ova of lungworms are ovoid to round in shape, thin-shelled, and contain a developing larva (see Fig. 160B, p. 205). Failure to demonstrate the adult parasite, larvae or ova is not conclusive because they are not constantly present in the respiratory mucus from affected animals. A faeces examination (see pp. 198–201) usually gives more reliable results. In the dog, *Filaroides osleri* infestation can be identified by bronchoscopical examination.

Microscopical examination of suitably stained smears is very important in the diagnosis of pulmonary tuberculosis in animals with clinical manifestations suggestive of the disease. A negative result should not be regarded as being conclusive. Bacteria of primary or secondary significance in relation to infections of the lower respiratory tract, such as *Corynebacterium pyogenes, Pasteurella* spp. streptococci, etc., may be observed, but specific identification would necessitate cultural and other methods of examination. Elastic fibres appearing in respiratory mucus may be of diagnostic significance when pulmonary gangrene is suspected. Fungi (*Aspergillus* spp., *Candida albicans*) may be of significance in association with clinical manifestations of respiratory disease, a situation which occurs occasionally in the horse and ox.

9

The Thorax

The thorax is the second largest and most anteriorly situated of the body cavities. It is shaped somewhat like a truncated cone, compressed laterally over its anterior part, with the base cut off obliquely at the costal arch where it adjoins the abdominal cavity. The roof is made up of the thoracic vertebrae and the associated muscle masses and ligaments. The lateral walls consist of the ribs and intercostal muscles. At its anterior, narrow portion the thorax is overlaid, on each side, by the scapula and humerus, and the mass of muscles comprising the upper part of the forelimb, above the elbow, which is attached to the lateral aspect of the ribs in this region. The posterior part of the thoracic cavity is shut off from the cavity of the abdomen by the diaphragm, which is attached at its periphery to the medial surface of the ribs and is strongly convex on its anterior aspect.

Internally the thorax is divided longitudinally by the mediastinal septum into two lateral chambers, the pleural cavities, which are lined by a serous membrane. The mediastinal septum is not median in position because the heart is placed more on the left side than on the right, so that as a consequence the right pleural sac is larger than the left. The important structures in the thorax include the pleura, mediastinum, lungs, heart, trachea, bronchi, oesophagus, major blood and lymph vessels and nerve trunks.

THE LUNGS AND RESPIRATION

Descriptively the respiratory system is divided into an upper and a lower portion, the greater part of the latter, comprising some of the trachea, the bronchi and the lungs, being accommodated within the cavity of the thorax. This arbitrary division has relatively little clinical merit because many of the diseases involving the upper respiratory tract have a marked tendency to spread and involve the lungs. In suspected cases of respiratory disease, the need to include all the associated structures in the clinical examination is patently obvious. Following a superficial appraisal of the clinical signs exhibited by an affected animal, confusion may arise as to which part of the respiratory system is involved in the disease process, e.g. acute pneumonia is not infrequently associated with bilateral nasal discharge of varying character, suggestive of rhinitis.

The physical aspects of respiration and the clinical methods for assessing them have been discussed in Chapter 6, along with some of the more important effects of disturbed respiratory function.

Regional Anatomy of the Lungs

The lungs occupy the major part of the thoracic cavity, where they are intimately related to the boundary structures and other organs situated within the cavity. In the horse the trachea, which is large in cross-section (5–7 cm), is slightly flattened dorsoventrally. It occupies a median position in the thorax and the bifurcation occurs opposite the fifth rib, about 15 cm ventral to the sixth thoracic vertebra, or at the midway point between the roof and floor of the thoracic cavity. The right lung is larger than the left, which is reduced in surface area and thickness by reason of the mediastinum being towards the left of the median plane of the body, to accommodate the heart. The dorsal border of the lungs, which is thick, extends posteriorly to the second last (sixteenth) intercostal space and lies in the angle formed by the bodies of the thoracic vertebrae and the ribs. The ventral border is thin and is insinuated into the narrow angle formed between the mediastinum and the ventral parts of the sternal ribs. Opposite the heart it is indented by the cardiac notch, which extends on the left side from the third to the sixth rib and on the right side from the third to the fourth intercostal space. At these points the pericardium comes into contact with the chest wall. The basal border is also thin and is situated between the diaphragm and the costal ribs, being on a level with the costochondral junction of the seventh rib, and approximately at the midway point of the twelfth rib. The position of this border varies during the different phases of respiration.

The trachea is relatively small in diameter (4 cm) in the ox, as compared with that of the horse. The accessory bronchus to the apical lobe of the right lung originates from the trachea at the level of the third rib, while the bifurcation is opposite the fifth rib about 10 cm below the vertebral column.

In the ox the size of right lung compared with the left is proportionately even greater than in the horse. The basal border of both lungs extends upwards and backwards from near the lower extremity of the sixth rib, in a straight line, to the upper part of the second last (eleventh) intercostal space where it meets the dorsal border. The trachea and lungs in the sheep are proportionately smaller than in the ox and, apart from the lungs extending slightly further back at the base, the regional anatomical relationships are broadly similar to those in cattle.

The trachea in the pig is relatively short; it supplies a supplementary bronchus to the apical lobe of the right lung. The dorsal border of the lung extends posteriorly only to the third last intercostal space (eleventh or twelfth according to the number of ribs). The basal border forms an almost straight line, running from the lower end of the sixth rib to the dorsal border at its posterior extremity.

In the dog the trachea is almost circular in cross-section at both ends, but the middle part is slightly flattened dorsoventrally. The bifurcation, which is opposite the fifth rib, forms a very wide angle. The costal surface of the lungs is more convex than in other species, conforming to the contour of the thoracic wall. The right lung is much larger (25%) than the left. The pericardium is in contact with the chest wall at the ventral part of the fourth and fifth intercostal spaces opposite the cardiac notch of the right lung. On the left side, the pericardium is in contact with the chest wall along a narrow area at the ventral part of the fifth and sixth intercostal spaces; there is no distinct cardiac notch in the left lung. The dorsal border of the lung extends posteriorly to the second last (eleventh) intercostal space. The basal border forms a shallow cavity and extends upwards from the ventral extremity of the seventh rib to the dorsal border near the upper part of the twelfth rib.

Physical Examination of the Thorax (Lung Area)

Consideration has already been given to respiration in respect of frequency, rhythm, and types of respiratory movements in the different species of domestic animals. Abnormal sounds that are associated with respiration, and which have already been discussed, include sneezing, wheezing, snoring, roaring and whistling, grunting, coughing and yawning.

More accurate information about the condition of the thoracic portion of the respiratory system can be obtained by means of physical examination of the lung area. This consists of palpation, percussion and auscultation, which should be routine procedure when the evidence obtained during the general clinical examination of the patient suggests the presence of respiratory disease. The information obtained by means of physical examination varies in value according to the particular method, the experience of the clinician, and the conformation and species of animal.

Palpation

Palpation of the lung area is of limited value because very little worthwhile evidence is obtained by this means. Increased sensitivity of the chest wall might suggest a pain reaction arising from pleurisy. Differentiation between a pain reaction and that evinced by a nervous animal is essential. Palpation may reveal the presence of a pleuritic thrill arising from the movement of fluid, in which case the intercostal spaces are bulging in character. Decreased rib movements, with narrowing of the intercostal spaces, which occur in the early stages of pleurisy, in tetanus and in extensive collapse of a lung, are recognizable by palpation.

Percussion

Percussion is a useful diagnostic procedure to

apply to the chest wall, more particularly in relation to the lungs. By this means some of the anatomical relationships and position of the normal lung, and the presence of abnormal states, can be recognized by noting the variations in the percussion sounds (resonance) so produced.

Types of Resonance

Percussive resonance is the sound that is produced at the place percussed by the blow itself, by the vibration of the body wall and by the column or body of air or gas contained beneath the point of impact. Any of these three factors may influence the percussive resonance and so change the nature of the sound produced by percussion.

Resonant sound (*ringing*). This usually indicates the presence of a large volume of air or gas beneath the site of percussion. It is the sound produced during percussion over a normal large lung (a smaller lung normally gives a tympanic response, see below). The thinner the wall of the thorax and the larger the lung, the more resonant the sound, and the smaller the lung and the thicker the wall, the less ringing the sound.

The ringing sound is exaggerated when there is an excessive quantity of air or gas present at the site of percussion. Such a sound, therefore, is induced in conditions such as pulmonary emphysema, pneumothorax (air or gas in a pleural cavity), subcutaneous emphysema, when a gas-filled viscus occupies a diaphragmatic hernia and over an area limited to the left posterior part of the thorax in ruminal tympany.

When the percussion sound is less clear and loud than the ringing sound it is said to be abbreviated. It represents the transition to the next type.

Dull sound. This is heard when there is no air or gas beneath the part percussed. If dull sounds are heard on percussion over the lung they must be taken to indicate the presence of disease; it is not possible, however, to decide by means of percussion alone which structure (lung, other thoracic organ, chest wall) is diseased and what type of disease (inflammation, neoplasia, fluid effusion) is present. In order to ascertain these points, other signs and findings (fever, cough, findings on auscultation, etc.) have to be taken into consideration. The dull sound itself indicates only that, in that particular part, air-containing tissue is absent or reduced in amount. Dull sounds can be recognized only when the airless area of the lung is at least as large as the palm of the hand, and is superficially situated.

Dull percussion sounds occur when there is an increase in density of pulmonary tissue as a result of congestion, neoplasia or collapse; in hydrothorax and effusive pleurisy; with thickening of the chest wall or pleura; in subcutaneous oedema when it impinges on the lung area; or because of a thick subcutaneous layer of fat.

Tympanic sound. This is distinguished from the preceding types of percussion sound by its characteristic musical ring (like a kettle-drum). It occurs only as an accompaniment to the foregoing types of sound, when it is known as a ringing tympanic sound or a dull tympanic sound. It occurs when, in addition to the conditions necessary for the production of ringing or dull sounds, there exists any comparatively small column of air, or a very large column that communicates with the air outside the body through a large opening. This type of percussion sound is produced from very small lungs, and may be noted in miniature breeds of dogs and in cats. Depending upon the musical tone, the tympanic sound is described as being high—or low—pitched.

Tympanic percussion sounds are associated with the early and late stages of pneumonia, pulmonary cavitation (rare in animals), pneumothorax, subcutaneous emphysema and the presence of loops of gas-distended intestine in the thoracic cavity (diaphragmatic hernia or rupture).

Metallic ring. This is similar to the tympanic sound, but its musical character is more pronounced. The tone is a very high-pitched tympanic one, and resembles the response obtained on striking an empty metal jug. It occurs in diseases similar to those in which the tympanic sound is obtained, particularly where there are small cavities containing air or gas under pressure.

The 'cracked pot' sound simulates that produced by striking a cracked pot. It arises when air escapes through a narrow opening, and is produced during percussion where there are cavities communicating with a bronchus through a narrow aperture (a very rare circumstance in animals), in subcutaneous emphysema and sometimes in pneumonia if an air-containing portion of lung has been surrounded by other areas devoid of air; it also occurs at the margin of the dull areas in exudative pleurisy.

Tracheal Percussion

In addition to the methods of performing percussion already described, certain other methods may be of value when applied to the thorax and some other parts of the body. Tracheal percussion, one of these procedures, is a combination of percussion and auscultation. In its performance an assistant places the pleximeter on the skin overlying the trachea in the mid-neck region and strikes it with the hammer, using single blows of medium strength. Immediate percussion with the fingers of one hand will serve the same purpose adequately. Simultaneously, the clinician auscultates the lungs in turn, and observes the manner in which sounds produced in the trachea are heard in the respiratory area. An air-containing lung is a poor conductor of sound, hence in a normal lung the percussion sounds are distant and indistinctly heard. Over consolidated areas, on the other hand, the sound of the percussion impact is loud and distinct, because dense tissue is a good conductor of sound. The value of the method is that its application makes it possible to distinguish between dullness caused by inflammatory infiltration of the lung and that resulting from the presence of free fluid in one, or both, pleural sacs. In pneumonia the referred sound is very loud and distinct, and seems to originate from directly beneath the chest-piece of the stethoscope. In exudative pleuritis, hydrothorax and other similar conditions the sound, although in fact equally loud, seems in comparison to be coming from a remote point.

Tuning fork–stethoscope method. The advantage of this method is that it can yield very accurate information concerning the underlying organs. With experience it is possible, in an extensive dull area, to distinguish the dullness of the lungs from that caused by the heart, and also from that caused by the liver, whereas in the more usual methods of percussion the area of cardiac, pulmonary and hepatic dullness appear to be continuous. The method is also particularly suitable for determining the exact limits of individual organs.

The instruments used are a stethoscope and a long-handled tuning fork. The procedure is to place the vibrating fork against the skin, where its tone is picked up by the stethoscope. When both instruments lie over the same organ or medium the tone is loud and distinct, but as soon as the tuning fork passes beyond the border of the organ or medium over which the stethoscope is placed, the tone becomes soft and indistinct. If a tuning fork is not available, a process of continuous scratching with the fingers may be substituted for the vibration of the fork (frictional auscultation).

Percussion of the Lung

In most species, percussion of the healthy lung evokes a resonant (ringing) sound, but in very small animals, e.g. miniature dogs, cats and rabbits, the sound is normally somewhat tympanic on account of the short length of the vibrating column of air in the lung. It should be appreciated that changes in the character of the percussion sound are detectable only when any lesion present is of considerable size and is superficially situated. It therefore follows that a lung which evinces normal percussion sounds is not necessarily healthy or free from consolidated foci. If such foci are small, as in bronchopneumonia, or deep-seated, as is often the case in the early stages of contagious bovine pleuropneumonia, tuberculous bronchopneumonia and metastatic pulmonary neoplasia, their presence cannot easily be demonstrated by percussion. The limitation applies, therefore, to the lungs of large animals as well as to those of small animals such as the dog, cat, etc. In the latter species, pulmonary lesions are frequently undetected during percussion, because in the small lung even relatively comprehensive changes are seldom extensive enough to produce a recognizable change in resonance.

It is not possible to examine the whole lung by percussion. That part of the lung situated beneath the shoulder is inaccessible on account of the heavy musculature overlying the area. Here, on percussion, only the completely nonresonant response of muscular tissue is obtained. Neither is it possible, in a large lung, to obtain a satisfactory percussion response from the deepseated areas surrounding the bifurcation of the trachea, because the thickness of the lung in this and in similar areas prevents the penetration of the percussion impulses.

Immediately posterior to the shoulder, above the heart base, the pulmonary tissue extends, except for the intervening mediastinum, from one wall of the thorax to the other. Farther back,

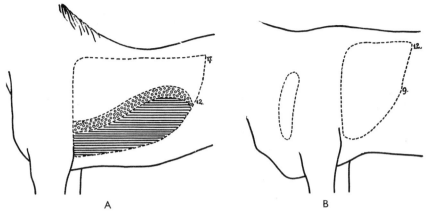

Fig. 120. *The areas of percussion and auscultation in the horse and ox. The changes in sound occurring in pneumonia are also indicated.* Dotted line, *boundary area;* hatching, *dullness;* circles, *tympanic sound.*

behind the mid-point of the seventh rib, this situation no longer prevails on account of the dome-like anterior projection of the diaphragm. The posterior border of the lung is normally situated a variable distance in front of the line of attachment of the diaphragm to the ribs. During inspiration, of course, and more markedly in the horse, the border of the lung moves closer to the anterior surface of the diaphragm at this point. This can be demonstrated occasionally by percussion, since at inspiration, percussion immediately anterior to the attachment of the diaphragm evokes a ringing sound, whereas during expiration the sound is dulled, because

the posterior border of the lung moves away from the insertion of the diaphragm.

In the horse, the area of the thorax suitable for percussion of the lung comprises a triangle, the points of which are situated at the posterior angle of the scapula, the olecranon process of the ulna, and the second last intercostal space at a point on a horizontal line from the scapula to the external angle of the ilium. The ventral boundary of the area extends upwards and backwards from the olecranon process of the ulna to join the dorsal one at the second last intercostal space, forming a shallow concavity on its antero-dorsal aspect (Figs 120, 121), The part of the

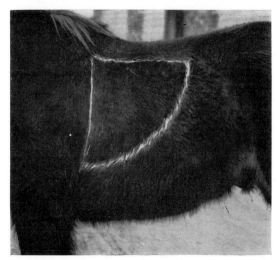

Fig. 121. *The area of percussion and auscultation of the lungs in a pony. As the animal is in fat condition, the area over which a distinct percussion sound could be elicited is relatively smaller than that in Fig. 120.*

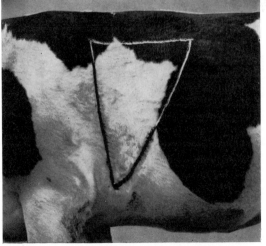

Fig. 122. *The area of percussion and auscultation of the lungs in a cow. The prescapular percussion area was too poorly defined in this well-nourished animal to be clearly indicated.*

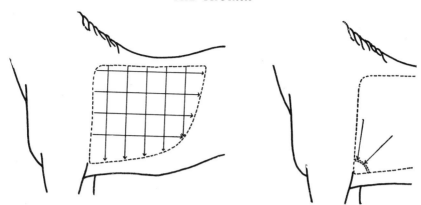

Fig. 123. *Direction of percussion of the lungs* (left) *and the heart* (right) *in a horse.*

chest wall within the limits of these boundaries is frequently referred to as the respiratory area.

In the ox, the ventral boundary of the area is a straight line extending from the point of the elbow to join the dorsal border at the second last intercostal space (Fig. 122). In addition to the thoracic percussion area, there is also a smaller prescapular area, more or less oval in shape with its long axis roughly perpendicular, which is situated in the lower part of the neck in front of the shoulder (Fig. 120). Percussion in this area normally gives an abbreviated sound. In adult cattle in good physical condition the area is roughly 3 cm wide, but in lean animals it is twice as wide. In this area it is possible to percuss the lungs in the region of the first, second, and even the third rib, particularly when the foreleg is drawn backwards.

In the dog and cat, the area available for lung percussion has the same general outline as in the horse. The area in the pig shows some variation in that the ventral boundary, which forms a straight line, joins the dorsal border at the third or even fourth last intercostal space.

The posterior boundary of the respiratory area, as indicated, is the approximate position of the posterior border of the lung midway between inspiration and expiration. To determine the position of this boundary, the thorax is percussed at various levels, along horizontal lines extending from the central or most resonant part of the respiratory area towards the abdomen (Fig. 123). By drawing the foreleg well forwards, it is possible to extend the area of percussion anteriorly. Care must be taken that percussion is uniform, and not too vigorous, particularly in the area approximating the posterior border of the lung, on account of the reduced thickness

of the organ at that part. The point at which a distinct change in sound occurs is the margin of the lung. A finger is placed at this point while, with the other hand, the intercostal spaces are counted from the last space forward to the point indicated. As a general rule it is sufficient to determine the posterior margin of the lung only in the upper and middle thirds of the respiratory area; it is only in special cases that determination of the lower part of this boundary is of importance. As the number of ribs in a particular species (see Table 9) is not always applicable to the individual animal—more (supernumerary) or fewer ribs may be present—accuracy is better served by recording the number of ribs posterior to the ventral border of the lung (counting anteriorly from the last rib).

TABLE 9. POSTERIOR BOUNDARY OF PULMONARY PERCUSSION AREA (MEASURED IN INTERCOSTAL SPACES)

Species	No. of Ribs	At Level of External Angle of Ilium	Middle of Thorax	Inferior Border
Horse	18	16	11	6
Ox	13	11	9	5
Sheep, goat	13	11	7	6
Pig	14–15	11–12	8–9	4–5
Dog, cat	13	11	9	6
Rabbit	12	10	—	7

The change in sound at the periphery of the normal lung consists usually of a transition—in some instances this is sudden—from a ringing sound to one that is dull. This occurs in those parts of the respiratory area where the thin border of the lung overlies organs such as the liver, heart, spleen and rumen, stomach and intestine when filled with food material. If, however, the adjacent parts of the rumen, stomach or intestine are distended with gas a tympanic sound or, more rarely, even a ringing sound, simulating that of the lung, may be obtained in the vicinity of and behind the normal respiratory area, thus rendering it impossible to determine the lung boundary (e.g. in the ox, on the left side in the upper posterior part of the thorax over the rumen, and at an intermediate point over the abomasum on the right side).

An increase in the size of the area over which lung percussion sounds can be evoked occurs in overdistension of the lung (pulmonary emphysema), and in accumulation of air in the thoracic cavity (pneumothorax). In large animals this increase in size, or backwards displacement of the lung, may amount to between 2 and 10 cm. In established cases of pulmonary emphysema characteristic expiratory dyspnoea will be observed, and in pneumothorax both inspiration and expiration are obviously laboured.

A reduction in size of the area over which lung percussion sounds are heard exists when the lungs are prevented from being fully inflated during inspiration because of increased intra-abdominal pressure. This occurs in pregnancy, tympany of the stomach, intestines or rumen, large abdominal tumours, ascites, etc. Enlargement of the heart, caused by hypertrophy or dilatation, and fluid distension of the pericardium will also, locally, reduce the area of lung resonance as determined by percussion. This reduction may only be detectable in large animals.

Changes in the percussion note at the posterior margin of the area must always be interpreted with caution, since they may result from changes elsewhere than in the lung itself. Gas-filled loops of intestine in this area will evoke a confusing tympanic sound, and a full rumen, stomach or intestine a correspondingly dull sound.

A general reduction in the resonance of the percussion sound occurs when, because of extensive pulmonary disease, the volume of air in the lungs is reduced. This situation prevails in acute congestion of the lungs, pneumonia associated with consolidation, collapse of the lung and chronic tuberculous pleurisy with adhesions. Local reduction in resonance may be caused by bronchopneumonia, congestion of dependent parts of the lung, or neoplasia. There may be a unilateral reduction in resonance as the result of hypostatic congestion which often follows from prolonged lateral recumbency. In many small

animals, percussion yields disappointing results because any area of dullness is too small to be readily defined.

A pain reaction produced by percussion is indicated by the animal becoming restive, withdrawing the body, biting or kicking, e.g. in fracture of a rib, acute pleurisy and other painful conditions of the parts percussed. Percussion may also induce coughing, more usually when there is acute disease of the lung and/or pleura, e.g. in pneumonia, bronchitis and acute pleurisy.

Loops of intestine that have moved forwards into a pleural cavity following rupture of the diaphragm, give a tympanic percussion sound that may change position during the course of the examination as a result of the motility of the largely gas-filled loops.

Differentiation between the reduced resonance caused by increased density of the lungs and that resulting from the presence of fluid in the pleural sacs, is determined as follows:

1. Increased density of the lung, as in pneumonia: the area of dullness has an irregular outline; the cardiac impulse is palpable; heart sounds are clearly audible outside the cardiac area; abnormal bronchial or other sounds are often heard during auscultation (râles or frictional sounds); on percussion over the trachea, strong, loud sounds are heard directly beneath the chest-piece of the stethoscope when it is applied to the chest wall.

2. Presence of fluid in the pleural sac (e.g. exudative pleurisy, hydrothorax); the area of percussion dullness has a horizontal delimitation; the position of the area of dullness changes when the posture of the animal is altered (the fluid always gravitates to the lowest possible site); as the heart is pushed away from the chest wall, the cardiac impulse is correspondingly less distinct; no râles or frictional sounds are heard during auscultation; on percussion over the trachea, the sounds heard on auscultation are distant, but strong and loud; fluid can be obtained by exploratory puncture.

Auscultation of the Lung

The area of auscultation is the same as that of percussion (Figs 120–122, p. 117). Auscultation requires much practice and application in order to yield worthwhile results. The chest-piece of the stethoscope should be held firmly against the thorax to minimize the crackling sounds caused by friction against the hair of the animal's coat.

When the coat is long or matted together it is necessary, before applying the chest-piece, to expose the skin by separating the hair or wool so that they do not form a barrier to sound waves. The whole of the respiratory area should be methodically auscultated, commencing in the upper, anterior part and moving horizontally backwards, and then forwards again, at a slightly lower level, until the entire area has been explored. The stethoscope should be applied to each point on the chest wall for the duration of at least one complete respiratory cycle. It is advisable to compare obviously diseased areas with those that are healthy, because this makes it easier to identify any lung abnormality. Comparing corresponding portions of lung on both sides, in the same animal, or in different animals of the same species with similar physical characters, may assist in recognizing relatively minor abnormalities. It should be remembered that the respiratory sounds may be masked by the thickness of the chest wall, and by the presence of subcutaneous oedema or emphysema involving the thoracic region.

Intrinsic (Normal) Respiratory Sounds

The normal respiratory sounds consist of the vesicular sound and the bronchial sound.

The vesicular respiratory sound. The vesicular murmur resembles the sound produced when the letter 'V' is whispered softly in a drawn-out manner. Its presence indicates that the lung contains air and that the alveoli are patent, since it originates from the air vortices that are formed where the terminal bronchioles open into the alveoli. This sound is normally heard throughout the respiratory area, except in the part where it is masked by the bronchial sound. The vesicular murmur is more clearly heard during inspiration; during expiration it may change its character and resemble the sound of the letter 'f'. In large animals, when resting, the rate of air movement is reduced so that even the inspiratory vesicular sound is submerged. In the dog and cat, and in all young animals, the vesicular murmur is readily heard.

When respiratory frequency and/or amplitude are increased (hyperpnoea), or the breathing is laboured (dyspnoea), the vesicular sound is exaggerated and is readily audible during both inspiration and expiration, as in excitement, painful conditions and following physical exertion, etc. The vesicular sound is attenuated when the chest wall is thick, and when the air content of the lung is locally or generally reduced, e.g. in the early stages of pneumonia, passive congestion of the lung or when the lung is compressed by fluid in the pleural sac. When air is not entering a portion of lung, so that not only the alveoli but also the bronchioles are devoid of air, the vesicular murmur is entirely absent, as in the later stages of pneumonia, pulmonary oedema and collapse of the lung. Shrill vesicular sounds are heard in active pulmonary congestion and hoarse sounds in early bronchitis, because swelling of the bronchial mucous membrane causes narrowing of the terminal bronchioles.

In cog-wheel respiration, the vesicular sound is interrupted and is heard in two or more parts, giving rise to a characteristic clicking sound, It is heard, as might be expected, when there is visibly jerking respiration, and may occur also when there is irregular expansion of lung due to either loss of elasticity of tissue, or where the bronchial mucous membrane is swollen to such an extent as to cause transitory obliteration of the lumen of the bronchioles during the late phase of expiration and the early phase of inspiration. Jerking respiration may be induced by fear, in which case the interrupted vesicular sound is heard on both sides throughout the area of auscultation. Localized interrupted vesicular sound occurs in tuberculous bronchopneumonia, and in fibrosis of the lung. Cog-wheel respiration is differentiated from chronic alveolar emphysema by being recognized during auscultation, as opposed to inspection.

Bronchial respiratory sound. This is blowing in character and resembles a long drawn-out guttural 'ch', which commences and terminates abruptly. Normally it is always audible over the larynx and trachea. In small animals, and in very lean large animals, it is heard clearly, and in other large animals less distinctly, in the anterior part of the respiratory area where the larger bronchi are relatively near the surface of the body (so-called bronchial area). At this site it is known as a physiological bronchial sound. Apart from this, only the vesicular murmur is heard during auscultation of healthy lung. The bronchial sound has an inspiratory and an expiratory component which are of approximately equal duration. In the so-called bronchial part of the respiratory area, the inspiratory bronchial sound terminates briefly before inspiration is completed, so that a short pause precedes the subsequent expiratory bronchial sound, which is continued to the end of expiration.

When the lung contains less air, along with an increase in structural density, it acts as a better conductor of sound, so that the bronchial sound tends to supersede the vesicular sound over a variable extent of the respiratory area. Bronchial sounds are therefore heard beyond their normal situation in pneumonia, effusive pleurisy, hydrothorax and pulmonary neoplasia. (They do not extend beyond the normal area in bronchitis.) Bronchial sounds are heard also over air-containing cavities in the lung. In small breeds of dogs and in the cat, if the respiratory rate is increased because of excitement, even in the healthy animal, the bronchial sound will be superimposed on the vesicular sound throughout the respiratory area.

An amphoric sound is a type of bronchial sound resembling that produced by blowing into a large vessel possessing a small mouth. It is heard when a bronchus communicates with a large cavity in the lung (e.g. in gangrene of the lung), and also occasionally in pneumonia, if air in one bronchus rushes past the orifice of another that is not functioning. This sound is rarely heard in animals.

An indeterminate respiratory sound is one that is too faint to be classified as being either vesicular or bronchial. Any condition causing attenuation of the vesicular murmur or bronchial sound may give rise to indeterminate sounds.

As opposed to this, respiratory sounds are said to be indistinguishable when they are difficult to hear for some other reason such as excessive environmental noise, bronchial râles or loud peristaltic sounds.

Alternating respiratory sounds, i.e. vesicular during inspiration and bronchial during expiration, are occasionally encountered.

Adventitious (Abnormal) Respiratory Sounds

Abnormal respiratory sounds heard over the respiratory area originate from diseases of the bronchi, lungs, pleura or diaphragm, and include râles, emphysematous sounds, frictional sounds and peristaltic sounds.

Râles are sounds indicating the presence of secretion or fluid in the bronchi and bronchioles (exudate, transudate, blood, aspirated fluid). According to the viscosity of the secretion, râles may be moist or dry. They are inconstant, i.e. they may disappear for the duration of a few respirations and reappear later. This is the result of movement of the mucus within the bronchial tree by coughing.

Moist râles occur when mucus of relatively low viscosity, or other fluid, is set in motion by air passing through it. They are bubbling in character (as when air is blown from the end of a tube under water). Accordingly as the râles originate in an alveolus, bronchiole or bronchus, they are classified as fine or coarse moist râles. The fine sounds are more unfavourable prognostically than the coarse sounds, because they indicate that the terminal parts of the respiratory tract are involved in disease. Moist râles occur in various forms of bronchitis, pulmonary haemorrhage, bronchopneumonia and inhalation of fluid.

Dry râles are heard when air is being forced through a bronchial tube which is partially constricted, either by dry tenacious mucus or by severe swelling of the mucous membrane. Fine threads of secretion or mucus are formed, which are set vibrating by the current of air. Dry râles vary in pitch according to the diameter of the bronchial tube in which they originate. They are heard as humming, rattling, whistling, crackling or squeaking sounds, or those produced by movement of a tightly stretched piece of paper. Dry râles occur in the early stages of acute bronchitis, in chronic bronchitis, spasm of the bronchial muscle and pulmonary neoplasia or tuberculosis when there is distortion of the bronchi.

Râles are occasionally very loud, strong, ringing and clearly audible. They originate in severely infiltrated tissue, which explains the good conduction of the sound. As opposed to this, râles that originate in air-containing pulmonary tissue, e.g. in bronchitis, are considerably softer in tone and therefore more difficult to hear.

In order to make occasional or very faint râles audible, it may be necessary to induce hyperpnoea by occluding the animal's nostrils for a short period, and then to auscultate during the deep breathing that follows the removal of the obstruction.

Crepitant râles (crepitations) are crackling sounds heard only during the later part of the inspiratory phase. They are produced when the bronchial mucosa is sufficiently swollen, or exudation has affected the alveoli, so that the opposing walls become adherent to one another and have to be parted by the stream of incoming air.

The sudden separation of the adherent mucous membrane causes a low-pitched crackling sound, which can be simulated by rubbing a tuft of hair held between the fingers, close to the ear, or by separating the opposed, moistened tips of the thumb and forefinger close to the ear. Care is necessary to avoid friction between the chest-piece of the stethoscope and the coat of the animal, otherwise confusing sounds are produced. This can be largely avoided by using an instrument with a rubber rim on the chest-piece, which should be held firmly against the chest wall. Crepitant râles occur in bronchitis, in the early stages of pneumonia, during the resolution stages of inflammation, and in pulmonary oedema along with bubbling sounds.

Emphysematous sounds are harsh and crackling, and are heard during the whole inspiratory phase and to a less obvious degree during expiration. This sound simulates that produced by crushing a sheet of soft paper into a ball. It occurs in chronic alveolar emphysema, in which case it is widespread, and in acute alveolar emphysema and oedema, when fluid sounds may also be detected.

Frictional sounds in the respiratory area are associated with the pleura or pericardium. Normally during the movements which occur in respiration, the visceral and costal pleurae glide silently over each other, since both membranes are smooth and are lubricated by a clear lymph-like fluid. When the two opposing surfaces are dry and roughened, however, rasping or scraping sounds are heard, and these are constant, occurring with each respiration. They can be simulated by rubbing together two pieces of dry leather or by pressing a finger against the ear and scratching it with a fingernail of the other hand.

Frictional sounds are associated with the early pre-exudative stage of pleurisy and pericarditis. Pericardial friction sounds can be differentiated from those of pleural origin by noting their position of origin, and that they are not related to respiratory frequency and movements. In the respiratory area frictional sounds may easily be confused with dry râles. The following points will serve to distinguish between them: râles are inconstant, being heard first at one place and then at another; following a cough, which in this case is strong and not painful, they may disappear for a varying period. Frictional sounds are constant, although not continuous, being heard in the same phase of respiration, more usually during inspiration; following a cough, which is usually painful and suppressed, they are still present. Pleurisy is in many cases a complication of pulmonary inflammation, therefore, râles and crepitations may accompany frictional sounds. Because of the pain that is associated with the early phase of pleurisy, the respirations, particularly in the horse, will show altered features, becoming characteristically abdominal. The disappearance of frictional sounds may mean complete resolution, exudation of fluid which lubricates the inflamed membranes and separates them, or the development of pleural adhesions. Râles and frictional sounds may be so voluminous that their origin can be perceived as a rasping, or thrill, when the hand is placed on the thorax.

During auscultation of the lung, sounds unconnected with respiration may be heard. They have a distracting effect and are sometimes mistaken, particularly by the inexperienced clinician, for respiratory sounds. To this category belong, for example, sounds that arise from the swallowing of food, groaning, contraction of muscles, trembling, abnormally loud cardiac, and in particular peristaltic sounds. The last, on account of of their volume, are frequently heard during auscultation of the lung; they are sometimes mistaken for râles. Such peristaltic sounds are more normally heard over the lung area on the left side in horses and cattle; in the horse they are caused by movements of the colon and in the ox by movements of the reticulum. The basis of differentiation is that intestinal sounds are distant sounds, they are splashing and rumbling in character and they are not related to any particular phase of respiration but occur independently of it. Râles can be determined to coincide with the respiratory movements. The functional sounds, originating in segments of intestine that have passed forwards into the thoracic cavity as the result of hernia or rupture of the diaphragm are of particular diagnostic significance.

Succussion sounds are splashing sounds, caused by agitation of fluid which has a free surface at which movement can take place. They are heard in pyopneumothorax (pus, with overlying air, in the pleural sac). When such fluid is set in motion by lung movement, or when a small animal is picked up and gently shaken, the splashing may be audible. In the last instance movement of fluid and gas in the digestive tract will produce similar sounds.

Special Methods for Examination of the Thoracic Respiratory Organs

Radiological Examination

For diagnostic purposes radiological examination of the chest is a practical proposition in the dog and cat, also in calves, sheep, goats and pigs, and may reveal essential evidence of respiratory or thoracic disease. Similar results can be obtained in foals or larger animals only by the use of high-output X-ray machines, which are not in general use. Fluoroscopic examination of the chest region makes it possible, in suitable cases, to assess the functional movements of the various respiratory components in this area, including the ribs and diaphragm.

The value of radiological examination as an aid to establishing a diagnosis of chronic bronchitis, or bronchiectasis, in the dog or cat is uncertain unless a suitable contrast medium is used (bronchography). The introduction of a radio-opaque medium into the bronchial tree involves anaesthetizing the subject and inserting a polythene catheter into the trachea and each dependent bronchus in turn to a selected point during bronchoscopy. Adjusting the posture of the animal will then assist the distribution of the small quantity of radio-opaque material required. In this way the incomplete filling of some bronchi, along with dilatation of the terminal part of the trachea and main bronchus, which are characteristic of chronic bronchitis, are revealed.

In bronchopneumonia the radiograph may reveal a variable picture which may include patchy variations in density, distension of major blood vessels in the perihilar area and atelectasis, which may involve the base of both lungs or the ventral parts of the lobes. The radiographic picture in interstitial lung change, a frequent sequel to diseases such as canine distemper and specific pneumonias caused by virus infection, is one of either peribronchial cellular proliferation or thickening of interlobular septa with areas of collapse. Spontaneous or other forms of lung collapse are readily recognized by marked increase in density of the whole or part of a lung, which is also reduced in size and is seen not to fill the pleural sac. The presence of fluid within the pleural cavity, encountered in some types of pleurisy (nocardiosis and tuberculosis in the dog), neoplasia and hydrothorax, produces a characteristic radiographic picture. When exposures are made with the animal in standing posture, the main features revealed are partial collapse of the lung with increased density throughout the ventral portion. In pneumothorax, radiography will show an air pocket at the highest point of the pleural cavity, with the posterior aorta forming an arch at the upper posterior part. Mediastinal displacement is not a marked feature in unilateral lung collapse or pneumothorax in the dog, at least, because air passes through the mediastinum so that pressure tends to equalize on both sides.

Radiography is particularly valuable as a diagnostic aid in diaphragmatic hernia, making it possible to recognize an abnormal diaphragmatic shadow or, in some cases, its complete absence. Other possible radiographic features of this condition include areas of increased, or decreased, density within the thorax, resulting from the presence of the liver and/or portions of the digestive tract in this abnormal situation. The administration of a barium meal, although unnecessary in most instances, will confirm the abnormal position of the hollow viscus.

Radiological examination will ensure confirmation of intrathoracic neoplasia. Routine screening of small animals has led to re-evaluation in many unsuspected cases of respiratory tract tumours. Primary neoplasms involve either the lungs or the mediastinum, and when of moderate or large size produce an area of increased density and cause a variable degree of organ displacement. Secondary pulmonary neoplasms are more common and, originating from a variety of sources, may be associated with appropriate clinical signs. Radiographically it is usual to ascertain that metastatic tumours involve both lungs producing a variable number of localized areas of increased density throughout the lung fields (Fig. 124).

Direct radiography will reveal radio-opaque foreign objects when they obstruct the thoracic portion of the oesophagus. The presence of objects in a similar situation, which are not revealed in this way, is usually disclosed by means of oral administration of a barium-containing capsule or draught, the former will be retained immediately anterior to the object, while the latter will outline it by forming a surface film. Other oesophageal conditions which are revealed in this way include achalasia.

Paracentesis

Paracentesis of the thorax is of value when the

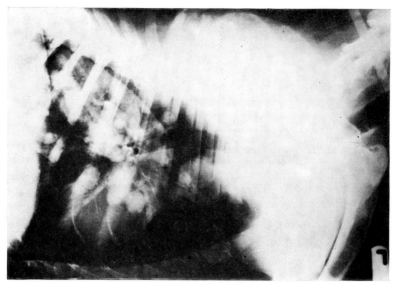

Fig. 124. *Multiple pulmonary tumours (metastatic) involving the diaphragmatic lobes of the lungs in a dog.*

presence of fluid in the pleural sac is suspected. The procedure is performed by means of a suitable sterile needle and syringe. The site for insertion of the needle is either the sixth or seventh intercostal space below the level of the fluid (it is best to select a point below the level of the costochondral junction). The needle should be inserted with care in order to avoid injury to the pericardial sac. Aspiration of fluid is effected by pulling on the piston and filling the syringe.

Examination of the aspirated sample of fluid will reveal its gross and microscopic features and thus assist in diagnosis. In haemothorax, the blood is fluid at the time of withdrawal but may clot on exposure to air unless an anticoagulant is added. As a rule haemothorax of significant proportions is accompanied by other clinical signs indicating the presence of acute haemorrhagic anaemia. In hydrothorax, the recovered fluid may vary in character from clear serous to opaque depending upon the number and types of tissue cells present. Clinical signs of general oedema, caused by congestive heart failure or hypoproteinaemia, or extensive pulmonary neoplasia, may be associated features. In cases of exudative pleurisy the causal organism may be revealed by microscopic or cultural examination (nocardiosis and tuberculosis).

THE HEART AND CIRCULATORY SYSTEM

Circulatory Dynamics

The cardiovascular system consists of two main structural units, the heart and the blood vessels, which are jointly concerned in maintaining the circulation of the blood and thereby ensuring normal exchange of oxygen, carbon dioxide, electrolytes, fluid nutrients and waste products between the blood and the body tissues. The autonomic nervous system acts as an important regulator of the two components. Either component may fail to function in an efficient manner independently of the other. Of the two forms of circulatory failure, that involving the heart is due to intrinsic factors, while in peripheral circulatory failure there is defective venous return, the heart itself being normal.

In heart failure two main effects are produced which are responsible for the clinical signs shown by the affected animal. Although both effects are produced simultaneously, one of them may be dominant, depending upon the speed at which failure occurs. These effects result from failure to maintain circulatory equilibrium and the nutrition of the tissues, most particularly the oxygen requirements of the brain. Circulatory equilibrium is deranged when the ventricular output is less than the venous return, and this persists for a significant period. If this occurs slowly, blood then accumulates in the veins and signs of congestive heart failure develop. If cardiac output is markedly reduced then the heart beat is suddenly arrested, producing acute heart failure.

Peripheral circulatory failure is brought about by reduction in blood volume, or by pooling of blood in the peripheral vessels as for example in splanchnic vasodilatation. The end results are similar to those of congestive heart failure although there is no primary defect of the heart itself, the venous return being effectively ejected.

In the majority of animals, the heart has a considerable functional reserve which maintains circulatory equilibrium under circumstances of increased demand, such as those created by exercise and to a lesser degree by pregnancy, lactation and digestion. The increased demands are immediately met with by an increase in heart rate and an increase in stroke volume. If the demands remain at an elevated level, a degree of compensation may also be achieved through the development of cardiac hypertrophy. Cardiac reserve can be eroded by many pathological processes, chemotherapeutic compounds and excessive physical exertion. Diminution of cardiac reserve, which may be detected by assessing exercise tolerance, is the first stage in heart disease. In the next stage, when the cardiac reserve is completely lost, decompensation occurs with inability to maintain circulatory equilibrium.

Regional Anatomy

In all species of domestic animals the chest is flattened laterally, usually to a more marked degree in the lower two-thirds. The heart, suspended at its base by the great vessels which traverse the mediastinum, occupies a considerable part of the middle mediastinal region. The apex of the heart is situated in the midline above the sternum.

In the horse the heart is asymmetrical in position, slightly more than half of the organ being on the left of the median plane. The base, which is directed dorsally, is situated on a level with the junction of the middle and dorsal thirds of the dorsoventral diameter of the thorax, and extends from opposite the second to the sixth intercostal space. The apex is positioned centrally about 1 cm above the last sternal seg-

ment, and about 2·5 cm anterior to the sternal diaphragm. The posterior border is nearly vertical and approximates to a position opposite the sixth rib or interspace. The left surface of the heart, consisting almost entirely of the wall of the left ventricle, covered by the pericardium, is in contact with the lower third of the chest wall from the third to the sixth rib. The relationship between the heart and chest wall on the right side extends from the third to the fourth intercostal space only, because of the relatively small cardiac notch in the right lung, and the degree of cardiac asymmetry. Enlargement of the heart from any cause will proportionately increase the area of contact between the organ and the chest wall on the right side. Internally the heart contains four chambers through which the flow of blood is directed, and regulated, by valves situated at the entry or exit from the cavities. The right atrioventricular orifice, guarded by the tricuspid valve, is situated opposite the fourth intercostal space about 7 cm above the lower extremity of the fourth rib. The pulmonary orifice, guarded by the pulmonary semilunar valve, is opposite the third intercostal space immediately above the level of the right atrioventricular orifice. The left atrioventricular orifice, guarded by the mitral valve is situated opposite the fifth intercostal space about 10 cm above the sternal extremity of the fifth rib. The aortic orifice, guarded by its semilunar valve, is opposite the fourth intercostal space on a line level with the point of the shoulder.

In cattle, the degree of cardiac asymmetry is slightly greater than in the horse. The base of the heart in this species extends from opposite the third to about the sixth rib. The apex, which is median in position and about 2 cm from the diaphragm, is opposite the articulation of the sixth costal cartilage with the sternum. The posterior border, which is almost vertical, is opposite the fifth intercostal space where it is separated from the diaphragm by the pericardium. On the left side, the heart and overlying pericardium are in contact with the chest wall from the third rib to the fourth intercostal space. On the right side the extent of the contact is limited to a small area opposite the ventral part of the fourth rib, and the adjacent third and fourth interspaces. The right atrioventricular orifice is opposite to the fourth rib almost 10 cm above the costochondral junction; the pulmonary orifice, which is slightly above this level, is opposite the third intercostal space; the left atrioventricular orifice is mainly opposite the fourth intercostal space, and the aortic orifice is opposite the fourth rib, about 12 cm above the sternal extremity.

The heart in the pig is small proportionately to the bodyweight; it is short and broad, and the blunt apex, which is situated medially, is about 0·5 cm away from the diaphragm. On the left side the pericardium is in contact with the chest wall from the second intercostal space to the fifth rib.

In the dog the heart is placed so obliquely that the base, which is opposite the ventral part of the third rib, faces mainly in an anterior direction. The apex is blunt and positioned near the diaphragm on the left of the median plane, opposite the seventh costal cartilage. The area of contact between the heart and chest wall, through the overlying pericardium, on the left side, extends from opposite the ventral parts of the third to the sixth ribs. On the right side the area of contact is limited to that extending between the fourth and fifth ribs.

Abnormal Types of Pulse

In order to extend and amplify the clinical information already obtained by determining the pulse frequency and quality, attention should now be directed towards detecting pulse abnormalities and interpreting their possible significance. It must be appreciated that many of the variations from the normal pulse reflect the functional status of the heart which is influenced in a variety of ways. It should be remembered, however, that pulse characters can also be significantly affected by extracardiac factors, e.g. decreased amplitude because of reduced venous return as well as from reduced contractile power of the myocardium. Reflex acceleration of the heart occurs in painful conditions, e.g. spasmodic colic, as well as in febrile diseases. In toxaemic and septicaemic conditions all the circulatory components, including the myocardium, blood vessels and medullary reflex centres, may be involved. The myocardium and medullary reflex centres may also be influenced by hypoxia in various forms of anaemia and in diseases, such as pneumonia, which depress the pulmonary gaseous exchange. Diseases having the latter effect will also cause cardiac disturbance because of the increased resistance which develops in the pulmonary circulation. Other important abnormalities of the pulse are due to primary heart diseases, which may be functional or organic in character. Functional disease of the heart occurs when no readily recognizable pathological lesion is observed, although it is probable that in many instances minute changes in structure or biochemical lesions exist.

When cardiac disease is sufficiently severe to permit failure of circulatory equilibrium along with inadequate oxygen provision to meet the nutritional requirements of the tissues, obvious clinical signs will be presented by the animal. The basic character of the cardiac disease varies somewhat according to the species of animal involved. In the horse, organic disease of the heart is infrequently encountered (examples are endocarditis caused by *Streptococcus equi, Actinobacillus equuli* and migrating *Strongylus* spp. larvae, and pericarditis in occasional cases of strangles and of generalized infection by *Strep. faecalis*); the commonest type in this species is functional in character. In cattle organic heart disease, including subacute bacterial endocarditis, post-vaccinal endocarditis in calves (*Mycoplasma mycoides*), traumatic pericarditis, tuberculous pericarditis and the pericarditis that occurs in pasteurellosis, is the most usual type, although functional defects occur, sometimes only temporarily, as in severe haemolytic anaemia, parturient paresis, etc. Endocarditis, caused in lambs by *Streptococcus* spp. and *Escherichia coli*, and in older sheep by *Erysipelothrix insidiosa*, and the pericarditis of pasteurellosis are the most commonly encountered types of heart disease. In pigs, endocarditis caused by *Streptococcus* spp. and *Erysipelothrix insidiosa*, and pericarditis occurring in pasteurellosis, enzootic pneumonia, salmonellosis and in Glasser's disease are the commonest forms of heart disease encountered. In the dog, functional and organic disease of the heart are of equal occurrence.

Disturbances of Pulse Rhythm

Irregular pulse. In this type of pulse the intervals between the individual pulse waves vary in length. Irregularity of the pulse rhythm is invariably associated with variations in pulse amplitude; it is particularly well marked in atrial fibrillation, atrial flutter, disorders of the cardiac intrinsic conduction mechanism and generalized myocarditis (true arrhythmia). During the course and convalescent phases of diseases such as pneumonia and other severe febrile and toxaemic conditions that impose increased work load on the heart, an intermittent pulse is often a transitory feature; it also occurs with atrial and ventricular extrasystoles (produced when impulses capable of stimulating myocardial contraction originate at points apart from the sinoauricular node) caused by focal myocarditis, also in digitalis and chloroform intoxication and sometimes in space-occupying lesions of the brain. In these circumstances the irregular ventricular contractions may not always produce a pulse wave because of inadequate strength. The detection of a pulse deficit enables extrasystolic arrhythmia to be differentiated from heart block.

During respiration the pulse rate in some species (particularly dogs) is appreciably more frequent during inspiration than during expiration (respiratory sinus arrhythmia). It is usually most marked when respiration is slow and deep. Sinus arrhythmia disappears on exercise or following the injection of atropine, if the animal is healthy, but if the pulse irregularity is the result of disease then it will, in many cases, become more obvious during severe dyspnoea.

Intermittent pulse. In this type of pulse individual waves are absent from an otherwise regular sequence. According to whether the waves are dropped at regular intervals (e.g. every fourth wave) or not, the condition is described as a regularly or irregularly intermittent pulse. If there is a corresponding intermission in the heart beat, the condition is described as deficient pulse. When, in spite of the pause in the pulse, the heart beat occurs, although not strongly enough to produce a perceptible pulse wave, the term intermittent pulse is applied; here, obviously, the pulse rate is less than the heart rate.

An intermittent pulse is caused by many of the same diseases as produce an irregular pulse, and is not infrequently encountered in apparently healthy animals, particularly thoroughbred horses in which it arises from partial atrioventricular node block (A–V block). If any irregularity in the pulse is abolished by exercise, excitement or following the injection of atropine (inhibition of the vagus), the full effect of which is obtained only some hours later, it may be concluded that the pulse deficit has no diagnostic significance unless it is accompanied by other signs of cardiac disease, when as a rule the pulse arrhythmia will be increased. Irregularity and intermission of the pulse may have various origins: irregular development of stimuli at the sino-auricular node

(S–A node block); irregular initiation of stimuli in the auricles (ectopic pacemakers) (atrial flutter and atrial fibrillation) and in the whole cardiac musculature (extrasystole) in focal myocarditis; and disturbances in the conduction of the contractile impulse from the atria to the ventricles (A–V block).

Disturbance in Pulse Quality

Changes in pulse quality are attributable to variations in the stroke volume of the heart, in the venous return and in the activity of the reflex centres in the medulla. Pulse quality is classified according to certain characteristics recognized by palpation:

Large strong pulse. In this pulse the artery is abnormally distended at each pulsation, the amplitude is greater than normal and the wave is not readily obliterated by digital pressure. It is indicative of persistent, or temporary, elevation of blood pressure (hypertension) and reflects increased cardiac stroke volume. This type of pulse may occur in athletic animals because of ventricular hypertrophy; it is also detected in the median artery of the horse in cases of acute laminitis, because of the inflammatory hyperaemia of the foot; and in dogs during the earlier stages of interstitial nephritis. It also appears transitorily after vigorous exercise.

Small weak pulse. Here the artery is only poorly distended, and the pressure wave is readily obliterated by finger pressure. It reflects reduced stroke volume and occurs in myocardial asthenia, mitral incompetence or stenosis, aortic stenosis and partial occlusion of the artery at which the pulse is taken. In the last two, the pulse will show other characters such as being slow and prolonged (see below).

Soft pulse. The pulse wave is poorly developed and easily obliterated. It occurs when the myocardium is debilitated by general septic or toxaemic disease.

Unequal pulse. The individual pulse waves vary in amplitude and, therefore, in strength, reflecting alterations in the stroke volume of the heart. It occurs characteristically in sinus arrhythmia and in extrasystolic arrhythmias.

Asymmetrical pulse. This is a pulse that has different qualities on the right side of the body from those of the left, e.g. in unilateral vasodilatation, and in iliac thrombosis. Slight differences of this type are not uncommon in small animals.

Alternate pulse exists when a strong wave alternates with a weaker one. Another form of alternating pulse occurs when there are groups of continually weakening waves interspersed by a few stronger waves. Both types of alternate pulse occur in severe cardiac weakness.

Water-hammer or Corrigan's pulse. The pulse wave rises rapidly until the artery is overdistended, and then collapses equally quickly (Fig. 25C, p. 31). The wave is not readily obliterated. It is pathognomonic of either insufficiency of the aortic valves or patency of the ductus arteriosus. A form of this pulse occurs in severe anaemia as a result of the very low arterial blood pressure.

Slow pulse. The pulse pressure wave rises slowly and collapses again in a similar manner (Fig. 25D, p. 31). The artery is only moderate distended. It occurs in stenosis of the aortic valve, complete A–V block and sometimes in space-occupying lesions of the brain. It should not be confused with infrequent pulse resulting from bradycardia.

Hard pulse. The wall of the artery is tense and hard, and the pulse wave is not readily obliterated. It occurs in diseases associated with hypertension (nephritis), pain, increased muscular tone (tetanus) and local hyperaemia (laminitis).

Wiry pulse. This pulse is hard and, at the same time, small. It occurs when there is some degree of vasoconstriction. A wiry pulse is associated with painful diseases such as acute pleurisy, acute peritonitis, acute and subacute endocarditis, the early stages of acute pericarditis and intestinal volvulus.

Thready pulse. The pulse wave is small and readily obliterated. Its significance is similar to that of wiry pulse although it may indicate that the disease may have an unfavourable termination. This indication is more clearly presented when repeated examinations reveal that the pulse rate is progressively increasing, and that the amplitude is decreasing, thus producing the so-called 'running down' pulse.

Dicrotic pulse. This type of pulse is appreciated only in very rare instances. Following closely upon the main pulse wave, a second wave is perceptible (caused by the slight, temporary rise in blood pressure following closure of the aortic semilunar valves). It occurs in prolonged and acute fevers, but sometimes occurs in the absence of demonstrable disease. In the vast majority of animals the dicrotic pressure wave is dissipated within a short distance of the heart.

Fremitus, i.e. a vibration or shaking of the arterial wall, instead of a pulse wave, occurs when the lumen is reduced (arterial thrombosis, congenital stenosis, stretching or kinking), in arteriovenous aneurysm of the spermatic artery of the bull, in parasitic aneurysm of the anterior mesenteric artery of the horse and in the middle uterine artery of the cow in late pregnancy.

Distension of the Veins

Jugular Pulse

In many animals, engorgement of the jugular vein produces movement which may be observed to involve that section of the vein which is situated subcutaneously in the jugular furrow. This is described as a jugular pulse. It may be negative or positive.

A negative jugular pulse occurs during the early part of cardiac systole when the blood, being temporarily unable to enter the contracted right atrium, is dammed back in the jugular vein. This type of jugular pulse takes the form of distension of the proximal part of the jugular vein, arising presystolically, i.e. before the heart contracts, and gradually extending from the lower part of the vein forwards. It is physiological, readily observed in lean animals and particularly common in cattle. Negative jugular pulse is exaggerated in tricuspid stenosis, heart block and exudative pericarditis.

Positive jugular pulse consists of true pulse waves which run forward from the shoulder towards the angle of the jaw. These regurgitation waves are not only visible but are palpable as moderately strong impulses. Positive jugular pulse occurs in tricuspid incompetence because, during cardiac systole, the blood in the right ventricle is forced backwards through the incompletely closed valvular orifice into the right atrium and the jugular vein. In lactating cattle affected with tricuspid valve insufficiency, a positive pulse may be detected also in the subcutaneous abdominal (mammary) vein. This type of jugular pulse is systolic and coincides with the arterial pulse; it is pathognomonic of tricuspid valve incompetence. The existence of positive jugular pulse is indicated if, following the application of digital pressure to the vein in the region of the larynx, the engorgement disappears only after two or more cardiac cycles.

In lean animals, the pulsation of the underlying carotid artery, noted particularly at the entrance to the thorax, may be transmitted to the overlying tissues and thereby simulate a positive jugular pulse. This condition, which is termed false jugular pulse, is not obliterated by compression of the jugular vein, whereas a true positive jugular pulse will disappear.

Venous Stasis

The state of the venous system can be assessed by observing the jugular vein, the smaller cutaneous veins, the auricular veins, the spermatic and the subcutaneous abdominal veins. In long-coated animals, venous distension is detected by palpation. In thin-skinned horses, such as thoroughbreds and hunters, when the coat is short, temporary distension of the superficial veins is readily seen after active exertion. Persistent dilatation of superficial veins occurs in all conditions in which there is obstruction to the flow of blood on the venous side of the blood vascular system. It is constantly present when the flow of blood into the right side of the heart is delayed by incomplete emptying of the organ during the preceding systolic contraction. It occurs in myocardial dystrophy, heart block and cardiac and mediastinal neoplasia; in endocarditis; in congenital defects including patent interventricular septum, patent foramen ovale, patent ductus arteriosus, and fibro-elastosis; in pericarditis and hydropericardium; and in pneumonia, chronic alveolar emphysema, overdistension of the abdomen, etc. (Fig. 125). In the broken-winded horse, the veins become distended after only a short period of exercise, and

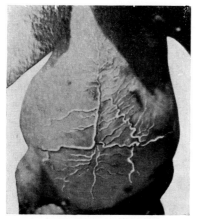

Fig. 125. *Distension of the abdominal veins in venous stasis in a dog. Tumour of the liver.* (After Schindelka)

remain dilated for much longer than in the healthy animal, indicating the severity of the dyspnoea and its influence on the pulmonary circulation and the heart. Occasionally, however, engorgement of the veins may be the result of a purely local condition, e.g. compression of a vein by a tumour or by a superficial inflammatory process.

In myocardial asthenia, if distension of the jugular and other large superficial veins is not already obvious, digital compression will rapidly produce very marked dilatation. In vasogenic failure, occurring in toxaemia and shock, the jugular vein is not engorged although the total blood volume is normal, and digital compression slowly produces only a slight distension of any of the superficial veins. In quiet dogs, the degree of venous stasis may be estimated by placing the animal in lateral recumbency, repeatedly raising the recurrent tarsal vein by digital compression and releasing the pressure with the leg held at various levels relative to the heart. If venous pressure is normal, and the animal is in a relaxed state, the vein should collapse rapidly when pressure is released with the limb at any level above that of the heart.

Cyanosis is bluish discoloration of the skin and mucous membranes caused by abnormally increased amounts of reduced haemoglobin in the circulating blood. In animals it is most readily detected in the conjunctival and gingival mucosae. In all cases the haemoglobin concentration shows little or no variation from normal, but the oxygen tension of the arterial blood is low. Cyanosis is present in all types of hypoxic hypoxia and in stagnant hypoxia, but not in anaemic hypoxia. The existence of cyanosis can be determined by noting that the bluish discoloration disappears temporarily when pressure is applied to the mucosae or skin and the blood flow is stopped. Methaemoglobinaemia is distinguished by noting that the discoloration of the mucosae and the skin is brown rather than blue.

A varying degree of cyanosis occurs in all forms of heart disease; it is most obvious in congenital heart defects and less so in acquired heart disease. In pulmonary disease, cyanosis is rarely very obvious because the circulation is impeded proportional to the degree of lung dysfunction.

When venous engorgement persists it will cause oedema, usually anasarca, ascites, hydrothorax and hydropericardium. The anasarca is limited to the dependent parts, including the ventral surface of the thorax and abdomen, the neck and the lower jaw. In severe congestion the liver is enlarged to a varying degree, so that in the dog and cat the thickened border of the organ can be palpated behind the right costal arch.

Diseases of the Blood Vessels

Other abnormalities of the blood vessels include arterial thrombosis and embolism, venous thrombosis and secondary defects in blood vessel walls. Arterial thrombosis frequently results from arteritis. Parasitic arteritis of the anterior mesenteric artery, the iliac arteries, the base of the aorta and occasionally the coronary, renal and cerebral arteries, caused by the migrating larvae of *Strongylus vulgaris*, is relatively common in the horse. Arteritis, to a varying extent, also occurs in onchocerciasis in cattle and elaeophoriasis in sheep. Arteritis is the most significant histopathological feature in bovine malignant catarrhal fever and equine viral arteritis. Ergotism is characterized by arteritis with vasospasm, producing thrombosis and proceeding to gangrene of the extremities. Frost-bite has the same total effect. Arterial embolism is, in most cases, only recognized at post mortem examination in the form of endarteritis. The lesions are most obvious in the lungs and kidneys and are found in association with a primary suppurative, or other inflammatory process elsewhere, e.g. vegetative endocarditis or arterial thrombosis at other sites. Non-infected arterial embolism caused by fat globules entering the pulmonary arteries is thought to occur, in rare cases, in the horse following castration in the cast position.

Venous thrombosis commonly arises from phlebitis, which may be caused by local extension of infection, by localization of a blood-borne infection, by bacterial invasion of the umbilical veins at birth or by injection of irritant substances in the case of the larger veins. Venous thrombosis may affect the jugular vein or the posterior vena cava in the horse when affected with strangles. In septicaemic diseases of the pig, phlebitis and venous thrombosis cause the development of purple discoloration, and later sloughing of the ears, which is a feature in many cases.

Defects in blood vessel walls usually involve the capillaries and smaller arterioles. They occur in septicaemic (or viraemic) diseases and in purpura haemorrhagica. The end effect is increased permeability leading to haemorrhages which are either petechial or ecchymotic. Spontaneous haemorrhage due to capillary damage, caused by bacterial action, is a feature of bracken fern poisoning in cattle, poisoning caused by trichloroethylene extracted soya-bean meal and radiation sickness.

The clinical manifestations associated with arterial thrombosis and embolism are a reflection of the interference with the function of the part supplied by the affected vessel. In parasitic arteritis the thrombi which inevitably develop may partially or completely occlude the artery. Obstruction of the anterior mesenteric artery causes recurrent colic or, in occasional cases, ischaemic necrosis of a segment of the intestine. Less commonly the origin of the iliac artery is occluded causing either mild or acute ischaemia of a hind limb. Occlusion of the coronary artery causes a varying degree of cardiac infarction. Embolic obstruction of the pulmonary arteries causes hypoxic hypoxia. Further consideration will be given to the clinical aspects at the appropriate point of the text.

Examination of the Heart

The examination of the vascular system, including taking the pulse and noting the condition of the peripheral vessels, is greatly supplemented by an examination of the heart. This is achieved by means of inspection, palpation, percussion, auscultation and, in selected cases, electrocardiography and phonocardiography. In order to interpret the results of these examinations to best advantage a knowledge of what comprises significant departures from normal is required.

Abnormal Variations in Heart Rate

Cardiac rhythm and, therefore, rate are influenced by extrinsic or neurogenic mechanisms and by local or autoregulatory mechanisms. The principal neurogenic mechanism, which is reflex in character, is concerned with regulation of blood pressure. Information about arterial blood pressure is generated by intravascular stretch receptors and transmitted by afferent nerves to the reflex centres in the medulla. Efferent discharges, arising from the processing of the information received, travel via autonomic nerves to the myocardium and arterial muscles, thereby adjusting cardiac output and peripheral resistance so that blood pressure is maintained within normal limits. The autoregulatory or intrinsic mechanism balances the output of the two ventricles; the basic principle involved is included in Starling's law. When venous return to the heart increases, autoregulation contributes to increased cardiac output.

Abnormalities of cardiac rate include tachycardia (increased rate), bradycardia (decreased rate), arrhythmia (irregularity) and gallop rhythms. Arrhythmia has been discussed in the context of abnormalities in the pulse.

Tachycardia

In interpreting the significance of heart rates the influence of age, temperament, presence or absence of exciting influences and of diseases, and the pattern of cardiac rhythm must be taken into account. In sinus or simple tachycardia the frequent heart rate reflects the pacemaker influence of the sino-atrial node, brought about by excitement, pain, hyperthermia, temporary hypotension, increased venous pressure or the administration of adrenergic drugs.

Paroxysmal tachycardia exists when there are sudden periods of tachycardia of short duration for which no known cause can be deduced. It is of rare occurrence in animals but has been observed in the horse. The cardiac rhythm is normal and the rate is more than twice the normal for the species. The heart sounds are of increased intensity but the pulse is small and weak reflecting marked reduction in the stroke volume. This form of tachycardia is usually an indication of myocardial disease, and affected animals exhibit poor exercise tolerance and are predisposed to acute heart failure or congestive heart failure if the paroxysmal attacks persist.

In some instances the frequency of the premature beats is very high (200–400/minute in adult large animals). Either the atria or the ventricles may be involved; the condition is called a flutter. In atrial flutter the ventricular rate, although increased, does not complement that of the atria. It is caused by an intrinsic cardiac defect such as myocardial disease. The cardiac rhythm is regular and the rate is not influenced by exercise or fear. Because it is persistent it is readily differentiated from paroxysmal tachycardia.

If the contractile impulses arise from a number of different foci the result is either atrial or ventricular fibrillation according to where the foci are situated. In atrial fibrillation the rate of contraction is very rapid and the ventricular rhythm is grossly irregular and the rate is much faster than normal. Exercise increases the heart rate and the arrhythmia tends to be exaggerated, pulse deficit being by no means uncommon. The condition, which is permanent, usually signifies severe heart disease and is often accompanied by congestive heart failure.

Ventricular fibrillation is incompatible with survival, but it may be converted to a sinus rhythm by electrical countershock (ventricular defibrillation) or cardiac massage. Ventricular fibrillation occurs in the terminal stages of lightning stroke, severe toxaemia, chloroform overdosage and most other diseases causing sudden death.

Bradycardia

Reduced heart rate is caused by reduction in the frequency of sino-atrial nodal discharge. It is essential to distinguish between sinus (simple) bradycardia and that form of reduced heart rate occurring in heart block. In the former there is the customary increase in heart rate with exercise and excitement, or following the administration of atropine. It occurs following stimulation of the vagus nerve (cardio-inhibitor), but most cases have an extracardiac origin and are caused by an increase in blood pressure (hypertension), and also in chronic acquired hydrocephalus and other space-occupying lesions of the brain, during the comatose phase of parturient hypocalcaemia, in neonatal hypoglycaemia of piglets, in coma generally, in association with jaundice, in those cases of traumatic reticuloperitonitis in cattle with extensive diaphragmatic adhesions, in some cases of displacement of the abomasum and occasionally in vagus indigestion and diaphragmatic hernia in cattle. It also occurs in normal athletic animals at rest because of improved myocardial efficiency.

Reduction of heart rate due to heart block is caused by interference with the initiation or transmission of the contractile impulse. In the first instance the block occurs at the S–A node, while in the second case it involves the A–V node. S–A block, which is a relatively rare condition (it occurs in the horse), produces irregular irregularity of rhythm. Its existence is confirmed by the electrocardiogram. In A–V block the ventricle is not stimulated to contract because of interference with conduction in this segment of the intrinsic nerve mechanism. The degree of A–V block varies, so that in some cases in the horse the irregularity disappears with exercise and an increase in heart rate. Unless other signs of heart disease are observed, this form of A–V block should be considered to have no diagnostic significance. When A–V block arises as the result of local myocarditis causing a lesion in the A–V bundle it is associated with degrees of arrhythmia which becomes accentuated on exercise.

Physical Examination of the Heart

Inspection

The anatomical relationship of the heart to the chest wall is such that contact between them is restricted to a nominal extent on the left side only. Visible evidence of this contact may be obtained by observing the so-called apex beat of the heart, causing movement of the chest wall, during cardiac systole. This is generally only possible in normal animals when the chest wall is thin and the coat short and in good condition. During the general inspection stage of the clinical examination such visible evidence of cardiac activity may be a reflection of the excitable disposition of the animal. Whenever the action of the heart becomes tumultuous, as in overexertion and haemolytic anaemia, the impact of the heart on the chest wall can be readily observed.

A significant increase in the size of the heart will enlarge the area of contact with the chest wall and, thereby, the cardiac impulse is more readily discovered. This is more obviously the case when the cardiac enlargement is caused by hypertrophy. Displacement of the heart may be associated with an increased, or decreased, area of contact with the chest wall, so that the pulsation may be exaggerated or completely absent.

Palpation

Palpation of the cardiac area provides an opportunity to assess the strength and extent of the cardiac impulse, and also to detect those occasional cases in which a palpable thrill exists. It is performed by placing the palm of the hand over the cardiac area on each side in turn. The tip of one finger can be employed to determine the exact site of the cardiac impulse (apical impulse) which is regularly palpable at the posterior boundary of the area. In the dog, the impulse is palpable, and in the narrow-chested breeds may even be equal in force and extent on both sides of the thorax, but in the other domestic animals it is normally detected on the left side only.

The point of maximum impact is increased in area and displaced posteriorly in cardiac hypertrophy or dilatation associated with insufficiency or anaemia, and anteriorly in ascites, hepatomegaly and distension of the stomach or intestines with food or gas, etc. It is imperceptible when the heart has been displaced away from the thoracic wall in effusive pericarditis or pleurisy, hydropericardium, hydrothorax and mediastinal or pulmonary neoplasia or hydatidosis. If such a condition is unilateral, the apex beat may be absent on one side and intensified on the other. In gross hypertrophy of the right ventricle the cardiac impulse may be equally strong on both sides (e.g. congenital pulmonary stenosis).

The rhythm of the cardiac cycle can be assessed during routine palpation of the cardiac area, and in extreme cases of vulvular insufficiency or stenosis, and developmental defects, an obvious thrill can be detected.

Percussion

Percussion of the heart is performed in the same manner and may be performed at the same time as that of the lungs. In any situation it is advisable, initially, to percuss from the more resonant towards the dull sounding areas. As the heart is a muscular organ which is air-free, it gives a completely non-resonant percussion sound (absolute cardiac dullness), which not infrequently, however, is perceived only as an abbreviated sound (relative cardiac dullness), since the thin lower border of the lung is interposed between the heart and the chest wall. Because of the wide variation in the thickness of the chest wall and, particularly in dogs, breed differences in the shape of the thorax, considerable experience is necessary to determine the area of cardiac dullness by percussion.

The heart is located, approximately, in the lower two-thirds of the thoracic cavity, between the third to the sixth pairs of ribs, and is so placed that the greater part is located on the left of the median plane of the body. The anterior part of the heart is covered by the muscles of the shoulder area. Less than half of the heart extends behind the muscle mass and, therefore, only this part is available for percussion. The area of cardiac dullness can be demonstrated if percussion is carried out in the direction of the arrows in Figs 123 and 126. This examination is greatly

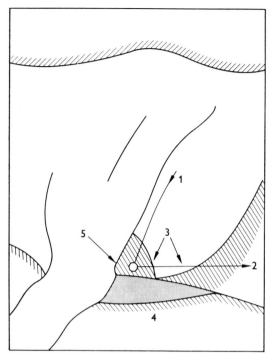

Fig. 126. *Direction of percussion in the examination of the heart in the ox. 1, First line of percussion, running downwards behind the shoulder to the area of cardiac dullness. 2, Second line, running horizontally backward from the area of cardiac dullness. 3, Approximate angle of the lung. 4, Area of absolute dullness caused by the sternum. 5, Area of relative dullness caused by the heart.*

area extending from the fourth to the sixth intercostal space, approximately a finger's breadth above the sternum. On the right side the area of cardiac dullness extends from the fourth to the fifth intercostal space, the upper border being rather less than a finger's breadth above the sternum. The area of cardiac dullness may be relatively larger in small dogs. Even in large dogs, accurate recognition of the position of the heart by means of percussion is often difficult; in very small dogs and in cats this method of examination is impracticable.

An increase in the area of cardiac dullness occurs in enlargement of the heart (cardiac hypertrophy or dilatation), in distension of the pericardial sac with fluid (pericarditis, hydropericardium, haemopericardium), in lateral displacement of the heart (unilateral pulmonary collapse, unilateral pneumothorax, rupture of the diaphragm with herniation of abdominal viscera into a pleural sac) and in neoplasia of the heart, pericardium, thymus or mediastinum. In the majority of such cases, the area of cardiac dullness may be more distinctly enlarged on the right side, the exceptions being those in which the heart is displaced towards the left side. Because of the anatomical relationships of the heart, any detectable increase in the size of the area of cardiac dullness involves the upper and posterior border, both of which are extended to a variable degree.

Reduction in the size of the area of cardiac dullness occurs in overdistension of the lungs (emphysema), when more lung tissue is insinuated between the heart and the chest wall. If fluid is present in quantity in the pleural sacs, definition of the area of cardiac dullness may be impossible because of lack of variation in the tone of the percussion sound. The upper part of the area of cardiac dullness may yield a tympanic sound when there is an accumulation of gas in the pericardial sac; this is found chiefly in the ox, as a feature of traumatic pericarditis.

A pain reaction during percussion of the cardiac area suggests the presence of acute pericarditis.

Differentiation between Cardiac and Pulmonary Dullness

If an area of dullness in the lung directly adjoins the area of cardiac dullness, it is extremely difficult to recognize whether there is enlargement of the latter, or consolidation of the neighbouring

facilitated when the foreleg is drawn well forward by an assistant; this applies particularly to the ox.

The cardiac area in the horse evinces absolute dullness, which is readily demonstrable on the left chest wall over an area approximately the size of the palm of the hand, situated behind the shoulder, above the level of the elbow. in the region of the third to the fifth intercostal spaces. On the right side of the thorax, the area of cardiac dullness is normally much smaller than that on the left, being demonstrable only in the fourth intercostal space; the right foreleg must be drawn forward.

The ox and small ruminant species reveal only relative cardiac dullness to percussion. On the left side the area is situated in the third and fourth intercostal spaces; cardiac dullness cannot be demonstrated on the right side in these species.

In the dog, percussion evokes absolute cardiac dullness. On the left side it is located over an lung tissue. To differentiate between the conditions, the following points are noted: in dullness of cardiac origin, the cardiac impulse, if detectable, occurs at the most posterior part of the area of cardiac dullness, the respiratory sounds are normal and a negative result is obtained by the tuning fork–stethoscope method of percussion. When the dullness is of pulmonary origin, the cardiac impulse does not involve the most posterior point, the pulmonary sounds are abnormal and the tuning fork–stethoscope examination yields a positive result.

Auscultation

Careful auscultation will yield more valuable information concerning the functional status of the heart than any other clinical procedure.

The cycle of cardiac activity is divisible into two phases, systole and diastole, which predominantly involve the ventricles. The cycle is measured from the onset of one ventricular contraction to the beginning of the succeeding contraction. Ventricular systole commences with the onset of rising pressure in the ventricles and terminates with the closure of the semilunar valves. Its clinical duration extends from the onset of the first heart sound to the beginning of the second heart sound. Ventricular diastole commences with closure of the semilunar valves and terminates with the initiation of the succeeding presystolic rise of blood pressure at the moment the auricles contract. Clinically it can be considered to extend from the onset of the second heart sound to the commencement of the succeeding first heart sound. Under resting conditions, in normal animals, the phase of contraction is shorter than that of relaxation.

Auscultation of the heart is carried out in the same manner as for the lungs, i.e. by the direct or indirect method (with the aid of a stethoscope or phonendoscope; Fig. 127). In large animals auscultation of the heart is readily performed with the animal in the standing position; it may assist to have the left foreleg drawn forwards. Small animals are best placed on a table of convenient height with a non-slip surface. In dogs with noisy respiration, it may prove helpful to close the mouth for a few moments in order to obtain the necessary quietness while auscultation is carried out. It should be appreciated, however, that this procedure may cause transient retardation followed by acceleration of the heart rate. (A similar effect is sometimes produced by

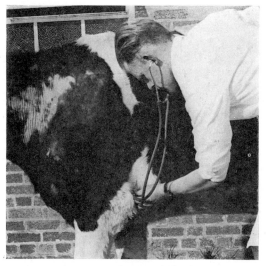

Fig. 127. *Indirect auscultation of the heart in a large animal using a stethoscope. The chest-piece can be placed medially to the point of the elbow at varying points directly over the heart.*

applying firm pressure, through the closed eyelids, to one or both eyeballs for 5–10 seconds—oculocardiac reflex.)

The purpose of auscultation is to determine the character of the heart sounds, and detect the presence of abnormal sounds. The best sites for routine auscultation are the fourth and fifth intercostal spaces. Because a fluid medium is a good sound conductor, the various sounds are heard at maximum intensity where the fluid in the heart chambers is closest to the chest wall, and not at points where the heart valves are most superficially situated. The first, or systolic sound is maximal over the cardiac apex, and the second, or diastolic sound is maximal over the base of the heart. A degree of isolation of the sounds associated with closure of individual heart valves is possible, more particularly in large animals with a relatively slow heart rate.

In auscultation of the heart, it is important to devote sufficient effort and time to ensure that all aspects are reviewed. Points to be noted are the rate, rhythm, intensity and quality of the sounds, and also whether abnormal sounds are associated with the functional activity of the heart.

Heart Sounds

The basic properties of sound are frequency (pitch), intensity and quality. The pitch is determined by the number of vibrations occurring within a unit of time, and intensity depends upon the amplitude of the vibrations. The quality of a sound depends upon the frequency and amplitude of the vibrations composing the sound.

Because human auditory perceptivity is largely restricted to sounds above 30 cycles/second, unless they are of great intensity, the vibrations associated with cardiac activity are, in great part, not audible. Cardiovascular sounds of increasing frequency are subjectively greater in volume than sounds of the same intensity but of lower frequency. The intensity of cardiovascular sounds of 500 cycles/second, or above, is generally so low that they are inaudible. There is a degree of variation between species in the relative intensity of the various components of the normal heart sounds.

Cardiovascular sounds are classified in two groups, transients and murmurs. The transient sounds, which are of short duration, include the normal heart sounds (first, second, third and fourth), diastolic 'gallop' sounds and systolic 'extra' sounds. The first heart sound is dull, loud and prolonged; it is followed immediately by the second sound which is short and sharper. The first sound is generated by several agencies, including tensing of the atrioventricular valves following their closure with vibrations of the contracting myocardium, opening of the semilunar valves and vibrations in the aorta and pulmonary artery arising from surges in blood flow during early systole, being of lesser importance. It corresponds to the phase of cardiac systole and is referred to as the systolic sound. In the dog the first sound is described as being more intense than the second.

The second heart sound is produced by closure and tensing of the semilunar valves; the intensity appears to be related to the arterial pressure. In the horse the intensity of the second heart sound is greater than that of the first. The sound is synchronous with cardiac diastole and is termed the diastolic sound.

When the heart rate is slow, the first and second sounds are readily recognized by their characteristics, and by the fact that the first sound occurs after a pause, whereas the second sound follows immediately after the first. If, however, the heart rate is increased, or is ordinarily rapid, the heart sounds cannot readily be distinguished from one another. In such cases it may be possible, while auscultating the heart, to detect the cardiac impulse by palpation with the fingertips. The sound that coincides with the cardiac impulse is the systolic heart sound. The first and second heart sounds are represented phonetically 'lub-dupp'. It is necessary to realize that the heart sounds vary somewhat not only according to species but also according to the size of the animal; furthermore with increasing thickness of the chest wall the sounds become less clearly audible.

In a proportion of normal horses and mules a third heart sound, which is short, low pitched, and of low energy, may be audible in early diastole; it is most readily heard in the mitral area. The mechanics of its production are thought to be associated with transient atrioventricular valve closure and/or vibrations in the walls of the ventricles. Occasionally, in dogs with a slow heart rate and a thin chest wall, a weak third heart sound may be recognized to occur immediately following the second sound. In certain types of cardiac disease the third heart sound is magnified.

The fourth heart sound is a complex one related to atrial systole and usually only detected by means of phonocardiography. It sometimes has two components, the second of which may be audible in the horse in first degree heart block (prolonged A–V conduction) or in second degree heart block ('dropped' ventricular beats).

The heart sounds have an enhanced volume when there is increased myocardial activity. Abnormally loud heart sounds occur in cardiac hypertrophy and in anaemia. In the former condition cardiac efficiency is optimal, in the latter the degree of cardiac asthenia is indicated by the poor pulse quality. Exertion, certain diseases of the nervous system and the early phase of febrile affections cause overstimulation of the heart, during which the heart sounds are intensified.

Enlargement of the heart, by virtue of the increased contact between it and the chest wall, will increase the volume of the heart sounds, more obviously perhaps, on the right side.

The heart sounds are reduced in volume when cardiac efficiency is impaired by the effects of disease, in advanced cardiac insufficiency and in congestive heart failure. The heart sounds are weaker in all conditions in which the heart is displaced from the thoracic wall or fluid is present in the pleural or pericardial sac (obesity, anasarca, hydropericardium, exudative and proliferative pericarditis, hydrothorax and exudative and proliferative pleurisy, etc.).

A comparison should be made of the two heart sounds for the purpose of detecting any variation in the normal volume of either sound relative to the species. The intensity of the first sound is related to the force of ventricular contraction, so that it has increased volume in ventricular hypertrophy, and decreased volume in myocardial asthenia. The volume of the second sound is dependent upon the systemic and pulmonary arterial pressure at the commencement of diastole when the semilunar valves close.

Accentuation of the second heart sound is, therefore, usually the result of an increase in the back pressure of blood against the closed valves. This occurs when the blood is expelled from the ventricles with greater force and in greater volume than usual, thereby elevating the blood pressure. It involves the right side of the heart more frequently than the left, and has its origin in those conditions, including bronchitis, pneumonia and pulmonary emphysema, which cause increased resistance in the pulmonary artery. More rarely, the accentuated second heart sound involves the aortic valve, in which instance it is attributable to increased resistance in the systemic circulation. Reduction in the volume of the second sound occurs when the arterial blood pressure falls below normal.

Doubling or reduplication of the heart sounds may occur in healthy animals and involve the first or the second sound. Reduplication of the first heart sound is common in normal cattle, and in horses and dogs, when the blood pressure is elevated. It is caused by asynchrony of closure of the mitral and tricuspid valves, in that order. In very obvious cases the cause is usually a disturbance in the conductivity of one branch of the bundle of His, or severe damage to the myocardium (myocarditis) so that asynchronous contraction of the ventricles is marked. When the condition is severe, three heart sounds, instead of the usual two, are heard at approximately equal intervals ('gallop rhythm'). Reduplication of the second heart sound is caused by the semilunar valves not closing simultaneously. Normally, aortic valve closure precedes pulmonary valve closure. During inspiration the venous return to the heart is increased, so that the stroke volume and ejection period of the right ventricle are increased, thereby delaying the closure of the pulmonary semilunar valve. In cardiac diseases causing delayed closure of the aortic valve (aortic stenosis, left bundle-branch block) split-

ting of the second heart sound occurs during expiration. Splitting of the second heart sound can be detected in many horses and in dogs with cardiac disease.

In the dog and ox, protodiastolic (ventricular) gallop rhythm resulting from abnormal accentuation of the third heart sound is associated with advanced myocarditis and myocardial asthenia. Because the third heart sound is more usually audible in the horse, significant development of ventricular gallop rhythm is difficult to recognize in the species. Exaggeration of the fourth heart sound (see above) produces an atrial gallop rhythm.

Auscultation provides the opportunity to assess cardiac rhythm which, in the majority of normal horses, has a regular cyclical pattern. In the dog, and to a lesser degree in the horse, the rhythm is influenced to a variable degree by respiratory activity (sinus arrhythmia). Slight variations in cardiac rhythm may only be detected by prolonged, concentrated auscultation. With irregularity there are usually variations in the time intervals between successive cycles, and in the volume of the sounds, louder sounds occurring immediately after significant pauses, and softer than normal sounds after shortened intervals. Simultaneously taking the pulse and auscultating the heart will indicate when there is a deficit, i.e. fewer pulse waves than cardiac cycles (extrasystole). Extrasystolic cardiac contractions occur prematurely before the next regular contraction is expected. They are introduced in an arbitrary manner, by extrinsic stimuli, into the normal rhythm that originates in the sino-auricular node. Such premature contractions are usually followed by a prolonged compensatory diastolic period.

Well-established irregularities in the cardiac rhythm indicate a varying degree of dissociation of the action of the auricles from that of the ventricles, on account of disturbances in the function of the intrinsic conduction mechanism (S–A node and A–V node and bundle of His). The significance of any disturbance in cardiac rhythm can be investigated further by means of electrocardiography. Otherwise, in the horse and dog, auscultation before and after exercise will frequently reveal significant rhythm defects by reason of the obvious increase in their severity that occurs as the result of physical exertion. An estimation of cardiac reserve can be made by the same means in an animal with heart disease.

The criteria for making the assessment include the heart rate before and after exercise, the time required for the rate to return to the resting frequency, the intensity of the heart sounds and the characters of the pulse.

Adventitious Heart Sounds (Murmurs)

These may replace one or both heart sounds, or accompany them. They may originate in the cavities of the heart of from the pericardium. Those that arise from inside the heart are classified as murmurs, and are caused by endocardial lesions such as valvular vegetations or adhesions, by valvular insufficiency and by abnormal orifices such as ventricular septal defect or patent ductus arteriosus. Cardiac murmurs caused by these conditions may be hissing, humming, whirring or even markedly vibrant in tone. They are produced when blood flows rapidly through a restricted opening. Such narrow outlets for blood may be formed by stenosis (narrowing) of the valvular orifice, or by incomplete closure (insufficiency, incompetence) of the valve cusps. The murmur of stenosis is harsh and whirring in character, whereas that of incompetence is softer and hissing in tone.

Knowledge of the mechanisms concerned in the production of cardiovascular murmurs is not too certain. Turbulent blood flow is considered to be of primary importance, although more recently the concept of periodic wake fluctuations beyond a point of obstruction has been suggested as an alternative explanation. Irrespective of the cause, vibrations within the heart, secondary to altered blood flow, generate the murmurs.

It may be possible by appreciation of the character of the cardiac murmur to indicate the nature of the endocardial defect. In occasional instances, a valve may be both stenosed and incompetent. Theoretically, there are eight possible separate valvular defects, but several of the pathological possibilities are extremely rare in animals. The murmur arising from stenosis is produced when the valve is open, and that of insufficiency only when the valve is closed. Valvular endocardial murmurs are the result of acute and subacute bacterial endocarditis, chronic valvular endocarditis, valve fenestration, cardiac dilatation, neoplasia, and cardiac displacement.

Endocardial murmurs occur during either systole or diastole. Systolic murmurs indicate either stenosis of the semilunar valves or insufficiency of the atrioventricular valves. Diastolic murmurs suggest the opposite—either stenosis of the atrioventricular valves or insufficiency of the semilunar valves (Fig. 128).

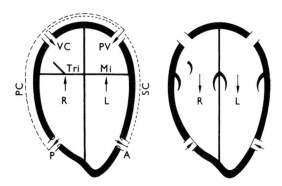

Fig. 128. *A diagram of the heart indicating the position of the valves and the direction of blood flow.* Right, *in systole*; left, *in diastole. R, right; L, left; Tri, tricuspid; Mi, mitral; P, pulmonary artery; A, aorta; PC, pulmonary circulation; SC, systemic circulation. VC, vena cava; PV, pulmonary vein.*

When the heart rate is relatively infrequent, as in the horse and ox, it is frequently possible to determine whether a murmur is systolic, or diastolic, in time. Simultaneous palpation of the pulse in the median artery, in conjunction with auscultation, may assist in determining the phase of its occurrence. The point of maximum audibility may suggest the valve which is affected (Fig. 129), but in addition other features, such as abnormalities of the pulse, may prove useful. Mitral murmurs in the horse are loudest on the left side in the fifth intercostal space; aortic murmurs are loudest on the left side in the fourth intercostal space, at the level of the point of the shoulder, and pulmonary murmurs on the left side in the third intercostal space, at the level of the olecranon process of the ulna. In ruminant species, mitral murmurs are loudest on the left side in the fourth intercostal space, and pulmonary murmurs similarly in the third intercostal space.

In the dog, identification of the origin of individual valvular murmurs is much more difficult than in the larger species because of the greater frequency of the cardiac cycle, the small size of the heart and its relatively more central position in the thorax. Mitral valve murmurs may be most intense in the fifth left intercostal space, at a point above the middle of the lower third of the thorax. Murmurs associated with lesions of the aortic valve may be heard most

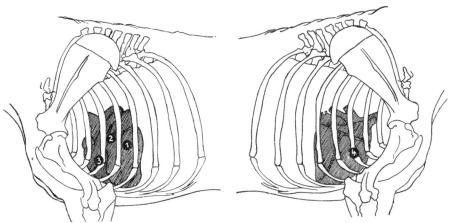

Fig. 129. *Sites of maximum audibility of organic endocardial sounds in the horse. 1, Mitral valve. 2, Aortic valve. 3, Pulmonary valve. 4, Tricuspid valve.* (After Marek)

distinctly in the fourth left intercostal space, just below a horizontal line through the point of the shoulder, and pulmonary valve murmurs are usually loudest in the third left intercostal space slightly below the point indicated for aortic murmurs.

Tricuspid valve murmurs are louder and clearer, on the right side, at the level of the costochondral junctions of the fourth intercostal space. When the heart is grossly enlarged or displaced the location of endocardial murmurs may vary considerably. Distortion of valve orifices by pressure on the heart, as in acute bloat or diaphragmatic hernia in cattle, is often associated with a loud systolic murmur.

In addition to endocardial murmurs of valvular origin, certain more or less distinctive murmurs originate from a variety of forms of congenital cardiac anomalies which cause clinical signs in young dogs more often than in other species. The continuous machinery murmur of patent ductus arteriosus may be heard, during both systole and diastole, over a wide area of the thorax but most intensely in the third left intercostal space in the region of the pulmonary valve. A murmur of this type occurring in young pigs during the first few days of life is thought to be caused by delayed closure of the ductus arteriosus. Shunting of blood from the left to the right side of the heart occurs in atrial septal and ventricular septal defects. In atrial septal defects, blood flows from the left to the right atrium, thereby increasing the right ventricular loading and producing relative pulmonary stenosis and a systolic murmur. In interventricular septal defect,

a relatively rare condition in animals, a harsh systolic murmur may be detected with, in large animals, a varying degree of vibration, which is most obvious towards the base of the heart.

Although murmurs are usually associated with valvular or developmental defects, they can occur in the absence of such lesions. Murmurs that originate in abnormalities of the valves or other cardiac structures are classified as organic, whereas those that occur in the absence of primary heart disease are termed functional or non-organic murmurs. Functional (haemic) murmurs, which are associated with debility, toxaemia or anaemia, wax and wane in intensity during the respiratory cycle, being loudest at the peak of inspiration. In anaemia, on account of the reduction in haemoglobin and erythrocyte population, the oxygen-carrying capacity of the blood is greatly reduced along with its viscosity, with the result that the circulation time is shortened in an attempt to prevent tissue hypoxia. The resulting increase in the rate of blood flow through the heart valve orifices produces audible sounds. Myocardial asthenia is also a significant cause of haemic murmurs.

The two types of murmurs can be differentiated in many instances. Functional murmurs are usually systolic, rather faint, are audible above the base of the heart and sometimes cannot be located within the cardiac area, and in the majority of cases disappear during convalescence. Organic murmurs, in contrast, are loud, either systolic or diastolic, audible at a precise phase in each cardiac cycle, can be located in the cardiac area, at least in large animals, and are usually accompanied by demonstrable enlargement of the heart with, in some cases, other signs of heart disease, e.g. congestive heart failure.

Pericardial Frictional Sounds

These sounds are caused by roughening of the pericardium and are not related to any particular phase of the cardiac cycle. In normal circumstances, movement of the heart within the pericardial sac produces no audible sound. When, however, two roughened, dry areas rub together, a 'friction' sound is created. Such sounds, which simulate those associated with roughening of the pleural membranes, are not very loud and occur during the early stages of pericarditis. The sounds are transient, usually disappearing when exudation separates and lubricates the dry, inflamed pericardial membranes. Rather obvious pericardial friction sounds are sometimes detected in tuberculous pericarditis in cattle, prior to adhesions developing. Frictional sounds originating in the pericardium are distinguished from those arising in the pleurae because the former can be related to the action of the heart, whereas the latter are synchronous with respiratory movements. Difficulty will arise concerning the source of origin when the respiratory and cardiac rates are about equal. It should be appreciated that friction sounds may originate from both membranes simultaneously when they are involved in an inflammatory process. Succussion (fluid) sounds will originate in the pericardium when the sac contains sufficient fluid so that it is set in motion by the movements of the heart. In this situation the normal heart sounds are muffled. Tinkling sounds in the cardiac area indicate the presence of gas on the surface of fluid in the pericardial sac. This situation exists in traumatic pericarditis in cattle; gas production results from the presence of certain bacteria introduced following the entry of a foreign body.

Circulation Time and Cardiac Output

The efficiency of the heart and blood vessels in maintaining the circulation within the limits of normality can be assessed by estimating the circulation time, which is the interval required for blood to complete the circulatory circuit of the body. Although acceptable techniques for this have been developed in man, none of the tests are suitable for general clinical use in animals. Similar tests have been used to measure cardiac output, which may be expressed as stroke volume

or as minute volume. The simplest method consists of introducing a known quantity of a foreign substance into the venous circulation; at the same time blood is sampled continuously from an artery, and the samples analysed for the marker substance at 1-second intervals. Suitable marker substances include chromium-tagged erythrocytes, Evans blue (horses and cattle) and indocyanine green (sheep). The cardiac output is increased, with a corresponding decrease in the circulation time after exercise, during pyrexia and in anaemia. The reverse will be the case in congestive heart failure.

Blood Pressure

Determination of blood pressure in animals has not been adopted as a routine procedure for a number of reasons. Firstly, it is virtually impossible to cause animals to relax so that satisfactory basal pressure readings can be obtained. Secondly, the clinical significance of elevated blood pressure has not been satisfactorily established. In certain states, including shock and heart disease, and in surgical subjects, determination of the blood pressure would be of value in prognosis.

Two methods are available: the indirect method employing a sphygmomanometer with a modified pneumatic cuff, and the direct method consisting of the insertion of a needle into a suitable superficial artery. Blood pressure can be determined, indirectly, in the horse by applying the pneumatic cuff at the base of the tail, where the middle coccygeal artery is available, or to the foreleg for the median or the dorsal interosseous artery. For the dog, the brachial or the femoral artery may be chosen and the cuff wrapped around the upper part of the fore- or hindleg respectively, with the animal in lateral recumbency. The short length of the limb in small dogs, and the sudden decrease in the thickness of the hindleg between the hip and stifle regions, which is particularly marked in some breeds, e.g. dachshund, makes it difficult to apply, satisfactorily, even the cuff designed for young children. Variously modified cuffs are available for dogs.

The procedure for obtaining a blood pressure reading is similar to that for man. After application the cuff, attached by rubber tubing to a mercury or anaeroid manometer, is inflated by means of the pressure bulb until the lumen of the artery and the pulse wave have been obliterated beyond the point of applied pressure. With the fingers applied over the distal portion of the artery, the pressure is reduced very slowly until the pulse wave just reappears, at which point the manometric reading is noted. This can be regarded as the systolic pressure. By employing the stethoscope further information can be obtained. For this purpose the stethoscope is placed over the artery beneath the distal portion of the cuff, or preferably beyond this point. When the pressure of the cuff is reduced to the point at which blood is forced through the constricted vessel, distinct tapping sounds are heard which coincide with the arrival of the pulse pressure wave. The manometer reading at this point gives the systolic pressure. Further reduction in the pressure allows more blood to flow through, and the tone of the sounds becomes lower pitched and finally, before disappearing altogether, they are blurred and muffled. A pressure reading at this point gives the diastolic pressure. Special apparatus has been devised to increase the accuracy, or overcome some of the difficulties associated with blood pressure determinations in animals. These include Grant's capsule and photo-electric cell and capacitance microphone manometers.

Blood pressure readings obtained by indirect methods in the standing horse differ from the arterial pressure at the base of the heart. The specific gravity of mercury is about 13·6, and that of blood is between 1·05 and 1·06. For every 13 mm above or below the heart base that a blood pressure determination is made a figure of 1 mm Hg is added or subtracted by the weight of blood in the artery. Recordings obtained at the middle coccygeal artery indicate that the systolic pressure range is 85–135 mm Hg and the diastolic range is 40–70 mm Hg. In the median artery the corresponding figures are 145–195 and 105–150 mm Hg.

In untrained dogs, by the indirect auscultatory method, the diastolic pressure range extends from 60 to 125 mm Hg and the systolic pressure from 100 to 185 mm Hg. In trained dogs, these pressures are from 50 to 65 diastolic and 95 to 135 systolic.

The direct method of determining blood pressure involves inserting a suitable needle, connected to a mercury or an anaeroid manometer, into a suitable artery. This system, because of inbuilt inertia, is only sufficiently accurate to provide mean blood pressure estimations.

Through the medium of the largest possible size of needle, and more sensitive recording equipment, such as an electromanometer or pressure transducer, reasonably accurate systolic and diastolic pressure readings can be obtained.

A technique for needle insertion into the brachial artery in the horse and ox has been described. The site in the horse is located by detecting a pulse wave at the base of the neck. Otherwise, the point of needle insertion is established, according to the size of the animal, as being 7–10 cm medially from and the same distance dorsal to the point of the shoulder (Fig. 130). Following infiltration of the selected area with a local anaesthetic solution, arterial puncture is effected by means of a 14 or 15 WG needle, 20 cm long, with a very sharp point, and which is directed parallel to the long axis of the animal, at about 5° to the horizontal, to a depth varying from 10 to 18 cm. In lean cattle, the

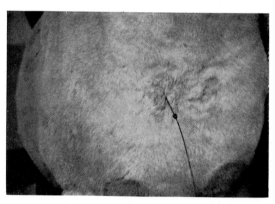

Fig. 130. *The site for percutaneous brachial artery puncture in the horse, showing the needle in the brachial artery* (E. W. Fisher (1961) Br. vet. J., *117*, 143).

brachial artery can be palpated by placing the hand, with the fingers extended in a vertical direction, immediately below the point of the shoulder. Following suitable preparation an 18 WG, long-pointed needle, 10 cm in length, is directed backwards at the point of arterial pulsation, or just medial to the point of the second finger and at about 15° to the horizontal (Fig. 131). The needle will penetrate to a depth of between 2 and 8 cm before the artery is reached. If venous blood is obtained, withdraw the needle for a short distance and reinsert it in a slightly more upward direction. In the dog the femoral artery is generally employed in making direct blood pressure determinations.

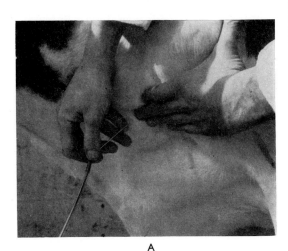
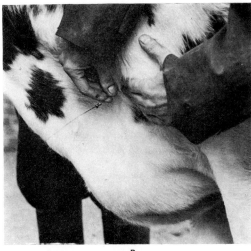

A   B

Fig. 131. *The site for percutaneous brachial artery puncture in the cow. Note the position of the hands and the direction of the needle.* (E. W. Fisher (1956) Vet. Rec., *68*, 691)

Cardiac catheterization is comparatively easily performed in unanaesthetized horses, cattle and dogs. The right heart and pulmonary artery are approached via the jugular vein, the blood pressures being determined, at appropriate points, by means of a pressure transducer coupled to the catheter. With a flexible catheter, the directional blood flow will readily carry the end of the instrument into the pulmonary artery. The left side of the heart in the horse is entered via the carotid or brachial artery; the former artery is also employed in the dog, and in both species a cut-down technique under local anaesthesia is necessary. A method of entering the left atrium has not yet been devised. During catheterization procedures, blood samples can be obtained from each of the blood vessels, and the heart chambers, for determination of oxygen saturation. This information, in conjunction with the blood pressure readings, may be of diagnostic value in recognizing the specific character of congenital vascular defects causing arteriovenous shunts, such as patent ductus arteriosus, septal defects, etc.

Venous pressure can be determined by the direct method at any point where a suitable superficial vein exists.

Radiological Examination of the Heart

Radiological methods of examining the heart are only practicable in small animals. The techniques that may be applied include fluoroscopy, radiography and angiocardiography. Standard data have not been produced in respect of heart size, but this lack does not preclude recognition of gross enlargement or significant displacement by these methods.

Fluoroscopy assists in the assessment of the position, silhouette and movements of the heart. Screening should be undertaken with the animal in the dorsoventral position; lateral viewing is generally not so informative. In cases of pericardial effusion, fluoroscopic examination will reveal an almost circular cardiac silhouette, with little or no movement of the heart shadow.

Radiographs provide a more accurate method for determining the cardiac outline, in the form of a reasonably permanent negative film from which prints can be made. In order to ensure a reasonable degree of accuracy in making such measurements, and for purposes of comparison, it is important to ensure that the X-ray tube is positioned at a constant distance, vertically above the central point of the heart for lateral exposures, and that the animal rests squarely on its sternum for dorsoventral exposures. Failure to subscribe to these requirements will result in varying degrees of distortion of the cardiac image on the film.

In heart disease the radiographic cardiac outline is quite often abnormal. It is unlikely, in many cases, however, that the nature of the cardiac disease could be recognized from the abnormal silhouette. In right-sided enlargement, which can be associated with pulmonary stenosis or tricuspid incompetence, a dorsoventral radiograph will show enlargement of the right sector of the cardiac shadow. In advanced myocardial asthenia with general cardiac dilatation, in patent ductus arteriosus and in pericardial effusion, the cardiac silhouette is circular. The information obtained by radiological means should be correlated in all instances with the condition of the pulmonary circulation as revealed by the lung fields and, most important of all, the clinical condition of the animal.

Radiological methods of examination are also of value in assisting diagnosis in certain types of congenital heart disease in dogs. In persistent right aortic arch (Fig. 132), following the administration of barium sulphate suspension, the

most cases results from incomplete medial closure of these structures. Loops of intestine, or other structures, may become displaced into the pericardial sac. Radiographic examination reveals what appears to be an abnormally enlarged cardiac silhouette, and oral administration of a contrast medium will assist identification when intestine is present.

Angiocardiography involves introducing a suitable radio-opaque substance into the blood entering the right atrium—this can be achieved by cardiac catheterization—and then exposing a series of radiographic films in rapid succession. The purpose of this technique is to study the condition and functional state of the heart valves

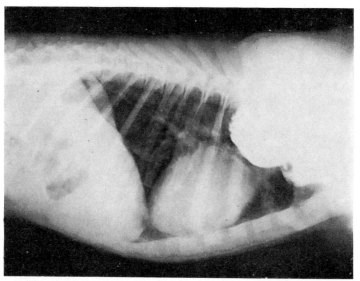

Fig. 132. *A radiograph of persistent right aortic arch in a dog. Note the pooling of the contrast medium in the grossly distended oesophagus, anterior to the point of constriction above the base of the heart.*

istration of barium sulphate suspension, the dilated oesophagus, anterior to the point of constriction caused by the pulmonary artery on the left, the base of the heart ventrally, the persistent right aortic arch on the right and the subclavian artery dorsally, is readily visualized fluoroscopically or radiographically. Pulmonary stenosis is a fairly common congenital cardiac defect in the dog; in this case the heart shadow shows enlargement of the right atrium and ventricle. A rare condition involving the heart has been recognized in dogs and cats; it occurs in conjunction with diaphragmatic pericardial hernia, which in

and cavities. It is generally only adopted for research investigations and is rarely employed in veterinary clinical work

Electrocardiography

Electrocardiography (Fig. 133) provides for very accurate diagnosis of certain functional abnormalities of the heart. The method has been most extensively employed in the horse and dog; although it has been applied in other species, including cattle, sheep and goats, the necessity to do so is rather limited. Electrocardiography is not to be regarded as a substitute for an adequate

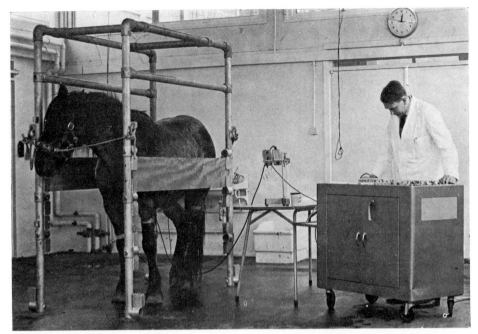

Fig. 133. *Electrocardiography in the horse. The animal is restrained in stocks. Plate electrodes are attached to the legs above the knees and hocks. The leads from these are shown extending to the electrocardiograph via a preamplifier.*

clinical examination, but rather as a supplementary method of examination in selected cases, when a cardiac defect, which merits further investigation, is so identified. The resulting electrocardiogram (Fig. 134) should be interpreted by the clinician and correlated to the clinical picture presented by the animal. It is advisable, therefore, for the clinician to possess some knowledge of the principles involved in electrocardiography and to be conversant with the main features of the normal and abnormal electrocardiogram.

By means of amplifiers and very sensitive electronic measuring devices coupled to a direct writing, recording apparatus, the electrocardiograph reveals, in a magnified form, the differences in electrical potential which are generated by the waves of depolarization and repolarization which traverse the atria and ventricles during cardiac systole and diastole. These electrical potentials radiate to points on the surface of the body. In general, a positive or upward deflection on the electrocardiogram occurs when depolarization causes a wave of electric potential to travel towards an electrode on the surface of the body. A negative (downward) deflection is recorded when the depolarization wave is

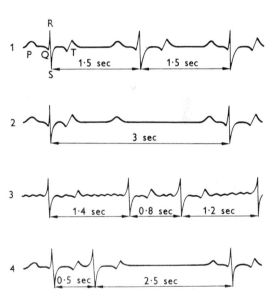

Fig. 134. *The electrocardiogram of the horse. 1, Three normal cycles. P, auricular; QRS, ventricular; T, termination of ventricular contraction. 2, Heart block, second grade. In the second cardiac cycle the whole of the ventricular contraction is absent, only the auricular contraction being shown. 3, Auricular fibrillation; numerous contractions of the ventricle. 4, Extrasystole immediately following the first heart beat, with a subsequent compensating pause.*

travelling away from the electrode. Changes of potential arising from a wave of repolarization are negative when recorded while travelling towards an electrode and positive when moving away.

A primary difference in electrical potential is created when myocardial contraction commences in the atria and is later repeated in the case of the ventricles. When the whole of the component area is in a state of contraction, an isoelectric state intervenes, but as the contractile state disappears from that part of the myocardium first involved, a secondary difference of electrical potential occurs. As these differences in electrical potential correspond to each wave of depolarization and repolarization they will produce a deflection which is opposite in direction. The electrocardiograph provides a time/distance recording (electrocardiogram) of the changes in electrical potential generated in the heart during any arbitrary period. The currents are collected and directed to the measuring device by means of electrodes which are applied to selected parts of the body surface.

Reliable results, providing for more accurate interpretation, can only be obtained when a standardized electrocardiographic technique is employed. This involves ensuring that the animal remains quiet and is not subjected to excitatory stimuli and, in the case of the dog, employing a uniform posture, preferably right lateral recumbency. The use of sedatives should be avoided and gentle handling practised. Positioning the animal on a thick rubber mat ensures that interference will be minimized. It is also essential to use recognized sites on the surface of the body for the application of the electrodes. The sites should preferably be clipped, and, following the application of an electrode paste, the metal electrode plates are fixed in position by means of suitable rubber bands (needle electrodes may be preferred). The standard bipolar limb leads are attached to the two forelegs and the left hindleg. For electrocardiographic purposes the three electrodes may be selected for use in the following manner: Lead I is derived from the right and left forelegs; Lead II from the right foreleg and the left hindleg; and Lead III from the left foreleg and left hindleg. In addition to the standard bipolar limb leads, so-called unipolar limb leads, augmented unipolar limb leads and precordial leads of the semipolar or unipolar variety may be found useful. Unipolar limb leads,

which are not commonly employed, are obtained by connecting three of the limb electrodes to one pole of the galvanometer and the fourth electrode to the opposite pole. Augmented unipolar limb leads are obtained by pairing any two of the three limb leads used in the standard bipolar limb leads against the third limb which is also connected to the opposite pole of the galvanometer. In the precordial leads an exploratory electrode is placed on various locations on the chest and paired with an electrode, or group of electrodes, located at some distance from the heart. The lead selector switch on the modern electrocardiograph enables records of the bipolar limb leads and augmented unipolar limb leads to be readily obtained once the limb electrodes are attached. Provision is made to earth the animal by means of an electrode attached to the right hindleg, and connected to the electrocardiograph.

By convention the various component waves in the electrocardiogram, which can be related to specific events in the cardiac cycle, are labelled P, Q, R, S and T (Fig. 134). Furthermore the use of graph-type recording paper, which can be made to travel at a range of selected speeds, permits study of the rate, rhythm, elapsed time sequence and electrical potential variations occurring in relation to the heart cycle. It is, however, necessary to remember when interpreting electrocardiographic recordings that the direction taken by the waves of electrical potential is determined by the anatomical position of the heart and the course of excitation throughout the myocardium. These factors vary as between species, so that although the direction of the P waves is similar in the horse and dog, the form of the ventricular complex in comparable leads is not the same in these two species.

The P wave corresponds to the process of excitation (depolarization) spreading from the sino-atrial node and causing contraction of the atria. In the horse, ox and dog, it is positive and pointed at the summit, but even in normal animals of these species it may be diphasic (notched or slurred). The P wave sometimes shows changes in amplitude, and even in form, with respiration (sinus arrhythmia) in the dog. It is always positive during inspiration in lead II; if it remains inverted during all phases of respiration with this lead it is abnormal. The duration of the most significant electrocardiographic intervals is given in Table 10. The data relate to recordings obtained from lead II. The P interval corres-

TABLE 10. DURATION OF ELECTROCARDIOGRAPHIC INTERVALS IN ANIMALS, LEAD 11*

Species	P	P–R	QRS	Q–T
Horse	0·08–0·16 (0·12)	0·19–0·39 (0·28)	0·07–0·14 (0·10)	0·34–0·57 (0·45)
Cattle	—	0·10–0·30 (0·19)	0·06–0·12 (0·09)	0·29–0·47 (0·39)
Dog	—	0·06–0·13 (0·10)	0·04–0·07 (0·05)	0·14–0·21 (0·18)

* Range in seconds; average shown in parentheses.

ponds to the time taken for depolarization of the ventricles to occur and is followed by the QRS (ventricular) complex. The Q wave is usually small and negative, R is usually more pronounced and positive, S is a negative deflection similar to Q. The P–R interval, which extends from the beginning of P to the commencement of the QRS complex, corresponds to the period during which the contractile stimulus spreads from the sino-atrial node to the bundle of His and the musculature of the ventricles. The QRS complex is followed by an isoelectric period which is succeeded by the T wave representing repolarization of the myocardium during the last stages of ventricular systole. The Q–T interval extends from the commencement of QRS to the end of T and corresponds to the time during which ventricular excitation and recovery takes place.

Electrocardiographic studies enable precise determinations to be made in respect of heart rate and rhythm, while at the same time providing a written record which will permit further study in order to detect any departure from normal. It is necessary to appreciate, however, that an abnormality in an electrocardiogram is not a disease; it may suggest the presence of disease which can only be identified on a clinical basis. Electrocardiographic examination before, and again after, exercise may provide more helpful information in some instances.

The rate of conduction of the excitation stimulus for cardiac contraction can be assessed by measuring the duration of the P–R interval. In first degree (incomplete) heart block, the P–R interval may be extended to one and a half times its normal duration, and failure of the ventricles to contract, which may only occur at irregular intervals, can be correlated to the absent QRS complex. In incipient cases of first-degree heart block in the horse, the condition may be more readily revealed during electrocardiography by applying a nose twitch, or exercising the animal, and then taking another recording. When heart block is almost complete (second-degree) the P waves occur more frequently and regularly in the ECG than the QRS complexes, which are usually irregular. In many such instances 2, 3, or 4 P waves may occur to each QRS complex. In third degree or complete heart block there may be a rapid sequence of small P waves indicating atrial flutter, or displacement of the P waves by a very rapid, continuous sequence of small modulation in atrial fibrillation. The QRS complex, in the ECG obtained from a case of atrial flutter, frequently appears at regular intervals, being one-half to one-third of the P wave frequency. In atrial fibrillation, contractile impulses occur at the rate of several hundred per minute, and the electrocardiogram indicates that the ventricular contraction rate is less than normal, with rhythmic irregularity, and on exercise shows a disproportionately reduced increase in rate. Atrial premature beats are characterized in the electrocardiogram by a P wave occurring earlier than would occur in normal sinus rhythm. If the contractile impulse originates in the atrium outside the sino-atrial node, then the P wave is abnormal; indeed if it originates from within the left atrium it will be negative in those leads in which it is normally positive.

The excursion of the waves in the electrocardiogram is a measure of the electropotential of the myocardium and, therefore, it is related to muscular effort. Ventricular hypertrophy, which occurs most commonly in racehorses, is indicated when, in lead II, the R wave shows increased amplitude, thereby extending the period of duration of the QRS complex. The potentiality for left ventricular hypertrophy to develop is much greater than that of the right-sided variety.

In bundle-branch block the contractile impulse is delayed or blocked in one or other branch of the bundle of His, so that there is a delay in contraction of the ventricle supplied by the defective branch. When the block is extensive, the ventricles contract asynchronously. The electrocardiogram in bundle-branch block reflects the delayed transmission of the excitation impulse in that the R wave may be bifurcated, or notched, on the down stroke. Otherwise the condition may be detected by comparing the P–R intervals obtained by the different leads. Ventricular premature beats give rise to QRS complexes of increased magnitude and prolonged duration, and may be followed by a compensatory pause.

Phonocardiography

By means of phonocardiography a graphic recording of the heart sounds can be obtained for visual comparison with known normal phonocardiograms. The basic constituents of a phonocardiograph include a microphone, audio-amplifier and recording galvanometer, in association with a time recording system which produces a pulse curve, or an electrocardiogram. Filter systems are included in order that the higher frequency components are sufficiently amplified to be visible, and the lower ones attenuated in comparison with a linear phonocardiogram. Without the inclusion of appropriate filters the linear record will also contain a high proportion of waves produced by sounds outside the range of average human hearing.

10

The Abdomen and Associated Digestive Organs

The abdominal cavity, the middle one of the three, is the largest of the body cavities. Externally its anterior part merges with the thorax at the costal arch where, internally, it is separated from the thoracic cavity by the diaphragm. It is continuous posteriorly with the structures comprising the pelvis; internally the demarcation line between the abdominal and pelvic cavities is formed by the brim of the pelvis, comprising the base of the sacrum dorsally, the iliopectineal lines laterally and the anterior border of the pubes ventrally.

Comparatively, the abdomen has a greater capacity in ruminant species than in the horse. The cavity of the abdomen, which is slightly compressed laterally, is ovoid in general form with its greatest axis extending from the concavity of the diaphragm to the pelvic inlet. The roof is formed by the upper part of the diaphragm, the lumbar vertebrae and the lumbar muscles. The wall is comprised of the transverse and oblique abdominal muscles, the abdominal tunic, the upper, anterior parts of the ilia, the parts of the posterior ribs which extend below the attachment of the diaphragm and the costal cartilages of the retrosternal ribs. The floor consists of the xiphoid cartilage of the sternum, the two recti muscles, the aponeuroses of the transverse and oblique abdominal muscles and the abdominal tunic. The anterior boundary is formed by the diaphragm, the convexity of which projects forward limiting the size of the thoracic cavity.

The abdominal cavity is lined by a thin serous membrane, the peritoneum, which is continued to a somewhat variable extent into the pelvic cavity. The peritoneum is reflected from the internal surface of the abdominal cavity on to the visceral organs, which are thereby covered to a greater or lesser extent.

Alimentary Tract Dysfunction

Some of the primary functions of the alimentary tract, including prehension, mastication and deglutition of food and water, have already been considered. Other major activities, such as digestion, absorption and excretion, which are the normal functions of the stomach and intestines, must now receive consideration. The significance of these functions, which are related to stabilizing the internal environment of the animal, can be realized by appreciating that almost without exception all its nutritional and functional requirements are processed by the digestive tract.

Alimentary tract dysfunction is an expression of derangement of one or more of the following: motility, secretion, digestion, absorption. In clinical diagnosis the primary consideration should be to recognize which of these functions is or are deranged.

Gastrointestinal motility, consisting of peristaltic movements and segmentation movements, and of which sphincter tone is an important component, depends upon balanced functioning of the sympathetic and parasympathetic nervous systems, together with that of the intrinsic nerve plexuses. Imbalance of the autonomic nerves, which can result from stimulation or damage to any of the component parts, is manifested by hypermotility or hypomotility. The change in the pattern of motility may be widespread or segmental in extent. Hypermotility causes diarrhoea; hypomotility is responsible for constipation. In segmental hypermotility there may be a reversal of the normal downward gradient from the stomach to the rectum, so that retroperistalsis is produced, proceeding to vomition.

Abnormalities of motility lead to distension of the stomach and/or intestine because of ineffective eructation of gas (more likely when gas accumulates rapidly), occlusion of the tract lumen by obstruction or displacement, or engorgement on solid or liquid foods. Overdistension of the gastrointestinal tract causes pain with reflex spasm and increased motility of adjoining segments. The distension is exaggerated because it leads to increased secretion of fluid into the lumen of the affected part.

Secretory dysfunction by the alimentary tract is a rare event in large animals. Recognizable syndromes arising from defective gastric and pancreatic secretion occur occasionally in dogs and cats.

Digestion is dependent on both the secretory and the motor functions of the alimentary tract. In herbivorous animals the activity of the microflora (in the forestomach compartments of ruminant species, or the caecum and colon of equine species) plays a significant role in the digestion of cellulose and nitrogenous substances. Impairment of microbial digestion can result from dietary imbalance, inadequate food, inappetence, derangement of ruminal pH or oral administration of antibiotics or specific antibacterial drugs in ruminant animals.

The absorptive functions of the intestinal tract will be impaired to a variable degree by hypermotility or by damage to the mucous membrane. These two states not infrequently coexist, but significant degrees of damage to the mucosa may occur, without hypermotility, in some forms of intestinal helminth infestations.

General Clinical Examination

Diseases of the digestive system are of frequent occurrence in domestic animals and, with the development of even more intensive production methods, or their wider application, may increase in incidence still further. Because many of the organs concerned, more particularly those situated within the abdominal cavity, are of relatively large size and are inaccessible, recognition of the situation and nature of any disease process is usually more difficult to establish

than when other parts of the body are involved. As a consequence, it is necessary to give careful consideration to all aspects of behaviour associated with digestive function. In this context, attention has already been directed to such features as physical condition, appetite for food and fluid, the oral cavity, deglutition and vomiting. Furthermore, the enquiries made when the history was being elicited included consideration of the excretory functions of the intestine, as indicated by the volume and character of the faeces. Correlating the history and behavioural signs with the clinical findings, and assessing the information so obtained on the basis of the disturbances of function mentioned earlier will assist diagnosis.

The clinical examination of the abdomen consists of external examination, comprising inspection, palpation, percussion and auscultation, and internal examination, which includes rectal exploration, exploratory puncture, peritoneoscopy and, in small animals, radiography.

Inspection provides an opportunity to assess the relative size of the abdomen and determine the presence of localized conditions. In the upper part of the flank, in the normal abdomen, it is usual to note a depression in the so-called paralumbar fossa or 'hunger hollow'. This is particularly obvious in ruminant species, including cattle and goats, and is slightly larger on the right side than on the left. Undulating movements, corresponding to the motility of the underlying rumen, may be observed on the left side.

The abdomen may appear distended, of normal size or reduced in capacity. An increase in the size or circumference of the abdomen (Fig. 135)

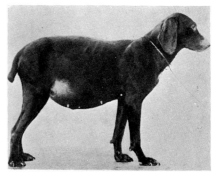

Fig. 135. *An increase in the circumference of the abdomen as a result of accumulation of fluid in the peritoneal cavity. Dropsy (ascites).*

occurs from varying causes, including advanced pregnancy, flatulence, distension of the rumen or stomach, tumours of the liver, spleen, lymph nodes, etc., diseases of the uterus (hydrometra, pyometra, etc.), urinary retention and accumulation of fluid in the peritoneal cavity (ascites, ruptured bladder, exudative peritonitis). In gaseous distension, the increase in size is more or less uniform, although in ruminal bloat the distension is greatest over the left flank. When gaseous distension of the intestine is severe the affected loops of bowel may cause distinctive bulging in the flank region.

In advanced pregnancy, and when there is fluid accumulation, the distension is most noticeable in the dependent part of the abdomen, the paralumbar fossae being considerably deepened. Fetal movements may be observed through the abdominal wall in advanced pregnancy—on either side in the mare and on the right side in the cow. Ruminal movements are often quite obvious by their influence on the left flank, but the frequency and quality of the movements are not readily assessed by inspection. If fluid is free in the peritoneal cavity, changes in the posture of the animal alter the position of the fluid, the altered conditions being appreciated by means of percussion, which reveals, by the production of a non-resonant sound, that the fluid always gravitates to the most dependent part. When the fluid causing abdominal distension is enclosed in a sac, or a hollow organ, percussion indicates that changes in posture have no influence on its relative position.

The degree of abdominal distension associated with faecal or urinary retention is, even in extreme cases, of moderate degree only. Enlargement of the abdomen caused by neoplasia involving the spleen, liver, ovary or other organ is generally only recognized in the advanced stages, and then usually only in the dog and cat. With tumours, more particularly when superficial structures are involved, hernias, abscesses and haematomas, there may be a frankly localized swelling (Fig. 136). Oedematous swelling of the ventral abdomen occurs in congestive heart failure, acute gangrenous mastitis, infectious equine anaemia, rupture of the penile urethra due to obstructive urolithiasis or malapplication of a crushing type castrator, and as an expression of hypoproteinaemia in the terminal stages of pregnancy, particularly in young mares and heifers.

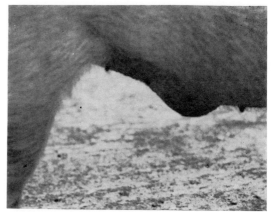

Fig. 136. *Localized swelling of the abdomen in a pig. Umbilical hernia.*

A decrease in the circumference of the abdomen, resulting in a tucked-up, 'herring-gutted' or gaunt appearance, is observed in prolonged malnutrition, in many chronic diseases with reduced appetite and in diseases associated with prolonged, severe dehydration (enteritis) or marked disturbance of the tissue fluid balance of the body, notably subacute grass sickness of horses (Fig. 137). Note should also be taken of any

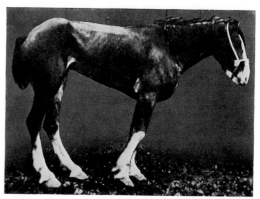

Fig. 137. *A decrease in the circumference of the abdomen, giving a 'herring-gutted' appearance. Subacute grass sickness.*

change in the anatomical conformation of the bony prominences such as 'knocked-down' hips —a possible indication of calcium or phosphorus deficiency (Fig. 138).

External palpation of the abdomen provides limited information in the horse. Its object is to ascertain the size and shape of the various organs, the character of the intestinal contents and the detection of any pain focus. As a rule horses

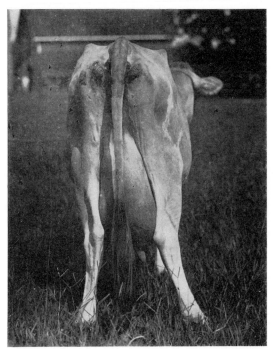

Fig. 138. *Knocked down hips as a result of calcium deficiency.* (Florida Agricultural Experiment Station Bulletin No. 262)

abdomen in peritonitis, and over the upper half of the last 3 or 4 ribs, on the right side, in various forms of subacute and acute hepatitis. In traumatic reticuloperitonitis, the existence of a painful lesion can often be demonstrated by applying firm, upward pressure in the hypogastric region at the point where the diaphragm is attached to the upper surface of the xiphoid cartilage (Fig. 139), whereupon the animal arches its back slightly, moves sideways, kicks and groans. Pal-

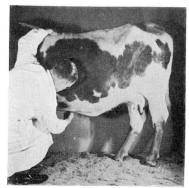

Fig. 139. *Testing for pain by applying pressure in the xiphisternal region of the ox (traumatic reticuloperitonitis).*

intensify the tone of the abdominal musculature during the examination and this together with the thickness of the abdominal wall, prohibits deep palpation of the abdomen. The whole hand, or closed fist, should be placed firmly in contact with the abdomen and held in place until a degree of muscular relaxation occurs, and then either a firm punch or jab applied for the purpose of detecting superficial pain. When deep-seated pain is suspected a firm, even application of pressure is required. This examination is made on both sides.

The abdominal musculature is much less tense in cattle, and palpation over the rumen in the left flank yields much useful information concerning motility and the amount and consistency of the rumen contents. Large tumours, or extensive areas of mesenteric or omental fat necrosis situated near the abdominal wall, and in advanced pregnancy parts of the fetus may be recognized by this means. In cattle in lean condition the upper right border of the liver, when the organ is enlarged, may be detectable by palpation behind the upper part of the right costal arch. A pain reaction may be elicited generally over the

pation of the abdominal wall is painful also in rumenitis and in inflammatory conditions of other abdominal organs.

In sheep and pigs, a suitable degree of relaxation of the abdominal musculature to permit palpation can not be obtained; in the latter species, the thickness of the abdominal wall is a further obstacle. Both species will, however, evince a pain reaction to palpation of any part of the abdomen in peritonitis.

Palpation of the abdomen is most satisfactorily performed in the dog and cat by reason of it being possible to identify many of the intra-abdominal organs. The examination should be made with the animal standing on a table with a non-slip surface; muscular tension is greatly increased and is difficult to overcome if the animal is apprehensive by reason of uncertain footing. If the dog is too large, or it is considered undesirable to place it on a table, the examination is made with it on the floor, the clinician sitting on a stool behind, and slightly to one side. During palpation, both hands, with the fingers firmly extended together, are placed one on each side of the abdomen, the thumb of each hand

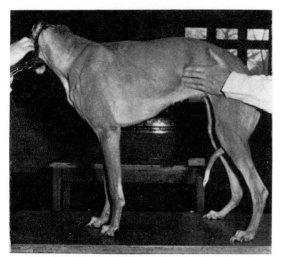

Fig. 140. *External palpation of the abdomen in the dog.*

pointing upwards (Fig. 140). Gentle pressure is applied and then gradually increased until the tension of the muscles disappears and the underlying organs can be identified. The procedure should be applied in a methodical manner over the whole area of the abdomen. Generally speaking, the gentler the palpation, the more readily the organs can be recognized and the more expeditiously the examination is made.

In obese animals abdominal palpation is unrewarding and in those with a nervous disposition it may be resented. A long period of continuous gentle palpation may prove successful, otherwise administration of a sedative or tranquillizing drug may be required. In such circumstances it must be appreciated that the animal may not react when pressure is applied over a pain focus. Abdominal pain occurs in a variety of inflammatory conditions including peritonitis, hepatitis, splenitis, nephritis, lymphadenitis, etc. Its presence is indicated by greater than usual tension of the abdominal musculature which is suddenly greatly increased when the painful area is approached. Observation of the animal may have revealed that the back is arched, and that it made voice sounds indicating pain when defaecating or urinating and during palpation.

Undulation ('fluid wave') can be demonstrated by a combination of percussion and palpation when the peritoneal cavity contains a large volume of fluid, as in ascites, exudative peritonitis, and rupture of the urinary or gall-bladder.

For the dog and cat, the palm of one hand is placed firmly against the side of the abdomen, and the opposite side is percussed at various levels with the fingertips of the other hand. The impact of any wave currents produced in the fluid by the finger taps is detected when they impinge on the palm of the hand that is applied to the abdominal wall. In large animals an assistant is required to generate the wave currents by strong percussion. A combination of finger percussion and auscultation may be employed for the detection of fluid motion in place of the more orthodox method. Wave motion of this type can be demonstrated only when there is sufficient volume of fluid present, and it does not completely fill the peritoneal cavity.

Percussion of the abdomen generally provides limited information of diagnostic value. It is, however, possible to distinguish areas where the percussion note is loud or tympanic, from those where it is dull, and thus determine whether the underlying structure is a gas-filled portion of the alimentary tract, or a solid organ. A dull sound is obtained over the impacted stomach or intestine, over the spleen and liver, over neoplasms and where there is an accumulation of fluid in the peritoneal cavity. In the last condition, the upper margin of the dull area is horizontal and, if the posture of the animal is changed, the dullness is always located at the most dependent part of the abdomen.

The sounds produced by the functional motility of the intra-abdominal portion of the digestive tract are detected by auscultating over the wall of the abdomen. When examining the larger animals in this way, the clinician should face caudally and run the hand along the dorsal part of the neck over the withers and back and down over the abdominal wall, pressing lightly, to prepare the animal for the application of the stethoscope. When the instrument has been applied to the abdominal wall (Fig. 141) it is necessary to listen for at least 30 seconds because the motility sounds (borborygmi) are not continuous at any one point, but occur at intervals of from 10 to 20 seconds or longer. Normal peristaltic and segmentation sounds have gurgling, murmuring or rumbling characteristics. They are often loud enough to be audible some distance away from the animal. The type of sound reflects the character of the intestinal contents, which may be solid, semi-solid, liquid or gaseous, and the pattern of motility. According

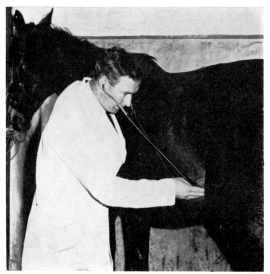

Fig. 141. *Auscultation of intestinal sounds (borborygmi) in the horse.*

to the frequency of the sounds, motility is described as active, sluggish, infrequent or absent. The activity of the rumen and reticulum, which can be investigated by means of palpation and auscultation, will be considered during the detailed examination of the abdomen in the ruminant species.

Rectal Examination

Rectal examination is the process of palpating the interior of the pelvis and posterior abdomen by means of a hand or finger introduced into the rectum through the anus. For aesthetic and hygienic reasons, a shoulder-length rubber or plastic glove or a finger-stall should be worn. In large animals, the examination may necessarily involve introducing the whole length of the arm into the rectum. The protective glove or finger-stall should be thoroughly lubricated with soap, bland oil, petroleum jelly or a suitable proprietary obstetrical cream; some of the last have the advantage of being readily removable, even in cold water. This last is of no account in the case of disposable plastic items. Suitable restraint should be used which, in the horse, may consist of lifting up a foreleg or applying a twitch. For obviously fractious horses more effective safeguards, consisting of side lines, service hobbles or stocks, are essential. Rectal examination in cattle can usually be performed with the animal tied in a stall and further restrained by an

assistant standing against one side and holding the tail.

The prepared, glove-covered hand is introduced through the anal sphincter by extending the fingers, which are held together to form a cone with the thumb directed towards the base of the middle finger. The tone of the anal sphincter is reduced by gentle insertion of the fingers, and the hand is then inserted with a rotatory movement. Many horses resent this action but once the hand passes beyond the anal sphincter, manipulations which do not engender pain, cause no resentment. Force must be avoided, and forward pressure applied with considerable caution. When the animal strains, no resistance must be offered; the arm should relax immediately and allow itself to be pushed backwards by the mounting intra-abdominal pressure, as otherwise it is likely that the intestinal wall will be perforated. This catastrophe is invariably fatal in the horse. Palpation is performed with the open hand, the extended fingers being maintained in close apposition, or with the closed fist. If, on introducing the hand, the rectum is found to be filled with faeces these should be removed before proceeding.

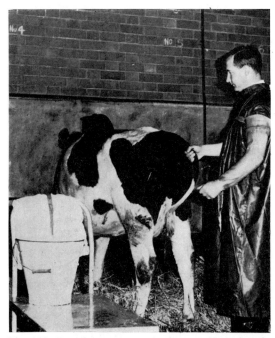

Fig. 142. *Rectal examination in the cow. Note that the operator is wearing a shoulder-length rubber glove, protective gown and rubber boots.*

Irrespective of whether a protective glove is worn or not, it is advisable to clip the fingernails quite short and, as a further safety measure, to fill the free edges with soap. In all cases, to avoid soiling the clothing, and in the interests of personal hygiene and disease control, the clinician should don a sleeve protector and a rubber apron or gown, which can be washed and disinfected immediately after use (Fig. 142; see also Fig. 172, p. 246).

To reduce excessive straining during rectal examination the following expedients can be adopted: enemas of lukewarm water; elevating the animal's head; applying pressure with the thumbs in the lumbar region; administering a sedative or tranquillizing drug; induction of low epidural anaesthesia.

In small animals, rectal exploration involves the same principles as in the larger species. It is obvious that, with this method of examination the information obtained in the large animals is much more extensive than that obtainable from the small species in which, at best, only the pelvic inlet is reached with the finger. The deficiencies of rectal examination in the small animal are, however, more than made good by the results obtained from external abdominal palpation.

General Anatomical Considerations

At this point in the clinical examination procedure it is expedient to consider the anatomical character and topographical arrangement and relationships of the organs and viscera situated within the abdominal cavity in the different species of domestic animals. Some of the important organs are the stomach, intestines, liver, spleen and their supporting structures the omentum and mesentery, in which are situated the associated lymph nodes, as well as the kidneys, uterus and pancreas. The bladder, when distended with urine, extends for a variable distance into the abdomen. Externally, in male animals of all the domestic species, with the exception of the cat, the prepuce, accommodating the free portion of the penis when retracted, is situated in the posterior part of the ventral abdomen. The testes in the stallion, bull and ram are situated in the inguinal region of the abdomen, as is the mammary gland in the mare, cow and ewe. In the sow, bitch and female cat the mammary glands, which vary in number, form two rows parallel to and a short distance away from the midline of the ventral abdomen.

The anatomical relationships, and in certain instances the physiological function of the organs within the abdominal cavity vary as between the different species of domestic animals. The difficulties in clinical diagnosis that arise from these factors become obvious during the physical examination, and are increased by the limiting influence of the abdominal wall and, in some species, the large size of the organs.

ABDOMEN OF THE HORSE

Internal Regional Anatomy

In the horse the stomach, even when distended with food, is relatively small; it is situated mainly to the left of the median plane of the body, in the concavity of the diaphragm immediately behind the liver. The major portion of the small intestine, with the exception of the duodenum and terminal segment of the ileum, is supported by relatively long folds of mesentery, so that its loops vary greatly in position; the major part is usually situated in contact with the abdominal wall on the left side, a few coils may reach the floor of the abdomen. The supporting mesentery originates from the roof of the abdomen beneath the first and second lumbar vertebrae. At no point is it possible to recognize small intestine by palpation through the abdominal wall. The various parts of the large intestine, comprising the caecum, the large colon, the small colon and the rectum, with the exception of the small colon which has a long supporting mesentery, are usually found to occupy a relatively static position. The rounded base of the caecum is situated in the right iliac and sublumbar region while the comma-shaped body which extends downwards and forwards, almost entirely fills the right flank area. The blind apex of the caecum reaches the abdominal floor to the right of the median plane, behind the xiphoid cartilage. The ileocaecal orifice is situated on the anterior concave curvature of the base, with the caecocolic orifice placed about 5 cm away in a lateral direction.

The first part of the large colon, the right ventral colon, originates from the concave base of the caecum opposite the lower extremity of the last rib or intercostal space. It then passes downwards and forwards, contiguous to the right costal arch, and continues along the floor of the abdomen where, above the xiphoid cartilage, it turns medially and then backwards on the abdominal floor, on the left of the right ventral colon, until it reaches the pelvic inlet. Here it bends acutely upwards and forwards, forming the pelvic flexure, and continues as the left dorsal colon, the lumen of which is greatly reduced in size compared with that of the two ventral segments. The left dorsal colon is immediately dorsal to the left ventral segment; it passes somewhat downwards and forwards opposite the middle section of the left flank to run medial to the costal arch, and reach the diaphragm and left lobe of the liver, where it bends medially to the right, and then backwards to form the diaphragmatic flexure. The terminal part, the right dorsal colon, extends backwards dorsal to the right ventral segment, until it reaches the medial aspect of the caecum where it bends to the left and dorsally, to a point below the left kidney, where it becomes reduced in diameter and becomes confluent with the small colon.

The small colon, which is about 3–3·5 m in length, commences behind the stomach, ventral to the left kidney, where it is attached in the sublumbar region by a long mesentery. The coils lie mainly between the stomach and pelvic inlet, dorsal to the left segments of the large colon, in which situation they mingle with loops of small intestine, and make contact with the abdominal wall in the left flank area. The small colon continues as the rectum at the pelvic inlet. The rectum, which is about 30 cm in length, is often situated slightly to the left of the median plane in the pelvis, where it is related anteriorly to the pelvic flexure of the large colon, and loops of the small colon. The retroperitoneal part of the rectum is related dorsally and laterally to the pelvic wall. Ventrally, in the male, it is in contact with the urinary bladder, the seminal vesicles, the terminations of the vasa deferentes, the prostate gland, the bulbo-urethral glands and the pelvic portion of the urethra. In the female this relationship is with the uterus, vagina and vulva.

The structurally important features of the gastrointestinal tract in the horse are the relatively small size of the stomach, the situation of the entry and exit orifices of the double blind-ended caecum, the sudden reduction in the diameter at two points in the large intestine and, in the case of the last, the longitudinal muscle bands in the wall of the caecum and colon. This feature can be recognized during rectal exami-

nation, particularly in relation to the sacculated character of both the large and small colon.

Digestion in the Horse

In the adult horse the stomach accounts for 12% of the total capacity of the digestive tract. Under normal feeding practices the stomach is never completely empty and secretion of acid gastric juice occurs continuously. Emptying of the stomach normally commences very soon after the horse begins to feed due to the development of powerful peristaltic contractions, probably initiated by vagal stimulation, which ensure the rapid onward passage of the ingesta from the stomach to the small intestine and into the large intestine. When eating stops the stomach contractions cease.

The precise mode by which the stomach functions in digestion is not conclusive; it has been suggested that maceration and bacterial breakdown, particularly of food with a high fibre content, may be of greater significance than enzymic digestion. The appearance of significant amounts of lactic and butyric acids in the stomach, when a hay diet is fed, favours this view. Enzymic action in the small intestine is responsible for the elaboration of protein and soluble carbohydrate which are absorbed before they can be subjected to attack by the flora of the large intestine. When the ingesta reaches the large intestine it is subjected to fermentation reactions by the microflora with the production of volatile fatty acids which are absorbed. Water and electrolytes are also absorbed, mainly from the colon. The motility of the large intestine in the horse is more frequent than in other species.

Clinical Examination of the Stomach and Intestines

The position of the stomach in the concavity of the diaphragm at the anterior part of the abdomen, where because of its relatively small size it does not come into contact with the abdominal wall, except to a limited extent in certain circumstances, causes difficulty in the diagnosis of gastric disorders in the horse. In considering the possibility of gastric disease the clinician must of necessity, therefore, take into account all the available indirect evidence that can be obtained.

Dilatation of the stomach in the horse is accompanied by clinical signs indicating acute, continuous pain consisting of elevated temperature, increased pulse frequency and, because of voluntarily restricted diaphragm movement, shallow breathing, with congestion of the mucous membranes. The intensity of the pain reaction in the individual animal is indicated by the degree of sweating, which is usually profuse. When gastric distension is severe, the horse assumes the dog-sitting posture in an attempt to relieve pressure on the diaphragm.

Gastric dilatation is caused by impaction, excessive gas production or consumption of excessive quantities of fluid, e.g. cold water, whey, etc. The most common cause of gastric impaction is unrestricted feeding on ground grains such as wheat, barley, cornmeal, etc. Dilatation as a complication of impaction may follow pyloric obstruction due to compression by a neoplasm or stricture of the pylorus. Excessive gas production in the stomach commonly follows the ingestion of succulent, rapidly fermentable foods such as growing oats, corn and legumes. Consumption of excessive amounts of cold water is more likely to occur when the horse is fresh from work and likely to be overheated. Dilatation in such cases is usually of temporary duration due to the low level of intestinal motility and the tendency to pyloric spasm.

Gastric tympany, occurring without intestinal flatulence, may be associated with tympanic resonance in the anterior abdomen on the left side. In this event, impaired intestinal motility is indicated by early reduction, followed by complete cessation, of defaecation. Periodic eructation of gas may be observed, and passage of the stomach tube permits the escape of large quantities of gas. When fluid causes distension of the stomach, regurgitation of small amounts of food admixed with liquid occurs, followed by its passage down the nasal cavities, which causes irritation, snorting and coughing. In this situation, fluid escapes in large amounts when the stomach tube is passed. When the stomach is impacted with food, eructation of gas or fluid does not occur, and introduction of the stomach tube does not lead to the return of any of the gastric contents. Here, occasional vigorous eructation movements occur which coincide with periodic bouts of intense pain and discomfort.

When eructation is associated with evacuation of fluid or gas from the stomach, the animal obtains relief, the pain reactions subsiding until gastric distension recurs. A check test which reveals the presence of hydrochloric acid will confirm that the regurgitated material originated in the stomach. In grass sickness the reaction of the mainly fluid vomitus is usually alkaline. If gastric distension persists for some hours, exhaustion and toxaemia will reduce the intensity of the animal's reaction to pain and, superficially, it may appear that clinical improvement has occurred. Closer examination will reveal that the pulse frequency has increased with considerable deterioration in pulse quality, the general reflex and toxaemic effect on the vascular system being revealed by the cold clammy state of the body surface.

If, following a severe bout of pain with retching, terminating in free vomiting, the horse appears to show sudden relief of pain, the likelihood that rupture of the stomach has occurred should be considered. In this event retching ceases and the animal stands quietly, but very soon signs of shock appear, consisting of tremors, cold sweating, subnormal temperature, severely congested mucous membranes with a pulse rate in excess of 120/minute and having running-down characteristics. Auscultation of the abdomen will reveal that peristaltic activity has ceased.

Gross distension of the stomach causes the spleen to become displaced medially and posteriorly within the abdominal cavity. The degree of displacement may be sufficiently great to permit the sharp, firm posterior border of the spleen to be readily recognized during rectal exploration. In small horses, the swollen mass of the stomach may be palpated just below the roof of the abdomen, near the kidneys. When rupture of the stomach has occurred the visceral peritoneum will have a dry, roughened feel, because of the presence of ingesta and developing peritonitis. In this condition manual exploration will be readily performed because of the flaccid state of the intestines.

The proportionately small size of the stomach in the horse, relative to the food requirements of the animal, imposes greater demands for intestinal efficiency. This is provided to some degree by the anatomical complexity of the large intestine. Because of this situation the incidence of intestinal maladies is quite high. The most important of these include spasm, tympany, impaction and inflammation or enteritis, in all of which distension and modifications of motility occur. As in the case of the stomach, the

distension may be static when there is an accumulation of ingesta, gas or fluid, or transient when
it is the result of periodic, segmental spasm and
hypermotility. These several conditions will be
associated with abnormal behaviour typical of
the colic syndrome, although the intensity and
character of the pain manifestations are related
to the severity of the malady. In the more acute
states, e.g. tympany, enteritis, acute obstruction,
etc., systemic effects (shock, dehydration) will
influence the character of the pulse and respirations. To aid understanding of the basic situation, static distensions are classified as causing
physical colic, and transient distensions as causing functional colic.

The modifications in intestinal motility consist
of increased or decreased function. Hypermotility, characterized by diarrhoea, occurs in enteritis and peritonitis. The causes of enteritis in
horses are many and varied. The young foal is
similar to neonatal animals of other species in
being highly susceptible to bacterial, protozoan,
mycotic and possibly even viral infections which
are directly or indirectly responsible for intestinal inflammation. The more common diseases
include colibacillosis, salmonellosis, shigellosis,
aspergillosis, equine viral arteritis (in a proportion of cases), 'colitis-X' (the cause of which is as
yet unidentified), strongylosis, ascariasis, etc.
Chemical agents and poisonous plants may occasionally cause intestinal irritation, as also may
physical agents such as sand or soil. Peritonitis
develops as the result of penetrating wounds of
the abdominal wall which may arise either
accidentally, in the course of hunting, riding or
working in harness, or intentionally as for
instance following intra-abdominal surgical procedures or trocarization of the caecum or colon.
Perforation of gastric ulcers caused by the larvae
of *Gasterophilus* spp. or *Habronema megastomum*
is an occasional cause of peritonitis. In conditions such as gastric rupture, intestinal torsion
or intussusception, mating accidents and over-
vigorous rectal examination, acute fatal peritonitis develops. Death, however, is usually the
result of shock and in some cases internal
haemorrhage.

Reduction in intestinal motility may develop
gradually, as in impaction of the large or small
colon or the caecum. In intestinal obstruction
caused by torsion, intussusception or incarceration, there is sudden, virtually complete cessation
of motility. Impaction of the ileocaecal valve is

associated with an initial period of hypermotility
of about 12 hours duration, followed by complete
cessation of peristalsis.

Inspection of the abdomen will reveal general
distension in primary tympany, which is usually
the result of recent feeding on rapidly fermentable, lush green food. In secondary tympany,
which develops following acute intestinal obstruction, the segmental distension is usually
insufficient to give rise to an externally recognizable increase in the size of the abdomen.
External palpation is unlikely to reveal clinical
evidence of any great value, apart from pain and
tension, in respect of the abdomen in the horse.
Percussion will indicate the presence of tympany,
the increased resonance being general throughout the area in the primary form, and localized
in cases of secondary origin. Segmental intestinal
impaction is, however, not invariably revealed
because of the uncertainty of eliciting a significantly dull percussion note at the appropriate
point on the abdominal wall.

Auscultation of the abdomen in the horse is of
considerable value because it will provide an
opportunity to assess the degree of functional
activity of the intestines from the peristaltic
sounds. Loud gurgling or rumbling sounds
suggest enteritis, spasmodic colic or the early
stages of acute obstruction arising from volvulus,
intussusception, strangulation or impaction of
the ileocaecal valve. Peristaltic sounds are reduced, or absent, in impaction, atony and after
a few hours in acute obstruction. Tinkling
sounds are heard when there is general intestinal
tympany or local retention of gas, because of
segmental spasm. The quality of the intestinal
sounds is also related to the character of the diet,
being loudest when the food contains relatively
large amounts of water. Loud bowel sounds may
reduce the audibility of the functional sounds
produced by other organs such as the lungs. In
rupture of the diaphragm, when segments of
intestine pass forwards into a pleural sac, peristaltic sounds can be detected during auscultation over the lower part of the respiratory area
on the affected side. The degree of intestinal
motility is reflected in the quantity of faeces, the
character of which will provide further evidence
of clinical value.

Rectal Examination

Prior to commencing the physical procedures
involved in rectal examination the condition of

the anal region is considered, noting the presence of neoplasms (melanosarcomas), or greyish-white deposits, signifying infestation with *Oxyuris equi* (because of the intense irritation caused by the parasite loss of hair at the base of the tail is a usual feature), and the tone of the anal sphincter, which is reduced in old age and in paralysis of the rectum.

When the hand reaches the ampulla of the rectum the quantity of faeces present should be assessed, also the tone of the musculature; ballooning or contraction of the rectum, paralysis of the rectum (most common in the mare approaching parturition, occasionally in encephalitis and in some cases of paralysis of the tail) and laceration and perforation of the wall can be recognized. Traumatic injury to the rectum, resulting from injudicious rectal exploration, sadism or in mares from mis-service or accident during foaling (rectovaginal fistula), if extensive, is readily recognized, and even where the damage is slight, or of recent origin, it is possible to detect a break forming a depression of the normally smooth mucous membrane, and which contains blood and faeces. The extent and the depth of the injury are determined by careful digital exploration, noting whether the finger, or the whole hand, can be introduced into the wound or, in some cases of perforation, even into the peritoneal cavity where segments of intestine are directly palpable. The condition of the pelvic bones and sacrum can be determined by palpation. Fracture of the pelvic bones may be recognized by hearing and feeling the grating (crepitation) of the opposing parts of the damaged bone during movement (over-riding), induced by an assistant rocking the hindquarters of the animal from side to side. The presence of calculi in the bladder or of neoplasms involving this and other organs and tissues in the pelvic cavity is easily determined.

Only a few parts of the normal intestines can be readily identified by palpation during rectal exploration. Definition is possible, however, when a portion of intestine is distended with gas or is the site of obstruction as in impaction, intussusception, volvulus or incarceration, provided the affected part is palpable.

The small colon is disposed in irregular loops distributed across the posterior part of the abdominal cavity and may even be found within the pelvic cavity. Almost consistently a segment of small colon can be palpated in front of, and below, the brim of the pelvis; it is as thick as the forearm of a man and usually contains balls of faeces (balled faeces occur only in the small colon and rectum), and is also recognizable because of the longitudinal muscle bands and sacculations of the wall. It can be grasped and moved easily in all directions on account of the long supporting mesentery. In impaction of the small colon, the offending faecal mass, which is very firm, varies in size from that of a turkey egg to that of a large coconut, depending to some extent on the size of the animal. Careful exploration and assessment may be required before the nature and situation of the condition, which is readily confused with impaction of the ileocaecal valve, are recognized. The character of the clinical signs and course of the disease will be of great significance.

In many horses, about 40–60 cm of the left ventral and the left dorsal sections of the large colon, together with the pelvic flexure, are easily palpated and recognized. These sections of the large intestine are abridged by a fold of mesentery varying from 5 cm to almost 15 cm wide at the pelvic flexure, but the united segments lie freely in the abdominal cavity. Although their normal position is along the left side, in contact with the abdominal wall, extending back to the pelvic inlet, these left divisions of the large colon may be situated medially, or even on the right of the median plane. The ventral portion differs considerably in certain anatomical features from the dorsal part, the former is about 20–30 cm in diameter, and its surface bears narrow, longitudinal, ribbon-like thickenings comprised of smooth muscle layers, and transverse constrictions and projecting pouches (sacculations); the latter segment, on the other hand, is about 7–10 cm wide, its surface is smooth and only a single longitudinal muscle band is present in the vicinity of the attachment of the abridging mesenteric fold. The left dorsal colon is often situated slightly medial to the ventral division. The pelvic flexure and contiguous parts of the large colon can be readily grasped with the hand, in their normal situation towards the left side, just in front of the pelvic inlet. The transverse and right sections are not ordinarily palpable— they are out of reach of the hand. In rare instances, in medium to small horses, the stomach-like dilatation of the right dorsal segment can be palpated, medially and anterior to the base of the caecum as a large balloon-like object, which can only be reached with the fingertips.

The commonest malady affecting the large colon is impaction with food residue or entero-liths. It commences in the left ventral colon and extends towards the sternal flexure. The impac-ted mass is firmest at the pelvic flexure which, in well established cases, is displaced posteriorly on the floor of the pelvis, and may be palpated immediately the fingers pass beyond the anal sphincter. In moderate impaction the mass can be indented by finger pressure, whereas in more severe cases the consistency is such that this is difficult to achieve. A horse affected with impac-tion of the large colon may stretch, or strain as if to relieve the condition, and may periodically adopt abnormal postures such as kneeling, 'dog-sitting' or standing with the hindquarters pushed into a corner. Torsion of the left seg-ments of the large colon is recognized by noting the absence of faeces in the rectum, gaseous distension of the intestines anterior to the point of occlusion, and the rotation of the pelvic flexure, which may occur either to the left or the right. In occasional cases these segments may be turned forwards on themselves, the displacement occupying a dorsal or ventral position, so that the pelvic flexure cannot be reached. In all forms of colonic displacement the clinical signs usually develop suddenly and are those associated with acute abdominal pain.

On the right side, in the upper anterior part of the abdominal cavity the immobile, rounded base of the caecum is accessible to the fingertips. In many instances, when in a normal state the caecum cannot be recognized; it is only readily identified when it is distended with solid or gaseous contents. Of the body of the caecum, only those parts contiguous to the base are normally palpable and then only readily identifiable when it is also distended. If the caecum is displaced and kinked backwards, its apex is sometimes within reach; it may even be found in the pelvic cavity. Distension of the caecum arises from impaction or tympany. General clinical signs are acute in gaseous distension, which usually involves neighbouring parts of the small and large intestine. The two conditions can be readily differentiated during rectal examination.

The terminal portion of the small intestine, which is distinguished anatomically from the remaining thin-walled parts of the intestine by reason of its thick muscular wall, can occasionally be palpated, more particularly when it is dis-tended. It is situated anteriorly in the upper area of the abdominal cavity, and it is recognizable as a firm tube 5–8 cm in diameter when normally distended, running horizontally, or obliquely, from left to right towards the base of the caecum. Towards the left it is mobile, near its termination with the caecum, on the right, it is fixed.

Impaction of the ileocaecal valve region, a not uncommon cause of colic in the horse, is indi-cated during rectal examination by the con-tracted state of the large intestine and the considerable distension of the small intestine by gas and fluid, which latter makes the examination difficult. This condition may be confused with volvulus of the small intestine because tightly stretched folds of mesentery may be palpable. Intestinal intussusception in the horse, a rela-tively rare condition seen most often in foals, often involves the ileum, more usually near its termination. In this case rectal examination reveals an empty rectum and reduction in the size of the large intestine, with a crepitant mass anterior to the brim of the pubes.

The more anterior parts of the abdominal cavity, which are within reach of the hand, are occupied by loops of small intestine, which during palpation give an impression of vague, indefinite objects which cannot be grasped. When distended with gas, the loops may then be more readily identified as resilient, cylindrical objects which are smooth, readily mobile and 7 cm or more in diameter. Gaseous distension is most marked if a segment of small intestine is the site of volvulus when, even if the affected part cannot be palpated, the folds of supporting mesentery, which are twisted into rope-like struc-tures extending downwards in varying directions from the roof of the abdomen, can be recog-nized.

Although not usually palpable during rectal exploration, the duodenum may be identified in some small horses. Even then it is only the terminal part that it is possible to palpate; it is recognized as a smooth-walled, compressible, pliant tube about 5–8 cm in diameter, emerging between the base of the caecum and the right abdominal wall, and passing to the left above the base of the caecum, in close contact with the dorsal wall of the abdomen and the right kidney, towards the anterior origin of the mesentery beneath the left kidney. It crosses the median plane ventral to the second or third lumbar vertebra.

The relative size and situation of the stomach in the horse ensures that it is not usually palpable. Exceptionally, when acutely dilated, it is within reach of the hand near the dorsal part of the abdomen. If palpable, the tense or firm sac-like character of the affected organ makes identification an easy matter.

The spleen is not regularly palpable in normal horses. Its location is sought by advancing the hand, with the fingers extended, forwards from the pelvis along the left wall of the abdomen above the left dorsal segment of the large colon. The posterior border of the spleen approximates to the left costal arch, so that if the fingers reach this point they will pass between the abdominal wall and the spleen. When palpable the normal spleen is recognized by its usual, but not invariable, position in contact with the abdominal wall, its soft, yielding texture and its sharp, vertical, posterior border. The position of the spleen is influenced by the degree of distension of the stomach. When the stomach is dilated, the spleen is displaced medially and backwards. Segments of intestine may insinuate themselves between the spleen and the abdominal wall either from above, over the lienorenal fold of mesentery, or from below. In such circumstances the spleen is situated away from the abdominal wall towards the median plane.

When enlarged the spleen may be more readily palpated during rectal examination. Splenic enlargement is most marked in congestive heart failure, portal obstruction or neoplastic involvement. In the last condition the disproportion may be local. Circumscribed enlargements of varying size also occur in tuberculosis. In general enlargement of the spleen the posterior border is thicker than normal.

The left kidney is situated well forward on the dorsal aspect of the abdomen beneath the last rib and transverse processes of the first two or three lumbar vertebrae, a little to the left of the median plane. It is usually held firmly in position by fascia and it is only rarely suspended by a mesenteric fold. Only the posterior pole of the left kidney is palpable, and then only in small horses. In such circumstances the fingertips impinge on a firm, semi-spherical body, some 15 cm in diameter, with a smooth surface. Very occasionally the renal artery can be recognized at the hilus. The right kidney is situated further forward than the left and is therefore out of reach. The ureter, in each case, can be identified only when it is grossly distended or thickened. A pain reaction to reasonable pressure on the kidney should be related to the general clinical picture in suspected cases of nephrosis or nephritis.

The abdominal aorta is identified as a strongly pulsating tube about 2·5 cm in diameter, situated under the vertebral column. It is located by introducing the arm into the rectum as far as the elbow, and then rotating the hand until the palm can be pushed upwards against the lumbar vertebrae and psoas muscles. By following the vessels backwards with the fingers, its division beneath the sixth lumbar vertebra into left and right external iliac, left and right internal iliac (hypogastric), and coccygeal arteries, is reached. Thickening and irregularity in the arterial wall are palpable over a variable distance in iliac thrombosis, which causes a mild or acute syndrome with a corresponding degree of lameness.

The anterior mesenteric artery and some of its branches can be identified by tracing the abdominal aorta forwards; in the position of the first lumbar vertebra a pulsating vessel, running vertically downwards, is palpable. If affected with a verminous aneurysm, the arteries, at their origin, are thickened, have a rough, uneven surface and may be the site of a pain focus. The condition arises from the migration of the larvae of *Strongylus vulgaris*; it may be followed by secondary bacterial infection with *Streptococcus equi, Actinobacillus equuli* or *Salmonella typhimurium*. In either case there is segmental atony of the large intestine which is expressed clinically by recurrent attacks of spasmodic colic, or persistent diarrhoea.

If, during palpation of either of the paired iliac arteries or the anterior mesenteric artery, a vibration thrill (fremitus) is found to replace the individual waves of the pulse, this indicates the presence of a thrombus (clot) in the artery concerned. In aneurysm there is an increase in the diameter of the artery, although this does not imply an increase in the size of the lumen in all cases.

The urinary bladder is palpated beneath the rectum, on the floor of the pelvis, by moving the palm of the hand backwards and forwards in the rectum. The empty bladder is recognized as a small, slightly yielding body, roughly the size and shape of a small coconut. When fully distended it is easily and distinctly identified as a fairly firm, globular, smooth-walled structure, the anterior extremity (vertex) of which projects from the pelvis to reach the abdominal floor in its posterior part. In urinary retention, caused by obstructive urolithiasis, the bladder may reach enormous dimensions. Cystic calculi, in the form of moderately large, firm objects, are usually easily identified by palpation of the bladder. Thickening of the bladder wall, which occurs in chronic cystitis, can also be appreciated.

The intrapelvic urethra in male horses can be palpated on the floor of the pelvis, immediately the fingers pass through the anus, as a firm, cylindrical structure about 2·5 cm or less in diameter which runs horizontally in an anterior direction. In urinary retention associated with pain, caused by cystitis, urethritis, calculi in the urethra and sebaceous concretions in the coronal fossa of the glans penis, palpation of the pelvic portion of the urethra produces spasmodic jerking of the penis.

In the stallion, a possibly important aspect of rectal examination concerns the abdominal inguinal ring (more correctly the vaginal ring), which is located in the following way: the anterior border of the pubic bone is identified with the extended fingers; the palm of the hand is placed upon it and the fingers then flexed until their tips come into contact with the abdominal wall. If the abdominal wall is now palpated for a distance of about 15 cm by moving the hand to the left or right of the median plane, a slit-like opening about 8–15 cm long is located on each side extending forwards and laterally. It is usually wide enough to admit only the tips of one to three fingers. In addition, the spermatic cord, the constituent parts of which unite together at the vaginal ring, is distinctly palpable as a cord-like structure as thick as the thumb, running downwards and outwards through the inguinal canal. If a segment of intestine has entered the inguinal canal and become incarcerated in the tunica vaginalis sac, it will be recognized as a thick cord, traction on which causes a pain reaction.

In the mare, the uterus is palpable (beneath the hand) as a short body interposed between the rectum and bladder, and continued anteriorly by the diverging cornua which are slightly concave towards the dorsal aspect. Although the body of the uterus is situated directly beneath the rectum, partly in the pelvis and partly in the abdominal cavity, considerable experience is necessary in order to recognize it; the more usual procedure is to locate one of the ovaries and slide the hand under the anterior extremity of the corresponding uterine cornu, so that the whole uterus can then be systematically palpated. In early pregnancy a bulge is recognizable in one horn towards the body; this increases in size as gestation progresses until the weight of the gravid organ is such that it is pulled down into the abdomen. Metritis causes a variable degree of general increase in the size of the uterus so that it is more readily identified.

The ovaries are located, one on each side, in the sublumbar region ventral to the fourth or fifth lumbar vertebra, in contact with the dorsal aspect of the abdominal cavity. They are recognizable because of their firm consistency, relationship to the uterus and relative immobility, the mesovarium being only 8–10 cm long. Their size is variable, being on average 5 cm long and 2·5 cm or more thick.

The lymph nodes of the abdominal cavity, including the iliac and lumbar groups, are palpable when normal or when enlarged as variously sized, more or less spherical nodular bodies, situated in the appropriate position. Lymph node enlargement, in occasional instances, is caused by neoplastic states such as malignant lymphoma, which is multiple and involves lymph nodes in various parts of the body, including the abdomen, and melanoma which is most common in old grey horses, often originating in the perineal and perianal region, from where it metastasizes to the pelvic lymph nodes. A group of lymph nodes just within reach of the fingers can be palpated in the vicinity of the anterior mesenteric artery. In certain diseases (strangles) the group may be enlarged and painful (abscessation).

The peritoneum, both visceral and parietal surfaces, is palpable only in its posterior area. Normally it is smooth and not painful on palpation. In inflammatory and neoplastic conditions, it becomes rough or nodular, and palpation causes pain. In rupture of the stomach or intestines, particles of food cause recognizable roughening of the peritoneum, or emphysema can be identified. The mesenteries are the site for rare cases of lipoma which, because they cause no obvious clinical signs although they are in most cases multiple, are usually only diagnosed on post mortem examination. Individual tumour masses are pedunculated and vary in size.

ABDOMEN OF CATTLE AND SHEEP

The abdominal cavity of the ox is absolutely and relatively more capacious than that of the horse. The larger capacity arises from the greater transverse and longitudinal diameters. The compound stomach, consisting of the rumen, reticulum and abomasum, occupies almost three-quarters of the abdominal cavity. It fills the left half of the abdomen (the spleen and a few coils of small intestine are situated in this part) and extends considerably over to the right side. The absolute volume of the stomach compartments varies according to the age and size of the animal. In average-sized adult cattle the capacity is between 136 and 180 litres, in large animals 180–270 litres, and in small animals 115–160 litres. In the newly-born calf the reticulum is very small, and the capacity of the rumen is less than half that of the abomasum; when the calf is 10–12 weeks old the rumen has become twice as large as the abomasum. The omasum remains functionless during this period. In the 4-month-old calf the capacity of the rumen and reticulum together is four times that of the omasum and abomasum together. At around 18 months the four compartments each have attained their final relative capacities.

The rumen, comprising about 80% of the total stomach capacity, occupies almost the whole left half of the abdominal cavity, except for the small area occupied by the spleen and reticulum and an occasional loop of small intestine. The middle and ventral parts of the rumen extend beyond the median plane. The antero-posterior long axis of the rumen extends from opposite the ventral part of the seventh or eighth intercostal space to the pelvic inlet. The left surface of the rumen is in contact with the diaphragm, spleen and posterior ribs, at its anterior part, and with the abdominal musculature elsewhere. This relationship enables the rumen to be subjected to all the physical methods of clinical examination over the whole extent of the left side of the abdomen. The external surface of the rumen is marked by grooves corresponding to the pillar-like projections on the internal aspect which divide the lumen into a dorsal and ventral sac, and dorsal and ventral blind sacs.

The reticulum has a capacity approximating to about 5% of the total stomach volume. It is the most anterior compartment, being opposite the sixth to the seventh, or even the eighth ribs,

mainly on the left of the median plane. The anterior surface is in contact with the liver and diaphragm. The posterior surface, which lies above the xiphoid cartilage, ends dorsally where it joins the rumen, forming the internally, upward projecting ruminoreticular fold. The reticulum is somewhat pyriform in shape with the lesser curvature facing to the right and dorsally, and the greater curvature to the left and ventrally. The right extremity forms a rounded sac which is in contact with the sternal part of the diaphragm, the liver, omasum and abomasum, opposite the ventral part of the sixth intercostal space. The mucous membrane of the reticulum has projecting folds about 1 cm high enclosing spaces which are four-, five- or six-sided. The oesophageal groove commences at the termination of the oesophagus in the dome-like vestibule common to the rumen and reticulum which is situated dorsal to the ruminoreticular fold. It passes in a ventromedial direction to reach the reticulo-omasal orifice.

The omasum constitutes about 7 or 8% of the total stomach capacity. It is situated mainly to the right of the median plane. The left surface is in contact with the rumen, reticulum and abomasum, while the right surface is mainly related to the diaphragm, liver and a small area of the abdominal wall towards its lowest part opposite the seventh to eleventh ribs. The omasum is situated above the main mass of the abomasum. Internally the cavity of the omasum is almost filled by about a hundred intimately related, longitudinal folds of varying length, which originate from the dorsal aspect and sides. A groove about 10 cm long on the floor of the omasum, extends from the reticulo-omasal orifice to the omaso-abomasal opening.

The abomasum, or glandular stomach, comprises 8% of the capacity of the stomach compartments in adult cattle. It forms an elongated sac, in the shape of a shallow tube, lying on the abdominal floor on the right side of the body. The anterior blind extremity is related to the reticulum above the xiphisternum, and the posterior end, which is much narrower, terminates in the pylorus at the duodenum, opposite the lower part of the ninth or tenth rib. The greater curvature of the abomasum is mainly in contact with the abdominal wall; it gives attachment to superficial layers of the great omentum; the lesser curvature is in contact dorsally with the omasum to which it is attached by a fold of peritoneum.

The left, or visceral surface comes into contact with the ventral sac of the rumen and the omasum, and the right (parietal) surface is related to the abdominal floor from the seventh to tenth ribs.

Internally the mucous membrane of the abomasum shows a distinct zonal arrangement. In the first part (fundus) it forms a series of spiral folds; the more distant (pyloric) region has a uniformly flat surface.

The position and bulk of the rumen, reticulum, omasum and abomasum in cattle cause the intestine to be accommodated almost entirely on the right side of the body.

The duodenum commences approximately opposite the ventral part of the tenth rib, and first passes dorsally and forward to reach the visceral surface of the liver where it forms a sigmoid curve beneath the right kidney. It then extends backwards almost to reach the level of the external angle of the ilium, where it again turns forward in company with the terminal part of the colon and continues as the free, or mesenteric, portion of the small intestine, which is suspended in short, close coils from the roof of the abdominal cavity in the vicinity of the right kidney. The range of movement of the small intestine is restricted as it occupies the space bounded medially by the ventral sac of the rumen, anteriorly by the omasum and abomasum, dorsally and laterally by the colon and ventrally by the abdominal wall. The ileum joins the colon opposite the ventral part of the last rib; at its terminal part the ileum is located between, and is attached to, the caecum and colon.

The large intestine of cattle has a much simpler anatomical arrangement than that of the horse. The caecum extends backwards from its junction with the colon near the ventral part of the last rib along the right flank, to end blindly at the pelvic inlet. It is separated from the abdominal wall by the greater omentum; on the left its main relationship is with the rumen. The average length is about 75 cm and the diameter about 12 cm. The colon extends forwards from its junction with the caecum for 5–10 cm and then turns dorsally and backward opposite the lower extremity of the last two ribs. It continues backwards in the sublumbar region in contact with the right flank, to near the last lumbar vertebra. At this point it turns forward and runs parallel to the preceding part, to reach the level of the second lumbar vertebra, where it turns backwards and continues as the spiral portion

which consists of a double loop coiled into a flat spiral and maintained in position between two layers of mesentery. The coils of the spiral are alternately centripetal and centrifugal. The spiral mass of the colon is parallel to and in contact with the right abdominal wall. At its terminal part the colon emerges from the spiral section, extends forward to near the origin of the anterior mesenteric artery, and then turns backward dorsal to the terminal part of the duodenum. In proximity to the ventral surface of the right kidney the colon passes towards the right, and near the pelvic inlet it forms a sigmoid curve and becomes confluent with the rectum. The average length of the colon in adult cattle is about 11 m. At its origin it is about 12 cm in diameter but it later becomes reduced to about 5 cm.

The rectum in cattle is shorter and has a smaller diameter than that of the horse. The peritoneum covers the rectum as far back as the first coccygeal vertebra. The retroperitoneal part is surrounded by a variable quantity of fat.

The general anatomical arrangement of the stomach compartments in the sheep follows that of cattle. The capacity of the reticulum is relatively larger, and that of the omasum relatively much smaller, than in cattle. The abomasum is relatively larger and longer than in cattle. The main part passes backwards somewhat ventral to and parallel with the right costal arch, and terminates at the pylorus opposite to the ventral extremity of the eleventh or twelfth intercostal space. The anatomical character and disposition of the small and large intestines in sheep are similar to those in cattle.

Digestion in Ruminant Species

The main features of digestive action in ruminant species are microbial fermentation and physical maceration which results from contraction of the stomach walls. Both features occur on a massive scale in the first two compartments of the stomach. The capacity of the rumen and reticulum is such that the passage of food is slowed down and this, together with an almost neutral, buffered fluid environment, ensures efficient fermentation.

Consequently dietary protein is degraded by bacterial action, and the simpler starches and sugars are utilized so that they are not directly available to the animal. A proportion of the microbial population is continuously passing with the food residues to the abomasum, from where the animal derives almost all its amino acid requirements from the digestion of the micro-organisms. Fermentation of cellulose in the rumen is a relatively slow process; it is seldom complete, and the residue undergoes secondary fermentation in the large intestine. The results of the fermentation of even complex carbohydrates comprise simple mixtures of volatile fatty acids with carbon dioxide. In animals fed on hay and other roughages the major VFA are acetic 60–70%, propionic 15–20% and butyric 10–15%, with small amounts of others derived from amino acid deamination.

The gas mixture produced by the fermentative processes in the rumen consists mainly of carbon dioxide and methane, along with some nitrogen and traces of oxygen and sometimes hydrogen. A not unimportant function of the bacterial flora in the alimentary tract, more particularly that of the rumen, is synthesis of B complex vitamins.

Clinical Examination of the Stomach and Intestines in Cattle and Sheep

Examination of the Stomach in Cattle

Changes in behaviour are much less obvious in cattle affected with painful conditions of the abdominal organs, compared with the horse in similar circumstances. In spite of this apparently reduced reactivity, careful clinical examination will usually provide rewarding results in many cases of intra-abdominal disease. If not already determined at an earlier stage, an enquiry should be made regarding the state of the animal's appetite, rumination and defaecation because these functions reflect the general condition of the digestive system. Other points of importance in this respect include the condition of the abdomen in respect of shape, size, etc., and whether the animal is actively evincing any noise or behaviour which might be interpreted to signify the presence of pain. The significance of grunting in cattle is not always related to disease of the digestive system. Cattle when replete grunt continuously because of slight respiratory embarrassment. Furthermore, grunting is a frequent accompaniment of severe respiratory disease in cattle, in which instance its frequency is the same as that of the respiration, occurring usually in relation to each expiration.

Grinding of the teeth in cattle is also an expression of abdominal pain, more especially perhaps in severe inflammatory states of the abomasum. Behavioural manifestations of abdominal pain in cattle, approximating those of equine colic, usually signify a serious situation, such as partial or complete obstruction of the urinary tract in lithiasis of the urethra or ureter, physical obstruction of the intestine such as exists in intussusception and certain forms of acute enteritis, e.g. anthrax or salmonellosis.

It has already been mentioned that the stomach compartments occupy almost 75% of the abdominal cavity. Because of the very intimate physical and functional relationships which exist between the various component parts, disease of one compartment will modify the activity of the others to a variable degree. By reason of its comparative size and its situation in relation to the left abdominal wall, the rumen compartment is the one most readily examined by the usual clinical methods. An assessment of its functional state obtained in this manner may reflect the condition of the other stomach compartments and that of the intestines. The two main functions of the stomach compartments, which are intimately interdependent, consist of microbiological degradation and synthesis and physical maceration. The latter involves motility, the periodicity and vigour of which are readily ascertained in respect of the rumen. The contractions of the stomach compartments are organized and controlled through the medium of the vagus nerve and the ruminorecticular motor centre in the medulla oblongata.

The cyclical movements, which ensure thorough mixing of the contents of the rumen and reticulum, occur at the rate of 1–3/minute, the greater frequency being related to recent ingestion of food. The cycle of motility commences with a double contraction of the reticulum, the second phase being associated with a simultaneous, strong contraction of the anterior dorsal sac of the rumen. As a result of these movements the fluid contents of the reticulum are spilled over the reticuloruminal fold and onto the surface of the dry food mass in the rumen. A sequential contraction of the ventral sac of the rumen then returns the fluid to the reticulum.

Eructation contractions, which are independent of the mixing contractions, mainly occur following the mixing cycle, their frequency being related to the gas pressure in the rumen. The contraction is initiated in the dorsal sacs of the rumen, from where it passes anteriorly to the oesophageal groove. Relaxation of the reticulum and cardia follows, depressing the level of the fluid so that the gas is freely expelled. Frothiness of the fluid will prevent clearing of the cardia so that eructation is impossible.

Regurgitation movements are an essential prelude to rumination; the associated ruminal contractions occur immediately prior to the normal mixing movements of the rumen. The function of the specific movements is to flood the oesophageal cardia with fluid. The next stage in rumination necessitates voluntary action by the animal, consisting of an inspiratory effort with the glottis closed, whereby the intrathoracic negative pressure is greatly increased. As a result some of the reticular fluid, containing solid material, enters the oesophagus and after initiating antiperistalsis is carried up to the pharynx. At this point a movement of the tongue directs the solid material between the tables of the molar teeth on one side of the mouth, the jaws are brought together and the base of the tongue is retracted into the pharynx, so that the regurgitated fluid is reswallowed. The mastication of the bolus then commences and is continued on the same side of the mouth.

In the healthy ox the periods of rumination vary in length from a few minutes to more than an hour and may occur at any time of the day. Although the animal usually lies down to ensure greater comfort for the purpose, rumination in the standing position is not abnormal. When ruminating, cattle present an appearance of comfort and placid contentment. Each bolus is methodically chewed some 50–80 times—the number of masticatory movements depending on the character of the food—before being reswallowed; the next bolus is regurgitated into the mouth within a few seconds. Generally, in any given period of rumination, the number of masticatory movements per bolus varies very little in healthy animals. Normally there are about 60 jaw movements per minute, which is a slower rate than that for ordinary mastication. The total time devoted to rumination on a daily basis is related to the character of the food; sheep fed on poor quality rough hay may spend up to 9 hours or more ruminating in comparison with less than 5 hours for ground dried grass and 2·5 hours for concentrates alone.

The healthy calf usually commences to ruminate for short and irregular periods at about the tenth day of life. By the time it is 6 weeks old the calf is ruminating regularly, but at a compara-

tively rapid rate (about 80 jaw movements per minute). The adult rate of mastication is not established until the animal is about a year old.

Rumination in sheep and goats is performed at a faster rate, the jaw movements being about 100/minute, otherwise the procedure is broadly similar.

Rumination ceases abruptly when the animal is influenced by excitement or fear. The absence of coarse fibre in the rumen of cattle fed on a diet of finely ground, or pelleted foods will cause diminished rumination. In many specific febrile diseases, and in ruminal atony, acute impaction of the rumen, traumatic reticuloperitonitis, vagus indigestion, actinobacillosis of the rumen and reticulum, rumenitis, impaction of the omasum and displacement and torsion of the abomasum, rumination may be infrequent or completely suppressed, or it may be performed slowly, with a low rate of mastication. In painful conditions affecting abdominal or other organs (traumatic reticuloperitonitis, ulceration of the abomasum, acute hepatitis) rumination is irregular and often associated with a grunting sound.

Rumen. Clinical examination of the rumen is achieved by inspection, palpation, percussion and auscultation. In addition, in selected cases, laparotomy or even rumenotomy may be undertaken. Inspection is of value in that it reveals evidence of gaseous distension by the presence of a bulge in the left paralumbar fossa. Visible movements of the abdominal wall, initiated by ruminal contractions, are rarely sufficiently obvious to be regarded as an accurate index of rumen activity.

Palpation of the rumen is performed with the extended fingers, the flat of the opened hand or the back of the closed fist, applied to the abdominal wall on the left side. Sufficient pressure should be exerted to overcome the tone of the abdominal musculature (Fig. 143) and thus bring it into more intimate contact with the rumen at the point of palpation. A methodical procedure should be adopted, commencing at the dorsal part of the abdominal wall beneath the extremities of the lumbar transverse processes, and continuing down towards the ventral aspect of the abdomen. In the upper part of the left flank, where rumen motility is most readily appreciated in healthy cattle, palpation reveals resilience of the rumen musculature. If moderately firm pressure is applied at this part, it will be found possible to push the abdominal and

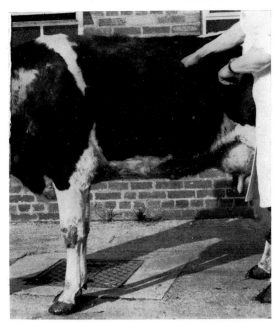

Fig. 143. *Palpating the rumen. Note that the examiner is pressing his fist firmly against the animal's flank, in order to be able to distinguish between the deeper movements of the rumen and the more superficial respiratory and adventitious movements of the abdominal wall.*

ruminal walls inwards under normal conditions, when the rumen is neither excessively full of foodstuff nor distended with gas. Palpation of the normally functioning rumen will enable the frequency, strength and cyclical pattern of the ruminal movements to be assessed. In the more ventral areas of the left flank the abdominal wall is more resistant to pressure because of the weight of the rumen contents, and the motility contractions are much less obvious.

Ruminal contractions are reduced in frequency and force or are entirely absent in simple indigestion, acute impaction, traumatic reticuloperitonitis and in other diseases of the stomach compartments such as vagus indigestion, rumenitis, actinobacillosis or neoplasia of the rumen and reticulum and ulceration, displacement or torsion of the abomasum. In simple indigestion caused by slight overfeeding on concentrates, sudden changes in diet or minor dietary abnormalities such as poor quality roughage, inadequate protein, mouldy, overheated and frosted foods, the rumen is not overfilled—if the period of ruminal stasis is prolonged the left paralumbar fossa may be more obvious, and palpation suggests that the abdominal wall and rumen wall

are not in normal close apposition—or distended, is firm and doughy and no pain reaction can be engendered by palpation.

Acute impaction of the rumen is caused by the ingestion of large amounts of highly fermentable, carbohydrate foods which produce excessive amounts of lactic acid, and is associated with a moderate degree of ruminal distension and, very occasionally, slight tympany, and the rumen contents are firm and doughy throughout the area. During palpation, evidence of pain may be elicited by the animal showing signs of restlessness and grunting. The pain is caused by inflammatory changes of varying severity and extent which develop in the mucous membrane and proceed to necrosis and gangrene in extreme cases. In traumatic reticuloperitonitis, ruminal movements are absent or reduced to a rate of one every 2 minutes or so, with decreased vigour. The rumen is mildly tympanitic and the left flank may be moderately distended. Palpation in the dorsal flank area reveals the presence of a gas cap overlying the firm doughy mass of solid ruminal contents.

In displacement of the abomasum to the left, there may be an initial bulge in the anterior part of the lower left paralumbar fossa caused by tympany of the displaced organ, followed later by deepening of the fossa and separation of the abdominal wall and rumen, due to reduction in the size of the latter because of capricious appetite. The medial displacement of the rumen gives the animal a somewhat 'slab-sided' appearance. Ruminal movements are decreased in frequency and vigour.

The rumen is situated some distance away from the left abdominal wall in intraperitoneal tympany, in which condition the paralumbar fossa is less, rather than more, obvious. Intraperitoneal tympany is a rare condition in cattle; occasional cases result from continued escape of rumen gases following trocarization for the relief of severe bloat, or when there is extensive necrosis in traumatic reticuloperitonitis with invasion of the damaged peritoneal tissues by gas-producing bacteria.

Percussion of the rumen adds little of value to the results of physical examination except, perhaps, to confirm the findings of other methods. Because of the thickness of the abdominal wall, and the limited degree of change that can occur in existing conditions, percussion must be vigorous in order to produce recognizable variations in the sounds evoked. In a normal state, the rumen, at its upper part, contains little or no food material. This is reflected in the slightly tympanic note obtained from percussion in this area. About one-third of the distance down the left flank the percussion note is dull in tone, and this state is determined to exist throughout the remainder of the rumen area. When the rumen is overfilled with foodstuffs, as in acute impaction, the percussion note is dull in the paralumbar fossa. In mild gaseous distension, when the gas forms a cap over the solid and liquid rumen contents, percussion evokes a tympanic sound which, if tympany is severe, becomes ringing in character. In frothy bloat, i.e. when the gas in the rumen is finely dispersed throughout the ingesta, the percussion sound is abnormally resonant much lower down the abdominal wall than in the normal animal.

In left displacement of the abomasum, when tympanitic distension occurs, percussion gives a resonant note over the area from the centre of the paralumbar fossa to the ventral parts of the last three ribs. Intraperitoneal tympany would be indicated by the elicitation of a tympanic sound over almost the whole of the left abdominal wall.

Auscultation of the rumen in the left flank (Fig. 144) gives rewarding results. By this

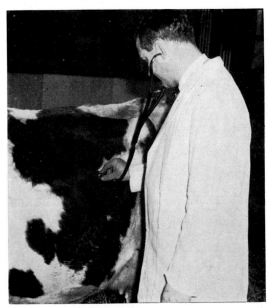

Fig. 144. *Auscultation of the rumen. The chest-piece of the stethoscope can be used to explore the whole area of the left flank.*

means the functional status of the rumen, and to a varying extent that of the other stomach compartments, can be assessed. The contractions of the rumen produce gurgling fluid and booming gassy sounds as the result of the movement of fluid and solid material on which a gas layer is superimposed. Reduction in rumen activity is accompanied by a decrease in the frequency and volume of the sounds. Diseases which modify rumen function in this way include acute impaction, simple indigestion, vagal indigestion, neoplasia and others not primarily involving the rumen, such as displaced abomasum, traumatic reticuloperitonitis and actinobacillosis of the reticulum. In animals severely toxaemic from these and other causes, there may be complete cessation of rumen activity and, therefore, of rumen sounds. High-pitched, splashing sounds are sometimes detected in the upper part of the left flank when ruminal atony has persisted for some time. They are produced by movement of the diaphragm causing variations in intraruminal pressure resulting in fluid motion. Similar fluid sounds at a lower, slightly more anterior point may signify displacement of the abomasum. Variations in the frequency and intensity of ruminal sounds will be noted in any febrile disease.

Reticulum. Palpation of the abdomen at selected points can reveal, by reason of the application of indirect pressure, when the reticulum is the site of pain in traumatic reticuloperitonitis. The pain reaction, which in these circumstances consists of a grunt, or groan, with an associated attempt by the animal to strike out with the horns or hind leg, is moderately severe, but the focus is rather localized. Pressure, producing an indirect effect on the reticulum, can be applied at several areas over the abdomen. The most suitable include moderately strong upward pressure in the sternal region at a point corresponding to the attachment of the diaphragm to the xiphoid cartilage (Fig. 139), whereupon the affected animal slightly arches its back, moves away from the direction of pressure application, strikes out with the head and hindleg and groans. Other methods of demonstrating the presence of pain in association with circumscribed peritonitis include pinching the skin of the withers (Fig. 145)—a healthy animal immediately depresses the back without discomfort, whereas an affected animal catches its breath or grunts, and depresses the back unwillingly or not at all—pressing the

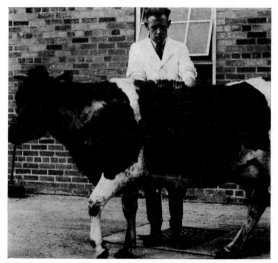

Fig. 145. *Testing for pain in the xiphisternal region by pinching the skin over the withers (traumatic reticulo-peritonitis).*

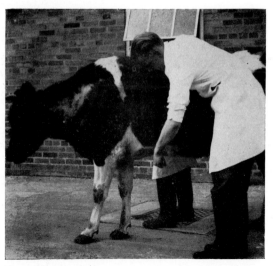

Fig. 146. *Testing for pain in the xiphisternal region by momentarily raising the body wall of the area with a pole, and then allowing it to drop suddenly.*

thumbs firmly into the left intercostal spaces where the diaphragm lies in contact with the ribs, and momentarily raising the ventral aspect of the trunk by means of a pole held under the posterior part of the sternal area between two assistants who rapidly elevate then suddenly drop the pole (Fig. 146). Cattle with traumatic reticulitis exhibit signs of abdominal pain during defaecation, urination or rumination. Palpation of the abdominal wall is painful in diffuse peritonitis, acute impaction of the rumen and in a variety of other inflammatory conditions of the abdominal organs.

The somewhat unselective eating habits of cattle contribute materially to traumatic reticulitis. Foreign objects ingested with the food, and which have a high specific gravity, drop into the reticulum. Those which are sharp-pointed may sooner or later penetrate the wall of the reticulum to a variable depth. The factors which bring about penetration are not clearly determined. Changes in size of the reticulum during its cyclical activity are of considerable importance— during its characteristic biphasic contraction it is reduced to less than one-half of its resting size— otherwise increase in intra-abdominal pressure appears to be significant because of the relationship between late pregnancy, or recent parturition, and the development of clinical signs. The functional disturbance of the reticulum which occurs is responsible for the clinical signs of impaired digestion which vary greatly in inten-

sity. In mild cases, when the circumscribed peritonitis is very limited in extent, the symptoms are likely to be confused with those of ruminal atony, indigestion or actinobacillosis. More severely affected animals exhibit a mild febrile reaction with sudden loss of appetite, an obvious or readily induced grunt and reduced gastro-intestinal activity involving all segments. In all cases there is rigidity of the back, which may be arched, and also of the abdominal muscles to some degree, so that walking is restricted and turning movements are precisely performed.

The majority of foreign body penetrations in the reticulum occur in the lower part of the anterior wall, but occasionally perforation may occur laterally towards the spleen or medially in the direction of the liver. If penetration is followed by progressive onward movement of the object, other organs are likely to become involved in the disease process. The most common complications are traumatic pericarditis, acute diffuse peritonitis, vagus indigestion and more rarely diaphragmatic hernia or abscess, splenic abscess and hepatic abscess.

Auscultation of the reticulum requires considerable experience to be able to detect those sounds which are specifically related to its functional activity, altogether apart from being able to interpret the significance of any departure from normal. The most informative point for auscultation is over the costochrondral junction of the seventh left rib, which is approximately 10 cm behind the point of the elbow. The cycle of mixing movements commences with a biphasic contraction of the reticulum which pours the liquid contents of the reticulum over the reticuloruminal fold, thereby producing a soft fluid sound, adequately described as having a swishing character; it persists for several seconds. A somewhat similar sound is heard when fluid is returned to the reticulum by the succeeding contraction of the ventral sac of the rumen. Fluid sounds are also detectable at the same point in association with eructation contractions and those for rumination; the former occurring immediately after, and the latter just prior to, the mixing sounds. The usual, readily observable signs associated with both these actions will indicate that the origin of the sounds is distinct from that of the mixing cycle.

Although in normal animals the rhythm of reticuloruminal and ruminal waves of contraction does not follow a strictly regular sequence, the variations in sequence are limited. The frequency of reticular contraction in all instances is reduced in primary diseases of the reticulum, in diseases of the rumen and other parts of the digestive tract, and in all febrile and toxaemic conditions. The diseases involving the reticulum which influence its function include traumatic reticuloperitonitis, actinobacillosis, vagus indigestion, etc. The infrequent contractions of the reticulum which occur in traumatic reticulitis have been associated with the production of a grunt, indicating pain. If a sound of this character can be correlated with the second phase of contraction of the reticulum and the dorsal sac of the rumen, in cattle evincing other suggestive signs of this condition, a more positive conclusion can be reached.

Metal detector units, although they have received considerable attention, have not been found entirely satisfactory in the differential diagnosis of traumatic reticulitis and its major complications. Such instruments will only react to ferrous metallic bodies, which under certain circumstances may exist in the reticulum of the majority of dairy cattle. Positive reactions, therefore, must be very carefully correlated to the clinical condition of the animal, and negative responses almost entirely disregarded. Experienced operatives can frequently determine the location of a penetrating metallic body with considerable accuracy. This degree of exactitude may assist consideration of the differential diagnosis.

Haematological determinations, in the form of total and differential leucocyte counts, can provide data helpful in regard to diagnosis and prognosis of traumatic reticulitis. It must be appreciated that the increase in total leucocyte and total neutrophil numbers may be transient, and in all cases is the result of a moderately strong pyogenic stimulus. At least two total and differential white cell counts, made at an interval of 12–24 hours, should be performed in order to observe the fluctuations which occur, particularly in the earlier stages of penetration of the reticular wall. As a corollary, it is essential to interpret the significance of the haematological findings in the context of the clinical findings in order to differentiate infective pyogenic processes in other parts of the body, e.g. kidneys, lungs, uterus, etc. Probably the haematological feature of most significance in relation to traumatic reticulitis is a sustained increase in the relative proportion of immature neutrophils. In cases in which penetration by the foreign body persists, and the peritoneal reaction remains localized, the neutrophil proportions remain abnormal, but probably the most diagnostically significant feature is a persistent increase in monocyte numbers. If acute diffuse peritonitis should develop, the total leucocyte count will show a rapid fall, followed later, in animals that survive this phase, by a sharp rise in total leucocyte and neutrophil counts. This latter feature is also characteristic of traumatic pericarditis, in which condition pronounced leucocytosis and neutrophilia occur (see Chapter 13).

Actinobacillosis of the reticulum, which usually also involves the oesophageal groove and rumen to a variable degree, is exhibited clinically as a persistent disturbance of digestive function. The main clinical features include partial anorexia, depressed rumination with reduction in rumen motility and subacute recurrent ruminal tympany. Neoplasia of the same structures will produce identical symptoms. The application of pressure at the recommended points, by failing to elicit a pain reaction, will exclude traumatic reticuloperitonitis in the diagnosis. Auscultation will also reveal reduced frequency and volume of the functional sounds, and no grunt will be heard.

Herniation of a portion of the reticulum into

a pleural cavity through a rupture in the diaphragm, which may arise from weakening of the latter by lesions of traumatic reticuloperitonitis or some other cause, as well as developmental defects, produces a syndrome consisting of initial hypermotility, capricious appetite, loss of bodily condition and a moderate degree of ruminal tympany. Auscultation is of little assistance in the differential diagnosis of this condition because, even in normal animals, reticular sounds are audible immediately posterior to the cardiac area. The condition is afebrile and, if cardiac displacement exists, a systolic murmur can be heard and the heart sounds may be more intense, suggesting that the heart has been displaced anteriorly or to the left.

In vagus indigestion the nerve supply to the stomach compartments may be impaired, giving rise to a variable degree of paralysis which is characterized clinically by ruminal distension, anorexia, retarded passage of ingesta and the evacuation of soft, pasty faeces in small quantities. The major form of the condition appears to result from achalasia of the reticulo-omasal and the pyloric sphincters. Food material accumulates in the rumen; this is often accompanied by a syndrome of pyloric obstruction, which becomes complicated by the development of pyloric ulceration. The major clinical aspects of achalasia of the reticulo-omasal sphincter occur as either of two syndromes. These are ruminal distension with hypermotility or ruminal distension with atony. In the former the heart rate is reduced and there may be a systolic murmur which waxes and wanes, reaching its peak at the termination of inspiration.

Omasum. The location of the omasum within the abdominal cavity is such that direct examination by physical methods is possible only to a limited degree. Fortunately, therefore, the omasum is only somewhat infrequently the site of primary disease. Generally its functional status is, in the main, determined by reference to the activity of the other stomach compartments and that of the intestines.

Enlargement of the omasum, which is then excessively hard, occurs in chronic impaction. The condition has been described in cattle fed on tough, fibrous foods such as dry lucerne stalks or loppings from fodder trees, and in sheep fed on dry, bare ground during drought conditions when accumulation of soil occurs in the omasum. The main clinical features consist of mild, re-curring bouts of depressed appetite and ruminal motility. Firm pressure palpation under the right costal arch, or in the seventh to ninth right intercostal spaces, may evoke a pain reaction and enable the firm mass of the distended organ to be recognized. Secondary atony of the omasum with impaction has been noted as a post mortem feature in piroplasmosis, parturient paresis and post-parturient haemoglobinuria. In such cases no obvious clinical indication that the omasum was involved, is determined during life, the clinical features consisting of complete anorexia and subacute abdominal pain due to local peritonitis which arises from patchy necrosis of the wall of the omasum. The omasum manifests pathological effects in a variety of specific diseases which also affect other parts of the alimentary tract. The most obvious of these include mucosal disease, malignant catarrhal fever, rinderpest, chlorinated naphthalene intoxication (hyperkeratosis) and trichlorethylene-extracted soya meal poisoning.

Abomasum. The position of the abomasum, the parietal surface of which is related to the abdominal wall on the right side ventral to the seventh to the tenth ribs, enables it to be subjected to physical examination by means of firm pressure with the closed fist (Fig. 147). In calves, because

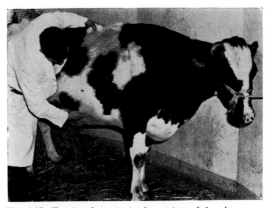

Fig. 147. *Testing for pain in the region of the abomasum by applying pressure with the hand.*

of the relatively low intra-abdominal pressure, this form of palpation will produce more informative results than in older cattle, in which the tension of the abdominal wall is usually so great, because of the weight of the digestive organs and their contents, that even strong pressure only produces a limited effect. A pain reaction, indicated by a grunt or groan, originating in the abomasum may be elicited by this method. As a rule in painful or inflammatory conditions of the abomasum, the presence of pain is indicated by the affected animal grinding its teeth. Invariably, when the functional activity of the abomasum is disturbed, rumen motility is reduced to a variable extent. Extension of abomasitis to the small intestine in a significant degree leads to the appearance of diarrhoea as an expression of the resulting hypermotility which follows.

In young calves, distension of the abomasum develops following pyloric obstruction from eating quantities of indigestible substances such as baling twine, wood-shavings or rags, and impaction, which is likely to occur when calves are fed at irregular intervals on excessive quantities of milk, thereby causing the formation of a rubbery, indigestible curd which gradually increases in size. In the terminal stages of impaction the calf is emaciated, with a pot-bellied appearance, and rattling fluid sounds can be heard in the abdomen on ballotement or when the animal is shaken.

Impaction of the abomasum has been recognized as a syndrome in adult cattle during periods of very cold weather when they have been maintained on a diet consisting entirely of chopped straw. Following maceration, some of the inadequately fermented straw passes into the abomasum and accumulates there because it is unable to pass through the pyloric sphincter. The main clinical features consist of complete anorexia, dullness, a slight degree of abdominal distension, with some pain causing discomfort. Palpation over the area of the abomasum will increase the discomfort, and it may possibly reveal the ill-defined mass of the distended viscus. Rectal examination will occasionally provide confirmation that the abomasum is enlarged and impacted.

Distension of the abomasum also occurs as the result of pyloric obstruction in vagus indigestion. The distended abomasum is unlikely to be recognized by palpation through the abdominal wall, and because most cases of vagus indigestion occur in late pregnancy, its palpation during rectal examination is also unlikely. The main clinical features consist of anorexia and a reduced volume of pasty faeces, with a marked rise in pulse rate in the late stages, by which time rumen motility has ceased.

By reason of the character and location of its anatomical supports, and its physiological functions, the abomasum, more particularly in adult dairy cattle, is liable to become displaced from its normal position on the floor of the right anterior abdomen. The most common form of displacement is that in which the greater curvature passes beneath the rumen and is retained between it and the left abdominal wall, sometimes reaching beyond the costal arch in the mid-flank area. In anterior displacement the abomasum is retained in a situation between the reticulum and the diaphragm. The condition is observed at or very shortly after parturition, and there appears to have been a real increase in its incidence in recent years, altogether apart from a greater awareness of its existence. Heavy grain or concentrate feeding in late pregnancy has been suggested to have a predisposing influence on its development.

The main clinical features are sudden reduction in appetite, which may become capricious, and moderate ruminal tympany. In left displacement an obvious bulge, caused by the tympanitic abomasum, sometimes develops in the anterior, left mid-flank area and may later extend upwards, almost to the upper limit of the paralumbar fossa. After a variable period the appetite returns and rumination may recommence, but the desire for food is quickly satisfied. The faeces are pasty, lack normal colour and are reduced in quantity. A mild degree of secondary (starvation) ketosis is present. Milk production is rapidly and severely curtailed.

Physical examination over the normal area of the abomasum reveals nothing of significance. Ruminal movements are reduced in frequency and vigour and in many cases can only be recognized, at least in the upper flank, when the abdominal wall is pushed inwards into contact with the slightly medially displaced rumen. If the distended abomasum reaches as far as the left flank it may be possible to palpate the bulging, cylindrical mass just behind the costal arch. Auscultation over an area below a line extending from the centre of the left paralumbar fossa to the costochondral junction of the seventh rib may reveal high-pitched tinkling (pinging) or splashing sounds. The abomasal sounds are not a constant feature and, although they may be frequent, quiescent intervals of up to 15 minutes duration can occur. In such circumstances, simultaneous ballotement and auscultation of the area may initiate the production of a high-pitched resonant note, typical of abomasal displacement. In established cases medial displacement of the rumen can be recognized during rectal examination, and in some instances the distended abomasum may be palpable on its left side.

The clinical signs associated with anterior displacement of the abomasum are similar, but ruminal sounds of varying intensity can be detected throughout the usual areas. Gurgling, fluid sounds can be heard behind and above the heart on both sides of the chest wall. Exploratory laparotomy may be necessary to confirm a diagnosis of displaced abomasum.

Varying degrees of dilatation of the abomasum, which is classified as right abomasal displacement, produce a syndrome of subacute intensity, suggestive of alimentary tract obstruction. It occurs mainly in adult dairy cows. The onset is insidious and the clinical indications of abdominal pain are not marked. There is inappetance, ruminal movements are depressed with slight tympany and the faeces are dark in colour and pasty. Within 3–4 days right-sided distension of the abdomen becomes obvious, and the presence of fluid and gas in the grossly distended abomasum can be detected by palpation, ballotement and auscultation. Rectal examination will reveal that the distended abomasum almost completely fills the right side of the abdomen, being comparable in size to the rumen. It is differentiated from the rumen by the tenseness of the wall.

Torsion of the abomasum is a much more serious condition than dilatation. Most cases of torsion occur in the period 3–6 weeks post partum. The twist is usually of the order of 180–270° and occurs in a vertical plane around a horizontal axis passing transversely across the body in the region of the omaso-abomasal orifice. When viewed facing the right side of the animal the torsion may be clockwise or anticlockwise. In some cases lesser degrees of rotation exist so that the blood supply to the part is not obstructed although only small quantities of ingesta can pass into the intestine. The clinical features indicate that there is a sudden onset of abdominal pain with kicking at the belly, restlessness and distress. The pulse rate increases to over 100/minute, the temperature may be subnormal and ruminal motility ceases. The faeces are usually passed in moderate quantity, are soft, occasionally very fluid, dark in colour and

become blood-stained within 1–2 days. Although thirst is exhibited no food is eaten. Distension of the abdomen occurs as the result of abomasal tympany. It sometimes causes bulging in the right flank. The tympanic state of the abomasum is revealed by evoking resonance during percussion in the vicinity of the last rib. Vigorous palpation of the abdominal wall on the right side, in the vicinity of the costal arch, will frequently produce succussion sounds. Auscultation reveals high-pitched, tinkling sounds simulating those heard in left displacement of the abomasum. Distension of the abomasum is not detectable on rectal examination in all cases of torsion. Death is almost the invariable outcome and follows in 2–4 days from severe shock and dehydration.

Ulceration of the mucosa of the abomasum is relatively common in young calves at the time when their diet is changed from milk to solid foods. The incidence is said to be particularly high in calves which have been subjected to the stresses of transport and of sale yards. Although in the majority of such cases no obvious, or only vague, symptoms have been described, occasionally fungal invasion (*Aspergillus* spp.) occurs producing severe diarrhoea, acute illness and rapid death. Specific recognition of the condition is not possible during life, and a post mortem examination is necessary to demonstrate a relationship between the fungus and the ulcers. In occasional cases abomasal ulcers may perforate and produce clinical signs of peritonitis and shock. In rare instances the inflammatory reaction heals when localization occurs as the result of peritoneal adhesions developing between neighbouring tissues. Ulceration of the abomasum has been noted in some cases of displacement, and in a few such cases perforation has occurred when the organ was in the abnormal position, giving rise to peritoneal adhesions Ulceration of the mucosa has been observed in a small number of cases of vagus indigestion.

Superficial erosions develop in the mucosa of the abomasum during the courses of rinderpest, mucosal disease, malignant catarrhal fever, hyperkeratosis and in poisoning by bracken fern, trichloroethylene-extracted soyabean meal and arsenic. The major clinical manifestations in these several conditions are not such as would suggest involvement of the abomasum. In fact it is likely that, at best, signs of visceral pain and diarrhoea only would be observed.

Examination of the Stomach in Sheep

Physical examination of the stomach compartments in sheep is carried out in the same manner as for cattle. The relative value of the different techniques is about similar although, in the case of adult animals, a heavy fleece presents a considerable interference, limiting the extent to which they can be applied. Thorough examination of the abdomen by means of deep palpation is possible in young lambs because of comparatively low intra-abdominal tension.

It will be readily ascertained that in sheep, the rate of jaw movements during rumination are more frequent than in cattle. The pattern of rumen motility is also faster, but basically similar.

Under natural grazing conditions the incidence of diseases primarily affecting the stomach compartments is rare in sheep. Improved pastures, particularly when they contain a large proportion of leguminous plants, have been associated with cases of ruminal tympany. Sheep, however, appear to be much less susceptible to this malady than cattle, probably because of more selective grazing habits and better opportunity for acclimatization.

The more general adoption of intensive method of sheep production will, no doubt give rise to an increase in the incidence of digestive disturbances. Acute rumen impaction, arising from excessive carbohydrate or protein feeding, could become a problem in feedlot sheep. Because of a high degree of oral discrimination, traumatic reticulitis is a rare event in sheep. Acute pyloric obstruction has been observed to occur in young lambs after eating indigestible material such as rags and wood shavings, in the same manner as in calves.

A specific haemorrhagic abomasitis known as 'braxy', caused by *Clostridium septicum*, occurs in weaned lambs and yearling sheep when heavy frost and snow occur in various European countries, including Britain and Ireland, and in Australia and North America. The disease is an acute toxaemia with a high mortality rate, consequently clinical signs are rarely observed. There may be gaseous distension of the abdomen and signs of abdominal pain with complere anorexia, depression and marked fever (42°C, 107°F). The diagnosis can only be made with certainty by finding lesions of abomasitis at post mortem examination and identifying the causal bacterium by cultural or fluorescent antibody techniques.

Examination of Intestines in Cattle

Physical examination of the right side of the abdomen is of little value in the investigation of diseases affecting the intestines in cattle. The character of the faeces is a fair indication of the functional status of this part of the alimentary tract. Intestinal motility may be increased or decreased in frequency and vigour as the result of inflammation or autonomic nerve imbalance which may be the result of derangement at any point in the control system. The sounds resulting from intestinal motility are rather faint and of low intensity in normal cattle and often masked by ruminal sounds.

Reduction in the tone of the intestinal musculature, causing constipation, occurs in association with general debility and in severe inflammation of the abdominal organs, such as is associated with acute peritonitis. In less severe, local inflammatory conditions, such as mild abomasitis and enteritis, there is increased motility, expressed by diarrhoea of varying severity. When intestinal motility is reduced, the prolonged fluid absorption time causes the faeces to be drier, firmer, reduced in bulk and passed at less frequent intervals, giving rise to constipation. In cattle so affected the faeces are characteristically coated with mucus so that they have a glazed appearance. Other causes of constipation in cattle, apart from severe general debility, include dehydration, deficient dietary bulk and partial intestinal obstruction.

Obstruction of the intestine arises from volvulus, intussusception and strangulation, in all of which there is virtually complete absence of defaecation, except for the passage. of blood-stained mucus, severe shock and acute abdominal pain. Torsion of the mesentery is the commonest form of intestinal obstruction in calves. In adult cattle intussusception is most frequent, although herniation through a rent in the mesentery has been observed. Organization of a blood clot following manual expression of a corpus luteum from an ovary has been noted occasionally to give rise to constriction of the intestine as the result of adhesions. Similar effects may arise in lipomatosis or fat necrosis of the mesenteries and omenta. Rotation of the coiled colon on its mesentery and torsion of the caecum are also recognized causes of intestinal obstruction. Torsion of the caecum develops under circumstances somewhat similar to those associated with dilatation and torsion of the abomasum, so it is recognized most frequently in cows in advanced pregnancy or immediately after parturition.

In those forms of obstruction which develop suddenly with complete occlusion, there is usually an initial attack of acute abdominal pain during which the animal is restless, depresses the back, kicks at its abdomen and grunts or groans—all signs indicating severe pain. This and even more violent behaviour, including rolling, continues spasmodically for between 6 and 12 hours in conjunction with anorexia and retention of faeces. During this period the temperature and respiratory rate are not significantly affected, and the pulse rate is only increased in frequency if occlusion of medium to large diameter blood vessels has occurred. Palpation or even percussion of the right wall of the abdomen during this phase will induce a pain reaction in the form of a groan or grunt, or even more obvious behaviour.

When the period of acute pain is past, the signs of shock become more evident and the animal is more depressed, with complete absence of ruminal and intestinal movement. Careful rectal examination is important in order to identify the nature of the intra-abdominal catastrophe.

When intestinal obstruction develops slowly, or is incomplete, as in torsion of the caecum, the signs indicating pain are not so acute. The faeces are passed more frequently and in small amounts, are diarrhoeic and may contain blood-stained mucus. In the absence of strangulation and necrosis, the animal survives for about 7 days, by which time moderate abdominal enlargement, somewhat pendulous in character, is apparent, along with severe toxaemia and significant deterioration in the character of the pulse. Dilatation and torsion of the caecum give rise to an appearance of fullness in the right paralumbar fossa, with a tympanic or fluid sound on percussion and ballottement. Generally, recumbency occurs at this time and death is inevitable within 24–48 hours.

With increase in intestinal motility, from whatever cause, because of reduced absorption, and in the majority of inflammatory states involving the intestines, actual increased secretion, the faeces are usually more fluid and bulkier, necessitating more frequent defaecation than in normal animals. This clinical sign of diarrhoea is a constant feature in enteritis, but intestinal hypermotility also occurs when the food eaten by the animal contains irritant substances. Func-

tional diarrhoea occurs in excitement and is also an expression of disturbed motor nerve control. The passage of soft faeces persists for a variable period in the majority of stalled cattle when turned out to graze lush pasture in the spring season. The high water and protein content of the herbage are probably the important factors in the situation. In chronic fascioliasis and molybdenosis, the mechanism whereby diarrhoea is produced is not clearly understood.

The clinical manifestations of enteritis, in addition to diarrhoea, include abdominal pain and, sometimes, dysentery. The signs vary considerably in severity according to the specific nature of the causal agent. In a number of acute systemic diseases, enteritis is less obvious than in some others in which it is a prominent feature from the commencement. Acute diarrhoea with dysentery, indicating intestinal involvement, occurs in a proportion of cases of anthrax. Affected animals evince signs of abdominal pain with slight straining. It is needless to point out the inadvisability of undertaking a rectal examination in a cow which is febrile and showing the aforementioned signs.

Other bacterial forms of enteritis in which dysentery may occur include colibacillosis, salmonellosis, pasteurellosis, vibrionic dysentery and enterotoxaemia. Colibacillosis or 'white scour', caused by a variety of serotypes of *Escherichia coli*, is a potentially septicaemic disease affecting young calves during the first few weeks of life. The incidence is highest in purchased calves kept in groups in unhygienic surroundings. The greyish-white, or yellow, fluid faeces, which in severe cases contain blood, suggest the diagnosis, confirmation being obtained by means of bacteriological examination of rectal swabs. Resort to this method is necessary because of the similarity between *E. coli* infection and salmonellosis in young calves.

In addition to the more obvious signs indicating enteritis, calves affected by salmonellosis may show signs of involvement of the nervous system including incoordination and nystagmus. The common species of salmonellae causing disease in calves are *Salmonella typhimurium* and *S. dublin*, but many other serotypes may be responsible. Adolescent or adult animals whose resistance has been reduced by intercurrent infection or stress may become similarly affected. When infection occurs in healthy adult cattle, localization in abdominal viscera is likely so that the animal becomes a chronic carrier. Identification of the species of *Salmonella* in suspect clinical cases requires the use of both bacteriological and serological examinations, which can also be applied to detect adult carrier cattle.

Intestinal involvement in bovine septicaemic pasteurellosis (caused by *Pasteurella multocida* Type 1 or B) occurs in the later stages of the disease, so that other features such as those indicating septicaemia, should indicate its nature which can be specifically identified by microscopic examination of blood smears and confirmed by bacteriological techniques.

perfringens types A, B and C has been identified in calves and adult cattle. The disease occurs in young calves up to 10 days of age and in adult cattle is most common in the period shortly after calving. The signs include diarrhoea, dysentery, acute abdominal pain associated with bellowing or moaning and marked restlessness. In most cases profound toxaemia develops and death occurs in from a few hours to about 4 days. Faecal smears may be subjected to examination by means of fluorescent antibody techniques and provide a diagnosis prior to death in affected animals. Diagnosis, otherwise, is made by the

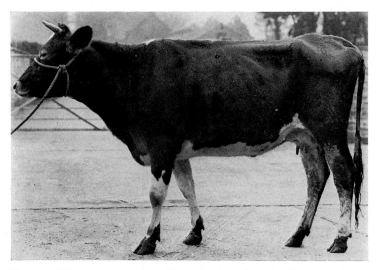

Fig. 148. *Diarrhoea in the cow. Note that the tail and hindlegs are splashed with faeces, whereas the forelegs are clean. The diarrhoea is of fairly recent origin, since the hindquarters are not yet caked with faeces. Johne's disease breakdown in a young Guernsey cow.*

Vibrionic (winter) dysentery is thought to be caused by *Vibrio jejuni*, although a primary virus agent is suggested by some authorities; it is a sporadic cause of severe diarrhoea of brief duration in adult dairy cattle, particularly those which have recently calved. General clinical signs include mild fever with a precipitate fall in milk yield and transient anorexia. The faeces are thin and watery, and are dark green to almost black in colour; they are often discharged with considerable velocity without any premonitory signs. Diagnosis depends on the exclusion of other causes of diarrhoea, in combination with the demonstration of the *Vibrio* in faecal material.

Haemorrhagic enteritis caused by *Clostridium*

detection of specific toxin in intestinal contents obtained after death.

Bacterial enteritis of chronic intensity occurs in Johne's disease caused by *Mycobacterium paratuberculosis* (Fig. 148). The main clinical features of Johne's disease are a long incubation period—even when exposed to infection early in life, cattle do not show clinical signs until they are at least 18 months of age—fluid faeces which contain gas bubbles, loss of condition (this and reduction in milk yield may precede all other signs in milking cows) and in the later stages, anaemia and oedema which more usually involves the intermandibular space. Clinical signs often develop within a few weeks after calving

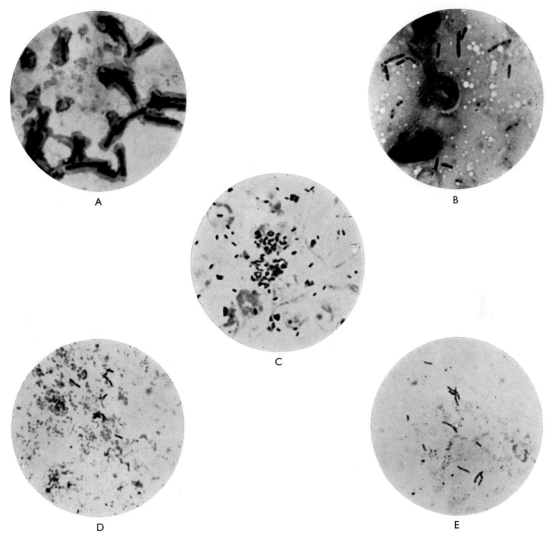

Fig. 149. A, Bacillus anthracis *in a thick blood smear. 1% aqueous methylene blue.* B, *Post mortem invaders in the blood.* C, Mycobacterium paratuberculosis *in bovine faeces. Ziehl-Neelsen.* D, *Non-specific acid-fast bodies in faeces. Ziehl-Neelsen.* E, Mycobacterium tuberculosis *in sputum. Ziehl–Neelsen. All* ×1000.

or following removal to another area, particularly if the diet is deficient in any essential factor such as phosphorus. Confirmation of the diagnosis is obtained by demonstration of *M. paratuberculosis* (Fig. 149c) in faecal smears. Failure to find the organism in smears does not justify a negative diagnosis. In occasional cases of generalized tuberculosis in cattle, chronic enteritis may appear following the spread of the infection to the intestinal mucosa with the development of ulcerated areas. At this stage of the disease affected cattle will usually exhibit other clinical signs of tuberculosis so that recognition

of the cause of the enteritis should not offer an insuperable problem.

Viral enteritides, in which diarrhoea is a prominent sign, include rinderpest, mucosal disease complex and malignant catarrhal fever. These are severe acute or mild acute diseases with febrile features. Rinderpest is highly contagious with erosive lesions which are largely confined to the alimentary tract. Salivation and nasal discharge, along with diarrhoea or dysentery, are characteristic features which, when exhibited by a number of animals in a group, should arouse suspicion of this disease. Mucosal disease possesses many of the clinicopathological features of rinderpest, although to a much less marked degree of severity in most cases. It is important because the characteristically shallow erosive lesions, which occur on the mucosa throughout the digestive tract, are likely to be confused with those of foot-and-mouth disease. The absence of large vesicles and the presence of diarrhoea help in excluding foot-and-mouth disease. The morbidity and mortality rates in mucosal disease vary widely; two main syndromes occur with some variations. The main clinical signs in the epidemic form are fever, excessive salivation and mucopurulent nasal discharge associated with the development of necrotic erosions on the buccal and pharyngeal mucosae and sometimes on the muzzle. The faeces are watery, foul-smelling, may contain blood or mucus and are increased in amount. Lameness, due to laminitis, may be common in some outbreaks. The morbidity rate may be 100%, recovery occurring in from 2 to 20 days. In the sporadic form anorexia and high fever are the initial signs. Later erosive lesions develop coincident with the onset of watery diarrhoea. Defaecation may be accompanied by straining. Lameness occurs in about 10% of affected animals, but there are no nervous signs. The moribidity rate is usually low (2–20%) but the mortality rate is of the order of 90%; death usually occurs in 4–15 days. Diagnosis depends upon recognition of the clinicopathological features; specific confirmation may be achieved by serological methods.

Malignant catarrhal fever, although acute and highly fatal, appears to have a low degree of infectivity so that the incidence is sporadic in most instances. Clinical features of diagnostic significance include catarrhal inflammation of the upper respiratory mucosa, as well as that of the alimentary tract, along with keratoconjunctivitis, and lymph node enlargement. The consistency of the faeces varies from constipation to profuse diarrhoea with dysentery. In acutely affected animals there is marked dejection, anorexia, pyrexia, nasal and ocular discharge, blepharospasm and dyspnoea. Discrete areas of superficial necrosis become evident on the nasal and buccal mucosae, and the muzzle may be similarly affected, along with the coronary band area of the feet. Incoordination and muscle tremor indicate nervous involvement; head pushing, paralysis and convulsions may occur in the final stages.

Diarrhoea, arising from enteritis, is a clinical feature in coccidiosis and in intestinal parasitism. Both of these diseases are most prevalent in young and adolescent cattle. The species of coccidia which are pathogenic to cattle include *Eimeria zurnii, Eim. bovis* and *Eim. ellipsoidalis*. The majority of cattle become infected with coccidia but only a minority show clinical signs; young animals kept closely confined in overcrowded conditions are most likely to be affected. The first sign of illness is the sudden appearance of severe diarrhoea, the fluid faeces, which are foul-smelling with shreds of mucus and streaks of blood, being passed in association with severe straining. Anaemia may be profound when the blood loss is severe. The duration of the illness is 5–7 days. Diagnosis is based on recognition of the nature of the clinical syndrome and identification of oöcysts in large numbers in the faeces (see Fig. 158E, p. 204).

The majority of clinical cases of intestinal helminth infestation occur in young cattle grazing pasture in groups. A variety of helminth species may be responsible (see Table 11, p. 203) causing loss of condition, unthriftiness, dehydration, anaemia and emaciation. In establishing a diagnosis of parasitic gastroenteritis in a group of young cattle, the results of faecal egg counts (see pp. 198–201) on samples from a representative proportion of the animals should be interpreted in relation to all the circumstances of the animals including age, physical condition, character of the faeces, nutritional status, time of year, prevailing weather conditions, stocking density and possible nutritional deficiency (cobalt, copper, etc.).

Chronic diarrhoea is a feature of liver fluke infestation (caused by *Fasciola hepatica* commonly and *F. magna* rarely in cattle). The reason for diarrhoea developing is not explained; the existence of a concurrent intestinal nematodiasis is a possible causal factor. Other clinical features of chronic fascioliasis consist of loss of weight, reduced milk production and anaemia. Epidemiologically important features include low-lying swampy land, which provides the conditions suitable for the survival of intermediate host snails and larval cercariae, and the propagation of the former during certain seasons, and suitable temperature conditions. The important host snails for *Fasciola hepatica* are *Lymnaea truncula* in Great Britain, Ireland and Europe *L. tomentosa* in Australia and *Galba bulimoides* and other species in the USA. The intermediate hosts for *Fascioloides magna* are *Galba bulimoides techella* and several other species of snails. The development of clinical signs in cattle, which may be affected at any age during the grazing season, should be taken to signify a fairly heavy infestation. Weather conditions are of considerable significance in relation to the extent and local density of the host snail population, periods of high rainfall during the relatively warm seasons assisting these ends. Diagnosis depends upon demonstrating fluke ova in the faeces of clinically affected animals.

Severe diarrhoea is a feature of enteritis caused by a variety of chemical agents including arsenic, inorganic phosphorus, mercury, copper, molybdenum, nitrates, etc. In subacute lead poisoning, foetid diarrhoea succeeds an initial period of constipation, but as a rule other signs dominate the clinical picture. Diagnosis in this particular instance would necessitate analysis of body tissues (blood, kidney, liver) and/or excretions (faeces). Recognition of the other forms of chemical enteritis is based on the history of availability to the animal, as well as the usually acute signs and, where applicable, response to specific antidotes. Molybdenum is of especial interest as a cause of diarrhoea in that it exerts its toxic effect in grazing cattle through mediating in copper metabolism. The incidence of molybdenosis is highest in areas where there is a naturally high soil level of the element, or certain industrial processes are in operation which cause pasture contamination (manufacture of ferro-molybdenum alloys or aluminium alloys). When soil copper levels are inadequate even moderate amounts of molybdenum (5–10 parts per million) are significant, especially if the herbage sulphate content is high. Molybdenosis, which has a geographical distribution, is expressed clinically by persistent diarrhoea—the faeces being light green—and dry, staring coat, with a tendency to depigmentation and hair loss (see Fig. 31, p. 41). Diagnosis depends upon demonstrating the presence of excessive amounts of molybdenum in the diet, although confirmation by therapeutic copper supplementation is frequently all that is necessary in the recognized geographical areas.

Many poisonous plants cause severe enteritis in cattle. The important species include *Pteridium aquilinum* (bracken fern), *Euphorbia* spp. (spurges), *Delphinium* spp. (larkspur), *Solanum* spp (nightshade), *Ranunculus* spp. (buttercup), *Umbelliferae* spp. (water hemlock, water dropwort). The signs of gastroenteritis which occur in poisoning by these plants are often accompanied by muscle tremors, incoordination and convulsions of varying severity.

Rectal Examination in Cattle

As an aid towards the diagnosis of diseases of the digestive system in cattle, rectal examination tends to be overlooked. This has largely resulted from the emphasis that has been given to the value of this procedure in relation to the investigation of diseases of the female reproductive organs. In addition, many of the alimentary tract diseases in large ruminants involve the rumen and reticulum. Rectal palpation, which is performed with due regard to anatomical relationships, provides confirmatory evidence in respect of the state of the rumen, the considerable mass of the dorsal blind sac of which is readily identified on the left side of the pelvic inlet. The strength and frequency of ruminal contractions, in addition to the nature of its contents which may be fluid, solid or gaseous, can be determined, as well as reduction or increase in size. Reduction in size, in conjunction with displacement towards the median plane, occurs when the abomasum is displaced to the left. Increase in size, so that the dorsal blind sac projects into the pelvis, occurs when the rumen is impacted or tympanitic.

The anterior parts of the rumen, the reticulum and the omasum are inaccessible during rectal exploration which, therefore, is of no direct value in assisting the diagnosis of actinobacillosis or neoplasia affecting these parts of the stomach, or in many cases of traumatic reticuloperitonitis, and in impaction of the omasum. In painful conditions of the rumen, e.g. acute impaction, a response is obtained on palpation of the posterior parts of the organ. When the abomasum has been displaced to the left there may be a feeling of emptiness in the right upper abdomen, with reduction in the size of the rumen, and the distended abomasum may be palpable on the left. Normally the abomasum is out of reach of the hand during rectal examination, but occasionally in torsion it becomes so distended that it fills the right half of the abdomen and reaches almost to the pelvic inlet. In this state the abomasum can be differentiated from the rumen on the left by the tense condition of its wall.

The behaviour of the animal during insertion of the hand into the rectum, and when the various organs are handled, should be noted. In intestinal obstruction, vigorous straining and pain result from the motility contractions which are induced. It is usual in obstruction to find the rectum empty except for a small quantity of blood-stained mucus which adheres to the hand and arm. In intussusception of the small intestine the affected segment is sometimes recognized, on being palpated, as a firm sausage-shaped mass, which when handled initiates a sharp pain reaction by the animal. Intestinal torsion may be recognized by finding a small, soft mobile segment attached to a tightly stretched mesenteric fold in the lower right abdomen. Rectal exploration is sometimes helpful in cases of intestinal incarceration arising from a rent in the mesenteric supporting fold, or through the development of peritoneal adhesions following injury or haemorrhage, provided that the affected segment is within reach of the hand. Gaseous distension of the small intestine is not a marked feature in obstruction because fermentative digestion is of minor significance at this point in the digestive tract in cattle. In torsion of the coiled portion of the colon, however, distension of loops of small intestine does occur and is readily appreciated; in torsion of the caecum, apart from the gross distension of the caecum itself, one grossly distended segment of intestine extends horizontally across the abdomen immediately anterior to the pelvic inlet. In anterior displacement of the caecum the organ will be missing from its normal position in the upper right posterior abdomen.

Extensive masses of fat necrosis and lipoma, which may surround the rectum, are readily recognized during rectal exploration because of their mobility and firm consistency. The small nodular lesions of tuberculosis may be found on the peritoneum, more readily perhaps over the dorsal blind sac of the rumen. Enlarged iliac and sublumbar lymph nodes, when recognized, suggest the presence of either lymphomatosis or tuberculosis; in the former the enlargement is usually bilaterally symmetrical.

In cattle exhibiting signs of abdominal pain, attention should be directed to the urinary tract. Rectal examination in male animals with urethral obstruction (urolithiasis) reveals distension of the bladder and pelvic urethra, with pulsation of the urethra when it is manipulated. A pain reaction may also be induced, and thickening of

the wall of the urinary bladder detected, in acute cystitis. Rectal examination may yield negative findings in the early stages of pyelonephritis, but later there is usually thickening of one or both ureters, making them readily detectable on the side wall of the pelvis, with concomitant thickening and contraction of the wall of the bladder. If the left kidney is affected, palpation will reveal enlargement, absence of distinct lobulation and pain. Enlargement of the kidneys to a variable extent occurs in hydronephrosis and amyloidosis.

Rectal exploration in cattle has its greatest application in relation to the female reproductive organs. By means of methodical palpation it is possible to determine when pregnancy exists, and when abnormal states such as fetal mummification, septic metritis, endometritis, salpingitis, certain ovarian disorders, neoplasia and developmental defects exist. Septic metritis usually develops shortly after parturition and causes a degree of toxaemia sufficiently profound to render the animal recumbent and even comatose. Detection of uterine distension is essential to differentiate the condition from clinical hypocalcaemia.

Examination of the Intestines in Sheep

Clinical examination of the right side of the abdomen in sheep only occasionally provides any information of significance in relation to the functional status of the intestines. Intestinal obstruction is an exceptional event, and constipation from other causes is also unusual. A history of food deprivation during drought or inclement weather or consumption of dry, fibrous food is usually ascertained. Intestinal hypermotility, expressed clinically by diarrhoea, has the same significance as in cattle. The most important bacterial causes of enteritis are, however, species belonging to the clostridial genus which survive in the soil; occasional episodes of colibacillosis and salmonellosis also occur. The disease syndromes are enterotoxaemic in character so that the signs of intestinal involvement are not always a prominent feature, especially if the course is short, as is the case with pulpy kidney disease and enterotoxaemia of older sheep, both of which are caused by *Clostridium perfringens* type D. In the acute form of lamb dysentery, which is caused by *C. perfringens* type B and affects lambs less than 1 week old, the faeces are fluid, brown in colour and sometimes contain blood. Other clinical features include severe abdominal pain, exhibited by grinding the teeth, arching the back, disinclination to move, failure to suck and recumbency, followed by coma and death within 24 hours. Because the clinical features are not sufficiently distinctive, the diagnosis of lamb dysentery depends upon the post mortem demonstration of haemorrhagic enteritis with mucosal ulceration, which in some cases is extensive, individual ulcers being 2·5 cm in diameter and penetrating almost to the serosa. In addition it is necessary to obtain confirmation of the diagnosis by means of laboratory biological toxin–antitoxin neutralization tests employing mice, or specific bacterial detection by fluorescent antibody techniques; the latter yields a more rapid result.

Dysentery in lambs 20–48 hours after birth is commonly ascribed in the USA to pathogenic strains of *Escherichia coli*. Unsanitary conditions in the lambing sheds and inclement weather conditions are considered to be important predisposing factors. The clinical signs consist initially of diarrhoea, the faeces being yellow and liquid; at this time the affected lamb is dejected, ceases sucking and stands with the back arched and the tail drooping. Within hours the diarrhoea becomes profuse, grey in colour and sometimes blood-stained. The mortality rate varies from 15 to 75%; death occurs within 24–36 hours.

Enteric salmonellosis in sheep is usually caused by *Salmonella typhimurium* or *S. dublin*. Affected sheep are markedly depressed with loss of appetite, elevated temperature (40°C) and diarrhoea, the faeces being thin and watery and sometimes streaked with blood. As a rule up to 25% of the flock may be affected; the mortality is rarely more than 5%. A specific diagnosis in cases of acute bacterial enteritis is obtained by culturing the intestinal contents or the mesenteric lymph nodes.

Johne's disease, because of the long incubation period, assumes clinical proportions only in sheep over 18 months of age. The disease is usually manifested by emaciation and other signs of general debilitation, including shedding of the fleece and anaemia. Diarrhoea is a rather late development and is not severe, the faeces becoming soft and losing their characteristic pelleted form. Appetite is retained but loss of weight leads to extreme emaciation and weakness so that the animal becomes recumbent some days before death. Diagnosis is achieved by microscopic examination of suitably stained faecal smears, but it is usual experience to find that the disease is widely established in the flock before its presence is suspected because of the mildness of the diarrhoea. Material of greater diagnostic value can be obtained from affected areas of intestinal mucosa during post mortem examination of an emaciated carcase. Differentiation from intestinal parasitism may be made on the basis of a faecal worm egg count, although it is necessary to realize that both diseases may co-exist, and in fact the presence of one may predispose to the establishment and development of clinical signs of the other.

Coccidiosis is not a very important disease of sheep under free-range grazing conditions; under intensive production systems such as in feedlots it has been a cause of considerable loss in lambs. The species of coccidia found in the intestines of sheep are up to 10 in number, of which only two are known to produce clinical disease—*Eimeria arloingi* and *E. ninakohlyakimovi*. The disease mainly affects lambs and the first sign is that the faeces become soft and then watery. Later blood streaks may be noted and sometimes tenesmus is quite severe. Loss of appetite and dehydration cause considerable reduction in body weight. Eventually weakness leads to recumbency and finally death. The diagnosis is suggested by the blood streaked, diarrhoeic faeces and is confirmed by direct microscopic examination of a faecal smear which should reveal the presence of oöcysts.

Diarrhoea is a prominent feature of parasitic gastroenteritis in sheep which may be affected at any age in life beyond 3 months. The disease is usually most severe in the younger age groups. The species of helminths (see Table 11, p. 203) which cause the disease in various countries throughout the world vary according to the climatic conditions. In some forms of parasitic gastroenteritis the main clinical effects are attributable to anaemia (haemonchosis, ostertagiasis and hookworm infestation). Diarrhoea, with soiling of the wool in the perineal region and of the hindlegs and loss of weight, occurs in trichostrongylosis, nematodiriasis and threadworm infestation. In considering the diagnosis, consideration should be given to the circumstances of the animals as referred to in cattle. The limitations of faecal worm egg counts should be borne in mind, and whenever possible a worm count with specific identification should be undertaken in order to ensure correct anthelmintic therapy and control measures.

The later stages of cobalt deficiency are often associated with diarrhoea and anaemia. Stunted growth in lambs and loss of condition in adult sheep, with gradual reduction in appetite and eventual emaciation, are the more general signs of this disease (Fig. 150) which has a geographi-

a point on the abdominal floor midway between the xiphoid cartilage and the umbilicus. The long axis of the stomach is transverse. The pyloric extremity is in contact with the right lateral lobe of the liver, opposite to the middle of the thirteenth intercostal space; the left end is ventral to the upper part of the left thirteenth rib and intercostal space.

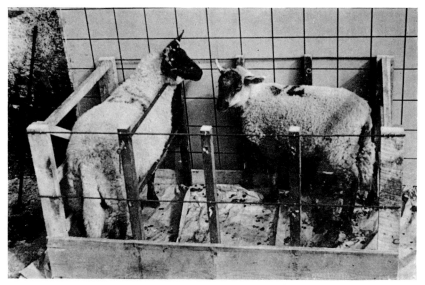

Fig. 150. *Worm-free lambs showing the result of cobalt deficiency. Two lambs of the same age were maintained on the same cobalt deficient diet, but the lamb on the left received cobalt supplementation. Note the difference in the appearance and the obvious difference in size.*

cal distribution, the incidence being fairly frequent on acid or peaty soils. The diarrhoea probably results from anaemia, or the concomitant intestinal parasitism which reaches significant proportions in the advanced stages. Confirmation of cobalt deficiency depends upon the results of soil and herbage analysis for the element, and the observed response to vitamin B12 therapy or dietary supplementation with cobalt.

Enteritis accompanied by diarrhoea can be caused by various chemicals and plant materials as in cattle; the incidence attributable to these factors is, however, considerably less in sheep.

ABDOMEN OF THE PIG

Regional Anatomy

The stomach of the pig is relatively large and when filled with food its greater curvature reaches

The small intestine, in adult animals, is between 15 and 20 m long. Its mesenteric portion is arranged in loops which lie above the colon and caecum, between the stomach and pelvis, mainly against the right wall, and on the posterior part of the floor of the abdomen. The supporting mesentery is 15–20 cm in length. The large intestine, comprising the caecum, colon and rectum, varies from 4 to 5 m in length in adult pigs. The caecum forms a cylinder about 20–30 cm long and 8–10 cm in diameter, which is situated in contact with the upper and anterior part of the left abdominal wall from where it extends downwards, backwards and medially. The blind apex is in contact with the abdominal floor, near the midline somewhere between the umbilicus and the pelvic inlet. The colon, which at its origin is of similar diameter to the caecum, gradually reduces in size. The major portion of the colon is accommodated in the mesentery in three closely opposed double spiral coils which are situated on the abdominal floor, being related to the liver anteriorly, the caecum and small intestine posteriorly and the small intestine on the right. The terminal part of the colon, when it emerges from the spiral coils, forms a rather shallow, irregular U-tube by passing forwards on the right side of the dorsal part of the abdominal cavity where, at a point behind the stomach, it turns towards the left until, ventral to the pancreas, it again turns backwards medially to the left kidney to reach the pelvic inlet where it continues as the rectum. The caecum has three rows of sacculations and three longitudinal muscular bands. The spiral colon has two series of sacculations and two muscular bands which do not reach the termination of the centrifugal part.

Clinical Examination of the Abdomen in the Pig

Clinical examination of the abdomen in the pig only occasionally provides rewarding results. Inspection readily reveals anatomical abnormalities such as umbilical or scrotal hernia (see Fig. 136, p. 149) which demand more detailed consideration when there is evidence suggesting intestinal obstruction. The laboured abdominal type of breathing ('thumps'), which occurs in acute pneumonia or pulmonary oedema when lung efficiency is markedly reduced because of pulmonary engorgement and infiltration and the accumulation of exudate in the bronchioles and alveoli, is readily audible.

Palpation of the abdomen is rarely worth while except that in cases of severe abdominal pain a response is obtained readily at almost any point; otherwise, because of the thickness of the abdominal wall, localization of a pain focus is impossible. Except in very young pigs, identification of abdominal organs or recognition of abnormal swellings is not practicable. As a consequence, the differential diagnosis of diseases involving the abdominal digestive organs in the pig is based on a consideration of the evidence of disturbed function. In this connection, appetite, vomition and defaecation are important.

Lack of appetite in the pig is a feature of any acute illness and is not to be taken to indicate a primary digestive disturbance in all instances. In fact in mild or chronic diseases of the alimentary tract, appetite may be retained to a variable degree. Acute diseases which cause redistribu-

tion of body fluids or disturbance of tissue fluid balance increase the appetite for fluid; consequently if clean water is not available in these circumstances, the pig will drink any other fluid, including urine, that is available.

Gastritis, which may be acute or chronic in intensity, can be caused by irritant substances in the food, including inorganic arsenic, sodium fluoride, sodium chloride and iron, by eating straw bedding, by foreign bodies, ascarid worms (*Ascaris suum*), especially in young pigs, and *Hyostrongylus rubidus, Ascarops strongylina, Physocephalus sexalatus* and *Simondsia paradoxa* in young pigs and lactating sows. Hyperaemia and infarction of the gastric mucosa occurs in acute colibacillosis, vibrionic dysentery, salmonellosis and swine erysipelas. Similar gastric lesions occur in swine fever, African swine fever and swine influenza. Gastritis is an important part of the pathological features of transmissible gastroenteritis. Similar, though less marked, gastritis occurs in vomiting and wasting disease.

In the pig, as in some other species of animals, acute gastritis causes increased motility, which is expressed clinically by vomiting of variable intensity. There is also an increase in peristalsis causing some abdominal pain. Appetite is always reduced, often completely absent, but thirst is excessive, so that affected pigs are almost continuously drinking whatever liquid is available. Vomiting recurs repeatedly with strong retching movements; the vomitus contains mucus, sometimes blood, and is voided in small amounts.

Chronic gastritis gives rise to increased secretion of gastric mucus which delays digestion and gastric emptying; this may lead to chronic dilatation of the stomach. The appetite is reduced or depraved, and vomiting, which is only occasional, usually occurs after feeding.

As is the case in other species, gastritis in the pig is frequently accompanied by enteritis of variable intensity. Parasitic gastritis in young pigs, caused by *Hyostrongylus rubidus, Ascarops strongylina* or *Physocephalus sexalatus*, produces a syndrome of anaemia, poor growth and diarrhoea with marked thirst. In adult sows occasional deaths occur as the result of heavy infestations causing gastric ulceration and then severe haemorrhage, or perforation and peritonitis. A specific diagnosis is possible only by post mortem examination of the gastric mucosa with, in the case of *H. rubidus*, careful examination of a mucosal scraping mixed with water on a glass slide held over a black background.

The specific infective diseases, including swine erysipelas, swine fever, African swine fever and swine influenza, although they may cause vomiting to a variable extent, are associated with other clinical manifestations such as patchy cutaneous erythema, febrile signs and in some instances convulsions.

Disturbances of intestinal motility in the pig, as is the case in other species of animals, are indicated by diarrhoea or constipation. Hypermotility with ensuing diarrhoea is a feature of enteritis, which is often associated with gastritis in a number of specific diseases including colibacillosis, salmonellosis, vibrionic dysentery, transmissible gastroenteritis and vomiting and wasting disease. Systemic infectious diseases in which enteritis is a part of the pathological picture include, swine erysipelas, swine fever and African swine fever. In many of these conditions there is usually a preliminary period of intestinal hypermotility before diarrhoea becomes evident. The clinical syndrome is also associated with fever and other systemic manifestations in a number of these diseases. Other causes of enteritis are heavy infestations with *Ascaris suum*, coccidia including *Eimeria debliecki, Eim. escabra* and *Eim. perminuta*, irritant foods such as frozen roots and chemical irritants such as arsenic, sodium fluoride or iron in excessive amounts.

Enteric colibacillosis of young pigs usually occurs in young animals of 8–18 weeks of age, although occasional cases are seen in piglets 24–72 hours old, in which the infection is generally septicaemic in character. The disease is caused by serotypes of haemolytic *Escherichia coli* similar to those causing gut oedema. The clinical features of the enteric syndrome include depression, anorexia, fever (40·5°C, 105°F) and diarrhoea. Dysentery is not a feature. The diagnosis depends upon appreciation of the clinical signs, history, post mortem findings of moderate to severe enteritis and isolation of haemolytic *E. coli* in almost pure culture from the caecum and colon or from rectal swabs in living affected pigs. Final assessment of the significance of any coliform bacterium isolated necessitates the application of serotyping methods.

Salmonellosis (paratyphoid) in pigs is generally a much more acute disease than colibacillosis. It is caused by *Salmonella choleraesuis* and *Salm. typhimurium*. Clinical disease appears, however,

to require the operation of a predisposing factor, or factors, such as sudden change in feeding, dosing with an anthelmintic, dietary deficiency, etc. In the acute enteric form of salmonellosis there is a marked, febrile reaction, 40–41°C (104–106°F), persistent watery diarrhoea, sometimes dysentery and, occasionally, tenesmus. Less severe cases give rise to a syndrome of rather persistent diarrhoea, with intermittent febrile periods and, eventually, marked emaciation. The diagnosis of salmonellosis is a matter of some difficulty in living pigs because a number of other diseases have similar clinical manifestations. The clinical and pathological findings for the enteric syndrome should direct attention to the need for bacteriological investigation. For this purpose samples of faeces (not less than 20 g) from living animals, or intestinal contents and specimens of spleen, mesenteric lymph node, liver and gall-bladder from carcases should be selected. Selective media are essential for primary isolation, and serological methods for specific identification of salmonellae.

Vibrionic dysentery of pigs is generally considered to be caused by *Vibrio coli*, although the possibility of there being some other primary factor has been postulated because of the difficulty of reproducing the disease with pure cultures of *V. coli*. Predisposing factors, such as fatigue and exhaustion arising during transportation, appear to have a significant influence on the development of clinical disease. The main clinical features consist of the sudden onset of severe diarrhoea with anorexia and mild febrile signs. The faeces are very fluid, contain mucus and are passed in an uninterrupted stream without physical effort. Initially they are yellow in colour but within 24–48 hours they become black or blood-tinged or whole clots of blood may be present. Affected animals are depressed and dehydration is severe. The morbidity and mortality rates may be high; acutely affected pigs may die within 24 hours but death may be delayed for up to 4 days. Apparently recovered pigs may relapse and die later. Occasionally the infection may be responsible for chronic persistent diarrhoea. Diagnosis is based on recognition of the severity of the diarrhoea associated with dysentery, and the absence of pulmonary and nervous system involvement which exists in some cases of salmonellosis. *Vibrio coli* can be demonstrated in stained smears from the mucosa of the colon.

Transmissible gastroenteritis of pigs is caused

by a host-specific virus. The initial clinical signs consist of the sudden onset of vomiting and diarrhoea; appetite, at least in young sucking pigs, is sometimes retained until shortly before death. The faeces are yellow-green in colour, watery in consistency and profuse in amount. Depression and dehydration are pronounced and weakness and emaciation precede death which may occur on the second to fifth day. The mortality rate is highest in very young pigs. The history and clinical signs form the basis for a presumptive diagnosis but specific confirmation depends upon the results of serological and biological tests.

Coccidiosis is a disease of young pigs. The initial sign of active infection is diarrhoea which may be followed by constipation. The appearance of blood in the faeces is exceptional. Other signs include anorexia, dehydration and emaciation. The disease is diagnosed by correlating the history and clinical signs with the results of a faecal examination for oöcysts. Specific identification is rather difficult and usually not necessary.

The significance of the protozoan unicellular ciliate, *Balantidium coli,* in relation to enteritis in the pig is not entirely clear. The infection rate varies from 20 to 100% but in cases of clinical disease bacteria such as streptococci or *E. coli* are frequently present. The disease affects pigs of all ages and is usually most severe in advanced pork and bacon pigs. The main signs are intermittent diarrhoea, anorexia, depression and loss of weight. Stunting is usual in young pigs. Diagnosis depends upon identification of the trophozoites or cysts in the faeces or in smears of mucosal scrapings from the haemorrhagic colon.

Vomiting and wasting disease of sucking pigs, which bears some resemblance to transmissible gastroenteritis, may be associated with diarrhoea in the older age range of the affected piglets. In this condition the diarrhoea is not severe and is overshadowed by other signs, particularly vomition.

Constipation is a sign of intestinal hypomotility, and is the result of the faecal contents of the gut becoming excessively dry, or of obstruction. Excessively dry faeces occur when there is insufficient water available with a dry-feeding system, when the fibre content of the diet is insufficient to ensure adequate bulk, and in sows in advanced pregnancy, in which lack of exercise is an important predisposing factor. The most important cause of intestinal obstruction is impaction with either inspissated faeces or large numbers of *Ascaris suum.* The clinical signs consist of failure to pass faeces, lack of appetite, slight to vigorous straining and depression. When restlessness, exhibited by lying down and standing up again repeated almost continuously and accompanied by vomiting with eructation of gas, is associated with constipation, then intestinal obstruction, caused by torsion, intussusception or strangulation, or peritonitis should be suspected. Intussusception more usually occurs in young pigs and frequently results from feeding unsuitable diets or from the presence of ascarid worms in the small intestine. In addition to the signs of abdominal pain there is the passage of blood-stained mucus and faeces in small amounts and tenesmus, which may lead to prolapse of the rectal mucosa.

Intestinal torsion is a relatively rare condition occurring in young pigs as a complication of hernial strangulation or of acute peritonitis with adhesions between neighbouring segments of intestine. Strangulation usually affects a loop of intestine in a hernial sac when the former becomes overfilled with food and is unable to escape from the sac. The majority of such cases are associated with an umbilical hernia, only exceptional instances occurring with scrotal or diaphragmatic hernia. In addition to signs indicating acute abdominal pain, local signs are recognizable consisting of inflammation of varying intensity in the skin over the hernial sac, and pain on palpation of the hernial contents which are somewhat firm and cannot be reduced.

Reduced intestinal motility also occurs, along with other signs in oesophagogastric ulceration and diverticulitis and ileitis in pigs. In the former the main signs are pallor due to massive haemorrhage into the stomach, anorexia and black pasty faeces, changing to mucus-covered pellets which are passed in small amounts. The condition is identified by finding ulcers confined to the oesophageal zone of the stomach at post mortem examination. The latter disease is usually associated with signs of acute peritonitis due to ulceration and, sometimes, perforation of the ileum. Post mortem examination reveals gross thickening of the wall of the ileum which may be perforated, with in this instance diffuse peritonitis.

Prolapse of the rectal mucosa occurs as the result of inflammation of the rectum (proctitis) which may arise as a stage of progression in enteritis, or follows prolonged and repeated tenesmus in severe constipation.

ABDOMEN OF THE DOG AND CAT

Regional Anatomy

Dog. The configuration of the abdomen in the dog varies somewhat according to the breed, being more rounded on cross-section throughout in some, compared with the somewhat laterally flattened, deeper abdomen existing in many of the sporting breeds.

The stomach is relatively large and when filled to capacity has an irregularly pyriform shape, the left, or cardiac, part being larger and rounded while the right, or pyloric, part remains small and cylindrical. The anterior or parietal surface of the stomach, when normally distended, is related to the posterior surface of the liver, the left section of the diaphragm and the abdominal wall on its left and ventral aspects as far back as a transverse line through the second or third lumbar vertebra. The greater curvature of the full stomach extends beyond the left costal arch and lies on the abdominal floor about midway between the xiphoid cartilage and the pubes. In these circumstances the long axis of the spleen approximates to the direction of the last rib beyond which it extends almost to reach the abdominal floor.

The pyloric extremity of the stomach is situated at a point opposite to the lower part of the ninth rib or intercostal space, slightly to the right of the median plane. The empty stomach is entirely accommodated within the concavity of the diaphragm, and is separated from the abdominal floor by the liver and small intestine.

The intestines in the dog comprise the small intestine, caecum, colon and rectum. The total length throughout is only about five times as long as the body. The duodenum commences at the pylorus from where it passes backwards and upwards, in contact with the upper part of the right flank, until near the pelvic inlet it forms a flexure by turning medially and then forwards along the medial aspect of the colon and the left kidney where it dips downwards and continues as the jejunum, or mesenteric portion. This part of the small intestine is arranged in loops attached to a long mesentery so that they reach to the abdominal floor. The terminal part, comprising the ileum, extends forward in the right

sublumbar region, contiguous to the medial surface of the caecum, and communicates with the proximal part of the colon opposite the lower extremity of the last rib.

The large intestine is about one-fifth the length of the small, and its calibre is only slightly larger. The caecum, which is sac-like and consists of a series of spiral flexures held together by the peritoneal covering, is about 8–15 cm in length. It is situated in the right sublumbar region midway between the median plane and the abdominal wall below the duodenum, and its anterior extremity opens into the colon lateral to the ileocolic orifice. The colon, consisting of three segments, is supported by a relatively short mesentery in the sublumbar region. The proximal segment, which is very short, extends forwards from the ileocolic confluence opposite the last rib on the medial aspect of the first part of the duodenum, until near the pylorus it turns left behind the stomach, forming the second section. The remaining segment extends backwards in the sublumbar region in the vicinity of the left kidney, at which point it inclines medially and is continued as the rectum. The rectum is almost completely covered with peritoneum, the retro-peritoneal portion being situated posterior to the second, or third coccygeal vertebra.

At the junction of the rectum and anus, the openings of the two lateral anal sacs are situated between the internal and external anal sphincters. The lining of the sacs and ducts consists of stratified squamous epithelium beneath which are situated numerous apocrine and sebaceous glands. The secretion of the glands collects in the sacs; it is light-grey to brown in colour, fluid to paste-like in consistency and has a rather noxious odour which is reputed to result from bacterial fermentation of cholesterol and its conversion into butyric acid, indole and skatol.

Cat. The abdomen in the cat is, in general, more rounded or barrel-shaped than in the dog. Because the concave depression of the diaphragm is relatively shallow and the stomach large the latter extends beyond the costal arch to a greater extent than in the dog. Otherwise the abdominal portion of the alimentary tract follows a similar general anatomic pattern to that of the dog. The disposition of the glands around the anus is not uniformly similar to that in the dog, although sac-like structures with a single duct are sometimes observed, more usually each individual gland has its independent opening.

Clinical Examination of the Abdomen

Clinical examination of the abdomen in the dog and cat is achieved through the media of inspection, palpation and percussion. Assiduous application of these methods elicits valuable information, not only relating to the state of the alimentary tract, but also to other organs including the kidneys, liver, pancreas, bladder, uterus, etc. For the purpose of the clinical examination the animal is best maintained quietly in the standing position. Small and medium-sized dogs, and cats, should be placed on a table with a non-slip surface, while large dogs are best kept on the floor.

Inspection provides the opportunity to assess the comparative size of the abdomen. The significance of any marked departure from normal has already been discussed in general terms. An increase in the circumference of the abdomen occurs in advanced pregnancy, gastric tympany, extensive neoplasia of the liver, pyometra, and accumulation of fluid in the peritoneal cavity. The latter can be the result of oedema (ascites) (see Fig. 135, p. 148). hepatic neoplasia, tuberculous peritonitis or rupture of the bladder. With an accumulation of fluid at this site, the distension is most noticeable in the lower part of the abdomen. A similar situation prevails in advanced pregnancy, except that the paralumbar fossae are not so obvious. Gastric distension, which occurs in both dilatation and torsion of the stomach, produces a generalized distension of the abdomen.

Percussion of the abdomen is of selective value, enabling accumulations of gas (tympany), hepatic enlargement or large tumours which are in contact with the abdominal wall to be provisionally suspected. The percussion responses elicited in tympany may indicate whether the condition is generalized or local and, in the latter event, it may be possible to identify the organs involved. A pain reaction is also likely to be produced in this disease and in others of an inflammatory character which involve any of the abdominal organs. Percussion, combined with simultaneous palpation, can be employed to identify the presence of fluid in the peritoneal cavity, a situation which occurs in ascites, exudative peritonitis, hepatic neoplasia and rupture of the bladder.

Palpation is of considerable value in the clinical examination of the abdominal organs. Even the more deeply situated organs may be satisfactorily examined by this method in many dogs and in all cats. It is best carried out with the animal in the standing position, but, in selected cases, more informative results are obtained with the animal in lateral recumbency. For large dogs the clinician should sit on a stool towards the rear and on one side of the animal. In most cases, both hands, with the fingers firmly extended together, are placed one on either side of the abdomen (see Fig. 140, p. 151), and sufficient pressure applied to overcome the natural resistance of the musculature, so that each organ is palpated. This is achieved by palpation of all appropriate parts of the abdominal wall relative to the position of the several underlying structures. The gentler the pressure applied during palpation, the greater the relaxation of the abdominal musculature and the more readily the internal structures can be recognized. The abdominal wall usually yields readily to pressure, except when the musculature is well developed, the dog is obese, in nervous animals and in those with a focus of pain in the abdomen. Resentment of the manipulative procedure is indicated by sudden tensing of the abdominal muscles. When this occurs a period of continuous gentle pressure may prove effective in obtaining the necessary degree of relaxation in order to continue the examination. To derive full value from palpation, the whole abdomen should be systematically examined with due regard to anatomical relationships, noting, by means of the animal's reactions, whether pain exists at any particular point. When the ventral part of the abdomen is palpated a cord-like structure, situated beneath the skin, can be felt slipping between the fingers. This is the edge of the double fold of the abdominal wall and it should not be mistaken for an abnormal structure.

Experience in palpating the abdomen of dogs of varying size, and of cats, is essential in order to avoid mistaking normal organs for some pathological condition such as tumour. This confusion arises most frequently with the kidney or distended urinary bladder. In the dog, only the posterior extremity of the left kidney is within reach of the fingertips, behind and below the last rib, on the left side, close to the vertebral column. It is not uncommon, however, in healthy dogs, for one or both kidneys to be 'floating'. The kidney is then recognized as a smooth, firm, freely movable, oval body with an indentation— the hilus—on its superior aspect. This anatomical feature helps to identify the kidney so that the possibility of confusion with a neoplasm is lessened. In the cat and rabbit both kidneys are normally of the floating type.

The urinary bladder, unless empty, is palpable anterior to the pelvic inlet as a firm, smooth-walled, globular structure the size of which varies between wide limits, according to its degree of distension with urine. In small animals the bladder may sometimes appear to fill a large part of the abdomen.

The liver, because it extends slightly beyond the costal arch on both sides, is fairly readily palpated in both dogs and cats, provided that in the case of dogs, the abdominal wall is not too tense or heavy. Palpation is achieved by placing the hands behind the costal arch, one on each side, and then pushing the fingers under the ribs, so that the fingertips are lying on the abdominal wall over the visceral surface of the lateral lobes of the liver. When normal, the border of the liver is smooth, even and thin. Examination of the liver by this means is more satisfactorily performed when the animal is in the lateral recumbent position.

Tumours and other gross abnormalities within the abdomen are only palpable when they are fairly large and have probably been established for some time. Although it is generally not very difficult to ascertain that an abdominal tumour is present, it may be extremely difficult or even impossible to determine its organ relationship and nature. In addition to the position and shape of the neoplasm, note is taken of any other signs of disease that may exist. For example in tumours of the pancreas, hypoglycaemia will be associated with hyperorexia, weakness, vomiting and spasticity, or even convulsions; in hepatic tumours, the urine may contain bile and there may be ascites; in neoplasia of the kidneys and bladder, the urine may contain red blood cells and other abnormal constituents, and the act of urination may be altered; in ovarian tumours, deviation from the normal oestrus cycle may be observed. Enlargement of the spleen may be local or general in extent. General enlargement (splenomegaly) occurs in lymphocytoma and congestive heart failure. If enlargement is great enough, the spleen can be palpated as a semi-solid mass extending backwards posterior to the left costal arch at the antero-inferior region of the abdomen. Localized splenic enlargement occurs in neoplasia and haematoma. The former may

be suspected following the detection of a firm, irregular swelling during palpation in the vicinity of the spleen area; the swollen mass in the latter is usually moderately soft in consistency.

Abdominal pain occurs in a variety of acute and subacute inflammatory conditions including peritonitis, gastroenteritis, hepatitis, nephritis, cystitis, acute pancreatitis and splenitis, as well as in acute gastric dilatation, and in intestinal obstruction, intussusception and torsion. The existence of pain is indicated by increased tension of the abdominal musculature, arching of the back and the fact that the animal cries out, with a sudden increase in abdominal tension, when the affected organ is palpated or during defaecation and urination. As a rule the pain is diffuse in peritonitis and gastroenteritis, but is usually localized, to a greater or lesser degree, in most other conditions, so that it is possible to define its precise situation. In addition signs, referable to the organ or part involved, might have been described by the owner or elicited during the clinical examination; such would prove extremely useful in aiding identification, not only of the site, but also the nature of the disease.

The stomach, particularly in the narrow-chested breeds of dogs, is more readily palpated when normally full or distended; in these circumstances it projects beyond the ventral part of the left costal arch. Elevating the forequarters of the animal may assist palpation in so far as it should allow the stomach to fall out of the concavity of the diaphragm, away from the liver. Pain induced by palpation of the anterior part of the abdomen should be related to any other clinical signs, bearing in mind the close anatomical relationship between the stomach and liver. Other helpful procedures that can be adopted for examining the stomach include gastroscopy and radiography.

The clinical signs of acute gastritis are variable but vomiting, to some degree, is a regular feature, with thirst and abdominal pain and in addition signs indicating enteritis are usually observed. A careful clinical examination may reveal that the gastric signs are part of a syndrome associated with a systemic infectious disease, e.g. distemper, viral hepatitis, leptospirosis, etc., are secondary to diseases producing toxaemia or uraemia or are local in origin. The causal factors which may act locally include overeating in puppies, ingestion of decomposing food, allergy (eggs, milk, horsemeat), irritants (arsenic, phosphorus, thallium, lead, mercury) and foreign bodies. In the infective diseases, vomiting is not persistent, febrile signs occur at some stage and in typical cases of distemper catarrhal inflammation involves some, if not all, of the mucous membranes. In the consideration of gastric signs of local origin it may be necessary to resort to gastroscopic or radiographic procedures in order to eliminate the possibility that a foreign body is responsible.

The incidence of foreign body in the stomach of dogs is greatest in animals up to 1 year of age. The clinical signs, of which vomiting is the most significant, are only likely to be severe when the condition has been present for some time or the foreign body is sharp-pointed and causes considerable irritation. It is unusual to identify the presence of a foreign body in the stomach by means of palpation because, in many cases in which it causes signs, it is lodged in the pyloric area. Furthermore, the appetite in dogs so affected is likely to be small, and this, along with a tendency to vomit, reduces the likelihood that the stomach is sufficiently distended to be palpable. If elevation of the forequarters of the animal does not assist the differential diagnosis, it may be necessary to resort to general anaesthesia in order to obtain sufficient relaxation of the musculature to enable the stomach to be palpated with the fingertips. Radiographic techniques, with or without a contrast medium, will provide confirmation.

Chronic gastritis gives rise to intermittent vomiting not related to eating. Other clinical signs are poor appetite and loss of bodily condition. The more common causes include smooth-surfaced foreign bodies, poor quality food, pyloric disease, mild uraemia, neoplasia and air-gulping which occurs in brachycephalic breeds of dogs. Diagnosis is based on a consideration of the history, clinical findings and the application of gastroscopic or radiographic techniques. Identification of uraemic states necessitates chemical investigations.

Acute gastric dilatation and gastric torsion usually develop very rapidly. Simple dilatation is the more common of the two conditions. It develops after eating food, more particularly following exercise, and when intestinal hypomotility slows down gastric emptying. Gastric torsion occurs in large, deep-chested dogs and takes place in a clockwise or anticlockwise direction, so that the oesophagus and pylorus become occluded and the venous return is prevented. The clinical signs develop suddenly and consist of restlessness, retching, without vomition being achieved, progressive distension of the abdomen, pain, signs of shock and lying down. The presence of gastric dilatation is recognized by the history of sudden development, by percussion of the abdomen and by radiographic examination.

Physical examination of the abdomen provides only negative evidence in cases of pyloric disease, which may occur as either pyloric stenosis or pyloric spasm. The latter is an expression of a functional imbalance because of dominance of the parasympathetic component of the nerve control mechanism. The condition is diagnosed by means of radiographic examination employing contrast medium coupled with the use of anticholinergic drugs.

Pyloric stenosis is seen most frequently in brachycephalic breeds of dogs; it can be congenital or acquired, the former type occurring in newly weaned puppies which have either hypertrophy of the musculature at the pyloric antrum, or a persistent gastrohepatic ligament. Acquired stenosis can result from post-inflammatory hypertrophy of the pyloric mucosa, fibrosis following trauma, e.g. by foreign bodies, or neoplasia. The severity of the signs depends on the degree of pyloric obstruction. As a rule appetite is good, the abdomen is often distended, but vomiting occurs only several hours after feeding unless the animal is excited by stimuli. Vomiting requires little effort and the dog frequently reswallows the vomitus. There is intestinal hypomotility. Diagnosis is made by consideration of the history and clinical signs in conjunction with radiographic examination employing a contrast medium to assess the rate of gastric emptying.

Because of the comparatively short length of the digestive tract in the dog, acute enteritis involves both the small intestine and the colon, and frequently the stomach as well. The intestinal hypermotility which is an inherent feature is manifested clinically by diarrhoea, with disturbance of digestion and absorption, and varying degrees of toxaemia.

Acute enteritis may be caused by bacteria, usually *Streptococcus* spp or *Staphylococcus* spp., and less frequently *Escherichia coli*, *Proteus* spp. or *Salmonella* spp.; by irritants in the form of foods to which the dog or cat are allergic, decomposed foods or, in occasional cases, poisonous agents such as heavy metals; or by systemic diseases such as canine distemper, infectious hepatitis, leptospirosis or infectious feline enteritis. Significant clinical signs include sudden onset, severe diarrhoea, transient vomiting, especially when irritants are responsible. Temperature is variable, usually being subnormal when shock effects appear. Abdominal palpation reveals general pain and atony of the intestine. Dehydration is usual; the accompanying electrolyte loss causes skeletal muscular weakness. Diagnosis is based on the history. The specific causal bacteria can be identified by bacteriological methods and the systemic diseases by detecting the existence of signs in other organs.

Chronic enteritis, which occurs in dogs of all ages, has a complex aetiology. The more important causes include foods which are irritant or initiate an allergic reaction, many of the bacterial species which cause acute enteritis (intestinal spirochaetes, *Borrelia canis, Spirillum eurygyrata,* and *Sp. minutum*, have been claimed to be common causal agents), intestinal parasites, particularly in young dogs (the species most frequently encountered are the hookworms, *Uncinaria stenocephala, Ancylostoma caninum* and *Anc. braziliense; Strongyloides stercoralis;* the large roundworms, *Toxocara canis, T. cati* and *Toxascaris leonina;* the tapeworms; and the whipworm, *Trichuris vulpis*), protozoa, including *Isospora bigemina, I. felis, I. rivolta* and *Eimeria canis, Giardia canis* and *Entamoeba* spp., chronic systemic states which affect the intestines secondarily including mild uraemia and congestive heart failure, and neoplasia of the bowel.

The main clinical signs include poor physical condition and dehydration with soft, watery and usually mucoid or blood-streaked faeces. It is often possible to detect thickening of the wall of the intestine by means of abdominal palpation. Diagnosis necessitates examination of the faeces by means of direct smears, worm ova concentration methods, enzyme tests and bacteriological techniques. The presence of hypertrophic changes or mucosal ulcers is revealed by radiographic examination.

The colon alone is involved in chronic ulcerative colitis which is observed in young dogs, particularly those of the boxer breed. The cause is obscure, but an autoimmune mechanism has been suggested. Affected dogs appear healthy but their faeces are voluminous, soft, light-coloured and evil-smelling, containing large masses of mucus and the terminal portion may contain blood. The disease is diagnosed by differential exclusion of other forms of chronic enteritis through consideration of the history, and radiographic and proctoscopic examinations. The last reveals that the colonic mucosa is friable, hyperaemic and haemorrhages readily; in established cases ulcers usually occur.

In addition to the factors already discussed increased intestinal motility in the dog can result from overfeeding or sudden changes in diet, defective intestinal absorption, defective pancreatic secretion and disorders of the nervous system, such as nervous temperament and anal sphincter paralysis.

Intestinal obstruction in the dog may be due to a variety of causes including foreign bodies, intussusception, neoplasia, hernia, etc. The clinical signs vary in intensity according to whether the obstruction is partial or complete, and its situation. Foreign body obstruction is more frequent in young dogs and is often associated with severe signs, particularly when the duodenum is involved. In this situation, vomiting occurs shortly after ingestion of food and defaecation is absent. Palpation of the abdomen will elicit a pain reaction, but it may not be possible to determine the site or nature of the obstruction. Elevating the forequarters of the animal, or the induction of deep narcosis or general anaesthesia, may help in resolving the difficulty, and finally radiography will reveal radiopaque foreign objects. When the ileum or even more distal parts are obstructed, vomiting is a usual sign but food retention occurs for a more prolonged period. It is possible, in the majority of low intestinal foreign body obstructions, to palpate and identify the situation if not the nature of the lesion. The pain reaction induced is severe, however, so that differentiation from intussusception may be difficult or impossible. The latter condition is usually associated with a cylindrical or banana-shaped swelling. In some cases, the intussusception is so extensive that it involves the colon to a greater or lesser degree, and in extreme cases it may protrude at the anus. When the obstruction of the intestine by a foreign body or intussusception is virtually complete, or irritation is severe, small amounts of blood-stained faeces or mucus are passed.

When intestinal obstruction causes obvious signs of pain the syndrome is defined as ileus, which may also be due to intestinal paralysis (paralytic ileus). This last may occur in peritonitis or cystitis, or develop following intra-abdominal surgery, in severe intestinal parasitism intussusception or other forms of intestinal obstruction of some duration. The clinical signs are most acute in obstructive ileus. In paralytic ileus, abdominal palpation may give the impression that the intestines, which are distended with gas, can be readily compressed. There is a slight degree of abdominal distension. Radiographic examination will confirm that both the small and large intestines are distended.

Neoplasms or strictures can cause progressive occlusion of the intestine, giving rise to signs of partial intestinal obstruction which gradually increase in severity until toxaemia develops. One of the common sites of tumour formation is the mesenteric lymph nodes, more particularly the group situated in the vicinity of the ileocaecocolic region which, when enlarged, is recognizable as an indeterminate mass in the posterior middle abdomen.

Hypomotility of the Intestine

Reduced intestinal motility which is associated clinically with constipation is a not infrequent condition in dogs beyond middle age. The main clinical features include straining (Fig. 151),

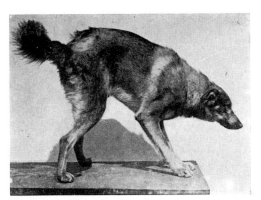

Fig. 151. *The posture adopted in severe constipation.* '*Straining*' (*tenesmus*).

anorexia, vomiting and posterior ataxia with paraplegia in some cases, or other signs of toxaemia if the condition persists. Abdominal palpation will cause pain and reveals the presence of a cylindrical mass of firm faeces in the colon. The degree of faecal retention reflects the period during which accumulation has been taking place. In the bitch, enlargement of the uterus, especially when caused by cystic endometrial hyperplasia (pyometra), is difficult to differentiate from faecal impaction of the colon. In old-standing cases the bilaterally distended uterine horns can be identified by palpation, as a moderately firm, cylindrical mass situated towards the anteroventral part of the abdomen. Digital rectal examination and abdominal radiographs will confirm the diagnosis; the latter also reveals the full extent of faecal retention. Elucidation of the primary cause will necessitate consideration of a large number of factors including the nature of the diet (dry food), exercising habits, amount of bone consumed, ingestion of hair, megacolon, matting of hair around the perianal region in long haired breeds of dogs, enlarged prostate gland, displaced and healed pelvic fractures, painful conditions of the anal sacs, perianal neoplasia or fistula and nerve dysfunction arising from spinal lesions.

So-called megacolon of dogs develops in later life and results from changes in the innervation of the colon. The resulting defect consists of a decrease in the number of the autonomic nerve fibres. The greatly increased tone of the muscle fibres inhibits the passage of faeces. The main clinical signs are those of chronic constipation with very low level toxaemia, usually in the form of dullness. The state of the colon is readily determined by palpation and can be confirmed by radiography.

Faecal incontinence, resulting in uncontrolled passage of soft faeces, is by no means a rare condition in dogs, affecting older dogs as the result of neurogenic failure. Otherwise it may arise following injury in the lumbar, pelvic or perineal region. Occasional cases may be due to trauma causing extensive damage to the anal sphincter muscle or to perianal neoplasia interfering with sphincter function. The clinical signs include the involuntary passage of soft or watery faeces during movement or whenever the dog becomes excited. On inspection the anal sphincter is seen to be relaxed.

Inflammation of the rectum (proctitis) is by no means an uncommon disease in dogs. The causal factors operate locally and include mechanical irritation by fragments of bone or sharp-pointed foreign bodies, as well as trauma arising from the use of forceps, enema tubes, etc. The most obvious clinical sign consists of repeated, unproductive straining. The rectum, which is usually empty and distended with air, is hyperaemic with a few ulcerated areas.

Rectal prolapse is more common in puppies in which it is often the result of severe tenesmus associated with diarrhoea. In adult dogs it may be caused in a similar manner by a foreign body or neoplasm. The condition is self-evident but the cause will require elucidation.

Another condition which is recognizable by inspection of the anal area is perianal fistula; it is observed in the Alsatian, Irish setter and cocker spaniel breeds. It is recognized by the presence of numerous small ulcers in the perianal skin which are thought to be caused by bacterial infection. The main clinical sign is constipation. Healing of the ulcers is associated with fibrosis which may lead to stricture.

Impaction and infection of the anal sacs are relatively common conditions in adult dogs. Impaction is due to failure to empty the sacs during defaecation, hypersecretion by the sac glands, pasty nature of the secretion and poor muscle tone in obese dogs. Affected dogs manifest pain during defaecation, which occurs less frequently than usual, lick the anal region and 'scoot', i.e. drag the hindquarters over the ground; this trauma may cause injury, and in protracted cases there is loss of hair over the base of the tail and tuber ischii. The distension, which may be unilateral or bilateral, is detected by digital examination. Many affected dogs will evince pain when the tail is elevated. Infection of the anal sacs usually follows impaction; the bacteria involved are usually either streptococci or staphylococci, although other species have been identified in some cases. The condition is painful, so that the clinical signs are similar to those of impaction. The contents of the affected sac are purulent and may contain blood. Spontaneous rupture with the establishment of a fistula is by no means unusual.

Perianal adenoma occurs in old male dogs. The neoplasms are usually multiple and they manifest a tendency to ulcerate and necrose. When the tumours encroach on the anal sphincter they may cause difficulty at defaecation, thereby giving rise to constipation, straining and prolapse of the rectum.

Rectal Examination

In dogs rectal examination is performed by introducing through the anus one finger (index or little finger) covered with a rubber or plastic disposable fingerstall, the surface of which should be lubricated. In order to avoid injury the fingernails should be cut short. Rectal exploration in small dogs and cats can be achieved by the use of a blunt thermometer or other suitable probe. The value of rectal examination is limited in small animals because, at best, only the pelvic organs and rectum are within reach of the finger.

Prior to inserting the finger through the anal sphincter, note should be taken of the animal's reaction to lifting its tail. In painful conditions of the anal sacs the animal will show some resentment to this part of the examination. When introducing the finger it is possible to confirm that a painful state exists. Disease of the anal sacs is frequently indicated by a visible, small, external bulge, ventrolateral to the anus, which is palpable when held between the thumb externally and the finger in the rectum. The contents of the sac, in the form of secretion or inflammatory discharge, can be evacuated by gently squeezing the swelling between the finger and thumb when in the position indicated. Bacterial infection of the anal sacs is associated with haemorrhagic or purulent discharge which, in the latter case, may escape through a fistula lateral to the anus.

When introducing the finger into the rectum the tone of the anal sphincter should be noted in conjunction with the degree of peristaltic activity produced. Flaccidity and absence of functional contraction indicate paralysis. The presence of faeces, which when hard and impacted would prevent the entry of the finger, a foreign body or spicules of bone in the rectum is readily determined. The width of the lumen of the rectum may be irregularly increased (diverticulum) or decreased (stricture). The latter may exist in the form of an annular constriction of the rectum which, if within reach of the finger, prevents deeper insertion and palpation of the area causes considerable pain. The pelvic bones can be palpated through the rectal wall, and fractures, exostoses, bone misalignment, hip-joint dislocation and advanced dysplasia can be recognized.

In male dogs the prostate gland can be palpated ventral to the rectum on the floor of the pelvis. When normal it is approximately the size of a hazel nut with a median longitudinal groove on its dorsal aspect. Enlargement of the prostate gland may be uniform or irregular in character.

Uniform enlargement due to hyperplasia occurs in old dogs; in some cases the enlarged gland is nodular because of cyst formation. In this situation digital pressure would reveal fluctuation, but the gland is invariably free of pain. In prostatitis, which is relatively common, palpation of the gland is resented. Irregular, nodular enlargement indicates carcinoma, in which case there is reduced mobility because the prostate gland has become attached to neighbouring pelvic structures. The intrapelvic part of the urethra is usually, and the neck of the bladder is occasionally, palpable. When the bladder is empty the presence of a calculus or neoplasm may be confirmed by digital palpation during rectal exploration.

Peritonitis

The peritoneal cavity consists of a sac-like potential cavity in the form of a thin serous membrane, the peritoneum, which lines the abdominal cavity and the pelvic cavity in part. The opposing walls of the sac, which in the male animal is completely closed, but in the female communicates indirectly with the exterior via the abdominal orifices of the Fallopian tubes and uterus, are separated by a thin film of serous fluid. This allows the essential movements of the viscera to occur without hindrance or pain.

Inflammation of the peritoneum brings about a change in the quantity and character of the serous fluid. The absence of the secretion, which may be local or diffuse in extent, is accompanied by abdominal pain of varying severity and extent, as the result of friction. Manifestations of abdominal pain can also occur when peritoneal exudation is excessive; in this situation the exudate itself is the factor which stimulates the pain receptors in the peritoneum.

In acute diffuse peritonitis the animal is observed to remain standing with the back arched, with lack of desire to move. During the procedure of lying down the movements are made with considerable caution, and groaning and grunting sounds are increased in frequency. Defaecation and urination are performed less frequently than normal. Appetite is completely suppressed. In dogs and pigs vomiting is an early sign which may persist if the appetite is retained to any degree. Palpation will elicit a pain reaction over the whole of the abdominal wall, which is rigid. Auscultation reveals absence of intestinal sounds because of paralytic ileus. Rectal exami-

nation reveals evidence of pain. The indications of systemic involvement include elevation of temperature with moderate increase in pulse and respiration rates, the last being the result of suppression of abdominal movement.

The clinical syndrome in acute local peritonitis is similar to the foregoing, but the signs are less obvious. In chronic peritonitis the clinical signs are not readily appreciated until the development of adhesions which interfere with intestinal motility, or peritoneal exudation is sufficient to cause abdominal distension. The adhesions are usually most advanced in the anterior abdomen, so are only rarely detected during rectal exploration.

The commonest causes of peritonitis in animals include traumatic and other perforating lesions of the alimentary or genital tract or of the abdominal wall. In horses, perforation of gastric ulcers produced by the larvae of *Gasterophilus* spp. and *Habronema megastomum* is occasionally observed, while traumatic reticuloperitonitis in cattle and goats, perforation of an abomasal ulcer in cattle and perforation of ulcers in regional ileitis in pigs are common causes in these various species. Rupture of the stomach or intestine following acute dilatation or obstruction by foreign bodies, or food masses, causes the immediate development of peritonitis in both large and small animals. Rupture of the rectum occurring during parturition, either assisted or non-assisted, in cattle, precedes the development of peritonitis. In this case the main clinical signs are those of shock and toxaemia; pain is not marked. Spontaneous rupture of the uterus at parturition produces the same effect. Traumatic perforation of the abdominal wall (from the exterior by stake wounds, horn gores, trocarization in the treatment of ruminal or caecal tympany in cattle and horses and automobile accidents and fights in dogs) is a common cause of peritonitis. Rupture of abscesses in the spleen, liver or mesenteric lymph nodes and infections of the female genitalia and of other abdominal organs are other causes. Less commonly, haematogenous and lymphogenous infections localize in the peritoneum; tuberculosis and actinomycosis may cause peritonitis in this way. In specific diseases such as serositis-arthritis of sheep and goats and Glasser's disease in pigs, peritonitis occurs as part of a more general syndrome involving all of the serous membranes.

The diagnosis of peritonitis is often difficult, especially when it has developed as a complication of some pre-existing condition. It should always be suspected when acute abdominal pain, paralytic ileus, absence of intestinal sounds and vomiting are observed, especially in association with any of those conditions which are known to precede the development of peritonitis. Haematological examination in acute or subacute cases will reveal an elevated neutrophil count, and in small animals radiographic examination may reveal the presence of fluid or air in the peritoneal cavity and in the intestinal tract, and evidence of paralytic ileus or obstructive foreign body. When peritoneal exudation occurs the inflammatory nature of the fluid can be determined by microscopic examination.

Special Methods of Examining the Abdominal Organs

Certain other methods, which are especially applicable to small animals, can be employed in selected cases to ascertain the condition of some of the abdominal organs. These techniques include those providing for direct or indirect visualization and radiographic examination.

Direct visualization of abdominal viscera, achieved by means of laparotomy, is a practical undertaking in all species of domestic animals. Usually this procedure is adopted only when the evidence obtained from the clinical examination indicates a disease of an abdominal organ, the nature of which cannot otherwise be ascertained. A modified form of exploratory laparotomy, peritoneoscopy, permits inspection of abdominal viscera by means of suitable illuminated specula. Gastroscopy can be performed in the anaesthetized dog and cat but should be undertaken only when the clinical examination indicates primary gastric disease. The technique is an exacting one because only a limited area of the gastric mucosa can be viewed at one time, and abdominal manipulation is required to ensure that the whole extent of the mucosa is examined. The flexible fibrescope is the best instrument for the purpose.

In those cases of abdominal distension in which the clinical examination indicates the presence of fluid in the peritoneal cavity, exploratory puncture (paracentesis) may assist the differential diagnosis. The operation is performed in compliance with surgical principles, the needle insertion being made at a dependent part of the abdominal wall taking care to avoid large blood vessels or other important structures. Samples of fluid obtained by this means can be submitted to chemical, microscopical and bacteriological methods of examination. The evidence obtained is likely to help in identifying the origin of the fluid which might be an exudate, transudate, haemorrhage, organ secretion or other body fluid.

Peritoneal exudation is a feature of tuberculous peritonitis in the dog and cat, and of acute peritonitis in cattle and horses, although in the large animals the volume of exudate is relatively small. Infectious feline peritonitis is also associated with varying volumes of peritoneal exudate. Microscopic examination of the deposit obtained by centrifuging a sample of the exudate reveals the presence of inflammatory cells including neutrophil leucocytes, lymphocytes, as well as erythrocytes, and possibly the causal bacterium.

In the early stages of peritoneal transudation (ascites), which develops as the result of portal congestion, chronic anaemia or congestive heart failure, the fluid is clear and straw-coloured and the deposit contains few cells. Later it becomes slightly turbid because epithelial and other cells, including erythrocytes and neutrophil leucocytes, are present in small numbers. Fluid with similar characteristics collects in the peritoneal cavity in the initial stages of rapidly growing neoplasms in the liver when the capsule is disrupted. This condition is observed with greatest frequency in the dog. Comparatively quickly, however, the fluid becomes turbid and brownish-red in colour owing to the presence of large numbers of erythrocytes, neutrophil leucocytes and tumour cells.

Haemorrhage into the peritoneal cavity occurs following rupture of the liver, spleen or major blood vessel, and occasionally following enucleation of a corpus luteum from the ovary in the cow. This kind of injury to the major abdominal organs occurs most commonly in the dog, and is usually the result of a forceful impact. The general clinical indications of haemorrhagic anaemia exhibited by the animal, and the appearance of the fluid on withdrawal, would reveal its nature. Haematological techniques provide the means for confirmation. Urine escapes into the peritoneal cavity following rupture of the bladder. In this case chemical examination is necessary to confirm the origin of the fluid which is suggested by the toxaemic

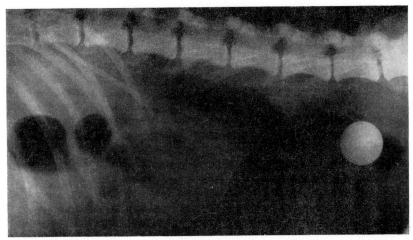

Fig. 152. *A radiograph showing a foreign body (a sponge-rubber ball) in the intestine of a young dog. Dark (i.e. gas-filled) loops of bowel are clearly seen.*

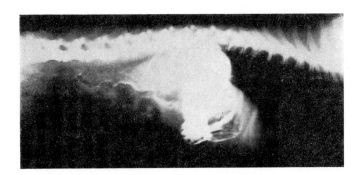

Fig. 153. *A radiograph showing a foreign body (a piece of thick string) in the small intestine of a dog. The string has been outlined by a contrast medium.*

state of the animal, the increasing size of the abdomen which may become obviously distended, and the absence of moisture on the floor if the animal is housed. Rupture of the gall-bladder or bile duct will allow bile to escape and collect in the peritoneal cavity. The nature of the fluid is determined by chemical tests. Fluid originating from a hydatid cyst in the liver, spleen or mesentery is recognizable by observing the scolices of *Echinococcus granulosus*.

Radiographic examination of the abdomen yields the most satisfactory results in small animals, having its greatest application in cases of suspected foreign body obstruction in the digestive tract and in obstructive urolithiasis, and as a means of assessing the functional state of the stomach and intestines. Radiopaque foreign bodies in the stomach or intestine are readily visualized by either radiography or fluoroscopy. Contrast media including air, non-toxic inert

gas, barium sulphate or bismuth carbonate are applicable when it is necessary to outline radio-translucent objects and the gastric or intestinal mucosa. If a plain radiograph is not conclusive, recognition of non-opaque objects can be speeded up by administration of a barium or bismuth suspension, followed in a few minutes by apomorphine administered parenterally in sufficient quantity to produce emesis. Sufficient radiopaque material will remain on the surface of the object to reveal its situation and possibly even its nature (Figs 152, 153).

The functional activity of the stomach may be assessed by means of a sequence of radiographs or by fluoroscopy following the administration of differential medium. In gastritis it will be noted that the rugae, or folds of the mucosa, are greatly increased in size and, when there is concomitant enteritis, hypermotility is indicated by the reduced gastric emptying time and the

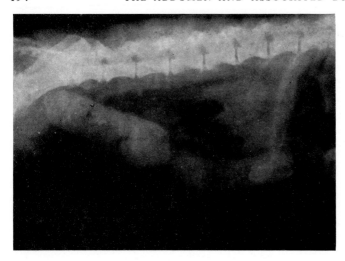

Fig. 154. *A radiograph showing gross dilatation of the colon (megacolon) in a dog. Note the degree of faecal retention.*

rapid passage of the medium along the digestive tract. The situation revealed in chronic gastritis is enlargement of the stomach, the cavity being mainly filled with gas, with thickening of the stomach wall. In acute gastric dilatation and torsion the grossly enlarged, tympanitic stomach, which almost completely fills the abdomen, will be revealed in plain radiographs. Radiographs from two planes may disclose displacement in the latter condition. A 'crater defect' or ulcerated area of gastric epithelium in the pyloric region, with diffuse thickening of the stomach wall, is revealed in carcinoma by radiographs obtained with barium or air as contrast media.

Retention of radiopaque substance in the stomach for protracted periods is a feature of pyloric spasm or stenosis. In severe cases of these conditions, radiography will often reveal marked gastric dilatation. In interpreting the significance of prolonged gastric retention of differential medium, the observations made by radiography or fluoroscopy must be related to the clinical condition of the animal because conditions other than those primarily involving the pyloric sphincter can influence the rate of gastric empty-ing, e.g. those arising from hypomotility of the intestine, early stages of enteritis, hyperexcit-ability and intestinal obstruction.

Compression stenosis of the intestine by neoplasms, incomplete obstruction by foreign bodies and other agents, including parasites, volvulus, etc., and intestinal stricture will slow down the onward passage of the radiographic marker material. It is desirable, when under-taking this method of examination, to withhold food for 8–12 hours before the radiopaque suspension is administered, and in all instances to obtain a plain radiograph as an initial step. In the fasting, normal dog, the time sequence for the onward movement of the administered material is fairly precise. Almost immediately the stomach will commence contracting, the pyloric sphincter will open and gastric emptying is initiated. This early movement is detected by making a radiographic or fluoroscopic examina-tion very soon after the contrast medium has been administered. A sequence of exposures will show that the stomach is cleared within about 1 hour, by which time the material is distributed along the duodenum and jejunum, and it will have reached the colon within 4 hours. When digestive tract function is normal the radiopaque substance is entirely cleared within about 24 hours.

Barium or bismuth enemas, in conjunction with radiographic examination, can be employed to assist in the diagnosis of megacolon, colitis and stricture of the colon or rectum. In mega-colon the gross dilatation of the colon, with faecal retention, is disclosed on a plain radio-graph (Fig. 154), and in colonic stricture seg-mental dilatation with a degree of faecal retention proximal to the point of stricture, will be revealed in the same manner.

THE FAECES

Faeces consist of the residue from the ingested food, in addition to certain products added during the digestive processes. They are composed of water, indigestible and undigested food residues, bile acids, bile pigments and mucin, cells from the intestinal mucosa, inorganic salts, bacteria in large numbers and bacterial fermentation products. The faeces are voided from the rectum through the anus by the act of defaecation. In assessing the functional status of the digestive system, note should be made of the frequency of defaecation and the manner in which it is performed—whether with difficulty, signs of pain, etc. The character of the faeces is then considered in relation to consistency, colour, smell and the presence of undigested food material or of foreign substances. When necessary, samples of faeces may be subjected to laboratory examination in order to detect the presence of helminth ova, occult blood, pathogenic protozoa and bacteria and certain enzyme deficiencies.

Frequency of Defaecation

The stimulus to defaecation is provided by the filling of the ampulla of the rectum which stimulates sensory nerve endings in the anal region. The external anal sphincter, which is under voluntary control, is innervated by sensory and motor nerve fibres in the pudendal nerves, while the colon and rectum are innervated by afferent and efferent nerve fibres in the pelvic nerves. The centres controlling the anal sphincters are situated in the posterior portion of the lumbar part of the spinal cord. Overall coordination of the events associated with defaecation with other gastrointestinal reflexes is achieved by a defaecation centre which is located on the floor of the fourth ventricle, close to the vomiting centre. The expulsion of faeces by the involuntary contraction of the colon and rectum is assisted, particularly in carnivores, by voluntary contraction of the abdominal muscles.

During the act of defaecation special postures or attitudes are adopted by the different species of animals with the object of aiding expulsion of the faeces by increasing intra-abdominal pressure. Animals of the large species usually abduct the hindlegs and may contract the abdominal muscles, while the glottis is closed; whereas carnivorous species squat down and may be noted repeatedly to contract and then relax the abdominal muscles. On completing the act of defaecation, carnivorous animals scrape the ground, with the hindfeet in the dog and a forefoot in the cat. Abdominal contraction is only obvious when the faeces are relatively dry.

The frequency of defaecation is related to the character of the food. Active healthy horses defaecate 8–12 times a day when they are stall-fed. When grazing, similar horses would defaecate 16 times or more each day. Cattle exhibit a similar frequency except that, when lactating, dairy cattle defaecate 12–24 times daily. When the diet consists mainly of flesh, carnivorous species defaecate 1–3 times daily, whereas if predominantly carbohydrate food is fed, defaecation occurs more often.

The length of time taken for ingested food material to pass through the alimentary tract is related to the anatomical complexity of the organs, the type of food, and the frequency of defaecation. The complex large intestine in the horse and the capacious stomach compartments in cattle prolong the sojourn for 1–4 and 2–4 days respectively, depending on the type of food ingested. In pigs, dogs and cats and other monogastric species, the alimentary sojourn varies between 12 and 36 hours.

Defaecation may be abnormal in respect of frequency and posture. It is relatively infrequent in diseased states that reduce peristalsis (hypomotility) and in paraplegia or painful conditions involving the abdominal wall or peritoneal cavity. Its frequency is increased in all circumstances causing increased peristalsis (hypermotility), including irritant substances in the food, and in nearly all forms of enteritis, including inflammation of the rectum (proctitis). When defaecation is accompanied by signs of pain such as groaning or grunting, with repeated tensing of the abdominal musculature, the condition is termed 'straining' or tenesmus (see Fig. 151, p. 189). This is a common sign of intestinal disease and it occurs in proctitis, colitis, megacolon and intussusception, as well as in prostatitis and other diseases of the organs situated in the pelvis including vaginitis, in placental retention, rabies and spinal cord abscessation.

Involuntary passage of faeces occurs when there is relaxation or paralysis of the anal sphincter, or loss of consciousness. Relaxation of the external sphincter is observed in severe general debility and in old age, while paralysis is usually the result of local trauma or a lesion of the posterior thoracic or lumbar segments of the spinal cord of sufficient extent to abolish or cause imbalance in the nerve control mechanism. Abnormal postures are assumed during defaecation by animals affected with painful and other conditions of the limbs which themselves induce postural changes, and in diseases of the vertebral column (ankylosing spondylitis) and of the spinal cord (ossifying pachymeningitis).

Character of Faeces

The consistency and form of normal faeces vary according to the species of animal and also in relation to the type of food. In the horse, during periods of stall-feeding, the faeces are yellowish-brown to brown and take on the form of relatively large balls of regular shape. The faeces of grazing horses are dark green and softer in consistency, so that the balls break on striking the ground. In grass-fed cattle the faeces are dark green and semi-solid and form flat cakes, but in house-fed cattle they are dark brown and firmer. In the goat and sheep the faeces are dark green to black and consist of large numbers of firm, somewhat spherical pellets. Those of the rabbit are of two types: firm pellets as in the sheep and goat, and soft, mucoid masses, each type being passed at particular periods during every 24 hours. The faeces of pigs are rather loose and break readily on hitting the floor. Those of the healthy dog and cat take the shape of firm, elongated, cylindrical masses.

The colour of normal faeces varies according to the diet. In herbivorous animals green fodder makes the faeces soft and green, beetroot makes them dark red and hay and cereal concentrates make them dark brown. In carnivorous species, when the diet contains meat, the faeces are dark brown, but they become firm and light grey when bone is included in any quantity. On a milk diet (young sucking animals and those being pail-fed) the faeces are yellow and semi-solid. The colour of the faeces is also influenced by the amount of bile present; this depends on the rate of bile production and release, and the length of time the ingesta are retained in the intestine. In all species the faeces assume a blackish-brown colour in continuing constipation, whereas while bile production is impaired, as in obstructive or toxic jaundice, the faeces become clay-coloured or pale, and hard in consistency, especially in dogs and cats. Certain medicaments can alter the colour of the faeces, e.g. calomel may give rise to greenish coloration, bismuth black and kamala blood-red. The administration of phenothiazine occasionally results in the appearance of reddish coloured faeces. Blood gives faeces a dark tarry or red colour.

The odour of the faeces depends largely on the character of the food eaten by the animal and, therefore, varies somewhat according to the species. The faecal odour in carnivorous species is offensive, whereas in herbivorous species it is only slightly unpleasant. The odour of the faeces in cases of intestinal disease is often particularly offensive. When the intestinal contents have undergone abnormal fermentation the faeces are usually lighter in colour than normal, have a sour odour and may contain gas bubbles. In herbivorous species the composition of the faeces in relation to the proportion of undigested fibre should be noted. Incompletely digested cereal grains or hay suggest the possibility of faulty mastication due to dental disorders. Similarly in dogs and cats, grey, putty-like, foul-smelling, loose faeces indicate inadequate digestion because of pancreatic insufficiency. Undigested meat in the faeces (creatorrhoea) is recognizable under the microscope by observing complete preservation of the transverse striation of the muscle fibres. Large amounts of fat (steatorrhoea) are recognized by the pasty consistency and fatty lustre of the faeces. The fat can be readily extracted from the faeces with ether; the ether extract leaves a greasy mark on filter paper.

Apart from the changes caused by dietetic and digestion factors, the consistency of the faeces is strongly affected by disease of the digestive system which may cause the faeces to be hard, soft, semi-liquid or watery. Abnormally firm faeces cause constipation and conversely unusually soft faeces cause diarrhoea. In impaction of the caecum in the horse the faeces, because of prolonged sojourn in the large intestine, are pasty and have a greasy appearance and an unpleasant odour. Pasty faeces also occur, for the same reason, in rumen stasis and abomasal displacement in cattle. Systemic diseases also influence the character of the faeces, e.g. in the initial phase of acute febrile diseases the faeces are generally firmer than usual; in primary ketosis they are firm and glistening because of an excessive coating with mucus; in toxaemic states they are soft and liquid in consistency and darker in colour.

Abnormal Constituents in Faeces

Abnormal faecal constituents which originate from within the alimentary tract or from elsewhere within the body include blood, mucus, parasitic helminths, their larvae or ova and shreds of intestinal mucosa. Foreign bodies ingested with food or at other occasions, such as sand, small stones, pieces of bone, wool and metallic objects may also be found.

When the faeces are admixed with blood that has originated from the upper part of the digestive tract they are uniformly dark and tarry because the haemoglobin has been reduced and also evenly mixed by the processes of digestion, whereas if the blood loss has occurred from the large intestine, it usually retains its normal colour and stains the faeces red. If the haemorrhage has taken place in the terminal portion of the colon or in the rectum, the blood is not mixed uniformly throughout the faeces, but is irregularly distributed on the surface in clots or in liquid form. In severe haemorrhage, solid blood clot only may be evacuated. Minor haemorrhage cannot be diagnosed from the gross appearance of the faeces. Gastric or intestinal haemorrhage may occur as a result of deep ulceration causing erosion of blood vessels (oesophagogastric ulceration of pigs), or from injury by foreign bodies, acute inflammation especially when the causal agent penetrates deeply into the submucosa and damages the vascular tissues, vascular engorgement caused by torsion, intussusception and embolic and thrombotic processes as in parasitic mesenteric arteritis. In cattle, the possibility that anthrax might exist must always be borne in mind when faeces containing unclotted blood are encountered.

When blood is present in faeces in such small amounts that it cannot be recognized macroscopically it is termed 'occult'. In such small quantities its presence may be revealed by chemical or microscopic tests. With the latter it is possible to recognize intact erythrocytes in appropriately stained smears. Because the chemical tests are not specific they will give false positive reactions with the faeces of carnivorous animals unless animal flesh has been excluded from the diet for at least three days. The clinical tests include the benzidine test (avoid this method if possible because benzidine has carcinogenic properties), the guaiacum test and a modified ortho-tolidine test (Occultest, Ames Co.). For the guaiacum test freshly prepared reagents are required otherwise a negative reaction will be obtained. On considerations of safety and convenience the ortho-tolidine test is the one of choice.

In performing the Occultest a small amount of the faeces is mixed with water to form a thin suspension, which is then boiled for a short time. One drop of the prepared suspension is placed on a piece of filter paper and the reagent tablet is placed in the centre of the moistened area. Then 2 drops of water are placed on the surface of the tablet. If blood is present, a blue colour will develop within 2 minutes. A similar colour reaction appearing after 2 minutes is of no significance. The test tablet contains ortho-tolidine, strontium peroxide, calcium acetate, tartaric acid and sodium bicarbonate.

Mucus is a normal constituent of the faeces which gives them a shiny appearance. This surface coating is increased in thickness when the alimentary sojourn is prolonged, as in constipation. Excessive amounts of mucus, which is admixed with copious fluid faeces, is a feature of intestinal diseases associated with extensive exudation from the mucous membrane. The excess mucus sometimes occurs in the form of shreds or even casts. The latter are roughly cylindrical structures consisting of mucus, fibrin, and epithelial components. Intestinal gas (flatus) is a normal byproduct of digestion and in small quantities is of no significance. Pathological quantities of intestinal gas give rise to tympany which is uaually caused, in monogastric animals, by the ingestion of rapidly fermentable fodder. The habitual swallowing of large quantities of air by horses addicted to wind-sucking, or cribbiting may also result in gas in the intestinal canal. In cattle affected with catarrhal enteritis, the soft faeces frequently contain numerous gas bubbles, e.g. Johne's disease.

Under traditional conditions of husbandry, all species of domestic animals harbour intestinal parasites, and evidence of infestation with many of these is to be found in the form of segments (cestodes), intact worms, ova or larvae (lungworms) in the faeces. The mere presence of helminth ova, however, is not to be taken as evidence of the existence of clinical parasitism. Moreover, owing to seasonal and other variations in the egg-laying activity of certain parasites, and to variation in resistance of the host caused by age, previous helminth infestation, nutritional status, intercurrent disease, etc., as well as variation in the consistency of the faeces themselves, the actual number of ova per unit quantity of faeces is not an absolute indication of the clinical importance of the parasites. Nevertheless, provided the results are interpreted in the light of all the clinical and other findings, parasitological examination of the faeces may be a valuable aid to diagnosis.

Another factor that should receive consideration in the interpretation of faecal helminth ova counts is the species of the parasites. As a rule blood-sucking nematodes such as *Haemonchus placei* and hookworms (e.g. *Ancylostoma caninum*), by their ability to produce severe anaemia, are capable of causing much greater damage to the host than an equivalent number of a species like *Trichostrongylus axei*. In addition some species of nematodes produce large numbers of ova, e.g. *Toxocara cati*, while others are poor egg producers, e.g. *Ancylostoma* spp. in cats. In the case of many nematode parasites, the species can not be identified from the eggs because they are indistinguishable on morphological grounds. For these species, faeces culture has to be undertaken and the resulting larvae then identified.

The stage of development of certain nematode parasites is also of significance in relation to their potentially harmful effects. Serious, even fatal, damage can be caused by the larvae of *Ascaris* spp., *Strongylus* spp. or *Nematodirus battus*, and by immature *Ostertagia* spp. or *Trichostrongylus axei* when the numbers are large. In such circumstances the absence of ova in the faeces may cause difficulty in establishing the diagnosis.

It should be remembered that, apart from the eggs and larvae of helminth parasites, a variety of non-pathogenic parasites may also be found such as amoebae, flagellates and ciliates. Coccidia, although potentially pathogenic, are almost invariably found in the faeces of healthy sheep, fowls and rabbits, and are common in the faeces of cattle. Other potentially pathogenic protozoa associated with faeces, and which are of public health significance, include species of the genera *Giardia, Globidium* and *Balantidium*. Vegetable structures such as pollen grains, fungal spores and plant hairs should not be mistaken for helminth eggs or larvae. Rabbit faeces, for instance, commonly contain large masses of saccharomycetes, which are small, oval or elongated, budding structures. The mites that occur in ground cereals, rice, cheese, etc. particularly tyroglyphids, are frequently ingested with food and can be demonstrated in the faeces. Mange mites may reach the faeces as a result of licking active skin lesions, as do the ova of *Linguatula rhinaria* by reason of the affected

dog licking away nasal discharge. Recognition of specific morphological detail will differentiate the mange mites from the virtually non-pathogenic forage mites (Figs 61–63, pp. 62–5).

Examination of Faeces

Samples of faeces for parasitological, bacteriological or chemical examination should be obtained from the rectum or at the time of defaecation, and not collected from the ground, in order to avoid contamination with soil which may contain free-living nematodes. Each sample should be collected into a small tin, wide-mouthed bottle or small self-sealing plastic envelope, which should be filled to capacity because the exclusion of air will retard hatching of the eggs. When sampling a group of animals, individual samples are taken from 20–25%, or equal quantities of faeces from a similar or higher proportion of individual animals are placed in one container. The samples should be examined in as fresh condition as possible so that, when it is necessary to send them to a laboratory, the containers should be adequately sealed and promptly dispatched.

Macroscopic Examination

Some of the larger intestinal helminths (ascarids, *Oxyuris* spp., etc.), certain larvae (*Gasterophilus*) and segments (proglottides) of several species of tapeworm can be recognized with the naked eye; final specific identification would, of necessity, involve microscopic examination. The freshly voided proglottides of the common tapeworms of sheep (*Moniezia* spp.) and horses (*Anoplocephala* spp.) have the general appearance of boiled rice grains. Segments of the tapeworms of the dog and cat—with the exception of *Echinococcus granulosus*—may migrate through the anus and become inspissated on the host's bed or coat, where they assume the shape and colour of dehusked barley grains. On being placed in water they quickly resume their normal shape and colour, whereby they are more readily identified. In small animals it may be necessary to administer a purgative to obtain tapeworm segments for diagnostic purposes. The eggs, especially those of *Taenia* spp., may, however, be free when passed in the faeces.

Microscopic Examination

Qualitative microscopic examination for helminth ova is performed by either a simple direct smear technique, or by flotation or sedimentation methods. In the first a small quantity of faeces is smeared onto a slide and diluted with water until newsprint can be read through the suspension. A coverglass is applied and the smear is examined under the microscope. This method is of little diagnostic value because, unless the parasite infestation is severe, it is unlikely that ova will be observed. Heavy infestations with adult ascarid worms in kittens or puppies, or with *Haemonchus contortus* in lambs, are most likely to be detected. Negative results should not be interpreted literally. The cysts of *Giardia* spp. can be identified in faecal smears from dogs on direct microscopic examination, but the addition of a few drops of Lugol's solution is required in order to curtail motility and reveal internal structure.

The flotation method separates the majority of the worm eggs from the faeces and concentrates them on the surface of the liquid. A level dessertspoonful of faeces is placed into 10–20 times this volume of saturated salt solution (660 g made up to 2·4 litres with water)—or alternatively a solution containing 450 g cane sugar in 360 ml water—in a stoppered glass jar containing small glass balls, thoroughly shaken or triturated, poured into a coffee-strainer type of sieve of approximately 1 mm mesh standing in a funnel in a centrifuge tube (duplicate samples should be prepared) and allowed to stand in a rack for about 30 minutes or spun in a centrifuge for a few minutes at 1500 rpm. Any ova at the surface of the solution may be recovered by filling the tube to the brim with the flotation solution, and then touching the meniscus lightly with the underside of a coverslip held horizontally, the resulting hanging drop and coverslip being then placed on a microscope slide for examination. This method is suitable for the detection of the eggs of ascarid species, *Strongyloides* spp., strongyles, trichostrongyles, ancylostomes and some tapeworms (*Anoplocephalidae*), and for the oöcysts of coccidia. Saturated zinc sulphate solution (331 g in 1·0 litre of water) may be used in the same way to float fluke ova and also those of many species of cestodes. In the case of fluke ova the examination should be completed as quickly as possible because zinc sulphate causes osmotic distortion and collapse.

The qualitative sedimentation method of faeces examination may be employed for the demonstration of trematode ova as an alternative to flotation with saturated zinc sulphate. A level dessertspoonful of faeces is thoroughly mixed with 30–40 volumes of water. The suspension is then poured through a fine sieve into a glass cylinder and allowed to stand for 20 minutes. The supernatant fluid is then poured off and the retained sediment resuspended in the same volume of water. The process of mixing, sedimentation and decantation is repeated at least twice, or until the supernatant fluid is clear. A small quantity of the final sediment is withdrawn into a pipette and transferred to a microscope slide. The preparation is ready for examination when a coverslip has been applied. This and the zinc sulphate flotation method are useful for the detection of fluke eggs, in respect of which it is virtually impossible to interpret the significance of numbers in relation to the severity of the infestation in the liver, or elsewhere. In ruminant animals *any* fluke eggs in the faeces are significant when clinical signs of fascioliasis exist.

Qualitative flotation examination of faeces for nematode ova is used mainly to detect subclinical helminth infestations of dogs and cats, in which species the presence of even a few worms of certain types is considered undesirable for public health and aesthetic reasons. In farm animals suspected to have clinical infestation with strongyloid nematodes, quantitative examinations are preferred; but a qualitative flotation investigation of the faeces in large animals is of value in detecting ascarid infestations.

Quantitative examination of faeces for the purpose of counting worm eggs and coccidial oöcysts is performed by either the modified McMaster or the modified Stoll method. These methods are particularly useful for routine diagnosis in suspected outbreaks of parasitic gastroenteritis in cattle or sheep, and strongylosis in horses. Because of the high range of faecal dilution inherent in the method, unless there are more than 100 eggs or larvae per gram of faeces, a negative result will be obtained. This is not altogether a disadvantage; egg counts of 100 g or less are generally considered as being unlikely to signify pathogenic adult intestinal worm infestation in the domestic animals. The other factors, already referred to, which influence the numbers of worm eggs in faeces should be borne in mind when interpreting the significance of ova counts. In this context clinical disease can be caused by helminth larvae when they exist in large enough numbers.

The McMaster technique is relatively simple and does not require very expensive equipment: 2 g of faeces are weighed out or measured with a special spoon made for the purpose, and placed in a 120 ml wide-mouthed, glass-stoppered bottle containing about four dozen small glass balls, and marked at 60 ml level. Saturated sodium chloride solution is added to the mark, the glass stopper inserted and the bottle and contents shaken for 2–3 minutes in order to break up the faeces. The mixture is then poured through a 100 mesh sieve into a small beaker and the debris discarded. The faecal filtrate is agitated, and with a Pasteur pipette sufficient is withdrawn to fill one chamber of the special counting slide (Fig. 155). The residue in the pipette is returned

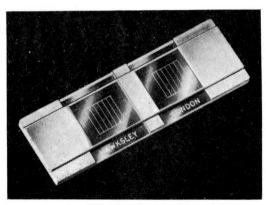

Fig. 155. *A McMaster worm egg counting chamber. Note the two sets of etched lines demarcating the counting area.*

to the filtrate which is then reagitated and a further quantity withdrawn to fill the second chamber on the slide. Filling of the chambers is facilitated by moistening the surface by breathing on the slide. The charged slide is then placed on the stage of the microscope, and after focusing a corner of the etched lines with the 1·6 cm objective, all the eggs are counted by moving up and down the columns of lines. The procedure is repeated for the second chamber; during the counting, when possible, species differentiation is performed. The total number of ova counted in the two chambers multiplied by 100 gives the number of eggs per gram of faeces (epg). Quantitative determination of the ova of *Fasciola* and those of many cestodes can be achieved by employing saturated zinc sulphate solution in the foregoing technique.

The modified McMaster method gives better results when egg counts are rather low, but it requires the use of a centrifuge. About four dozen glass balls are put in a 120 ml bottle and 42 ml water added; 3 g of faeces are weighed out and put in the bottle. After inserting the stopper the bottle is shaken until an even suspension is formed, which is then poured through a 100 mesh sieve placed over a beaker. The fluid collected in the beaker is stirred thoroughly and then poured into two centrifuge tubes to within 1 cm of the top. The tubes are centrifuged for 2 minutes at 1500 rpm and the supernatant is poured off. A little saturated salt solution is added and the sediment in the tube is loosened by means of a Pasteur pipette. The tube is then filled with saturated salt solution to the same mark as before and thorough mixing performed by means of the pipette which is then used to withdraw sufficient fluid to fill one side of the counting chamber. The second chamber is filled after further mixing of the tube contents. Counting is performed as already described and the epg number is obtained by multiplying the total number of eggs in the two squares by 50.

The Stoll technique is more time-consuming, but it enables a count to be made of all types of worm ova: 3 g of faeces are weighed from the sample, stirring well if they are fluid, and are placed in a 120 ml wide-mouthed, glass-stoppered bottle containing four dozen small glass balls. Water is added to the 42 ml mark etched on the bottle. Shake until a uniform suspension is obtained and pour this through a fine mesh sieve into a clean porcelain basin or beaker. With a McDonald pipette (Fig. 156), 0·15 ml of the well-mixed filtrate is removed, ejected onto the surface

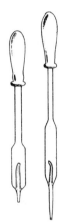

Fig. 156. *The McDonald pipette, designed to deliver 0·15 ml.*

of a microscope slide and covered with a square or rectangular coverslip. Examination is performed with the 1·6 cm objective, and for accuracy a mechanical stage is required. The whole area covered by the faecal suspension is examined, including any that may have flowed beyond the extremities of the coverglass, and all eggs are counted and differentiated. For convenience counting should start along one edge of the coverslip. The number of eggs obtained is multiplied by 100 to give the epg number.

Other more specialized methods of faeces examination are ordinarily only employed in the parasitology laboratory. They include the Baermann technique for detection of lungworm larvae, and cultural methods for the specific identification of the third stage larvae of the strongyle worms of the horse and the trichostrongyles of the ruminant species.

The Baermann method, which is also applicable in the demonstration of the larvae of intestinal helminths in any animal, provided the infestation is a patent one, consists of filling a glass funnel 20–25 cm in diameter, fitted with a short piece of rubber tubing and a metal clip, with water at 37°C. The apparatus is supported in a retort ring on a stand (Fig. 157). A metal sieve (15–20 cm in diameter) with about 120 meshes to the linear centimetre is moistened with water and then placed in the funnel. Water is poured into the funnel until it is about 1 cm above the mesh of the sieve. Then with a spatula 20 g of fresh faeces are spread over the surface of a filter paper about 12–17 cm in. in diameter, which is then inverted and placed, faeces side downwards, on the gauze of the sieve. The preparation is allowed to stand for 24 hours, during which time any motile larvae will have sedimented to the stem of the funnel from where they are recovered by running off about 15 ml of fluid into a collecting tube. After allowing sedimentation to take place, or centrifuging the tube and its contents, the fluid is syphoned off until about 0·1 ml remains. After being well mixed the residue is withdrawn and placed on a microscope slide. The bottom of the tube is rinsed out with 0·1 ml water which is also transferred to the slide and then a rectangular coverslip is applied and the larvae counted by means of the 1·6 cm objective. Dividing the total number by the weight of the faeces in grams will give the number of larvae per gram. (For details of more accurate methods of larval counting refer to a textbook on veterinary parasitology.)

Cultural techniques for detecting the presence of helminth larvae in faeces are readily performed by incubating appropriate samples in Petri dishes at 37°C in a bacteriological incubator. The faeces are spread evenly to a depth of at least 0·8 cm over the whole base of the Petri dish and four wells, one in each quadrant, about 0·5 cm in diameter, are made completely through the layer of faeces with a glass rod. The wells are filled with water and the preparation is incubated for 4–5 days. Samples of fluid are recovered from the wells by means of a suitable pipette and then ejected onto a microscope slide. The preparation is examined for larvae after a coverslip has been applied. Another method is to incubate the faecal sample for the requisite period in a Petri dish, or other container, and then to concentrate the larvae by means of the Baermann technique. Specific differentiation of larvae is achieved by noting particular morphological details including bursae, number of oesophageal cells, presence or absence of granules in the intestinal cells, etc.

Serum Pepsinogen

Certain other diagnostic and prognostic methods can be employed in living animals in order to extend the limitations of egg counting techniques. Some such as haematocrit and

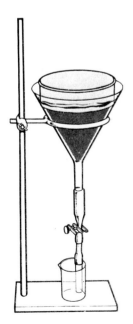

Fig. 157. *The apparatus for the Baermann method of examining faeces for the larvae of intestinal worms and lungworms.*

haemoglobin determinations have more value in prognosis than in diagnosis. In parasitic gastritis caused by *Trichostrongylus axei* and *Ostertagia ostertagi* because of mucosal damage in the abomasum, pepsinogen (a precursor of gastric pepsin) leaks away and appears in significant amounts in blood serum. Normal serum pepsinogen levels for cattle of different ages average from 0·2 milli international units/ml for 6–8-week-old calves, and 2·39 mIU/ml for adult cattle. Cattle infected with *T. axei* alone have raised values of the order of 1–1·2 mIU/ml and with *O. ostertagi* alone up to 4 mIU/ml. Serum samples from obviously clinically affected and from normal cattle in the same group should be tested in order to assist the interpretation of the results.

Worm Counts

In general the interpretation of faeces egg or larval counts must be finalized in relation to the clinical signs and history of the animals concerned. It well may be that one or more animals have died, or that the disease is far advanced, thereby providing the opportunity for post mortem examination, with particular reference to enumeration of intestinal parasites. By tying-off the appropriate portions of the gastro-intestinal tract it is possible to count the number of worms in the stomach or various segments of the small intestine. For this purpose selected specimens can be forwarded to a laboratory. The method for worm counting consists of emptying the stomach or intestinal contents into a suitable bowl. Then the exposed mucous membrane of the stomach is washed under a stream of tap water, the washings being collected in the same bowl. The intestinal contents are recovered into a separate receptacle by a milking-out process, and then each segment of intestine is filled with water by clamping one end and attaching the other end to the tap, the washings being collected with the contents. Formalin is added in the proportion of 50 ml/litre of collected material.

The collected material from either the stomach or the intestine is poured through a sieve with 32 meshes/cm (if immature larvae are suspected a sieve with over 40 meshes/cm should be used) and washing of the material in the sieve should be continued until no more food particles or coloured matter passes through. The contents of the sieve are then washed into a glass bowl.

Usually when the numbers of adult worms are high, direct examination at this stage will reveal their presence. The contents of the bowl are made up to the 1 litre mark with water and while the whole is kept vigorously stirred 10 ml are removed by means of a trumpet-ended pipette and transferred to a Petri dish. Small quantities at a time of this aliquot are placed in a cavity block, diluted further if necessary and examined with a dissecting microscope and the worms enumerated and differentiated. In order to expedite the counting, all the worms large enough to be readily visible to the naked eye should be counted and removed from the first aliquot, the whole of which should be examined. When performing a worm count on the contents of the digestive tract of large animals the volumes mentioned above should be increased by a factor of four. In all events the total number of worms obtained from the aliquot multiplied by 100 will give the worm population for the stomach or intestine. Table 11 includes the common intestinal worms of ruminants.

The interpretation of worm counts depends upon identification of species as well as the actual total number, some such as *Haemonchus contortus* being capable of producing clinical disease in sheep, when as few as 500 worms are present, whereas 5000 small trichostrongyle worms may be regarded as being necessary to cause disease in the same host. For cattle up to 15 000 small trichostrongyle worms may be considered to be of pathological significance in animals showing appropriate clinical signs.

The ova of some of the commoner types of parasitic helminths found in the faeces of animals are illustrated in Figs 158–161. A detailed description of these eggs can be found in textbooks of veterinary parasitology. For brevity, specific names have been avoided in most of the illustrated examples. Indeed, in those important nematodes of the superfamily *Strongyloides* that produce ova indistinguishable one from another, or which are identifiable only by the experienced parasitologist, the term strongyloid nematode egg has been used. Ova of this type are produced by a very large number of different nematode parasites in a variety of hosts. Certain other egg types also are common to several animal hosts. To avoid repetition of photographs, therefore, Fig. 158 is a comprehensive one for ruminant hosts. In the remaining plates, which relate to other animals, only those egg types that have not

TABLE 11. COMMON INTESTINAL HELMINTHS OF RUMINANTS*

Parasite	Cattle			Sheep		
	A	B	C	A	B	C
Haemonchus contortus				+		
Haemonchus placei	+					
Trichostrongylus axei	+			+		
Ostertagia ostertagi	+					
Ostertagia circumcincta				+		
Ostertagia trifurcata				+		
Trichostrongylus colubriformis		+			+	
Trichostrongylus vitrinus					+	
Cooperia curticei					+	
Cooperia onchophora		+				
Cooperia mcmasteri		+				
Cooperia punctata		+				
Cooperia pectinata		+				
Neoascaris vitulorum		+				
Nematodirus helvetianus		+				
Nematodirus battus				+		
Nematodirus filicollis				+		
Nematodirus spathiger				+		
Bunostomum phlebotomum		+				
Bunostomum trigonocephalum					+	
Strongyloides papillosus					+	
Moniezia expansa					+	
Moniezia bedenini		+				
Oesophagostomum radiatum			+			
Oesophagostomum venulosum						+
Oesophagostomum columbianum						+
Chabertia ovina			+			+
Trichuris ovis						+
Trichuris globulosa			+			+

* A, abomasum; B, small intestine; C, large intestine.

already been illustrated are shown; where ova morphologically similar to those shown in Fig. 158 occur, reference is made to the latter for morphological detail, but this does not imply that the helminths producing such ova are identical species.

Bacteriological Examination

The principal diseases in which bacteriological examination of the faeces is employed are Johne's disease, salmonellosis, coliform enteritis, winter dysentery and vibrionic dysentery.

In suspected Johne's disease the specimen of faeces is rubbed through a fine mesh wire gauze sieve to remove gross particulate matter, otherwise a mounted needle can be run through the faeces and any mucus recovered on the needle can be placed on a microscope slide. Smears are prepared by placing a small quantity of the strained faeces, or mucus, at one end of a microscope slide, and with the cut-off end of another slide it is then pushed along the surface

to form a film. The smear is air-dried and then fixed over a flame and after a strip of filter paper is placed over the smear, it is flooded with Ziehl-Neelsen's carbol fuchsin solution. Gentle heat is applied until steam rises from the staining solution, and the hot stain is allowed to act for 5 minutes. The preparation should not be allowed to become dry; further staining solution can be added as required with heating. Then the filter paper and moist stain are washed off and decolorization performed by flooding with a solution consisting of 3% hydrochloric acid in 70% alcohol. This is allowed to act for 1 minute and more acid–alcohol solution is applied to wash off the freed stain; this process is repeated until the colour remains clear (for about 3–4 minutes). After thorough washing the preparation is counterstained with 1% methylene blue for 1 minute. A final washing is carried out followed by drying, using fluff-free filter paper; then, after applying lens immersion fluid, the smear is microscopically examined

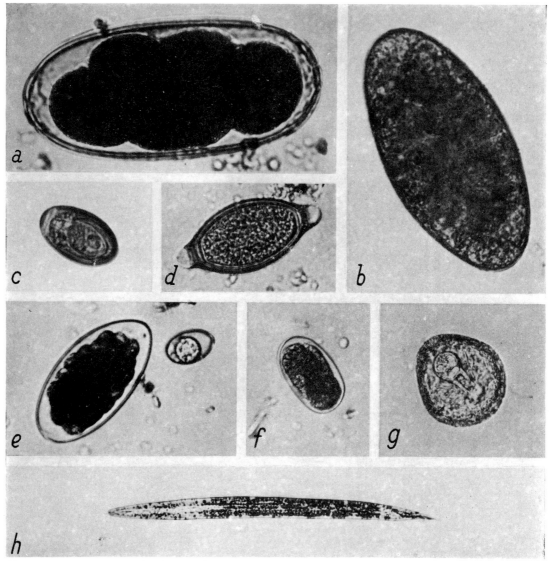

Fig. 158. *Parasitic ova etc. found in the faeces of ruminants.* A, Nematodirus *spp.* B, Fasciola hepatica. C, Dicrocoelium dendriticum. D, Trichuris *spp.* E, *Strongyloid nematode egg; a coccidial oöcyst is also shown.* F, Strongyloides papillosis. G, Moniezia *spp.* H, *First stage larva from a lungworm; this species is* Dictyocaulus viviparus *from a calf. The larvae of the predominant lungworms of the sheep and goat show certain differences in morphology.* A–G ×500; H ×300.

along one of the straight edges with the 0·2 cm objective.

    Examination of faeces for *Mycobacterium paratuberculosis* is best made when diarrhoea is obvious. In positive smears the causal organism is found in characteristic clusters of small red bacilli (Fig. 149C, p. 175), sometimes within the confines of extruded epithelial or other cells. Isolated individual bacilli should not be taken to indicate a positive infection because of the

frequency with which saprophytic acid-fast organisms are present in faecal smears. Neither should a negative smear be regarded as being conclusive and, in all suspect cases of this disease, it is advisable to obtain repeat samples for examination at intervals of 2–3 weeks.

    Cultural examination of faeces is of little practical value in the diagnosis of Johne's disease (allergic and serological tests will be considered in Chapter 16). This method is

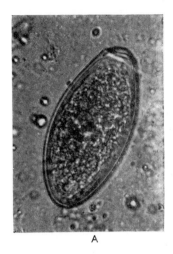
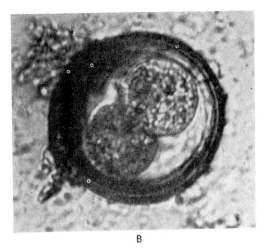

A B

Fig. 159. *Parasitic ova found in the faeces of the horse.* A, Oxyuris equi, *occasionally found in faeces but more usually on the perianal skin.* B, Parascaris equorum. ×*500. Other parasite eggs that may be seen include those of* Anoplocephala *spp.* (*similar to* Monezia, *Fig. 158*G), Strongyloides westeri (*Fig. 158*F) *and strongyloid nematode eggs* (*Fig. 158*E).

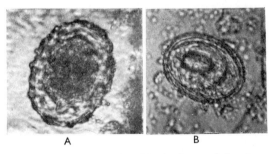

A B

Fig. 160. *Parasitic ova found in the faeces of the pig.* A, Ascaris suum. B, Metastronglyus *spp.* ×*500. Other parasite eggs that may be seen include those of* Fasciola hepatica (*Fig. 158*B), Strongyloides *spp.* (*Fig. 158*F), Trichuris *spp.* (Fig. *158*D), Hyostrongylus rubidus, Oesophagostomum *spp. and strongyloid nematode ova similar to that in Fig. 158*E.

frequently necessary, however, to establish the specific nature of the infection in the enteric forms of salmonellosis and colibacillosis. Isolation of *Salmonella* is more certain when at least 20 g of faeces from each of a number of affected animals are innoculated into a suitable transport medium such as 1% peptone broth, and then further isolation continued in tetrathionate broth at a temperature of 43°C. In the case of *Escherichia coli* isolation is, as a rule, readily achieved by means of MacConkey's medium. Slide agglutination tests are necessary for serotype identification of salmonellae and pathogenic *E. coli*.

Faecal smears, particularly if made from epithelial or mucus shreds, are of value in the diagnosis of winter dysentery in cattle. In positive cases large numbers of *Vibrio jejuni* are often present. Direct staining with dilute carbol fuchsin is all that is necessary, no counterstaining is required. In many outbreaks of swine dysentery *Vibrio coli* is found in faecal smears prepared in a similar manner. The significance of these two organisms as primary pathogens is open to question.

Chemical Examination

Relatively simple tests can be carried out on samples of faeces from suspected cases of pancreatic disease, the incidence of which is probably highest in dogs.

The existence of steatorrhoea is suggested when the faeces are pale yellow or clay coloured with a foul odour and a glistening appearance. Confirmation of the diagnosis is achieved by adding Sudan III to a homogenous mixture of the faeces and finding red or orange droplets in a smear when examined microscopically.

In creatorrhoea the addition of Lugol's solution (iodine 1 g, potassium iodide 2 g, water to 100 ml) or tincture of iodine to faeces will delineate the striations in poorly digested muscle fibres.

Deficiency of pancreatic trypsin is easily revealed by means of a film strip test; the tube

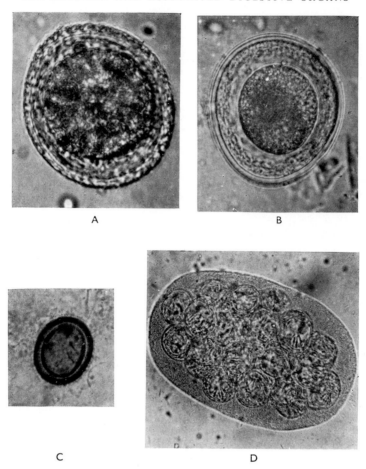

Fig. 161. *Parasitic ova etc. found in the faeces of the dog and cat.* A, Toxo-cara *spp.* B, Toxascaris leonina. C, Taenia *spp.* D, *Egg capsule of* Dipylidium caninum. A–C *×500;* D *×300. Other parasite eggs that may be seen include those of hookworms (a strongyloid nematode egg similar to that shown in Fig. 158E),* Trichuris vulpis, Capillaria aerophila (*Fig. 158D) and coccidial oöcysts (Fig. 158E).*

test is more accurate but somewhat more complex to perform. In the film test sufficient faeces are added to 9·5 ml of 5% sodium bicarbonate solution to bring the volume to the 10 ml mark. After adequate mixing one drop of the faeces suspension is placed on a strip of unexposed, or dark area of exposed X-ray film (alternately a strip of unexposed film can be partly submerged in the tube). The prepared film strip is placed in a Petri dish to prevent drying and incubated for I hour at 37°C, or 2·5 hours at room temperature. The strip is then washed gently in running tap water. A clear spot on the film or clearing of the lower part of the tube strip indicates the presence of trypsin. In the tube test 1 ml of the faecal suspension is added to 2 ml of 7·5% gelatin and the mixture incubated in the same manner as for the strip test. The tube and contents are refrigerated for 20 minutes and failure of gelatin to set indicates the presence of trypsin. Repeat tests should always be performed as the results of single tests are unreliable. Consistently positive results indicate normal trypsin production, whereas the reverse finding suggests pancreatic enzyme deficiency. Trypsin inhibitors and pro-teolytic enzymes of bacterial origin may give false negative and false positive results respec-tively.

THE LIVER

Regional Anatomy

In the domestic animals the whole of the liver, when normal, is situated in the concavity of the diaphragm, and it does not extend sufficiently beyond the costal arch, even on the right side, for its border to be palpable.

Horse. The greatest part of the liver is situated on the right of the median plane. The parietal surface is in contact with the diaphragm, and the visceral surface is moulded to some extent by the organs which lie against it. The highest point of the liver is level with the right kidney, and its lowest about 7–10 cm from the abdominal floor, opposite the sternal extremity of the seventh or eighth rib on the left side. The right border, which is thin, extends backwards to the sixteenth rib, just below its middle. At this point the liver is separated from the ribs by the diaphragm.

Cattle. The liver is situated almost entirely on the right of the median plane. The parietal surface is mainly in contact with the right portion of the diaphragm but a small area is in direct contact with the last two or three ribs, occasionally even with the flank.

Sheep. The liver is situated entirely to the right of the median plane. The right border may project beyond the costal arch at its lower part.

Pig. The greater part of the liver lies to the right of the median plane. A small part of the parietal surface is in contact with the abdominal floor in the xiphoid region and also at a point ventral to the right costal arch. The ventral border of the two central lobes extends 2–5 cm behind the xiphoid cartilage.

Dog. The parietal surface conforms to the concavity of the diaphragm and the contiguous parts of the ventral abdominal wall. The ventral border of the lobes is related to the abdominal floor a variable distance behind the xiphoid cartilage above the rectus abdominis muscle.

The internal structure of the liver comprises a large number of morphologically identical lobules each of which is capable of performing all the functions of the liver. Assessment of liver disease and of disturbed liver function is not only made complex by the many metabolic activities performed, but also because the organ possesses considerable powers of regeneration.

In the latter regard, clinical signs of hepatic dysfunction only appear when about 75% of all lobules have been rendered inactive, in spite of which complete regeneration can occur within a few weeks.

The main functions of the liver include secretion and excretion of bile, protein, fat and carbohydrate metabolism, detoxication, fibrinogen, prothrombin and heparin production, vitamin A formation from carotene, blood volume regulation and iron and copper storage.

Disturbance of hepatic function is much more likely to occur in diffuse diseases of the liver than with focal lesions, which produce their effects by locally formed toxins or by pressure on other organs, or on the liver itself. The majority of liver diseases in animals are secondary to generalized infection or spread from another organ; primary hepatic disease, which is rare, is usually the result of poisoning by toxic agents of chemical or plant origin. In any diffuse disease the various functions of the liver are disordered to the same degree, consequently the clinical manifestations vary in intensity according to the severity of the hepatic injury. There are some functions which, however, when disturbed are more likely to be responsible for clinical signs. These include the maintenance of normal blood sugar levels through the medium of glycogen, formation of some of the plasma proteins, maintenance of bile production and excretion, formation of prothrombin and detoxification and excretion of many toxic substances.

Clinical Examination

The evidence obtained during the general clinical examination may suggest disease of the liver. Special attention can be given to the liver through the medium of a physical examination coupled, when necessary, with biochemical tests, biopsy and occasionally radiographic examination.

The position of the liver in most species of animals is such that physical methods of examination are of limited value. In cattle, dogs and cats, gross enlargement of the liver (hepatomegaly) causes the right or the ventral border to project beyond the costal arch or xiphoid cartilage, and the edge is usually uniformly thickened and rounded, in contradistinction to the sharp edge of the normal liver. Local enlargement, such as occurs in neoplasia or hydatidosis, etc., when it impinges on the border, causes it to be irregular. Palpation of the liver is unrewarding in horses and pigs because of the rigidity and thickness of the abdominal wall.

Gross enlargement of the liver occurs as the result of severe congestion arising from chronic congestive heart failure, and also particularly in the horse, in those forms of plant poisoning in which fibrosis is a prominent feature, in multiple abscessation, in metastatic neoplasia and in occasional cases of hydatidosis. The increase in size of the liver in acute diffuse hepatitis is not sufficient to be appreciated by physical examination. In terminal fibrosis, the reduction in the size of the liver is often not appreciated unless the right or the ventral border is distorted, when palpation may reveal the rather rigid irregular line.

By means of percussion it is possible to obtain some idea of the extent of the dull area overlying the liver, although it is unlikely that hepatic enlargement would regularly be recognized in this way. Strong percussion or firm palpation over the liver area is of value in recognizing the presence and extent of hepatic pain. The entire area should be subjected to percussion in order to avoid missing focal pain associated with a discrete lesion.

Clinical Signs of Liver Disease

Jaundice

Secretion of bile is one of the most important functions of the liver. Bile is composed of bile salts (derived from the metabolism of cholesterol), bile pigments (excretory products derived from the catabolism of haemoglobin liberated from effete erythrocytes), alkaline phosphatase, water and various lipids (cholesterol, lecithin, etc.). Bile salts are involved in the digestion and absorption of fats; about 90% recycles from the small intestine back to the liver and is resecreted in the bile. The initially formed free bilirubin (indirect or unconjugated bilirubin) is conjugated in the liver cells with glycuronic acid thus forming bilirubin glycuronide (direct or conjugated bilirubin). When the liver is damaged, in primary and secondary diseases, the quantities of bile pigment in blood, urine, faeces and body tissues will change as the result of deranged excretion.

Jaundice, which is caused by the accumulation of bilirubin, is manifested clinically by orange-yellow discoloration of the mucous membranes, submucosal tissues, unpigmented skin and other body structures, often occurs in diseases of the liver and biliary system, but also in diseases in which these organs are not significantly damaged; conversely, it may not develop even when the liver is extensively involved as in acute hepatitis. The intensity of the tissue staining is much more pronounced with direct than with indirect bilirubin, so that jaundice is more severe in cases of obstructive jaundice than in haemolytic jaundice. The staining is due to accumulation of bilirubin in the tissues, especially elastic tissue, so that it is usually most obvious in the sclera.

Jaundice has been classified in many ways and for clinical purposes the most simple system is the best. Perhaps the most basic differentiation is between jaundice with and without biliary obstruction.

1. *Mechanical or obstructive jaundice.* This is jaundice arising from obstruction of the bile ducts or common bile duct (cholestasis). The discolored tissues are greenish yellow, and when biliary obstruction is complete bile pigments are absent from the faeces, the serum levels of direct bilirubin become markedly elevated so that large amounts are excreted in the urine which is free of urobilinogen because no bile pigment is available in the intestine for its formation. In partial biliary obstruction similar variations occur in the serum and urine, but some bile pigments occur in the faeces and urobilinogen in the urine.

Obstruction or compression occlusion of the larger bile ducts or common bile duct can be caused by nematodes, trematodes or inflammation of the ducts themselves. In pigs, *Ascaris suum* is an important cause of biliary obstruction and secondary cholangitis, especially in animals which have been subjected to transportation for prolonged periods. Cattle and sheep occasionally develop cholangitis and cholecystitis as the result of infestation by *Fasciola hepatica* or *Dicrocoelium dendriticum*. Occasionally, also, ascending cholangitis, developing secondarily to catarrhal enteritis, may be sufficiently severe to cause obstruction of the common bile duct at its termination. This form of obstruction has been observed in horses with parasitic enteritis. Obstruction of the bile ducts or common bile duct by calculi or compression by neoplasms is a rare event in animals. In all these conditions the cause is extrahepatic in origin.

Mechanical bile stasis can also occur when there is constriction and obliteration of the intrahepatic biliary canaliculi after hepatitis, and in certain forms of hepatic fibrosis. The changes in the blood, urine and faeces are the same as those which occur in extrahepatic biliary obstruction.

2. *Haemolytic or overproduction jaundice.* In this form the affected tissues are distinctly yellow and there is haemoglobinuria and anaemia. The urine contains no bilirubin but there is an increased amount of urobilinogen. The indirect bilirubin content of the serum is greatly elevated. This type of jaundice is caused by excessive intravascular haemolysis which results in an abnormally large quantity of bile being produced. Haemolytic jaundice is very common in animals and may be caused by bacterial toxins (bacillary haemoglobinuria, leptospirosis), protozoa (babesiasis, anaplasmosis, eperythrozoonosis), viruses (infectious equine anaemia), inorganic and organic poisons (chronic copper poisoning, phenothiazine poisoning in horses), vegetable poisons (rape and other cruciferous plants), snake venoms and immunological (iso-immunization haemolytic anaemia of foals, puppies and piglets) and other blood incompatability reactions.

3. *Jaundice due to hepatic cell degeneration* (*toxic jaundice*). This occurs when the parenchyma of the liver has been damaged to a sufficient degree to interfere with the normal formation and elimination of bile. The serum bilirubin level is elevated and the urine contains an increased amount of direct bilirubin and urobilinogen. The body tissues including the unpigmented skin areas are reddish-yellow or brownish-yellow in colour. The cause may be any disease associated with acute or chronic diffuse hepatitis.

In an animal with complete obstructive jaundice, because of the absence of bile, the faeces are light-grey, clay-like and firm (acholic or bile-free faeces). They also contain a proportion of undigested fat. In haemolytic jaundice the faeces are usually normal in colour, or otherwise somewhat yellow. The differences are explained by the fact that in obstructive jaundice, when occlusion is complete, the intestine is deprived of bile pigments which normally impart colour to the intestinal contents. In haemolytic jaundice,

in contra-distinction, an excessive quantity of bile is released into the intestine.

Neonatal jaundice, which is rarely, if ever, observed clinically in young animals, is probably caused by biliary retention rather than excessively rapid breakdown of fetal erythrocytes. Otherwise, severe jaundice developing in young animals, particularly foals and puppies, soon after birth, is usually caused by iso-immunization of the dam during pregnancy. The disease results from the natural occurrence of inherited blood groups with anti-erythrocyte antigens, in species such as horses, mules, pigs and dogs. In this situation the fetus has an equal chance, in matings between parents of incompatible blood groups, of inheriting erythrocyte antigens from the sire. The antigens may then traverse the placenta and, if not already part of the dam's complement of antigens, they will stimulate the production of erythrocyte antibodies. These antibodies, although they may be present in high titre in the blood of the pregnant mare from the eighth month of pregnancy onwards, are unable to reach the foetus because they are molecularly too large to diffuse across the placenta, but they are transferred to the newborn animal in the colostrum, causing massive destruction of its erythrocytes with severe haemolytic anaemia, haemoglobinuria and jaundice.

False jaundice. This is a situation in which yellow colouration of the body tissues occurs which is not caused by bile pigments but by other colouring substances, the commonest of which is carotene, a complex pigment found in young green plants. Deposition of carotene in the tissues is most marked in certain breeds of cattle, particularly the Guernsey; it also occurs to a moderate extent in horses eating green plant foods.

Nervous and Other Signs

In animals with diffuse hepatic disease, apart from jaundice, which is by no means a constant feature, other signs may be observed indicating involvement of the nervous system, or oedema and emaciation, deranged intestinal function, haemorrhagic diathesis and abdominal pain. The main nervous signs include dullness, anorexia, muscle tremor and weakness, compulsive walking, head-pressing, hyperexcitability, failure to respond to customary signals, and convulsions. Biochemical aspects which, it has been suggested, might be responsible for these changes in behaviour include hypoglycaemia, accumulation of excess amino acids or of acetylcholine due to failure of the usual hepatic detoxification mechanisms.

Oedema and emaciation are the result of failure by the liver to anabolize amino acids and proteins. This leads to a fall in plasma protein and thus a reduction in plasma osmotic pressure with loss of fluid into the tissues. The oedema is most marked in the intermandibular space. The alimentary tract syndrome consisting of anorexia and constipation with intermittent attacks of diarrhoea is the result of the partial, or complete absence of bile salts in the intestines (bile salts possess both laxative and disinfectant properties). In these circumstances absorption of fat-soluble vitamins, especially vitamin K, is seriously reduced. The formation of prothrombin, fibrinogen and thromboplastin is impaired in all severe, diffuse diseases of the liver. The deficiency of prothrombin, which along with other similar factors requires the presence of vitamin K for its synthesis, leads to prolongation of the blood clotting time and, therefore, the appearance of tissue haemorrhages. Abdominal pain in diseases of the liver arises from two mechanisms: tension of the capsule from increase in the size of the liver and lesions involving the capsule itself. Distension of the liver occurs in acute inflammation and in congestive heart failure, and is due to vascular engorgement. The pain results from stimulation of the subcapsular pain end-organs by inflammatory or neoplastic involvement of the capsule or the subcapsular parenchyma of the liver. Clinically, pain of hepatic origin causes arching of the back, disinclination to move and tenseness of the abdominal wall.

Liver Function Tests

An appreciation of the tests that would most effectively measure the degree of liver derangement in disease can be obtained from a consideration of those hepatic functions, which, when deranged, are responsible for clinical signs. The tests can be classified into five groups: those that measure secretory and excretory functions, those that measure the metabolic activity of the liver, those which measure protein, lipid and carbohydrate metabolism, those which test detoxification mechanisms and finally serum enzyme tests.

As yet, laboratory tests for assessing hepatic function, because they are exacting, time-consuming and somewhat expensive, have not been generally applied in clinical work; normal criteria for most of the selected parameters have been established, but the significance of the variations which can occur have not been exactly determined in all cases. The accurate determination of particular body constituents may supply much information relating to liver function, provided it is realized that they vary from other than hepatic causes.

Secretory and excretory functions. These are measured by determining whether there is any alteration in the quantities of bile pigment in blood, urine and faeces, and also by measuring the excretion rate of bile pigment, or more usually bromsulphalein, following intravenous injection. Bile pigments and bile salts are normally present in the blood in such low concentrations that none, or only a trace in the case of bile pigments, appears in the urine. Consequently the state of bile metabolism in an individual animal can be investigated by performing suitable tests on a urine sample. Unfortunately up to 25% of normal cattle have traces of bilirubin in the urine, so that the interpretation of positive results in this species requires careful evaluation, paying particular attention to the clinical examination and the results of other more meaningful liver function tests.

A variety of tests are available for the detection of bilirubin in urine, including Fouchet's test for which two solutions are required: (a) a 10% solution of barium chloride and (b) Fouchet's reagent which is made up as follows:

Trichloracetic acid	25 ml
Distilled water	100 ml
Ferric chloride 10% solution	10 ml

The urine should be boiled and filtered if protein is present and, in the event that the urine is alkaline, acidified with a little acetic acid. Add 5 ml of the barium chloride solution to about 10 ml of the urine, mix thoroughly and filter. The urine damped filter paper is then laid flat on a dry filter paper and one drop of Fouchet's reagent is placed on the precipitate. The presence of bile pigment is indicated by the appearance of a green or blue colour.

A proprietary tablet (Ictotest, Ames Co.), containing a stable diazonium compound, sulphosalicylic acid and sodium carbonate, will give a rapid result, but it may be more difficult to read the colour reactions. Five drops of urine are placed on an asbestos-cellulose fibre mat, and then one of the tablets is put on the urine-moistened area. Two drops of water are deposited on the surface of the tablet. A purple colour developing on the mat around the periphery of the tablet within 30 seconds indicates that bilirubin is present. Delayed colour reactions are of no significance.

The methylene blue test, which is easy to perform, can be made to give a quantitative result. In the presence of bilirubin, methylene blue is changed to a green colour; this is not a specific chemical reaction. Methylene blue solution at a concentration of 0·2% is added drop by drop to a measured quantity of urine with continuous mixing. Each milligram of bilirubin requires 200 drops of the methylene blue solution to bring about the colour conversion.

Changes in the quantities of bile pigments in blood can be measured by means of the diazo test for bilirubin (van den Bergh test). In performing the test an acidic diazobenzene sulphonic acid solution is added to serum. In obstructive jaundice a reddish-blue or violet colour appears at once; giving the so-called 'direct reaction'. With sera from cases of haemolytic jaundice, the colour only develops after the addition of alcohol following the diazo reagent—the 'indirect reaction'. In cases of hepatocellular jaundice, a biphasic reaction occurs consisting of the rapid appearance of a reddish colour which intensifies on standing.

Variations in serum bilirubin and, therefore, in the intensity of jaundice can be determined by measuring the 'yellowness' or icteric index. This is an empirical method and consists of adding saline solution to 1 ml serum until it matches a standard solution of 1 in 10 000 potassium dichromate. The icteric index is the volume of saline in millilitres. In animals, more particularly horses and cattle, the presence of lipochromes or carotenoids causes yellow colouration which reduces the efficiency of the test.

Of the tests measuring excretory efficiency that employing phenoltetrabromophthalein (bromsulphalein, BSP) has been extensively employed. It is of limited diagnostic value in cattle, but gives a fair indication of hepatic dysfunction in horses, and is regarded as being sensitive and reliable in dogs. Bromsulphalein, following intravenous injection of an amount proportional to bodyweight (5 mg/kg), is largely eliminated from the body through the liver, so that hepatic dysfunction is indicated by delayed blood clearance. The principle of the test in the dog is that a sample of heparinized blood is collected 30 minutes after the injection, the plasma is removed and treated with sodium hydroxide solution. The colour reaction is compared against a similarly treated sample of plasma collected prior to the injection of the bromsulphalein. The percentage dye retention is calculated by multiplying the 30-minute concentration (mg/100 ml) by the factor 10; in healthy dogs it is 5% or less. For large animals 1 g bromsulphalein is injected intravenously. Then two heparinized blood samples are taken at an arbitrary interval—usually 4 minutes—before 12 minutes have elapsed. The BSP clearance rate is determined by estimating the concentration of the dye in the two samples and plotting the results against time on semilog graph paper. The half clearance time can be read off.

Bile salts. In intrahepatic and extrahepatic biliary obstruction the bile salts, sodium glycocholate and sodium taurocholate, are returned to the blood and excreted by the kidneys. By reason of their detergent properties bile salts reduce the surface tension in the gut and in the urine. When a sample of urine containing a significant amount of bile salts is shaken a persistent foam is produced. Reduction in surface tension can also be recognized by means of Hay's sulphur test which is satisfactory for the urine of all species except cattle. For the test a small amount of sulphur is sprinkled on the surface of a motionless column of urine. If the sulphur immediately sinks through the urine it may be concluded that bile salts are present, provided that synthetic detergents can be excluded as a cause of a false positive reaction.

Metabolic functions. A large proportion (90–95%) of the serum proteins including albumin, globulin and fibrinogen are synthesized by the liver. Serum protein estimations, which may be carried out by empirical turbidity and flocculation tests or by electrophoresis, have been found to have a limited application in veterinary diagnosis because changes, which may not involve the liver, do not appear until a disease process is somewhat advanced. Measurement of the prothrombin time has been found of use in the diagnosis of liver disease.

Measurements of lipid metabolism, particularly cholesterol, provides a useful index of liver function in animals. The method is, however, a complex one. In the case of carbohydrates, liver function can be assessed by means of the galactose tolerance test. Galactose utilization is restricted to the liver and its metabolism appears to impose a considerable burden on the hepatic cells.

Detoxification mechanisms. The liver deals with toxic substances by biotransformation, conjugation and destruction. Conjugation is with amino acids and substances such as glucuronic acid. Substances such as benzoic acid and chloral hydrate are detoxified by this mechanism and, therefore, form the basis of a method for measuring liver function. The risk associated with introducing a toxic substance into the body of an animal considered to have severe or extensive liver disease should not be overlooked.

Serum enzymes. The concentration of certain serum enzymes varies as the result of three processes involving the liver: (*a*) elevation due to disruption of liver parenchymal cells because of necrosis, or greater membrane permeability, e.g. glutamic pyruvic transaminase (SGPT), glutamic oxalacetic transaminase (SGOT), arginase, isocitric dehydrogenase (SICD), sorbitol dehydrogenase (SD), glutamic dehydrogenase (GD), ornithine carbamyl transferase (OCT), and lactic dehydrogenase (LDH); (*b*) elevation because of lack of biliary excretion in obstructive jaundice, e.g. alkaline phosphatase (SAP); and (*c*) decrease due to impaired synthesis by the liver, e.g. choline esterase. Certain of these enzymes exist in high concentrations in hepatic tissue and might be regarded as being 'liver-specific', e.g. SGPT in the dog, cat and primates; SD and GD in sheep and cattle; SD in horses; arginase and OCT in all ureotelic animals. The other enzymes mentioned occur in high concentrations in other tissues than the liver so that unless the disease process is localized to the liver, measurement of these enzymes is likely to be confusing in diagnosis.

The techniques for measuring serum enzymes are, in most instances, complex; 'kit' tests are commercially available and are reliable and relatively simple to perform but they require a colorimeter or spectrophotometer on which to read the results. Serum enzyme values for various species of animals are given in Table 17 (p. 297).

Biopsy of the Liver

Biopsy of the liver provides material suitable for histological and chemical examination. In the former case the small proportion of tissue recovered may not reveal significant changes, except when the liver is diffusely affected. Chemical determinations of value include those for copper, glycogen and vitamin A. Success in performing the operation requires anatomical knowledge and experience, and is more easily achieved in cattle than in horses or other species. The essential equipment consists of a sharp-pointed, small-bore trocar and cannula about 30–40 cm long with a screw thread at the blunt end to which can be attached a syringe of sufficient capacity to produce the necessary negative pressure for withdrawing the sample of liver. The pointed end of the assembled instrument is inserted through the desensitized skin in the upper part of the intercostal space appropriate for the species, on the right hand side, directed towards the left elbow region and advanced across the pleural cavity. The instrument is inserted with a rotating action, until the point is considered to have reached the surface of the liver, when the trocar is withdrawn; the syringe is then attached and insertion continued for about 2–5 cm. Suction is then applied, the instrument vigorously rotated and slowly withdrawn, during which time strong suction is maintained. The syringe is useful in discharging the core of liver from the cannula when the biopsy has been successful. Although the technique has been repeated on many occasions in the one animal without untowards effect, it is not free from attendant risk. The main danger arises from misdirection of the instrument, causing damage to large blood vessels or bile ducts in the portal area. Other recognized sequelae include suppurative peritonitis as the result of penetrating an active abscess or fatal haemoperitoneum if there is a defect in the blood clotting mechanism. Failure to obtain a sample may arise when the liver is shrunken or the instrument not inserted at the correct point or in the right direction. The technique is suitable for horses, cattle, sheep and dogs.

Radiological Examination

The application of radiological examination to the liver and biliary system is almost entirely confined to the dog and cat although it is possible, on an experimental basis, to extend the method to some species of farm animals. The gall-bladder can be visualized through the medium of cholecystography following the oral administration of a halogenated phenolphthalein compound. Cholelithiasis is a rare condition in animals, occurring very occasionally in the dog. The concretions are usually soft in consistency, and would be unlikely to be revealed by direct radiography. Visualization of the intrahepatic biliary system cannot be satisfactorily achieved by means of intravenous injection of a radiopaque phenolphthalein compound. It may be stated that radiographic examination of the liver has a low level of diagnostic efficiency, frequently failing to reveal any abnormality even when hepatic disease is advanced. Distortion of the outline of the liver may be noted in radiographs when the organ is extensively involved in neoplasia, by which time the presence of the abnormality is usually indicated by clinical signs and may be palpable. Primary neoplasms of the liver include adenoma and adenocarcinoma; occasionally the gall-bladder is the initial site. Metastatic liver tumours are more common, consisting of a wide variety of types.

11

The Urinary System

Diseases of the urinary system in animals occur more frequently, perhaps, in the dog and cat. In the farm animal species diseases of the bladder and urethra are more common and of greater importance than diseases of the kidneys. Properly to understand the origin and effects of urinary disease a knowledge of the physiological mechanisms involved in urinary secretion and excretion is essential.

Basically the two main functions of the kidney are to excrete the waste products of metabolism (including urea or uric acid, creatinine, ammonia, and hydrogen ions and excluding carbon dioxide), and to regulate desirable constituents (including water and a variety of solutes including glucose, amino acids and 'fixed cations') by selective reabsorption in order to maintain the tissue fluid and electrolyte balance of the body. The first function is the province of the glomeruli and is achieved by simple filtration of the plasma; the filtrate, which varies in volume according to the number of functioning glomeruli, the plasma osmotic pressure and the hydrostatic pressure in the renal capillaries, normally contains little, if any, proteins or lipids. Selective action by the tubules ensures retention of those substances required for metabolic purposes and excretion of waste products. When the kidneys are functioning normally there is a wide variation in the volume of urine excreted and in the concentration of urinary solutes. Reabsorption of water from the glomerular filtrate by the proximal convoluted tubules is by osmosis and this reduces the volume to about 20%. Further concentration takes place in Henle's loops, in the distal convoluted tubules and finally in the collecting ducts which are under the influence of the antidiuretic hormone released by the posterior pituitary gland. This control is not absolute and can be overcome by the action of diuretic drugs. Other additional hormones which are of importance in controlling kidney function include the steroid secretions of the adrenal cortex and the hormone of the para-thyroid gland. Cortisol-like steroids are essential for maximum water excretion, while aldosterone regulates potassium. The parathyroid hormone regulates the rate of calcium and phosphate excretion into the urine. The kidney itself secretes two important endocrine substances: erythropoietin, which has a role in normal haematopoiesis, and renin, which regulates aldosterone secretion by the adrenal cortex.

Disease of the kidneys, and in some cases of the ureters, bladder and urethra, interferes with glomerular filtration and selective reabsorption by the tubules and thereby disturbs the excretion of metabolic waste products, and upsets protein, solute and water homeostasis. When loss of function is only partial it is described as renal insufficiency, complete loss is renal failure.

Renal Insufficiency

Primary renal insufficiency is due to intrinsic dysfunction of the kidney arising from deranged glomerular filtration rate or tubular reabsorption. Insufficiency may develop secondarily to significant alterations in circulatory dynamics, such as those associated with shock, dehydration and haemorrhage, all of which cause reduced glomerular filtration, but more important, because of protracted renal ischaemia, may cause necrosis of tubular cells in sufficient degree to produce renal insufficiency.

Although renal insufficiency of glomerular origin may occur independently of that of tubular origin, because both these constituent parts of each nephron share a common blood supply, damage to one part is invariably followed by damage to the remaining parts. The clinico-pathological course and termination of renal disease, therefore, tend to be rather similar. In nephrosis and interstitial nephritis the primary lesion involves the tubules but glomerular derangement is a common sequel, and the reverse chain of events tends to occur in glomerular nephritis.

When there is damage to the glomerular epithelium, plasma proteins (principally albumin because of its smaller molecular size) appear in the filtrate; extensive glomerular damage may be associated with complete cessation of filtration. When only a proportion of the glomeruli are damaged there is a compensatory response by the normal ones to such a degree that their associated tubules are capable of reabsorbing both fluid and solutes to give urine of normal composition. If tubular damage coexists this defect may be exaggerated. Lack of ability to concentrate urine (isosthenuria), irrespective of variations in fluid and electrolyte intake, is a measure of the degree of renal insufficiency. Coincident with reduction in glomerular filtration there is also retention of urea and other non-protein nitrogenous end-products in the blood. Sulphate and phosphate retention also occur; the latter eventually causes a secondary hypocal-caemia, due in part to increased secretion of parathyroid hormone and in part to increased urinary calcium excretion. The variations in serum potassium levels, which appear to be influenced by dietary intake, do not appear to have any significant influence. Hyponatraemia, consequent upon inability by the tubules to reabsorb sodium, is a feature in all cases of nephritis. Due to continued tubular dysfunction sufficiently large amounts of water are lost to give rise to incipient or actual clinical dehydration, with the attendant high risk of circulatory emergency such as shock or further critical fluid loss.

Renal Failure

If renal compensation fails, or nephron damage progresses to involve more and more units, then the terminal stage of renal insufficiency—renal failure—is inevitable. The excretion of gradually increasing amounts of urine of low specific gravity leads to a degree of clinical dehydration which is readily exaggerated, or that is likely to cause such circulatory emergency as will result in renal ischaemia followed by acute renal failure. Continued loss of protein leads to rapid decline in body condition and muscle weakness. Low serum sodium (hyponatraemia) and potassium (hypokalaemia) cause skeletal muscle weakness and cardiac asthenia. The risk of circulatory failure and reduction in skeletal muscle power may be increased by the hypocalcaemia, which may also intensify the nervous signs. The multiplicity of factors which is concerned in renal failure contributes to the development of a variety of clinical syndromes. In the final stages of renal failure the clinical syndrome of uraemia, which can also occur in urinary tract obstruction, is uniformly exhibited. The mechanism by which the clinical signs are produced has not been recognized, but as the chemicophysiological disturbances are of the character described above, the signs are simply an endpoint of depressed function in other important organs. Biochemically the degree of impaired renal function can be assessed by measuring the increase in blood levels of total as well as urea nitrogen (azotaemia), and of certain other solutes as already described.

Renal insufficiency, renal failure and uraemia may be caused by prerenal and renal factors. The important prerenal causes include congestive heart failure, and acute cardiac or peripheral circulatory failure when acute renal ischaemia occurs. Haemoglobinaemia and myoglobinaemia, when they cause severe nephrosis, are also in this category. Renal causes include interstitial nephritis, pyelonephritis, glomerulonephritis, embolic nephritis and amyloidosis. Complete obstruction of the urinary tract or internal rupture of any part will lead to uraemia.

Uraemia

The terminal stage of renal failure is associated with a clinical syndrome which is usually referred to as uraemia. The clinical signs include depression, muscular weakness and muscle tremor, deep, laboured respiration, and oliguria or anuria, the last occurring when there is complete obstruction of the urinary tract. If the primary disease process has been in existence for some time there has been considerable loss of bodily condition as the result of albuminuria, dehydration and gradually increasing anorexia. In the dog and cat, vomition is usual, the mucous membranes are hyperaemic and, in the case of the buccal mucosa, ulceration occurs. Myocardial asthenia and terminal dehydration are responsible for a marked increase in heart rate. The syndrome terminates with recumbency followed inevitably by coma and death.

Regional Anatomy

Anatomically the urinary system comprises the kidneys, ureters, bladder and urethra. The kidneys, which secrete the urine, differ in external appearance as between the various species of animals. In the majority of animals, however, they are almost symmetrical in position, one on each side of the vertebral column in the dorsal part of the abdomen. The tubular ureters, one on each side, provide for the conveyance of the urine from the kidneys to the sac-like bladder, which, because it is a reservoir for the urine, varies in position on the floor of the pelvis and posterior abdomen according to the volume of urine which has accumulated. The urethra is a single tubular structure, varying in length and direction according to the sex and species of the animal respectively, which provides for the periodic expulsion of the urine from the bladder to the exterior.

Horse. The right kidney is somewhat firmly fixed in position ventral to the upper parts of the last three ribs and the transverse process of the first lumbar vertebra. Its dorsal surface is related chiefly to the diaphragm and the ventral surface is contiguous to the liver, pancreas and caecum. The posterior extremity extends back to the first lumbar transverse process where it is related to the base of the caecum. The left kidney, because of its looser attachment, is more variable in position, and is usually situated more caudally than the right one, so that the posterior pole may correspond to the transverse process of the third lumbar vertebra.

The ureter, which originates at the renal pelvis and terminates at the bladder, is a collapsible tube less than 0·5 cm in diameter, situated towards the dorsal wall of the posterior abdomen, and deviating to the side wall of the pelvis near its termination, where it obliquely enters the dorsal wall of the bladder anterior to its neck. The urinary bladder, when empty, is a small rather fleshy body, about the size of a closed fist, lying on the anterior part of the floor of the pelvis. The vertex reaches further forward on the ventral abdominal wall as the bladder is increasingly distended with urine, and may be related to the small colon or small intestine. In the male horse, the dorsal surface of the bladder is related directly to the rectum and the genital fold; in the mare, the surface is in contact with the anterior part of the vagina and the body of the uterus.

The pelvic portion of the urethra, in the male horse, is about 10–12 cm long; at its mid-part, behind the prostate gland, it has a potential diameter of about 5 cm. The extrapelvic portion commences at the ischial arch, where the urethra forms a sharp bend and runs forwards in the corpus cavernosum in a shallow groove on the ventral aspect of the penis and, after passing through the glans penis, forms a projection, the urethral process, which is a membranous tube extending about 2·5 cm from the fossa of the glans penis. In the mare, the urethra is about 5–8 cm long and extends from the neck of the bladder to the external urethral orifice which is situated at the anterior extremity of the floor of the vulva. Ordinarily the urethral lumen will readily permit the introduction of one finger; following digital manipulation it can be considerably dilated.

Cattle. In the ox the kidneys are superficially divided into a variable number (20–25) of lobes. The right kidney, which is flattened against the roof of the abdomen, is related dorsally to the last rib and the transverse processes of the first two or three lumbar vertebrae. In some cases it may be some 8 cm further back. The ventral surface is related to the liver, pancreas, duodenum and colon. The left kidney is variable with regard to the position it occupies. When the rumen is partially filled with ingesta, as in the fasting animal, it may lie slightly to the left of the median plane. Following consumption of food, when the rumen is normally distended, it pushes the left kidney across the median plane so that it occupies a situation below and behind the right kidney, ventral to the third, fourth and fifth lumbar vertebrae.

The ureters are largely similar in structure and position to those of the horse. The urinary bladder occupies the same relative position as in the horse, but when it is distended it is longer and narrower, and extends further forward on the abdominal floor. In male cattle the pelvic part of the urethra is about 12 cm long and about 2·5 cm in overall diameter. At its commencement the lobulated seminal vesicles, which are 10–12 cm long in the bull and much smaller in steers, extend forwards on each side of the neck of the urinary bladder. The extrapelvic portion of the urethra follows the course of the penis through the sigmoid flexure posterior to the scrotum. It gradually diminishes in diameter to its termination at the external urethral orifice which is relatively small, and situated at the end of a groove on the bluntly pointed glans penis. The urethra in the female is about 5–8 cm long and the external orifice is on the floor of the vulva, about 10–12 cm from the ventral commissure. The orifice is a longitudinal slit about 2–5 cm long, and immediately beneath it is the blind pouch-like suburethral diverticulum; this structure is over 2 cm long and readily accommodates the end of one finger.

Sheep and goat. The kidneys in both sheep and goats are bean-shaped, have a smooth surface and occupy roughly the same position as in the ox. In the male sheep the extrapelvic urethra follows the sigmoid flexure of the penis, and the terminal part projects about 4 cm beyond the glans penis, forming the twisted urethral process. The external urethral orifice in the female sheep and goat, has the same general position as in the cow; there is a very small suburethral diverticulum.

Pig. The kidneys of the pig are smooth, bean-shaped and elongated. They are usually situated beneath the transverse processes of the first to the fourth lumbar vertebrae; in some pigs the left kidney is further forward than the right. The urinary bladder, when distended, assumes a large size and the greater part is accommodated in the abdominal cavity. The urethra, which has a pelvic part 15–20 cm long in adult boars, follows the course of the sigmoid flexure, which is prescrotal in position. The external urethral orifice is situated ventrolaterally near the pointed extremity of the penis; it is slit-like. In the sow, the external urethral orifice is bounded on each side by a thick fold which extends backwards. There is a depression lateral to each fold, and another behind the urethral orifice, so that it appears to project into the vulva.

Dog. The kidneys of the dog are bean-shaped, smooth and convex over both surfaces. The right kidney has a rather fixed location, ventral to the sublumbar muscles, opposite the bodies of the first, second and third lumbar vertebrae; in occasional cases the anterior extremity is situated beneath the last rib. The left kidney is more variable in position because it is loosely attached to the peritoneum and it is readily influenced by the degree of fullness of the stomach. When the stomach is empty the left kidney may occupy a position almost symmetrically opposed to the right one. Complete distension of the stomach causes the left kidney to occupy a position under the transverse processes of the third, fourth and fifth lumbar vertebrae.

The ureters follow the same general path from each kidney pelvis to the neck of the bladder, as in the horse. The urinary bladder varies considerably in position according to the degree of distension. When empty it is situated entirely within the pelvic cavity; in the fully distended state, the neck lies at the anterior border of the pelvic bones, and the vertex extends to the umbilicus. In the male, the neck of the bladder and proximal part of the pelvic urethra are surrounded by the relatively large prostate gland. The pelvic part of the urethra, which is relatively long, terminates at the urethral arch in a large bulb-like structure. Towards its termination, the extrapelvic urethra is accommodated in the ventral groove of the os penis where, because of the rigidity of the bone, it cannot be dilated. The urethral opening is situated just beneath the pointed extremity of the glans penis. In the bitch the external urethral orifice is situated on the floor of the vulva about 2–5 cm from the ventral commissure. A small depression on each side of the orifice causes it to project slightly upwards into the vulva.

Cat. The kidneys in the cat are relatively large and may occupy a somewhat variable position in the abdomen because they are loosely attached to the peritoneum and are influenced by the degree of distension of the alimentary tract. When the latter is empty the kidneys hang down to occupy the middle horizontal plane, in which situation they may be mistaken for tumour masses, or foreign bodies. The urinary bladder has the same general relationship as in the dog. When fully distended it occupies almost the entire posterior abdomen, and the vertex extends beyond the umbilicus. In male cats, because the penis is largely composed of fibrous tissue, the lumen of this portion of the extrapelvic urethra is relatively narrow.

Clinical Examination of the Urinary System

The principal clinical signs arising from diseases of the urinary system include those associated with the act of urination, changes in the quality and quantity of the urine itself, evidence of pain and the manifestations of toxaemia, affecting the function of organs outside the urinary system, which result from advancing renal insufficiency and involve, particularly, the cardiovascular system, the digestive system, and the nervous system. Other manifestations originate from rupture of the renal pelvis, bladder and urethra. Further signs may be elicited by physical examination of the accessible parts of the urinary system.

Urination

Aspects of the act of urination which may have significance include posture, frequency, and any evidence of pain.

Posture

The horse usually urinates at rest and the individual animal performs the act at rather precise times. This is noted, in the working horse, to occur when the animal is returned to its box or stall. Both horses and mares adopt a rather similar characteristic posture, which is achieved by extending both forelimbs and then lowering the abdomen, thereby increasing intra-abdominal pressure. This is assisted by the animal making an inspiration and holding its breath which, when slowly released, produces a groaning sound. Horses protrude the flaccid penis from the preputial cavity to a variable degree.

In female cattle the hindlegs are advanced, thus arching the back, and the tail is elevated. Male cattle urinate when moving, feeding or standing still, by allowing the urine to run into the preputial cavity, and then escape from the orifice. Sheep urinate in the same manner as cattle. Female pigs when urinating adopt a posture rather similar to that of female cattle. Male pigs void urine in a sequence of spurts, simulating ejaculation. Bitches flex the hindlegs so lowering the perineum to within a few centimetres of the ground when urinating. Male dogs raise one of the hindlimbs and appear to direct the discharged urine against a selected object (this characteristic behaviour appears to possess territory marking components).

The adoption of an uncharacteristic posture should invariably be considered to indicate abnormality. Evidence should be sought as to whether the particular animal has habitually adopted an abnormal posture when urinating. An abnormal posture during urination may arise from disease of either urinary or non-urinary origin. Cystitis often causes male dogs to adopt a squatting posture, and certain defects of the spinal cord, which interfere with muscular coordination, will cause the dog to micturate in the standing position.

Frequency

In normal animals the frequency of urination depends upon the quantity of water consumed and the amount lost by respiration, perspiration and defaecation; milk production is an important route of water loss in lactating animals, more particular dairy cows. Horses and cattle urinate 5–6 times daily, pigs urinate 2–3 times and sheep and goats 1–3 times daily. Adult male dogs urinate voluntarily at frequent intervals.

Abnormally frequent urination (pollakiuria) may occur with or without an increase in the volume excreted. An increase in volume (polyuria) occurs in diabetes insipidus and diabetes mellitus, in chronic interstitial nephritis, during resorption of exudates and transudates, following administration of diuretics, which either increase glomerular filtration or decrease tubular reabsorption, or of drugs which raise the hydrostatic pressure in the renal capillaries, after increased consumption of water and in cold weather. Increased frequency of urination without increase in urine volume occurs when alterations in the character of the urine render it irritant to the bladder and/or urethra. Such changes in quality are likely to occur in acute nephritis, pyelonephritis and cystitis. Irritation of the bladder may also arise from the presence of calculi or of residual urine if it should undergo decomposition. Abnormally frequent urination is also a feature of urethritis. Partial obstruction of the urethra, spasm of the external sphincter of the bladder and inability to adopt the normal posture for urination by preventing complete emptying of the bladder are also associated with increased frequency.

Abnormally infrequent urination is not readily recognized in animals. It occurs as the result of reduction in the volume of urine excreted (oliguria), and in all those conditions in which there is retention of urine. Complete absence of urine (anuria) occurs under similar circumstances. Oliguria may be due to increased loss of fluid by other means, such as the alimentary tract in diarrhoea, and in haemorrhage, shock, exudation, dehydration, peripheral vascular failure, congestive heart failure and the terminal phase of all forms of nephritis. Reduced urine excretion in dehydration results from the increase in plasma osmotic pressure which develops, and in both peripheral circulatory failure and congestive heart failure reduction in renal blood flow produces a similar fall in urine volume.

Retention of urine with apparent reduction in the frequency of urination occurs temporarily in partial obstruction of the urethra, in spasm of the external sphincter of the bladder and when there is inability to adopt the normal posture for the act. The gross distension of the bladder, which inevitably develops, overcomes the obstruction or forces open the sphincter, so that small quantities of urine are voided at frequent intervals or urine constantly dribbles from the external urethral orifice. Urinary retention, due to defects of the sphincter control of the bladder, may arise from those lesions of the lumbosacral segments of the spinal cord which cause posterior paresis or paraplegia. Loss of parasympathetic function, which normally contracts the detrusor muscle and relaxes the internal sphincter during urination, results in urinary retention which is followed in some instances by incontinence from overflow. With loss of sympathetic control, incontinence develops immediately because there is paralysis of the internal sphincter and the bladder is always empty.

Pain and dysuria. Diseases of the urinary tract may cause sufficient discomfort so that the animal evinces signs of abdominal pain and dysuria (painful urination). Acute abdominal pain, exhibited by depressing the back, paddling with the hindfeet and kicking at the abdomen, occurs in occasional cases of bovine pyelonphritis, and originates from renal infarction, or obstruction of the renal calices or ureter by products of inflammatory origin; in very rare instances similar behaviour appears in other animals as the result of sudden distension of the renal pelvis or ureter, or renal infarction. Subacute pain, manifested by tail-swishing, kicking at the abdomen and frequent attempts to urinate accompanied by groaning, is associated with overdistension of the bladder and urethral obstruction.

Urination is painful or difficult in cystitis, vesical calculus, urethral obstruction and urethritis. Groaning and straining may precede, and accompany, the act of urination when there is urethral obstruction and, if the obstruction is not readily overcome in this way, only a few drops of urine are voided (strangury). In urethritis, groaning and straining occur immediately after urination has ceased and gradually disappear and do not recur until urination has been repeated. Increased frequency is usual when dysuria is present. Defaecation may also be associated with pain when there is dysuria, so that faecal retention is a feature of some urinary tract diseases. Abdominal pain, originating from colic which, in the horse, makes the animal strain and adopt the urination posture, may be confused with disease of the urinary system in which, however, it should be possible to determine other signs including abnormal urinary characteristics.

Physical Examination of the Urinary System

Because of the considerable thickness and rigidity of the abdominal wall in the horse, the kidneys cannot be located by external palpation. Indirect pressure in the general area of the kidneys may, however, induce a pain reaction in animals with nephritis. When considering the significance of such behaviour, temperament and other clinical findings should be considered. Internal palpation of both kidneys may be achieved during rectal exploration in small horses, whereas only the posterior part of the left kidney is palpable in this way in horses of medium size, being recognized as a firm semi-spherical body about 15 cm in diameter. When normal the ureters are not detected during rectal examination.

In cattle of medium to small size the posterior pole of the right kidney may be palpated during rectal examination. The left kidney can be identified during this procedure in most cattle. Palpation of the kidney through the abdominal wall is not possible in adolescent and adult cattle. The normal ureters cannot be detected during rectal exploration.

The abdominal urinary organs are not directly available for physical examination in the sheep, goat and pig. The kidneys can be palpated through the abdominal wall in the majority of small and medium-size dogs (see Fig. 140, p. 151), and the left kidney even in some large dogs. Because the kidneys in the cat are proportionately large and pendulous they are generally easily palpable. Identification is aided by recognizing the indentation (hilus) on the attached border.

During palpation of the kidneys an attempt should be made to determine relative size, presence of pain, consistency and condition of the surface. Enlargement may be due to neoplasia, hydronephrosis or certain forms of nephritis. Renal tumours may cause irregular, firm enlargements in the kidney cortex, compared with fluctuating regular enlargements in hydronephrosis. In pyelonephritis in cattle the affected kidney may be obviously enlarged and firm, with absence of lobulation, and the animal shows a pain reaction on palpation. The ureter associated with the affected kidney is also sufficiently distended to be detectable during rectal examination as a flexible tube which may pulsate when pressure is applied with varying force. Similar changes in the ureter are not unusual in hydronephrosis. Variation in the size of the kidneys in the dog is not readily appreciated by means of abdominal palpation, unless it is considerable. Reduction in size, which is a feature of some cases of advanced chronic interstitial nephritis, usually cannot be appreciated by this means.

In large animals, examination of the urinary bladder during rectal exploration is expedited if, when the organ is distended, urination is effected by applying moderate pressure with the hand. Otherwise it will be necessary to catheterize the animal. When the bladder is grossly distended it should be palpated with care because of the risk of rupture. Overdistension occurs in urethral obstruction by calculus and, initially, in dysfunction of the parasympathetic nerve supply to the detrusor muscle and the internal sphincter of the bladder. The former condition may be suggested if, when the pelvic portion of the urethra is palpated, pulsation is detected. Manipulation of the bladder will reveal if it is a focal origin of pain and, if the organ is empty, any calculi of reasonable size can be recognized, as well as tumours and thickening of the bladder wall due to inflammatory changes. When the bladder is ruptured (a not unusual complication of urethral obstruction by calculus), it is permanently small and lacking in tone. In small animals the degree of distension of the bladder, the presence of pain and large calculi in the cavity of the organ can be recognized by means of palpation simultaneously applied on both sides of the abdomen just in front of the pelvic inlet. In male dogs, enlargement of the prostate gland, as the result of inflammatory involvement, hyperplasia or neoplasia, can be recognized by digital rectal examination. In prostatitis and neoplasia a marked pain reaction can be induced by palpation of the prostate gland.

Palpation of the penis at the point where obstruction by a calculus has occurred will produce a pain reaction. In the horse and dog, urethral patency is readily determined by catheterization. If perforation of the urethra has occurred as the result of obstruction, urine will infiltrate the connective and muscular tissues of the ventral abdominal wall and prepuce and cause obvious fluid swelling, with extensive superficial necrosis, involving the skin at a later stage in some cases. Infiltration of neighbouring tissues with urine will occur in cattle when the penis has been injured during mating, or more certainly by inclusion in a crushing-type castrator. Palpation of the penis is of value in revealing such abnormalities as paralysis, 'fracture' and neoplasia.

In male animals the preputial structures should be included in the clinical examination of the urinary system. Castrated male horses sometimes collect inspissated masses of sebaceous material in the coronal fossa of the glans penis which cause compression of the urethral process, thereby interfering with urination. In other instances this material collects in the preputial cavity in sufficient quantity to prohibit protrusion of the penis for urination. Both these states can be identified by inspection and palpation. Occasionally, in steers, calculi may cause obstruction of the preputial orifice with distension of the preputial sac and infiltration of the ventral abdominal wall with urine. Confusion with urethral perforation is excluded by recognition of the calculus during palpation. In castrated cattle, inflammation of the preputial orifice will produce a similar clinical syndrome, the nature of which can be ascertained by means of inspection and palpation which reveal swelling and pain with obstruction of the preputial orifice. In rams, ulcerative dermatosis and pizzle rot cause balanoposthitis which, by producing inflammatory swelling of the prepuce and pain, interferes with urination. Balanitis in the male dog is associated with a purulent discharge from the preputial orifice, in spite of which in the majority

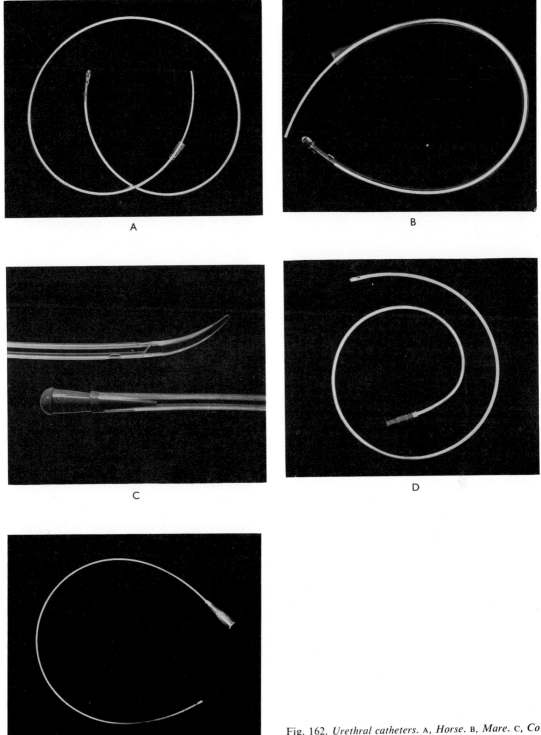

Fig. 162. *Urethral catheters*. A, *Horse*. B, *Mare*. C, *Cow or bitch*. D, *Dog*. E, *Cat*. (Portland Plastics Ltd).

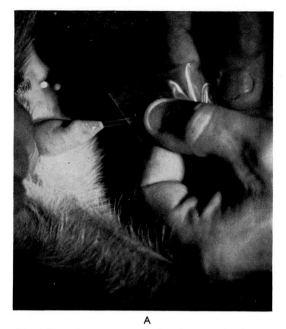
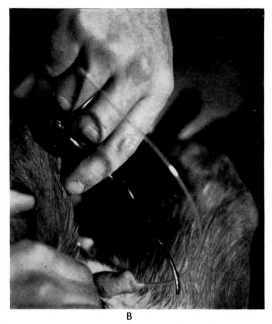

A   B

Fig. 163. A, *Passing a urethral catheter in the dog. Note that the penis is exposed and held in the left hand by pressure on the preputial skin. The catheter, retained in its sterile envelope, is inserted into the urethra with the right hand.* B, *The same procedure using sterile forceps.*

of cases the animal appears to suffer little or no discomfort.

Special Examination of the Urinary System

Rectal examination, which can be included under the above heading, has already been considered as an important part of the clinical examination of the urinary system in horses and cattle. Other special methods include catheterization, chemical and microscopic examination of urine, renal function tests and radiographic examination.

Urethral catheterization. A urine sample can be obtained by collection in a suitable vessel during spontaneous or induced urination, or by catheterizing the animal. In cows, gently rubbing the perineum a short distance from the vulva will often initiate urination; laying down straw bedding in the box or stall has a similar effect in horses; in male sheep urination is induced by occluding the nostrils for a few seconds.

Mares, cows and bitches can be catheterized with variable ease. In all cases a suitable sterile instrument (Fig. 162) should be employed, along with an appropriate speculum in the mare and bitch. Introduction of a catheter into the urethra in the cow necessitates inserting the end of one

finger into the suburethral diverticulum. The vulva in the ewe and sow are too small to permit easy access to the urethra, although suitable specula may help. The presence of a small suburethral diverticulum in the ewe makes it virtually impossible to direct the tip of the catheter into the urethra.

In the stallion and gelding it is necessary to withdraw the penis from the prepuce in order to introduce the catheter into the urethra. This is often difficult or impossible to achieve. The prior administration of a tranquillizing drug, by assisting relaxation of the retractor penis muscles, will frequently simplify this problem. Because of the considerable length of the urethra in the male horse, it is necessary to employ a catheter which possesses adequate rigidity but at the same time is sufficiently flexible to be directed around the ischial arch. The instrument should be well lubricated before use. In order, successfully, to pass a urethral catheter in the bull, or steer, it is necessary to relax the retractor penis muscles and, by withdrawing the penis from the preputial cavity, eliminate the sigmoid flexure. This requires the adoption of pudendal nerve block; ataractic drugs may be effective in some cases. A polyethylene catheter of the type employed for intracardiac catheterization is suitable, provided it is sufficiently long (290 cm), with a small diameter (2·5–3 mm) and has a rounded tip. Boars cannot be catheterized because the penis is inaccessible. In rams, the urethral process prevents introduction of the tip of the catheter into the urethra. There is no problem in passing a suitable polyethylene urethral catheter in male dogs because the penis is relatively readily accessible (Fig. 163). In male cats, catheterization is achieved by employing a rigid metal catheter of small diameter (0·5–1·0 mm), the tip of which is inserted into the urethral orifice after exposing the penis (Fig. 164). The free end of the instrument is then directed backwards until the penis is pointing posteriorly in line with the floor of the pelvis. The catheter can then be freely moved forwards into the bladder.

Care should be taken that infection is not introduced into the urinary tract by the catheter, and trauma should be avoided. Urine samples, when required for chemical and microscopical examination, should invariably be collected in clean, sterile containers. Passing a catheter is a useful method for determining the state of patency of the urethra. When it is reasonable to suspect the occurrence of obstruction with possible perforation, or urethritis, the further pain induced during catheterization can be controlled by prior administration of a suitable sedative or narcotic drug.

Urine Analysis

Interpretation of Results Relative to Urinary and Other Diseases

Routine urine analysis is an important first step in the evaluation of renal function. An appreciation of the character and constituents of normal urine in the various species of animals is essential to be able, correctly, to interpret the significance of any abnormal feature detected during routine analysis. The abnormalities that may be encountered include constituents not normally present, normal constituents in excessive or diminished amounts, and the presence of normal constituents in abnormal forms. Urine analysis alone should never be depended upon to establish a diagnosis, the results obtained should be, without exception, related to the history and clinical condition of the animal, so that the final interpretation is the responsibility of the clinician.

To demonstrate that an unknown fluid is urine, a drop of it is mixed on a slide with a drop of nitric acid, and the slide warmed. Hexagonal crystals of urea nitrate separate out (Fig. 165E); these can be identified microscopically. If the mixture of urine and nitric acid is evaporated the residue changes to a red colour on the addition of ammonia solution, or blue on the addition of

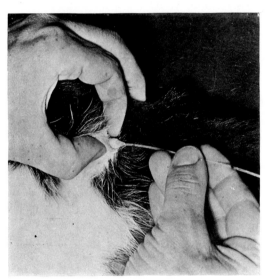

Fig. 164. *Passing a urethral catheter in the male cat. Note the direction to ensure free passage of the instrument along the intrapelvic urethra.*

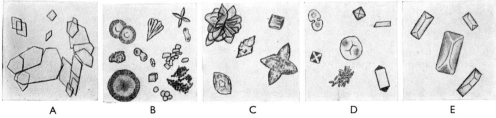

Fig. 165. *Crystals from urinary deposits.* A, *Calcium carbonate.* B, *Urate salts.* C, *Calcium oxalate.* D, *Triple phosphate.* E, *Nitrate salts.*

caustic potash or caustic soda solution, and these colours disappear on heating (uric acid test, murexide test).

Colour

Urine is usually a variable shade of yellow. Changes in colour do not always indicate abnormality. Concentrated urine, which is produced when the fluid intake is reduced so that water homeostasis is impaired, or there is excessive fluid loss from the body by other routes, is darker due to concentration of urochromes, and assumes a brownish-yellow colour. Dilute urine, which occurs following the administration of diuretic drugs and in diabetes insipidus, advanced chronic interstitial nephritis and renal cortical hypoplasia, has a lighter colour and may, in extreme cases, simulate water in appearance. Red, reddish-brown or blackish-brown urine usually indicates the presence of whole blood, free haemoglobin or myoglobin. A brownish-green colour suggests the presence of relatively large amounts of bilirubin; this characteristic is observed most readily in a narrow column of urine, or better still in the froth which is readily produced by agitating the urine in its container. The urine is brick-red or coffee-coloured when there is an abundant excretion of urates. This feature is associated with the urine of carnivorous species. In rare cases cattle, and very rarely other animals, void urine which, on exposure to air, becomes red or brown due to the presence of large amounts of porphyrin. This is an inherited trait transmitted via a recessive characteristic. Affected animals usually evince marked photo-sensitivity. The administration of certain drugs or chemicals may cause changes in the colour of the excreted urine; it becomes red with pheno-thiazine, certain anthracene purgatives, phenol-phthalein and pyridium, olive-green with phenol and green with methylene blue and acriflavine.

Clarity

The urine of carnivorous species is normally clear and transparent. When freshly excreted the urine of ruminant animals is clear, but it soon becomes turbid on standing because of precipi-tation of phosphates. The urine of the horse is turbid and opaque when excreted on account of the abundance of calcium carbonate crystals which are suspended in mucin. The carbonates precipitate in the bladder when the urine is concentrated by reabsorption. On exposure to air the turbidity is increased because carbon dioxide is released from soluble acid calcium carbonate which is then converted into insoluble calcium carbonate. Pathological turbidity is not un-common; it may be due to the presence of organized elements such as inflammatory cells, blood cells and cells from the parts of the urinary tract (kidney, bladder, urethra), which are recognized by microscopical examination. Un-organized elements (solutes), including various organic and inorganic salts, also produce turbidity in urine when present in excessive amounts. By means of chemical tests many of the solutes in urine can be specifically identified. Normal urine frequently contains a number of solutes at a supersaturated concentration, preci-pitation being prevented by the presence of colloids which, by converting urine into a gel, preserve the solutes in solution. Under certain influences or changes, however, the colloid capacity to maintain the solutes in solution is overcome so that precipitation occurs and the urine becomes turbid. The more important of these ancillary factors include concentration of urine, pH changes and, in herbivorous animals, the character of the diet.

Viscosity

The urine of the horse is viscid on account of its high content of mucus, derived from glands in the kidney, pelvis and ureter, and which can sometimes be drawn out in thick threads. The urine of the other domestic animals is of low viscosity, simulating water in this respect. When inflammatory products from the urinary system or protein of blood origin are present in urine the viscosity is raised.

Odour

Freshly excreted urine has an odour, derived from volatile organic acids, particular to the species of animal, that of the boar, tom cat and billy goat being somewhat offensive, whereas that of herbivorous species is not. Urine from an animal with cystitis has an unpleasant pungent odour when excreted owing to bacterial production of ammonia. A similar state is produced when urine is kept in a stoppered container for some time. The presence of certain drugs and endogenous substances in urine can sometimes be detected by the distinctive odour, e.g. oil of turpentine gives an odour like violets; acetone, which occurs in ruminant urine in

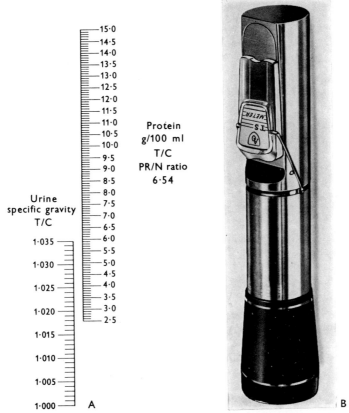

Fig. 166. *The Goldberg refractometer (total solids meter) with a built-in scale (shown enlarged) for measuring specific gravity and percentage protein content of body fluids.* (American Optical Company)

pregnancy toxaemia, ketosis and certain diseases of the digestive system, gives a fruity odour.

Specific Gravity

Specific gravity determination gives only an approximate measurement of the solute concentration in urine because it is influenced not only by the number of molecules present, but also by molecular size and weight. A determination of the osmolarity of the urine gives a much more meaningful indication of renal tubular reabsorbing function but for this purpose a crystalloid osmometer is required. For practical clinical purposes the correlation between specific gravity and osmolarity is sufficiently close to give the determination validity.

The measurement is made by means of a urinometer or a refractometer (total solids meter) (Fig. 166), the latter being slightly more accurate. The urinometer (Fig. 167) should be graduated from 1·000 to 1·060, 1·000 representing

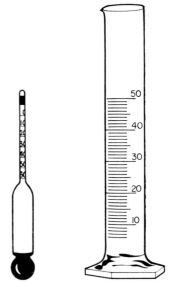

Fig. 167. *A hydrometer for measuring the specific gravity of urine.*

the specific gravity of pure water. Ideally the measurement should be made on a mixed 24-hour sample of urine, but this is rarely possible with animals. As an alternative, when there is clinical evidence of renal disease, it is expedient to repeat the measurement on a number of occasions. If the volume of urine is inadequate (30–50 ml) to float the urinometer, add an equal, or greater, measured amount of pure water and determine the specific gravity of the mixture. The specific gravity of the original urine can be calculated by multiplying the last two digits of the reading by the dilution factor. Urinometers for measuring the specific gravity of urine are usually calibrated at 15°C so that it is necessary to correct for temperature. This is done by adding or subtracting 1 for every 3°C that the temperature of the urine sample is above or below 15°C at the time the reading is made.

Too much significance should not be attached to the determination of the specific gravity of a single isolated sample of urine. The specific gravity of urine normally varies between wide limits (Table 12) and is influenced by the fluid

TABLE 12. SPECIFIC GRAVITY OF NORMAL URINE

Species	Specific Gravity
Horse	1·020–1·050
Ox	1·015–1·045
Sheep, goat	1·015–1·050
Dog	1·020–1·045
Pig	1·005–1·025
Cat	1·020–1·040
Rabbit	1·010–1·015

intake, the character of the diet, the environmental temperature, and the amount of physical exertion to which the animal is subjected. As a general rule in healthy animals, the specific gravity of urine varies inversely with the quantity produced each day.

High specific gravity occurs in all diseases in which the volume of urine excreted is significantly reduced, e.g. febrile states, and in diseases of the urinary tract in which plasma proteins and/or inflammatory products appear in the urine in significant quantities. In diabetes mellitus, a prerenal disease, the urine shows increased volume as well as an abnormally high specific gravity. The specific gravity is temporarily reduced when urine volume is greatly increased because of high fluid intake, and more persistently, or even permanently so, when renal concentrating ability is reduced, as in diabetes insipidus or chronic interstitial nephritis.

Hydrogen Ion Concentration (pH)

The kidney is of primary importance in maintaining the acid–base balance and electroneutrality of the body. From this it might be expected, contrary to what does occur, that urinary pH would vary over a very wide range. The pH of a sample of urine can be roughly determined by the use of red or blue litmus paper. Red litmus paper becomes blue when alkalis (bases) predominate; blue litmus paper becomes red when acids predominate. When neither the red nor the blue litmus paper is affected by the urine the reaction is described as neutral. If red litmus paper becomes slightly blue, and blue litmus paper slightly red, the reaction is said to amphoteric. An estimate of the pH can be obtained by the use of a universal colour indicator, varieties of which are available in liquid or paper strip form (Combostix, Ames Co.). Accurate pH values can only be obtained with a suitable potentiometer.

The pH of the urine of healthy animals is influenced by the character of the food. Healthy horses, cattle and sheep excrete alkaline urine; carnivorous animals including the dog and cat normally excrete acid urine, but not infrequently, dogs fed on diets consisting mainly of carbohydrate excrete alkaline urine. Omnivorous species such as the pig produce acid urine when the diet contains large amounts of protein and alkaline urine when mainly carbohydrate is fed. The alkaline reaction shown by the urine of herbivorous animals is largely due to the presence of soluble calcium bicarbonate which is derived from a variety of organic calcium salts in the food. Sodium and calcium acid-phosphates are responsible for the low pH of the urine of carnivorous animals. Determination of the pH should always be made on fresh urine. As a rule acid urine becomes alkaline when it is exposed to the air for some time.

Variations from normal in the pH of urine are not of great diagnostic significance. In febrile diseases, those which cause anorexia of some duration and nephritis, the urine of herbivorous animals becomes acid. The ingestion of acidifying salts such as ammonium chloride, ammonium mandelate, sodium acid phosphate and calcium chloride will lower the pH of the urine in all species. Respiratory or metabolic acidosis may cause the urine to be acid. Abnormally alkaline urine is usually the result of bacterial fermentation in the bladder with the production of ammonia from urea; this occurs in cystitis. The ingestion of sodium or potassium acetate, citrate, bicarbonate or lactate will raise the pH of urine. Persistent vomiting and continued hyperventilation may bring about the excretion of alkaline urine as the result of metabolic and respiratory alkalosis.

Protein

The healthy glomerular membrane prevents the loss of plasma proteins along with the normal filtrate, and any protein of small molecular size (predominantly albumin) which does filter across is reabsorbed by the renal tubules. Colloids (mucoprotein) may, however, be present in normal urine in small amounts; it is characteristically present in dog urine and in horse urine, along with carbonate salts, giving the urine a turbid appearance. The quantities present in such circumstances, however, are usually insufficient to produce a positive result, even with the most sensitive test method.

In the traditional tests for urinary protein, denaturation, and hence precipitation of protein, is achieved by heating and/or acidification. Heating alkaline urine which contains plasma proteins may cause the formation of alkaline metaprotein which is not coagulated, giving rise to the necessity to acidify the urine when this test method is used. A precipitate produced by heating urine, which is soluble in nitric acid is usually composed of phosphate or oxalate salts.

Salicylsulphonic acid test. This test is simple to perform and yields few equivocal results. Add, in drops, 0·5 ml of 25% solution of salicylsulphonic (or trichloracetic) acid to 5 ml of clear urine, (filtering if necessary). The presence of protein is indicated by the appearance of a greyish-white coagulum which sediments rapidly. The method gives positive results when the protein value is greater than 10 mg/100 ml. A false positive reaction may occur when the urea content of the urine is high.

Tetrabromophenol test. For this test strips of absorbent paper, which are commercially available (Albustix, Ames Co.), are impregnated at one end with tetrabromophenol blue in an inert base buffered with nitrate to pH 3. When the paper strip is immersed in urine containing protein, provided the pH is between 5·2 and 7·5,

a reaction will occur consisting of a change of colour from yellow to green, or even blue, depending on the amount of protein present. A colour chart, which provides a basis for measuring roughly the amount of protein present, is necessary to interpret the result of the test. Results are unsatisfactory with very alkaline urine, cat's urine and that of the dog if the sample is stale.

Normal urine contains an insignificant amount of protein which does not react in the standard tests for proteinuria; it is derived from desquamated epithelial cells. The proteins most commonly occurring in urine are those originating from the blood plasma, and are largely a mixture of albumin and globulin. Because plasma albumin has a smaller molecular size (60 000) than the globulin, it usually predominates, hence the term albuminuria. As a rule alphaglobulin also accompanies the albumin; beta- and gammaglobulin occur when glomerular damage is more serious. Specific identification of the various proteins can be achieved by electrophoresis.

Proteinuria occurs when the glomerular membrane becomes sufficiently permeable to permit the filtration of the plasma proteins along with the normal filtrate. This state occurs in acute renal failure arising from glomerulonephritis, suppurative nephritis and interstitial nephritis, nephrosis, renal infarction and pyelonephritis. A similar state exists in acute renal insufficiency resulting from chronic congestive heart failure, acute pancreatitis, intestinal obstruction and nephrotoxic poisoning. Also in many febrile and toxaemic diseases the degree of glomerular damage produced may permit the loss of variable amounts of plasma protein. Trauma, neoplasia, parasitism, convulsions, exposure to cold and prolonged recumbency, as in cows following parturition, are also associated with abnormal proteinuria. The virtual absence of formed elements and casts in the urine in the majority of the prerenal conditions assists differentiation from primary renal diseases.

In renal disease the concentration of protein in the urine may vary during the progress of the condition. This variation is a characteristic feature of the urine during the course of interstitial nephritis in the dog, in which the late stages are associated with traces of protein because of dilution, although the total protein loss is considerable. Protein is also added to the urine in such post-renal conditions as cystitis and bovine enzootic haematuria, urethritis, vaginitis, prostatitis and balanitis. Prerenal conditions causing proteinuria are haemoglobinaemia and myoglobinuria. In these conditions not all the urinary protein is derived from haemoglobin and myoglobin, however; both pigment proteins increase glomerular permeability as the result of the toxic damage they produce. In both these states, characteristic discoloration of the urine is noted, and the other clinical evidence of the diseases which produce them, may be recognized. Haematuria will be associated with protein in variable degrees according to the amount of blood loss.

Haemoglobin

Haemoglobin may occur in urine in free form or along with intact erythrocytes. The tests for the presence of blood or blood pigment include microscopic examination for erythrocytes, spectroscopic examination for haemoglobin in its various forms, and chemical tests for haemoglobin.

Microscopic examination. Large numbers of intact erythrocytes give the urine a characteristic red colour. Very small numbers are unlikely to be recognized by the unaided eye. When the specific gravity is less than 1·015 any erythrocytes present are prone to rupture because of osmotic influences. It is generally accepted that microscopic examination will detect erythrocytes when they are too few to be revealed by chemical tests or spectroscopically. The method consists of centrifuging a quantity of the urine, discarding the supernatant portion and resuspending the deposit, from which a smear is made. The preparation can be examined in the moist state, when the erythrocytes are seen as non-nucleated, pale yellow-coloured, biconcave discs. Osmotic effects usually produce changes in shape which make recognition difficult. Continuing the procedure as for a blood film may provide further confirmatory evidence.

Spectroscopic examination. This method of examination, in combination with chemical tests, provides useful evidence when haemoglobin is present in urine. Laboratory direct-vision or reversion spectroscopes are expensive, but a pocket-size direct-vision spectroscope will prove quite satisfactory. The size of the slit and the eyepiece distance are adjusted by observing ordinary bright light, and then the urine sample is placed in a 15 + 2 cm testtube and the position of the absorption bands noted. By reference to published tables the identity of haemoglobin, or any of its various derivatives, can be established.

Chemical tests: Ortho-tolidine test. The sensitivity of the *o*-tolidine test is related to the concentration of the reagent used. The reagents required for the test include 4% *o*-tolidine in ethyl alcohol (will keep for many weeks if stored at 4°C), hydrogen peroxide, 20 volumes per cent, and a working solution consisting of equal parts of the 4% *o*-tolidine solution, glacial acetic acid and water (will keep for 1 month if stored at 4°C). For the test, run four drops of the *o*-tolidine working solution and one drop of the hydrogen peroxide solution into a testtube. Allow to stand for 1 minute to ensure that no colour reaction ascribable to contamination develops. Then add one or two drops of urine. The appearance of a green to blue colour, which gradually intensifies, indicates a positive reaction.

There are a number of modifications of the *o*-tolidine test some of which, by employing filter paper, avoid the use of glassware. In addition a compressed tablet containing *o*-tolidine, strontium peroxide, calcium acetate, tartaric acid and sodium bicarbonate is available from commercial sources (Occultest, Ames Co.). In performing the test in this case, a drop of urine is placed on a piece of filter paper (Whatman No. 1) and a tablet is then placed in the centre of the moistened area. Two drops of water are run onto the upper surface of the tablet. The presence of haemoglobin, or any of its derivatives, is indicated by the development of a blue colour within 2 minutes.

The chemical tests generally used for the detection of haemoglobin are indirect and also react with myoglobin. When a positive reaction occurs it is necessary, therefore, to determine whether haemoglobin or myoglobin is present and, in the case of the former, to make further tests to differentiate between haematuria and haemoglobinuria.

Haematuria is caused by prerenal, renal and postrenal diseases. The prerenal conditions include septicaemic and viraemic diseases, renal and general trauma such as that occurring in automobile accidents, purpura haemorrhagica and idiopathic thrombocytopenic purpura in dogs, in all of which there is damage to the vascular endothelium. The number of erythrocytes present, in these circumstances, is not often sufficient to be readily appreciated, so that their presence may only be detected by microscopic examination of the centrifuged deposit. In more severe cases the urine may have a slight cloudy appearance, and a red deposit forms when the erythrocytes have sedimented. In very severe cases of this type of haematuria the red cells are uniformly distributed in the urine giving it a red to brown colour. Renal haematuria is caused by pyelonephritis, suppurative nephritis, acute glomerulonephritis, renal infarction and severe tubular damage, such as can arise from precipitation of certain sulphonamide drugs. Postrenal haematuria is caused by acute cystitis, urolithiasis, warfarin or dicoumarol poisoning, urethral catheterization, enzootic haematuria of cattle, cystitis and pyelonephritis of pigs and neoplasia of associated structures.

When the blood originates from the urinary bladder it is usually most concentrated in the urine passed towards the termination of urination, whereas in the case of haemorrhage from a urethral lesion it is usually most evident in the initial portion of the urine flow. In sexually mature female animals, blood from the reproductive organs may contaminate the urine, so that catheterization is essential in order to determine accurately whether the blood is derived from the urinary tract itself.

Haemoglobinuria occurs in association with those prerenal diseases which cause intravascular haemolysis. The urine, which varies in colour from bright to dark red, and even reddish-black, according to the concentration of haemoglobin present, is positive in chemical tests for haemoglobin and protein. In normal circumstances the reticuloendothelial system successfully converts the haemoglobin from senile and damaged erythrocytes into other pigments so that the blood-free haemoglobin level does not rise above the renal threshold and it escapes in the urine. When intravascular haemolysis occurs to an excessive degree the renal threshold is surpassed and free haemoglobin is excreted with the urine. The molecular size (64 000) is greater than that of some plasma proteins which do not ordinarily pass the glomerular filter. This anomalous situation arises because the anaemic hypoxia, which occurs with varying degrees of severity in all forms of haemoglobinaemia, gives rise to tubular nephrosis, the severity of which is increased by tubular deposition of iron. In addition the precipitation of haemoglobin in the form of casts which obstruct the renal tubules, contributes to increased glomerular permeability.

Haemoglobinuria is a clinical feature of many infectious and non-infectious diseases. In ruminant animals the important diseases include babesiasis (all species), piroplasmosis, anaplasmosis, eperythrozoonosis, leptospirosis, bacillary haemoglobinuria, post-parturient haemoglobinuria, rape and kale poisoning, blood transfusion reactions, poisoning by lead and snake venoms, and drinking a large volume of cold water. In horses, haemoglobinuria is a feature of infectious equine anaemia, iso-immune haemolytic anaemia and phenothiazine intoxication. Severe intravascular haemolysis causing haemoglobinuria occurs at the terminal crisis in chronic copper poisoning in sheep, pigs and cattle. In dogs, haemoglobinuria is a feature of iso-immune haemolytic disease, blood transfusion reactions, thermal effects in severe and extensive burns and certain types of neoplasia.

Myoglobin

Myoglobinuria, a relatively rare manifestation in animals, occurs in diseases in which there is rapid breakdown of muscle. These include azoturia, tetanus, crushing injuries and violent struggling. Unlike haemoglobin, however, myoglobin is not bound to plasma proteins and appears in the urine at much lower blood concentrations. As a result myoglobin appears in the urine, giving it a dark-brown to black colour, quite soon after muscle damage has occurred. Other conditions in which muscle damage occurs include enzootic muscular dystrophy of young calves and lambs. In this condition the urine is not obviously discoloured because the muscles do not contain large amounts of myoglobin in early life. Azoturia in most instances gives rise to other clinical signs which draw attention to the development of severe acute myopathy.

Bile Pigments

The chemical tests for bile pigments in urine are described on p. 210. Normal urine does not contain bile pigments in significant amounts. The yellow colour is due to the presence of urochrome, thought to be derived from the cytochrome pigments; the colour is enhanced by low concentrations of bilirubin. Unconjugated bilirubin is not water soluble and, therefore, cannot be excreted by the kidney. Conjugation with glucuronic acid and to a lesser extent sulphuric acid takes place largely in the liver by the action of glucuronyl transferase. In animals, the presence of conjugated bilirubin in the urine is regarded as indicating the existence of certain prerenal diseases which cause abnormally large quantities of bile pigments to build up in the blood and to be deposited in the tissues, giving rise to jaundice (see p. 208). In overproduction (haemolytic) jaundice there is complete absence of urinary bilirubin and an increase in urobilinogen as well as haemoglobinuria (see above). Jaundice due to hepatic cell degeneration (hepatitis), which may be caused by toxic chemicals and plants, specific infectious agents including viruses, bacteria, helminth parasites and congestive heart failure, is associated with a moderate increase in urinary bilirubin and urobilinogen. Cholestasis, due to mechanical and functional causes, gives rise to an increase in urinary bilirubin with complete absence of urobilinogen. In partial biliary obstruction the condition of the urine is similar to that occurring in hepatocellular jaundice. Because glucuronyl transferase occurs in the kidney of the dog, bilirubin appears in the urine, making it difficult to differentiate haemolytic and obstructive jaundice; indeed a high proportion of normal dogs show mild bilirubinuria and up to 25% of cattle show bilirubinaemia although an extrahepatic source of glucuronyl transferase has not been identified. When bile pigments are present in large amounts the urine has a brownish-green colour.

Bile Salts

The chemical test for bile salts is given on p. 211. The bile salts sodium glycocholate and sodium taurocholate are formed by combination with glycine and taurine respectively. In obstructive states the bile salts are excreted by the kidney concomitantly with bilirubin; in the dog they potentiate bile pigment excretion.

Reducing Substances

The chemical tests which are applied for the detection of glucose in urine may, in many instances, give confusing results because other reducing substances are present including lactose, galactose, glucuronates, uric acid, and creatinine. Other substances which have a reducing action include chloral hydrate, formaldehyde and antibiotics (penicillin, streptomycin, tetracycline). Glucose can be specifically recognized by means of yeast fermentation, the preparation of osazones, paper chromatography and various techniques employing glucose oxidase.

The carbohydrate-reducing substances present in urine are subject to metabolism by the multiplying microflora so that, in order to ensure reliable results, tests should be performed on fresh samples. The chemical tests which are most commonly used to detect reducing substances in urine are those in which alkaline copper solutions are reduced to cuprous oxide giving a green to orange colour.

Benedict's test. The reagents for the qualitative test consist of 173 g sodium citrate and 100 g anhydrous sodium carbonate dissolved by heat in 600 ml water; to this is added slowly and with constant stirring a solution containing 17·3 g copper sulphate ($CuSO_4$, $5H_2O$) dissolved in about 100 ml of water. Final preparation consists in cooling the mixture, and after it has been transferred to a 1 litre volumetric flask, in making up to volume with water. When made in this way the reagent will remain stable for an indefinite period.

The test is performed by adding 0·5 ml of the urine to 5 ml of the reagent in a testtube which is then immersed in a beaker or bath of boiling water for 5 minutes. Remove the tube and allow to cool in a rack. A positive reaction is indicated by the formation of a precipitate which varies from green to yellow or orange colour according to the total amount of reducing substance present. A green colour with no discernible precipitate should be regarded as a negative reaction, and a white precipitate may be taken to indicate that the urine contains large amounts of phosphates. An unequivocal positive result is obtained if reducing substances corresponding to 15 mg/100 ml or more of glucose are present. A quantitative form of the test can be performed but it is not specific for glucose. Fehling's test is not so satisfactory as Benedict's test.

Commercially prepared tablets (Clinitest, Ames Co.) are available which make it possible to perform tests for reducing substances outside the laboratory. The tablets contain copper sulphate, sodium carbonate, citric acid and a considerable amount of sodium hydroxide. For the test five drops of urine and ten drops of water are put into a clean testtube followed by one tablet. Sufficient heat is generated by the caustic soda to ensure rapid reduction of the copper. The colour chart provided enables any colour reaction to be interpreted.

It is recommended that for the purpose of these tests, horse urine should first be admixed with a small quantity of 10% lead acetate solution and then filtered.

Glucose oxidase test. In the presence of atmospheric oxygen, glucose oxidase will oxidize glucose to gluconic acid and hydrogen peroxide, which latter reacts with ortho-tolidine to give a blue colour if peroxidase is present. Paper strips, one end of which are impregnated with glucose oxidase, *o*-tolidine and a vegetable peroxidase, are available commercially (Clinistix, Ames Co.). In the test, the active part of the paper strip is dipped into the urine and then withdrawn. The development of a blue colour within 60 seconds indicates the existence of glucose. The test is fairly sensitive, positive reactions can be expected at all levels of glucose above 100 mg/100 ml of urine; the results can be quantified up to 2% of glucose. It appears, however, that temperature, pH, and concentration of other urinary constituents can influence the sensitivity, and although the test is specific for glucose it may occasionally give a false negative reaction.

Fermentation test. This test can be employed quantitatively with a graduated saccharometer, or qualitatively by means of a small beaker and suitable testtube. For either method mix a few grains of live yeast, which has been washed with distilled water to remove any residual sugar, with about 30 ml urine after the gases have been driven off by either boiling and then cooling or by the addition of dilute tartaric acid solution. In the qualitative method the testtube is filled with urine-yeast suspension and then the open end is closed with a fingertip and the inverted tube is placed in the remaining liquid in the beaker. The blind limb of the saccharometer is loaded by filling the open end which is then stoppered and the instrument inverted so that the suspension runs into the graduated limb of the U tube. It is advisable to include positive and negative controls, for which normal urine, boiled, cooled and then yeast added, both with and without added glucose, is satisfactory. Although yeast fermentation of glucose will take place at room temperature, to speed up the process the tubes should be placed in an incubator at 37°C where production of gas becomes obvious within one hour, and is usually complete in 24 hours. The introduction of dilute caustic soda solution will confirm that the gas, which has collected in the blind-ended tube, is carbon dioxide by its disappearance through the formation of water soluble sodium carbonate. The quantity of sugar present is indicated as a percentage on the scale of the saccharometer. The fermentation test is positive only with glucose and fructose.

Glucose is not normally present in urine because the plasma concentration rarely rises above the renal threshold (about 170 mg/100 ml blood) so that tubular resorption is complete. In occasional animals, especially dogs, the renal threshold for glucose is sufficiently low so that if the animal is fed a predominantly carbohydrate diet, renal glycosuria occurs. If such dogs are fasted for a period of 24 hours the glucose will disappear from the urine. In such cases the blood glucose level is normal. Otherwise, occasional cases are the result of a tubular transport defect which may be congenital or an acquired toxic tubular necrosis (thallium poisoning). In lactating animals, especially cows subjected to overstocking, lactose in variable amounts appears in the urine following its absorption into the blood. Pathological glycosuria is a relatively rare state in animals. It occurs in conjunction with ketonuria in diabetes mellitus, which is rarely observed in farm animals and only occasionally in dogs, and in pregnancy toxaemia. Otherwise glucosuria is associated with *Clostridium welchii* type D enterotoxaemia, rabies, and following parental administration of glucose solutions, glucocorticoids or adrenocorticotrophic hormones. In these circumstances the glycosuria is the result of hyperglycaemia.

Ketone Bodies

These include acetone, diacetic acid, beta-hydroxybutyric acid and related substances which are intermediary products of fat metabolism and therefore appear in the blood in relatively small amounts, traces of which are excreted in the urine. With the exception of acetone, they can be utilized by the kidney as an energy source, so that it is only when the supply is excessive that they occur in urine. Once this situation is established, however, because of tubular reabsorption of the glomerular filtrate the concentration of ketone bodies in the urine greatly exceeds the blood level. In lactating cattle the milk ketone level is, in general, a better reflection of the blood concentration. The tests used for the detection of ketone bodies do not react with beta-hydroxybutyric acid.

Rothera's test. For field use a modification of

Rothera's test has many advantages. The reagent in general use consists of:

Ammonium sulphate	100 g
Sodium carbonate anhydrous	50 g
Sodium nitroprusside	3 g

Each item should be ground separately to small particle size and then thoroughly mixed by shaking the bottle or container. If kept dry, the prepared reagent will remain potent for at least a year.

For the field test 1–2 g of the reagent are put into a dry testtube and then urine (diluted 1 in 10 with water in the case of cows) or milk is run down the inside of the tube so that it forms a layer on top of the reagent. Without mixing the contents, the tube is set aside for a few minutes. The presence of acetone and acetoacetic acid is indicated by the development of a violet colour. In the laboratory test, place about 0·25 g of the reagent on a white filter paper and add 1–2 drops of diluted urine (milk and serum can also be tested in this way). The immediate development of a permanganate colour indicates the existence of acetone and diacetic acid.

Acetest tablets. This test is based on a modification of Rothera's test and employs a commercially prepared tablet (Ames Co.). It is suitable for field use. The active ingredients consist of sodium nitroprusside, disodium phosphate, glycine and lactose. A tablet is placed on a white tile and one drop of urine is run onto the surface. The appearance of a purple colour within 30 seconds is indicative of acetone and acetoacetic acid. Impregnated paper strips (Ketostix, Ames Co.) similar to Acetest tablets are available.

Comparison of the sensitivity of the Rothera, Acetest and Gerhardt's test (the last reacts with acetoacetic acid only) has suggested that for urine they give positive reactions at 3, 15 and 50 mg/100 ml ketone bodies respectively. With the powdered reagent, serum gives a positive reaction when the combined acetone and diacetic acid content is about 10 mg/100 ml. This is rather useful because serum values below this figure, at least in ruminant species, may be regarded as normal. In addition an approximate estimation of the combined amount of these two ketone bodies in positive sera is possible, on this basis, by diluting to extinction.

Cattle normally have a low blood glucose level (40–60 mg/100 ml) so that they are incipi-ently hypoglycaemic. As a result any condition in which the carbohydrate demands of the body exceed the carbohydrate metabolism will result in ketosis and ketonuria. This situation may result from dietary carbohydrate deficiency, starvation, digestive anorexia arising from disturbance of function in traumatic reticulo-peritonitis, displaced abomasum, actinobacil-losis of the reticulum, and a number of other conditions including metritis, mastitis, pododer-matitis, etc. In sheep an intense ketonuria is a feature of pregnancy toxaemia, otherwise it occurs secondarily to similar conditions stated for cattle. Bovine ketosis and pregnancy tox-aemia are associated with hypoglycaemia. In small animals the principal cause of ketonuria is diabetes mellitus in which there is concomitant glycosuria and hyperglycaemia. Adult dogs and cats seldom show ketonuria from other causes; young puppies and kittens may do so when acutely febrile or after a period of starvation.

Indicanuria

Jaffe's test. Equal volumes of urine and concentrated hydrochloric acid are mixed in a testtube followed by a few millilitres of chloro-form and then a few drops of dilute calcium hypochlorite (bleaching powder) solution. Mix-ing is achieved by inverting the tube several times. Any indican present is converted by oxidation to indigo blue, which is soluble in chloroform and so forms a distinct layer in the tube. The intensity of the blue colour is pro-portional to the amount of indican present.

Potassium indoxyl sulphonate (indican) is a normal urinary constituent. It occurs in consider-able quantities in the urine of the horse, ox, sheep and other herbivorous animals, being derived from the blood following absorption of indole (a product of protein putrefaction in the intestine) which is conjugated to indican in the liver. Indican is present in very small quantities in the urine of the dog. Abnormally large quantities appear in the urine when intestinal putrefaction is increased. This occurs in intestinal obstruction, constipation, gastroenteritis, impac-tion of the stomach or large intestine, peritonitis and when there is rapid breakdown of body tissue, as in blackleg and malignant oedema. Because the reaction is non-specific and does not indicate the focus or nature of the lesion the test is no longer applied in clinical diagnosis.

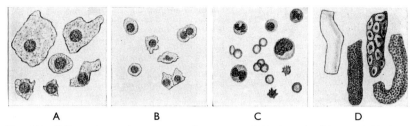

Fig. 168. *Cells and casts from urinary deposits.* A, *Cells from bladder.* B, *Cells from kidney.* C, *Red and white blood cells.* D, *Hyaline, granular, cellular and calcareous casts.*

Creatine

Creatine occurs in the body, particularly in muscle where it provides energy, as a phosphate compound. It is present in the plasma of adult animals at low levels, and in young growing animals at higher values. Dehydration of creatine gives the ring compound creatinine which is readily excreted by the kidneys. Relatively high levels of creatinine can occur in the urine of animals and as the sources are not identified, tests for its detection and measurement serve little purpose. Creatinine is, however, of value in renal function tests.

Deposits

Urinary sediments are of considerable value in the differential diagnosis of diseases of the urinary system. In all instances in which urine analysis reveals some other abnormal constituent suggesting renal or postrenal disease, an examination of a specimen of deposit, obtained by centrifugation, should be made. The sediments obtained from urine are of two types: the organized or cellular deposits and the unorganized or crystallized deposits. The cellular elements in the deposit are of most importance in the recognition of urinary tract disease.

Organized deposits. The cellular elements occur in urine irrespective of its pH; some, including bladder and urethral cells and vaginal cells in the bitch, when present in small numbers, are not indicative of a pathological process. Spermatozoa are quite commonly seen in dog urine, and so are erythrocytes in the case of the bitch when in oestrum. Otherwise large numbers of renal, bladder or urethral cells, erythrocytes, casts, parasite ova and bacteria (Fig. 168) indicate a pathological process. Spermatozoa occur as long-tailed cellular structures of characteristic morphology, and are often still motile. Although they occur most often in urine from dogs, they are occasionally found in the urine of sexually

mature male animals of other species, and in that of the very recently mated bitch.

Erythrocytes may be present in variable numbers; when few they are dispersed throughout the urine; in moderate numbers they give the urine a cloudy appearance, but if moderately severe haemorrhage has occurred into the urinary tract the urine is usually obviously red, and even blood clots may be present—specific identification in all circumstances depends upon recognition during microscopic examination of suitably stained smears. Their presence suggests haemorrhage from some point in the urinary system. (Contamination of the urine with blood from the reproductive organs may occur in female animals, more particularly the bitch.) The presence of neutrophil leucocytes indicates pyogenic inflammatory exudation into the urinary tract; this may occur at any point. The neutrophil cells can occur in variable numbers, sometimes in the form of visible pus clots, but they are particularly numerous in suppurative conditions of the urinary system including embolic suppurative nephritis, pyelonephritis and cystitis. Neutrophil leucocytes will contaminate otherwise normal urine voided by dogs with balanitis.

The epithelial cells which appear in the urine may vary in size, shape and numbers. The morphological characters of the cells may indicate their site of origin in the urinary tract. Such judgements must be made with considerable reserve because the cells are exposed to a considerable number of influences which can alter their morphology. These include the inflammatory process which brought their separation, chemical changes in the urine, the intracellular changes which result from the osmotic influences of the urine, and death of the cell. In addition, cells from the deeper layers of the epithelial tissues are generally smaller than those which are more superficially situated so that, in less recently established inflammation of such parts as the urinary bladder, the epithelial cells are uniformly small.

Renal tubular epithelial cells are polygonal or columnar, being somewhat smaller than the neutrophil leucocyte, with round, relatively large, distinct nuclei. Individual renal epithelial cells occur in very small numbers in normal urine, but the number is greatly increased in nephritis. The cells from the renal pelvis or calyx are roughly triangular, or are similar to those from the ureter, bladder and urethra, which are transitional. Cells from the superficial layers of the bladder epithelium are large and flat with small, rounded nuclei, and are often found in a sheet-like group. They are present in small numbers in all forms of cystitis. Cells from the middle layers of the mucosa are caudate and those from the deeper layers are small, cuboidal or rounded, and are readily confused with epithelial cells from the renal tubules.

Casts are cylindrical moulds of the renal tubules. The presence of casts in urine indicates the existence of an inflammatory or degenerative lesion in the kidney. The types of casts that occur in urine are epithelial, erythrocyte, granular, hyaline, amyloid and haemoglobin. Casts which are formed by the agglomeration of erythrocytes or desquamated epithelial cells in a matrix of coagulated plasma protein, vary in appearance according to their composition and the length of time the renal disease has existed.

Both epithelial and erythrocyte casts are indicative of acute nephritis or severe nephrosis. In epithelial casts the cells may show evidence of disintegration through being exposed to the macerating effects of the urine, or the primary degenerative changes prior to extrusion. Granular casts probably result from epithelial casts which have degenerated, the coarser the granules the younger the cast. Hyaline casts are homogeneous and transparent, and consist of protein (more globulin than albumin because the former is less soluble than the latter) and mucopolysaccharide; their presence is taken to indicate that renal disease has been in existence for some time. Erythrocyte casts are seen only occasionally; they progress rapidly to a homogeneous haemoglobin cast which has a copper colour. Because they exist longer in acid than in alkaline urine casts are rarely found in the urine of herbivorous animals.

The presence of parasite ova, or pathogenic bacteria in urine is demonstrated microscopically, either in unstained preparations or in stained smears, or by other methods such as dark-ground illumination and cultural or biological techniques. In order to avoid confusion regarding the origin and significance of the parasite ova, bacteria or yeasts, urine samples should be obtained from animal patients by catheterization, and then subjected to examination without delay.

Specific bacteria occurring in urine include *Corynebacterium renale* and *C. suis*, the causes of pyelonephritis in cattle and pigs respectively, and leptospirae (*Leptospira icterohaemorrhagiae*, *L. canicola*, *L. pomona*, *L. hyos*, etc.), which cause leptospirosis in dogs, cattle, pigs and man. The last group of bacteria can be visualized only by means of dark-ground illumination. The number of leptospirae excreted with the urine may be too few to be detectable, so that repeat examinations will increase the efficiency of the method. It must be realized that the examination should be carried out as soon as possible after a urine sample has been collected, because leptospirae quickly degenerate, especially in acid urine. Streptococci, staphylococci and other pyogenic bacteria occur in urine in suppurative nephritis, cystitis, prostatitis and urethritis. In the majority of cases in which yeasts and fungi are found in urine it is the result of extracorporeal contamination; occasional cases of yeast infection of the urinary tract do occur in animals.

Parasite ova which may occur in urine include those of *Dioctophyma renale* (dogs, more rarely horses, cattle and silver foxes), *Stephanurus dentatus* (pigs) and *Capillaria plica* (dogs, foxes). The larvae of *Dirofilaria immitis* may be found in the urine of the dog.

Unorganized deposits. These consist of amorphous or crystalline materials which vary somewhat according to the chemical reaction of the urine. The presence of unorganized deposits in the urine of animals is only significant when they occur in large amounts, and there are obvious indications of pain originating in the urinary tract. The urine of herbivorous animals, especially horses, normally contains relatively large amounts of calcium carbonate crystals (see Fig. 165A, p. 223) which are recognized as brown, radially striated spheres. Urinary carbonates are soluble in acetic acid with liberation of carbon dioxide gas in the form of small bubbles.

Phosphates, urates (see Fig. 165B), cystine and oxalates occur in the urine of carnivorous animals. Calcium oxalate crystals (Fig. 165C), which are relatively rare in the urine of domestic animals, are seen most frequently in cattle and sheep when they are grazing herbage with a high oxalate content; the incidence of urolithiasis is likely to be significant in these circumstances. Oxalates occur in various forms, including octahedral crystals having eight triangular faces, and a dumb-bell form. Triple phosphates (ammonium magnesium phosphate) (Fig. 165D) are deposited from alkaline urine either as an amorphous mass resembling carbonates, or in the form of elongated 'coffin lid' crystals. Phosphates do not dissolve in acetic acid. In freshly voided urine from animals with cystitis or pyelitis they occur in larger quantities than in normal fresh urine, because they are precipitated from solution when the pH of the urine rises during bacterial decomposition of urea. Deposits of uric acid in fairly large amounts occur in the urine of Dalmatian dogs. Urate crystals form reddish-brown granules with an amorphous quality while those of uric acid are thin, square sheets. Sodium urate is sometimes precipitated in relatively large quantities as a brick-red or coffee-coloured deposit when the urine of carnivorous animals is cooled. It redissolves on being heated and is of no pathological significance. Cystine crystals, in the form of hexagonal plates, are excreted in urine of male dogs with an inherited defect consisting of deranged tubular reabsorption of the amino acid from the glomerular filtrate. Sulphonamide crystals will occur in varying amounts in urine when they have been administered for therapeutic or other purposes.

Normally the unorganized sediments present in urine, which are derived from the dissolved inorganic and organic salts, are of no significance although many of the solutes are present in supersaturated concentration. Under certain poorly defined circumstances, including marked rise in urinary pH, concentration of urine which may occur particularly in hot climates in water-deprived animals, excessive intake of mineral matter in the form of phosphate or calcium and the ingestion of large quantities of oxalates in certain plants which may dominate in pastures at certain times of the year, there is a marked increase in the quantity of deposited matter. Such crystalline urinary deposits only become clinically significant if they cause obstruction through the formation of calculi. Urolithiasis may occur when conditions favour the development of a nidus in the form of a group of desquamated epithelial cells or a fragment of necrotic tissue. Sporadically, nidus formation results from local inflammatory involvement in the urinary tract (a correlation has been found to exist between *Staphylococcus aureus* infection of the urinary tract in dogs and triple phosphate calculi); more generally it can result from excessive epithelial desquamation associated with hypovitaminosis A, or the ingestion or administration of oestrogenic substances. Whenever possible the chemical nature of calculi should be determined otherwise effective treatment and control will not be possible.

Assessment of Renal Function

The first point to establish in determining the efficiency of kidney function is whether or not the particular animal is urinating. From this it is then possible to proceed to an assessment of renal function by examination of blood and urine with, where considered advisable, the application of a renal function study.

Perhaps the simplest and most direct test is to measure the potential of the kidney to increase the specific gravity of the urine under regulated conditions. This test is of particular importance when urine analysis reveals a low specific gravity near the 'fixed point', suggesting chronic nephritis with tubular damage. In these circumstances the specific gravity is not appreciably altered by either forced administration of large quantities of water by stomach tube, or water deprivation for a period of 12–24 hours. In the latter test the animal is allowed free access to water and food for 24 hours, at which time the bladder is drained and the specific gravity of the urine noted. All water is then withdrawn for the period of the test, after which the bladder is again emptied. After the lapse of a further hour the bladder is catheterized and the specific gravity of the final sample of urine is determined and a comparison made with the first reading. An obvious increase in the second reading indicates that endogenous antidiuretic hormone is being produced and that the kidney tubules are able to react to it; no significant difference between the readings suggests either absence of hormone or tubular failure.

Kidney function can also be assessed by

measuring the time of appearance, and persistence in the urine of substances such as inulin, para-aminohippurate or phenolsulphonphthalein following intravenous injection. These exogenous substances are principally excreted by the kidneys so that they are the most suitable for use in clearance tests for which purpose a measured amount is administered and then urine collected at intervals for 40–60 minutes by means of catheterization. The rate of disappearance of the selected substance from the plasma can be determined from blood samples taken prior to and then at regular intervals for 30 minutes following injection. Satisfactory standards for interpretation have not been determined in all animals but, as a general finding, the interval before the test substance appears in the urine, and the excretion time are prolonged in renal disease. Under well controlled test conditions, significant reduction in the clearance rate may be taken to indicate that over 50% of the nephron complement have been damaged. Because the kidney possesses considerable regenerative capacity, repeated clearance studies may be required before a final assessment can be made.

Renal function can also be assessed by measuring the blood concentration of certain metabolites which are normally excreted with the urine. For this purpose determination of the blood urea level has been commonly employed, although non-protein nitrogen and creatinine would serve the same purpose. When interpreting the results of such tests it is necessary to take into account the clinical condition of the animal, the character of the diet and such prerenal factors as dehydration and circulatory efficiency, and to appreciate that the ratio of exogenous and endogenous protein catabolism has a significant influence on the degree to which any of them may accumulate in the blood. Finally, a better appreciation of the value of such tests is obtained from the realization that the blood levels are not likely to be significantly affected until at least 60% or more of the functioning nephrons are destroyed. It is possible for an animal to survive on 25% of its full complement of nephrons if under good management and on a controlled diet.

In a proportion of dogs with advanced chronic renal disease a type of osteodystrophy termed 'rubber jaw' is not uncommon. Renal lesions which cause the condition include interstitial nephritis, congenital cysts, bilateral hydrone-phrosis and pyelonephritis. Although the exact mechanism for the production of renal osteomalacia is not known it has been suggested that failure of renal tubular ammonium synthesis leads to decreased calcium retention, increased amounts of the latter being excreted along with sodium and potassium in the urine. In addition deranged glomerular function causes increased retention of phosphorus. The resulting calcium and phosphorus imbalance is adjusted by mobilization of skeletal calcium which is mediated by the action of the parathyroid hormone; this engenders secondary parathyroid hyperplasia. Although demineralization will affect all the bones of the skeleton the flat bones are most severely affected. Determinations of blood calcium and phosphorus levels would, in conjunction with the clinical findings, the results of urine analysis and radiography, reveal the presence of the condition.

Radiological Examination

The value of radiographic examination of the urinary system is limited because the method is ordinarily only applicable to small animals. In this case it may be utilized to confirm the position of a renal neoplasm the presence of which has been suspected by recognition of a vague mass during abdominal palpation. Differentiation from a tumour of the adrenal gland is virtually impossible during life because no obvious indication of hormonal dysfunction develops, at least in the dog. Similar neoplasms of the bladder, which occur in the form of carcinomas, fibromas and sarcomas, are revealed by either direct radiography or the use of air or a solution of potassium iodide as a contrast medium. The contrast media are readily introduced by means of a urethral catheter.

The main value of radiographic examination is to reveal the presence of calculi, some of which may be composed of non-radiopaque substances such as cystine. The most common sites at which urinary calculi cause trouble by being held up are the renal pelvis, the bladder, and the urethra in the male animals. Moderate to large sized calculi are usually clearly visualized (Fig. 169) but small opaque calculi may be rendered more obvious by draining the bladder and then inflating it with air. A solution of sodium or potassium iodide may be employed to reveal cystine calculi. The use of contrast media by intravenous injection or retrograde pyelography

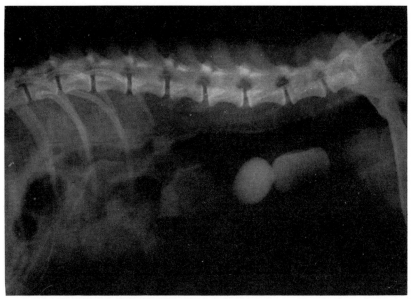

Fig. 169. *A radiograph showing calculi in the bladder of a 6-year-old bitch. Note also the dark (i.e. gas-filled) loops of intestine.*

has had a very restricted application in veterinary medicine. With the former method some appreciation of the functional state of the kidneys may be obtained from the character of the radiographs in relation to the rate of renal clearance of the contrast medium.

Urinary Abnormalities in Certain Diseases

Prerenal Diseases

Diabetes mellitus. Polyuria; usually a high specific gravity (1·035–1·060); glucose; ketone bodies; albumin and casts in severe or advanced disease.

Diabetes insipidus; Cushing's disease; dystrophia adiposogenitalis. Polyuria; low specific gravity (1·001–1·006); almost colourless; abnormal substances (albumin, casts, glucose) are absent; increased 17-ketosteroid in Cushing's disease.

Bovine ketosis. Specific gravity decreased; reaction acid; ketone bodies.

Diseases associated with jaundice. Brownish-green colour from increased urobilin in haemolytic jaundice; yellowish-green froth which foams readily in obstructive jaundice; bilirubin also in obstructive jaundice.

Diseases associated with haemoglobinaemia or myoglobinaemia. Red, brown or black colour; foams readily; albumin, haemoglobin or myoglobin; moderate amount of deposit containing few, if any, erthrocytes and renal cells; haemoglobin casts.

Enteritis and intestinal obstruction. Reaction acid; bilirubin; increased indican.

Renal Diseases

Interstitial nephritis, chronic nephrosis and chronic glomerulonephritis. Polyuria; low specific gravity; only traces of albumin; cellular elements scanty; urea and non-protein nitrogen increased.

Pyelonephritis. Discoloured turbid urine; alkaline reaction; albumin; abundant sediment containing neutrophil leucocytes, cells from renal calices, erythrocytes, blood clots, fibrin and bacteria (*Corynebacterium renale* in cattle and *C. suis* in pigs).

Acute nephrosis and acute glomerulonephritis. Oliguria; high specific gravity; acid reaction; albumin in quantity; erythrocytes and neutrophil leucocytes; renal cells and casts.

Suppurative nephritis. Acid reaction; albumin; microscopic haematuria; neutrophil leucocytes; specific pyogenic bacteria.

Postrenal Diseases

Cystitis. Frequent urination with strangury; turbid urine; reaction alkaline; ammoniacal odour; albumin; abundant deposit containing bladder cells, neutrophil leucocytes, erythrocytes, bacteria and triple phosphate crystals.

In chronic cystitis the abnormal features are not very well marked. Increased frequency with small volume are usual.

Bovine enzootic haematuria. Urine red; recognizable streaks or clots of blood; albumin and haemoglobin; deposit consists mainly of erythrocytes.

Postrenal haematuria of varying severity also occurs in urolithiasis when obstruction is partial.

12

The Reproductive System

The reproductive system consists of the external and internal genital organs with, in female animals, the mammary glands. The external genitalia and mammae of all species can be subjected to clinical examination by means of the visual and tactile senses, whereas the internal components of the genital system are generally only available for indirect palpation in various ways.

The objectives of clinical examination of the reproductive system are: (a) to recognize disease that may be presently affecting the general health of the animal, or which is likely to cause impairment of health in the future; (b) to diagnose venereal disease; (c) to assess fertility with, in sexually mature female animals, status in respect of pregnancy; and (d) to identify genetic defects. The first and last of these objectives require that a thorough, systematic clinical examination should precede the detailed examination of the reproductive system itself. It is not the intention in this text to give detailed consideration to venereal disease or to the assessment of fertility.

Male Reproductive Organs

The most important parts of the male genital system are the scrotum and paired testicles with their epididymes, the seminal vesicles, the prostate and paired bulbourethral (Cowper's) glands and the penis.

In the horse the testicles are situated in the prepubic region in the scrotum which is a diverticulum of the abdomen. They are ovoid in shape, being compressed from side to side, with their long axes almost longitudinal. The epididymis is attached to the dorsal border of the testicle with the head (caput epididymis) overlying the anterior and the tail (cauda epididymis) the

posterior pole of the testicle. Because the left testicle is quite frequently larger and more dependent than the right, and placed a little further back, the globular-shaped scrotum is commonly asymmetrical.

The penis of the horse, comprised largely of erectile tissue, encloses the extrapelvic part of the urethra. It extends from the ischial arch forward between the thighs on the ventral part of the posterior abdomen. It is compressed laterally and in the quiescent state—when it is normally accommodated in the prepuce it is about 50 cm long; during erection it increases 50% or more in length. The expanded free end (glans penis), which is convex, is surrounded by a prominent margin (corona glandis) and has a deep depression at its lower part (fossa glandis) in which the urethra protrudes for about 2 cm as a free tube (urethral process). The prepuce is a double invagination of skin which houses the prescrotal portion of the non-erect penis. The external part of the prepuce extends from the scrotum to within a few centimetres of the umbilicus where it invaginates forming the preputial orifice and is continued as the internal part.

The scrotum of the bull is situated a little further forward than in the horse. It is long and pendulous, with a distinct neck except when it is contracted. The testicles are larger than those of the horse; they are oval and elongated in shape, with the long axis vertical. The epididymis is attached along the posterior border with the head covering the dorsal pole. The penis is cylindrical and is longer and of much smaller diameter than in the horse. Immediately behind the scrotum it forms an S-shaped curve, the sigmoid flexure, which is effaced during erection.

The glans penis is about 8 cm long and has a pointed extremity which is twisted; the external urethral orifice being situated at the end of a groove formed by the spiral. The prepuce is long (40 cm) and narrow; the orifice, which is situated about 5 cm behind the umbilicus, is surrounded by long hairs.

The genital organs of the ram resemble those of the bull with one or two major differences. The testicles are proportionately much larger and the terminal part of the urethra projects beyond the glans penis for at least 3 cm, forming the twisted processus urethrae.

In the boar the scrotum is situated a short distance ventral to the anus. The testicles are very large, with the long axis extending upwards and backwards, the tail of the epididymis forming the highest point. The penis has a general resemblance to that of the ox, but the sigmoid flexure is prescrotal, there is no glans and the anterior part is spirally twisted, especially during erection. The external urethral orifice is slit-like and is situated near the pointed extremity in a ventro-lateral position. The prepuce is long and narrow and the orifice is surrounded by stiff hairs.

The scrotum in the dog is situated midway between the inguinal region and the anus. The testicles are proportionately small and have their long axes directed obliquely upwards and backwards. The free portion of the penis encloses the os penis which, in the large dog, may be up to 10 cm long. The glans penis is very long, the anterior part being cylindrical with a pointed extremity; behind this there is a rounded enlargement ('bulbus glandis') which is especially prominent during erection. The prepuce forms a complete sheath enclosing the free portion of the penis.

Clinical Examination of the Male Genital Organs

In the male animal it is essential to examine the skin of the prepuce and scrotum, the testicles, the internal aspect of the preputial cavity and the glans and the other parts of the free portion of the penis. Many animals resent palpation of the external genitalia, so it is necessary to perform this part of the clinical examination with some caution; administering a sedative drug invariably assists the application of the physical procedures. In the gelding and stallion the penis can be exposed by inserting the hand into the preputial cavity and grasping the organ behind the glans, or passing a loop of a broad bandage round it at

this position, and then applying gentle steady traction. The penis of the bull can be inspected briefly by allowing the animal to mount a teaser cow and then directing the organ into an artificial vagina. A similar procedure may be adopted for the boar and ram. For a thorough examination of the whole extent of the free portion of the penis in the bull it is necessary to make use of internal pudendal nerve block or epidural anaesthesia. With the latter, induced paraplegia frequently occurs and poses an obvious problem. The penis of the dog can be exposed for examination by restraining the animal in dorsal or lateral recumbency and then pushing the prepuce backwards with the fingers of one hand while pushing the penis forwards with the other hand (See Fig. 163, p. 222).

The entire length of the preputial cavity should be palpated in order that such abnormalities as adhesions, fibrous tissue proliferation, abscesses, painful states and sebaceous concretions are detected. Similarly the penis can be palpated through the sheath; by this means it is possible to recognize the existence of haematomas, adhesions to surrounding tissues and neoplasms.

Permanent protrusion of the penis occurs in paralysis of the pudic nerve (Fig. 170), and in

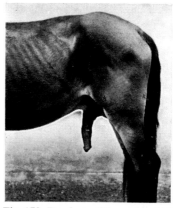

Fig. 170. *Paralysis of the penis, which is flaccid and hangs loosely from the prepuce and cannot be retracted. Loss of function of the pudic nerve.*

paraphimosis (constriction of the penis by a contracted or narrow preputial orifice so that retraction does not occur); both these conditions occur in the horse. Invariably the exposed penis soon becomes swollen because of the increased hydrostatic pressure arising from venous constriction. Swelling of the penis may also be caused by inflammation, but in such circumstances the penis does not necessarily protrude from the prepuce. In some cases of inflammation of the penis, more particularly when the glans and terminal part of the urethra are involved, erection persists for considerable periods (priapism). In the horse, in which species the penis is normally exposed during urination, intermittent protrusion of the organ, not associated with urination, suggests urethral obstruction. This may take the form of an impacted urinary calculus or compression of the urethral process by a sebaceous calculus. Localized swelling of the penis in the bull frequently results from 'fracture' followed by haemorrhage; the initial injury occurs in vigorous bulls during mating. When the free portion of the penis is affected in this way adhesions, developing in the preputial cavity, increase the size of the swelling. Bulls so affected are unable to protrude the penis to the normal extent; sometimes exposure cannot be achieved during erection.

The 'preputial calculi' that are occasionally found in the gelding and bullock are in reality concretions of sebaceous secretion. In the horse, urination may be prevented because the inspissated sebaceous mass interferes with protrusion of the penis, or when it collects in the coronal fossa of the glans penis, by compression of the urethra. Sebaceous concretions cause trouble in bullocks only when they obstruct the preputial orifice and cause retention of urine; they are usually torpedo-shaped and readily movable. Prolapse of the mucous membrane through the preputial orifice occurs occasionally in bulls, the incidence is highest in the beef breeds. Superficial lesions in the form of papules, vesicles, ulcers and small depigmented flecks may occur within the prepuce, and on the glans and other parts of the penis, not only in diseases affecting the skin, but also in specific diseases such as glanders and, more particularly, in venereal conditions such as dourine. Lesions in the form of small white pustules (2 mm in diameter) occur on the penis and prepuce of the bull when infected with infectious pustular vulvovaginitis virus. The associated oedema may cause phimosis or paraphimosis; severely affected bulls may develop adhesions. Bovine papillomatosis virus causes fibropapillomatosis of the penis in the bull. The lesions which consist largely of connective tissue

appear to be painful. In venereal disease of sheep the lesions of posthitis appear at the preputial orifice in the form of ulceration, which may result in phimosis or paraphimosis. The glans penis may also become extensively ulcerated. In inflammation of the preputial mucosa (suppurative balanitis), which is very common in the dog, purulent fluid is more or less constantly discharged through the preputial orifice. Occasionally small nodules develop on the mucosa of the prepuce and penis in this condition, in which case libido is increased. Balanoposthitis (pizzle rot, lip and leg ulceration), affecting young rams and wethers, is associated with ulceration of the skin surrounding the preputial orifice, followed by spread of the inflammatory reaction into the prepuce until eventually the penis becomes involved. The most important clinical signs are swelling of the affected parts, with pain on palpation, purulent discharge and interference with urination.

The inguinal region is of clinical significance, more particularly in colt foals and stallions, in which animals incarcerated or strangulated hernia is a cause of acute colic. Examination of the scrotal region should never be omitted in a case of acute colic in a stallion or a colt foal. Inguinal hernia gives rise to a unilateral, hot, painful scrotal swelling which may evince a tympanic sound when it is percussed, indicating the presence of gas in the incarcerated intestinal loops. Inherited scrotal hernia is very common in the pig, in which species it only occasionally gives rise to serious disturbance in health.

The testicles and epididymes are readily palpable in the normal animal, and the skin of the scrotum is freely movable over them. The examination will be resisted by the majority of farm animals, so that some degree of restraint will be necessary. By means of palpation the size, shape, position, consistency and sensitivity of the testes can be determined. At this stage it may be necessary to determine whether both testicles are present in the scrotum and, if one or both are absent, whether they are located in the inguinal canal or the abdomen (cryptorchidism). In this situation the sedative effect of a tranquillizing drug may be found useful. Cryptorchidism is considered to have an hereditary basis and in dogs is particularly prevalent in certain breeds, e.g. poodles and terriers. It is essential to appreciate that there is considerable disparity in the size of the testes in normal animals of the same species, and as a general rule a slight degree of testicular asymmetry occurs in individual animals. Marked asymmetry may be the result of unilateral orchitis or hypoplasia, testicular atrophy following orchitis or neoplasia. Bilateral enlargement occurs in acute and sometimes in chronic orchitis, and small testes in hypoplasia and advanced degeneration. The epididymis is generally involved in acute orchitis. A specific form of epididymitis is noted in *Brucella ovis* infection in rams. Palpation reveals that the epididymis is enlarged and firm, more frequently the tail, with oedema and inflammation of the scrotum occurring during the initial, more acute phase. A proportion of the affected rams excrete the causal bacterium in their semen.

The scrotum may be enlarged as the result of inflammation of the testicle (orchitis) which may extend to the scrotal tissues. The epididymis may or may not be involved. Palpation of the scrotum reveals warmth and causes the affected animal to manifest pain. When the orchitis is acute there will be systemic effects including elevation of temperature, and reflex increase in respiratory and pulse rates. Primary inflammation of the scrotum causes the scrotal wall to increase considerably in thickness. Enlargement of the scrotum may also be caused, particularly in the bull, by deposition of fat in considerable amounts. Acute orchitis may be caused by trauma or systemic infection, and in the dog infection of the prostate gland. Occasional cases of orchitis in the horse develop as a sequel to strangles. In the bull infection of the genital organs, in particular the testes, epididymes and seminal vesicles, by *Brucella abortus* is a not altogether unusual event. In infectious infertility of cattle (epivag) the initial physical sign consists of enlargement of the spermatic cord with, later, considerable swelling of the epididymis, followed by orchitis characterized by swelling and later fibrosis and atrophy.

Testicular neoplasia is most common in the dog, occurring particularly in animals over 5 years of age. In occasional cases the tumour is malignant. It appears that malpositioned testes are more likely to become neoplastic than scrotal testes. Because they can originate from any of the basic tissues, each of which has a distinctive function, testicular neoplasms produce varying effects on animals. The majority can be classified into three types, one of which produces large quantities of oestrogen-like substances; it is suggested that the others may produce androgen-like substances. As a consequence, a neoplasm of the testes in the dog is associated clinically with other recognizable signs, apart from the abnormal state of the testicle itself.

Interstitial-cell tumours, which are the most common type in the dog and bull, are generally small and of such little clinical significance that they are generally unobserved; the majority of cases are detected during autopsy. This type of neoplasm is said to produce androgens. The seminoma, which originates from the germinal epithelium of the seminiferous tubules is a less common testicular tumour. Dogs so affected may manifest pain by adopting a crouching posture, with lameness and abnormal gait. The Sertoli cell tumour, although comparatively rare in the dog, produces the most obvious clinical effects, all of which are attributable to the feminization action of the large amount of oestrogens produced by the tumour cells. This neoplasm has its origin in the sustentacular cells of Sertoli in the seminiferous tubules of the testes. The acquired female characteristics, which regress rapidly following removal of the tumour, include alopecia of the lateral aspects of the body, reduced libido, sexual attraction for other male dogs, gynaecomastia, enlargement of the prepuce, atrophy of the normal testicle and increased melanin deposition in the skin of the scrotum and abdomen (see Fig. 32, p. 42).

To a varying degree the internal sex organs of male animals can be examined by manual or digital rectal exploration. In the stallion and bull, the pelvic part of the urethra can be identified as a firm cylindrical structure about 2–5 cm in diameter, situated in the midline of the pelvic floor. The prostate gland in the stallion consists of two lateral lobes somewhat prismatic in shape which are directed forward and laterally from the neck of the bladder and origin of the urethra, ventral to the rectum; the connecting isthmus cannot be recognized. The seminal vesicles consist of two elongated, somewhat pear-shaped, blind sacs about 15–20 cm long and 5 cm in diameter at the widest point near the anterior end. In the gelding they are much smaller. The seminal vesicles extend forwards from the dorsal surface of the bladder, near its neck, where each one is situated medial to its corresponding lobe of the prostate gland. Infections of the seminal vesicles (vesiculitis) are occasionally observed in stallions. They may be the result of systemic infections such as strangles, but in many cases their origin cannot be determined. In cases of acute vesiculitis, one or both seminal vesicles will be found on rectal examination to be considerably enlarged and sensitive. As a rule in chronic cases, particularly those of long standing, the vesicles will not be obviously abnormal. Affected stallions may be impotent and unable to ejaculate, or capable of copulation but producing semen containing large numbers of neutrophil leucocytes. The causal bacterium, which is most often a streptococcus, less often a staphylococcus or coliform, can be isolated by bacteriological culture. The bulbo-urethral glands, two in number and each about 5 cm long and 2 cm wide, are situated on either side of the pelvic part of the urethra near the ischial arch.

The prostate gland in the bull surrounds the anterior part of the pelvic urethra; dorsally it forms a band about 4 cm transversely and about 1·5 cm wide, across the neck of the bladder and the origin of the urethra. The seminal vesicles comprise two compact glandular structures with a lobulated surface which measure 10–12 cm long, 5 cm wide and 3 cm or more thick. They extend forward from the anterior part of the pelvic urethra. The pelvic portion of the urethra and prostate are only occasionally involved in disease, the former sometimes being the site of obstruction by a urolith, which if unrelieved leads to rupture of the bladder. The seminal vesicles, however, are comparatively frequently the site of pyogenic infection by bacteria including *Corynebacterium pyogenes*, streptococci and *Brucella abortus*. The inflammatory reaction may be unilateral or bilateral; in the former case marked asymmetry is usual. In acute vesiculitis involvement of the surrounding pelvic tissues may cause general febrile signs with abdominal pain, and constipation. During rectal examination the affected bull manifests a severe pain reaction when the inflamed structures are palpated. When the condition is chronic the gland is of firm consistency, with absence of lobulation, and there are extensive pelvic adhesions. Very occasionally the terminal portion of the ductus deferens (ampulla) is involved in an inflammatory reaction, which may be recognized when digital pressure is applied over the neck of the bladder between the seminal vesicles.

The prostate gland in the dog is relatively large and forms a globular structure surrounding the neck of the bladder and the origin of the urethra.

A dorsal median groove indicates the division of the gland into two lobes. There are no seminal vesicles or bulbo-urethral glands. Examination of the internal sex organs in the dog is restricted to digital exploration of the posterior part of the pelvic cavity. The most important structure in this situation is the prostate gland, which may not be within reach of the finger in large dogs.

Abnormalities of the prostate gland which cause clinical disease in dogs include hyperplasia, prostatitis and neoplasia. Dogs with prostate hyperplasia, which usually occurs in animals of five or more years of age, frequently develop constipation, passage of characteristic ribbon-like faeces being accompanied by obvious tenesmus. Occasionally it is complicated by perineal hernia, in which case dysuria may develop because of retroversion of the bladder. Prostatic hypertrophy can be recognized by rectal palpation, the enlarged gland being smooth or nodular, but in either case the dorsal furrow is deeper; so a pain reaction is induced. Cysts are a frequent feature; in some instances they are very large, filling almost the whole extent of the pelvic inlet and projecting forwards into the abdomen.

Atrophy of the prostate gland occurs in occasional instances as a senile involutionary change in old dogs. The gland, which may be reduced to half or even a quarter its normal size, is shrunken and firm. Prostatic atrophy is thought to arise from deficient secretion of androgens.

Prostatitis is invariably an acute painful condition, so that the dog stands with its back arched, and cries out when the tail is elevated or a finger inserted into the rectum. Systemic involvement is indicated by raised temperature and increased pulse frequency. Some cases of prostatitis occur in association with hypertrophy of the gland. In many instances the inflammatory reaction develops following invasion of the prostate gland as the result of an ascending infection by a pyogenic bacterium. The formation of an abscess is indicated if small fluctuating areas are detected when the gland is subjected to digital palpation.

Neoplasia of the prostate gland in the dog is relatively rare, the most common tumour is a carcinoma; dogs over 10 years of age are most often affected. Clinical signs usually appear when the condition is well established and consist of discomfort with pronounced pain and straining preceding, and persisting after defaecation. An acute pain reaction is induced by palpation of the prostate which is firm, irregular in shape, with a propensity to infiltrate neighbouring structures so that it may be adherent to the pelvic bones. Large tumours may give rise to a perineal swelling. Urinary disturbances are unusual and when they occur take the form of retention, dribbling and dysuria. The terminal signs include cachexia, vomiting, anorexia and diarrhoea.

The sexual impulses (libido) may be increased or reduced in strength compared with the normal pattern in male animals. Increased libido is indicated by frequent erections (priapism), mounting other animals of the same species, masturbation, etc. Such behavioural patterns are most commonly associated, in young animals, with the development of sexual maturity. Inflammatory conditions affecting the preputial mucosa and/or the penile surface are a common cause of priapism. Reduced libido is indicated by slowness or unwillingness to copulate; other aspects of mating behaviour, such as the manner of mounting and thrusting, also reflect the vigour of the sex drive. It should be remembered, however, that painful conditions of the hind limbs, vertebral column or abdominal cavity (overgrown feet, arthritis, ankylosis, spondylitis, peritonitis), and genetic defects (neuromuscular spasticity in bulls and boars) may produce the same effect. In both male and female animals, abnormal libido is not infrequently the result of disease of the gonads, but it may also be caused by disease of other parts of the genital system and by certain nervous disorders.

Microscopic, cultural or other methods of examining preputial secretion may prove of value in diagnosis of those infective diseases which primarily involve the preputial cavity and penis. Preputial secretion can be obtained from the bull by inserting a plastic pipette fitted with a suitable rubber bulb or attached to a flutter valve into the deepest part of the preputial cavity. The secretion can be aspirated into the pipette by suction with the rubber bulb, or the preputial cavity can be flushed out by introducing a small quantity (30 ml for a bull) of sterile normal saline solution by means of the rubber bulb or flutter valve. In this way material is made available for the detection of specific pathogenic organisms including *Trichomonas foetus* and *Vibrio fetus*. Because *Tr. foetus* does not survive for more than a few hours in physiological saline, microscopic

examination should be made as soon as sedimentation of the sample has occurred. This can be expedited by centrifuging at 2000 rpm. The best material for examination is that immediately above the sediment, it is withdrawn by means of a capillary pipette and several preparations are made. A negative result is not conclusive. For transporting preputial secretions the use of sterile skimmed milk containing antibiotics to suppress bacterial growth is recommended. This medium can also be used for culturing the protozoan organism. In suspected cases of *V. fetus* infection the preputial washings should be examined within 12 hours of collection. For microscopic examination the sediment is separated by centrifuging and is then placed on slides and stained prior to examination. The sediment can be cultured on blood agar containing thioglycholate with anaerobic incubation, or it can be subjected to a fluorescent antibody test provided specific conjugates are available. It is now generally accepted that direct serological tests possess too many limitations to have any worthwhile diagnostic merit. In cases of doubt, test matings with a series of virgin heifers is the most certain method of determining the status of bulls in relation to these venereal diseases.

Examination of the semen is necessary when the fertility of a prospective sire is in question. A sample of semen can be collected from the majority of male animals of the domestic species by directing the penis into an artificial vagina during simulated copulation, or in a suitable container after artificial stimulation of the penis. This can be achieved in the bull by rectal massage of the seminal vesicles, which flushes the urethra, followed by firm massage of the ampullae of the ductus deferentes. In this way concentrated semen is obtained. The electro-ejaculator will achieve the same result in the bull and ram.

Gross examination of semen includes inspection for abnormalities of colour or volume, and the presence of foreign material. The colour of normal semen varies from white to yellowish-white, giving a milk- or cream-like appearance. Watery-looking semen may have few or no spermatozoa present. Naked eye examination of bull semen may reveal wave-like movements; microscopic examination of a fresh specimen will confirm the existence of wave motion and help to classify its character. Stained smears will often prove more satisfactory than fresh wet preparations in revealing the presence of abnor-

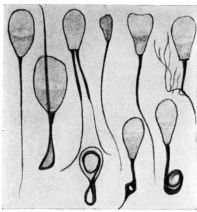

Fig. 171. *Spermatozoa of the bull. The one on the left is normal; the remainder show various pathological features.* (After Lagerhöf)

mal spermatozoa (Fig. 171), neutrophil leucocytes or bacteria. Full bacteriological examination of semen is recommended only when there are lesions in the testicles or in other genital organs, when the semen contains pus or blood and when naturally mated breeding female animals develop a purulent vaginal discharge within a few days.

Full evaluation of a sample of semen requires the services of a specialist working in this field, nevertheless an adequate assessment can often be made under field conditions, on the basis of an examination of a fresh unstained preparation. In all circumstances, several separate ejaculates of semen (four, in the case of a bull which has not been in recent use) are necessary for a satisfactory examination. If the samples have to be transported to a laboratory, special conditions should be provided in order to avoid temperature shock, rough handling, and delay in transit. In the laboratory, additional methods of determining semen quality include assessment of proportional motility, classification of degree and character of morphological abnormalities, sperm concentration, methylene blue reduction test, pH determination, variation in electrical impedance and bacteriological examination. The results of one series of tests should not be considered to give a correct reflection of the animal's potential fertility.

Female Reproductive Organs

The female genital organs consist of the two ovaries, the Fallopian tubes, the uterus, the vagina and the vulva. Because of the close physiological relationship which exists between them, the mammary glands are, as a rule, considered in the context of the organs of reproduction.

External Genitalia

In female animals the external genitalia comprise the vagina and vulva. In the mare the vagina extends horizontally through the pelvic cavity. It forms a tube about 15–20 cm long and, when slightly distended, about 10–12 cm in diameter; it extends from the neck of the uterus to the vulva. On its dorsal aspect it is related to the rectum, while ventrally the relationship is continuous anteriorly with the vagina and terminates posteriorly at the vulval cleft which is located 5–8 cm below the anus. The floor of the vulva is 10–12 cm long, while at its dorsal part it is considerably shorter. Dorsally it is related to the rectum and anus, ventrally to the pelvic floor and laterally to the sacrosciatic ligament, the semimembranosus muscle and the internal pudic artery. The vulvar cleft forms a vertical slit, 12–15 cm long and is bordered by the labia vulvae which meet dorsally at an acute angle (dorsal commissure) and below in the form of a thick rounded ventral commissure situated about 5 cm behind and below the ischial arch. The ventral commissure is occupied by a rounded body, the glans clitoridis, which is about 2·5 cm wide and lies in a cavity the fossa clitoridis. The external urethral orifice is situated on the floor of the vulva at its junction with the vagina, about 10–12 cm from the ventral commissure.

The vagina of the cow is much longer than that of the mare; in the non-pregnant animal it is 25–40 cm long, and in pregnant animals the length is increased. The two canals of Gartner are located in the submucosa towards the floor of the vagina; their ducts open near the external urethral orifice. The labia of the vulva are quite thick, and both commissures form acute angles; the ventral one has a tuft of long hairs. The external urethral orifice is about 10 cm from the ventral commissure.

The vagina in the ewe is about 7–10 cm long; while the vulva is 2 cm or more in length. The labia vulvae are thick and the ventral commissure forms an acute angle.

In the sow the vagina, which is of small calibre, is about 10–12 cm long. The vulva is about 7 cm in length; the labia are thick and the dorsal commissure is rounded, but the ventral one forms a long, pointed projection.

The vagina in the bitch is relatively long and the vulva has thick labia which form a projecting pointed ventral commissure.

Clinical Examination of the Female Genital Organs

Clinical examination of the external genitalia in female animals is performed by direct inspection. The mucous membrane of the posterior vulva is exposed to view by parting the labia with the hands. The deeper parts of the vulva along with the vagina are examined by introducing a suitable vaginal speculum (Figs 172, 173), which also enables inspection of the external os of the uterine cervix to be performed. The interior of the vagina can also be palpated following the introduction of a finger or hand, according to the size of the animal. In the mare and cow the condition of the internal organs of

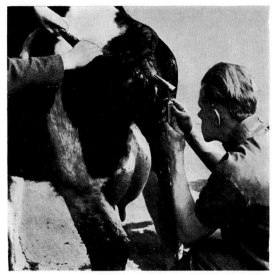

Fig. 172. *Examination of the vagina with the aid of an illuminated vaginoscope; the battery is in the handle. The operator is wearing a rubber gown suitable for rectal and vaginal examinations in large animals.*

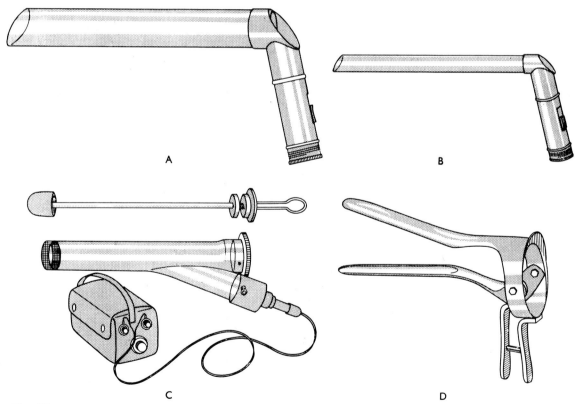

Fig. 173. *Instruments used for examining the vagina in large animals.* A, *Illuminated Perspex vaginoscope with battery handle (mare).* B, *Illuminated Perspex vaginoscope for the cow.* C, *Illuminated Perspex vaginoscope with detachable battery for the cow.* D, *A metal vaginal speculum.*

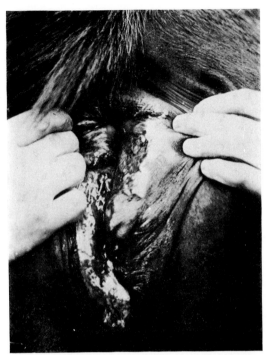

Fig. 174. *Rectovaginal laceration in a mare; a recent case. The condition is by no means a rare accident during foaling.*

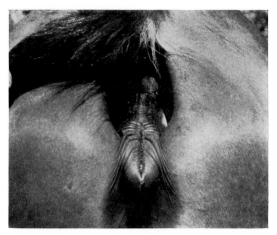

Fig. 175. *Horizontal or sinking vulva in a mare. This usually occurs in old mares and predisposes to pneumovagina.*

reproduction can be determined by means of rectal exploration.

By simple elevation of the tail, abnormalities of the vulva and vagina may be revealed, including severe rectovaginal laceration in the mare (Fig. 174), and horizontal or sinking vulva which predisposes to pneumovagina in old mares (Fig. 175). Developmental defects involving the vestibule are relatively rare in mares. Persistent hymen, which occurs very occasionally, is generally only recognized when a careful examination is made. This condition is more frequently observed in heifers, in which it may not be recognized until, during parturition, hymenal remnants impede the birth of the calf. Persistent hymen is commonly associated with failure of development of all or various portions of the genital tract, including occlusion of the external os of the cervix, absence of the cervix or anterior vagina, prominence of the Mullerian ducts and aplasia of the uterus to varying degrees. The various states are classified under so-called 'white heifer' disease, which is considered to be caused by a single, sex- and colour-linked gene.

The syndrome has been observed in all breeds of cattle.

At an early stage, after puberty has been reached, persistent hymen may be confused with freemartinism, which is indicated externally by a degree of hypoplasia of the vulva and vagina and a prominent clitoris. In the vast majority of freemartins the history indicates that the affected animal, which is essentially neuter rather than female, was born twin to a bull calf. Observations indicate, however, that in only 5% of heifers born twin to a male calf does the freemartin condition occur. Associated anomalies of the internal genitalia include hypoplasia of the ovaries, Fallopian tubes, uterus and cervix. The most acceptable theoretical explanation for the origin of the condition is that it arises from endocrine influence, brought about because in 95% of bovine heterozygous twin fetuses the chorionic blood circulations anastomose. The earlier development of the male gonads leads to the secretion of hormones which suppress the development of the female genital organs. The condition is of some economic significance because affected animals are sterile, so that it is useful to recognize it as early as possible. A simple method of achieving this is to measure the length of the vagina by inserting the closed end of an ordinary 15 × 1·5 cm testtube. In the freemartin the tube can usually only be inserted about half its length compared with almost the full length in the normal heifer.

Vaginal prolapse, which may be of varying severity, is readily observed, more particularly

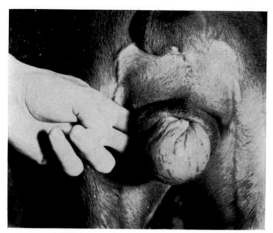

Fig. 176. *Vaginal hyperplasia in a bitch. The protruding mass consists mainly of oedematous mucous membrane.*

when the animal is lying down, and usually occurs during late pregnancy in cattle and sheep, less frequently in bitches. Imperforate hymen in the heifer may present a somewhat similar clinical picture. Vaginal hyperplasia (Fig. 176), which may be confused with vaginal prolapse, occurs in bitches and is frequently observed subsequent to oestrum. The dome-shaped mass arising from the floor of the vagina becomes so large that it protrudes between the lips of the vulva. In this case entry into the vagina is possible only over the dorsal aspect of the mass, whereas in prolapsed vagina entry is achieved through the centre of the mass.

The external parts of the reproductive system are examined for the presence of any indication of past or existing disease which might occur in the form of an eruption, depigmented areas or vaginal discharge. The vaginal mucosa is examined for evidence of hyperaemia, papules, vesicles, haemorrhage, signs of trauma, etc.

Acute vaginitis and vulvitis are comparatively rare conditions in the mare. They occur characteristically in coital exanthema (vesicular venereal disease) in which numerous small vesicles (3 mm in diameter) develop in the mucous membrane, later becoming pustules and then small ulcers. The vulva is congested, swollen and irritated so that the affected mare stands with elevated tail and arched back, swishes the tail, stamps the feet, strains and urinates frequently. The associated whitish discharge causes soiling of the buttocks and tail. Other causes of acute vaginitis and vulvitis include trauma which can occur during mating or parturition; in such cases the injury is located in the anterior vagina. Chronic

vaginitis is common in the mare, occurring in pneumovagina (wind-sucking) which is most prevalent in aged, multiparous animals. In affected mares it is usual to find that the vulva and pelvic ligaments are greatly relaxed during oestrus; otherwise a sunken anus with the lips of the vulva pulled into a horizontal position (Fig. 175), is a common clinical sign. Laceration, stretching and tearing of the muscles of the vulva or the perineum during parturition are other causes. The vestibular mucosa shows signs of irritation and a discharge is obvious at the ventral commissure of the vulva. In more severe cases ballooning of the vagina is usual, with some faeces in the vulva and vagina. A similar situation exists in rectovaginal fistula, in which condition faeces pass freely from the rectum to the vagina where they accumulate.

Female cattle affected with infectious pustular vulvovaginitis exhibit clinical signs similar to those occurring in coital exanthema in mares. In occasional cases the lesions extend from the vulva to the adjacent areas of the perineum. Granular vaginitis (granular venereal disease) occurs in cattle of all ages, but is generally most severe in heifers. The major clinical signs consist of small nodules (1–2 mm in diameter) composed of lymphoid tissue situated beneath the epithelium of the vulva. In severe cases the mucous membrane is uniformly congested, and there is a small quantity of mucopurulent exudate. The specificity of the condition is in doubt. A chronic, contagious venereal disease affecting the anterior vagina, with a tendency to spread to the uterus, occurs only in South Africa. The condition, known as infectious infertility or epivag, is caused by a virus, which is spread during coitus. The initial signs consist of an odourless, mucopurulent discharge from the vulva with reddish-purple areas in the mucosa of the anterior vagina. Although vaginitis occurs in the early stages of *Trichomonas foetus* infection, the clinical signs are never very obvious and do not appear in the majority of affected animals. Other causes of vaginitis in cattle include trauma, retained placenta and prolapse of the vagina. A severe form of vaginitis occurs in sheep affected with ulcerative dermatosis when the disease assumes a venereal character and is transmitted by the ram during coitus. In this case, the lesions commence at the ventral commissure of the vulva and may develop to involve the whole extent of the labia, giving rise to oedema. The vagina is not usually affected. Vaginitis is sometimes a feature in sows affected with pyelonephritis. Vaginitis and vulvitis are fairly common in the bitch; when the vagina is involved, so is the vulva, but the vulva can be affected alone. The inflamed mucous membrane is hyperaemic with small, red, elevated nodules present. The hyperaemia and exudation cause swelling of the vulva. In severe cases the animal is restless, strains after urinating, constantly licks the vulva, and may manifest a desire to copulate but not always permit its completion.

Internal Genitalia

The ovaries in the mare are bean-shaped being about 7–8 cm long and 2–3 cm thick. They are situated in the sublumbar region ventral to the fourth or fifth lumbar vertebra in contact with the lateral wall of the abdomen. The Fallopian tubes originate from the vicinity of the ovaries and are continuous with the uterus posteriorly; when normal they cannot be identified by rectal palpation. The uterus forms a hollow muscular organ consisting of two horns (cornua), a body and a neck. The uterine horns are situated entirely in the abdomen where they are most commonly pushed up against the sublumbar muscles by the intestines. They are cylindrical in cross-section and about 25 cm long. The dorsal or attached border is somewhat concave and is attached by the broad ligament (mesometrium) to the sublumbar region. The ventral border is convex and unattached. The body of the uterus is situated partly in the abdomen and partly in the pelvis; it forms a cylinder which is flattened dorsoventrally with an average length of 18–20 cm and a diameter of about 10 cm. The neck (cervix) is about 5–7 cm long and 2–3 cm in diameter, and at its posterior part it projects into the vagina. The body of the uterus is attached to the pelvic walls by the uterine broad ligament.

The ovaries of the cow are smaller than those of the mare, measuring 3 cm long and about 2 cm wide. They are situated near the middle of the lateral margin of the pelvic inlet, anterior to the external iliac artery, in parous animals they are usually further forwards. The Fallopian tubes have similar relationships as in the mare. The uterus, in adult cattle, lies almost entirely within the abdomen; the horns average about 38 cm in length and the body only about 3 cm long, although externally it appears to be 12–15 cm long because the posterior part of the horns are closely united by connective and muscular tissue. The free part of each horn forms a spiral coil deviating forwards and outwards from the body, then downwards and outwards and finally backwards and upwards. The cervix is about 10 cm long with a dense wall 2 cm thick. The lumen of the cervix (cervical canal) forms a spiral canal. The supporting broad ligaments are attached, one on each side, to the upper part of the flank about 10 cm below the tuber coxae. The internal genital organs of the ewe, in general, resemble those of the cow.

The ovaries in the sow are concealed in the ovarian bursae; their situation is near the lateral margin of the pelvic inlet, as in the cow, but in parous animals they may be located 2–5 cm behind the kidney. The uterine horns are long, flexuous and freely movable because of the long broad ligament. The non-pregnant uterus has an appearance like small intestine: it is arranged in coils and may be 120–140 cm long. The body is only 5 cm or so in length. The cervix, which is directly continued by the vagina, is 10 cm long.

The ovaries in the bitch are situated about 1–2 cm posterior to the corresponding kidney, so that they are about half-way between the last rib and the iliac crest, opposite to the third or fourth lumbar vertebra. Each ovary is concealed in its ovarian bursa. The uterine horns are 12–15 cm long, very narrow and lie entirely within the abdomen. The body is about 2 cm long and the cervix is very short.

In the larger species of domestic animals the necessity to examine the uterus and other internal organs of reproduction arises mainly in connection with reproductive performance, which may be impaired by reason of clinically recognizable organic, as well as functional, disease. There are several important principles which would be applied when it is necessary to undertake such examinations. Care should be taken to determine the health status of the stud, herd or flock in order that the existence of an infectious disease is not overlooked when dealing with individual animals. Then at all stages of the examination procedure, precautions are necessary to avoid spreading infection to healthy in-contact animals, or to those on other premises. These include the use of readily washable (see Fig. 142, p. 152) or disposable overalls, rubber boots and shoulder-length gloves, in conjunction with the liberal use of an effective antiseptic.

By means of rectal palpation the condition of

the uterus in the mare and in adult female cattle can be determined in relation to pregnancy and certain disease conditions. Prior to commencing the examination, details of the breeding history of the individual animal in relation to oestrum and mating should be obtained. The form of mating, whether natural or by artificial insemination, might also be pertinent. In the mare, the early phase of pregnancy is characterized by the appearance of a tangerine-sized bulge in the lower part of the uterine horn. At the end of the second month the enlargement, which is about the size of a football, involves the body of the uterus, and may be confused with the urinary bladder. Later, between the fourth and fifth months, the gravid uterus is pulled downwards and forwards to the floor of the abdomen. Changes in the vagina and cervix are of very doubtful value as an aid in recognizing pregnancy in the mare.

Numerous laboratory tests are available for determining pregnancy in mares. Two main types of test are in general use. That for the detection of serum gonadotrophins is a biological test, based on the response shown by the ovaries in a sexually mature animal, such as the rabbit. It is claimed to be 90% accurate between days 45 and 100 of pregnancy. The chemical tests in general use are various modifications of the Cuboni test which detects the presence of oestrogens in urine. An accuracy of 90% has been claimed for the period from 100 days after conception until near parturition.

Infection of the uterus and cervix is quite common in mares. A variety of bacteria can act as specific causes, including *Streptococcus genitalium, Klebsiella genitalum, Escherichia coli, Pseudomonas pyocyanea, Salmonella abortivoequina, Shigella equirulis, Corynebacterium equi* and others. The inflammatory reaction may be acute or chronic in intensity, but the metritis usually remains localized, and systemic signs are unusual. Discharge from the vulva is not a uniform feature. When the cervix is involved it is enlarged, bright red in colour and has a somewhat oedematous appearance. As a rule a discharge collects in the vagina below the cervix and may be observed seeping from the external os. The abnormal signs tend to be more pronounced during oestrum. Pyometra is a rare condition in the mare and is often associated with atresia of the cervix. It is differentiated from pregnancy by noting the thin, flaccid and atonic

state of the uterine wall, the indefinite shape of the organ and its dough-like consistency.

Early pregnancy in cattle is indicated by detecting the presence of a slightly turgid, somewhat spherical swelling in one uterine horn. This rapidly extends along the horn, so that there is an obvious disparity in size between the two horns. That the increase in the diameter of the cornu is the result of pregnancy is confirmed by gripping the uterine wall between the fingers and thumb and lifting it in an upwards direction. When a degree of tension exists and the grip is gently relaxed, the amniotic vesicle will be felt slipping away by the tugging movement it imparts to the uterine wall which is still being grasped. Distension of the uterus will occur when fluid collects under circumstances other than pregnancy. The fluid may be watery or thick in consistency; in the latter case it may be purulent. In these circumstances the wall of the uterus feels leathery, is less resilient and the cotyledonary excrescences of pregnancy cannot be palpated.

The freemartin state should be suspected when one or both ovaries are absent, and the uterus shows only partial development. Hypoplasia (infantilism) of the reproductive organs, although relatively rare, occurs most frequently in heifers of beef breeds. Abnormal development of the genitalia is a well-known state in so-called 'white heifer disease'. In typical cases, apart from the short vulva and vagina, the cervix is abnormal and the uterine horns tubular, with fluid-filled sacculations which could be confused with pregnancy.

Acute endometritis in cattle, occurring as a postparturient infection, is a cause of profound toxaemia. In the advanced stages the affected animal remains lying down, so causing confusion with parturient paresis. In all such cases it is pertinent, as an aid to differential diagnosis, to determine from the history the interval since parturition and to perform a vaginal and rectal examination, in order to ascertain the condition of the uterus. As a rule one horn is larger than the other. On inspection the cervix is usually inflamed, but the presence of discharge in the anterior vagina is not a constant feature. In less severe cases of endometritis the abnormal features are less obvious. Chronic metritis, which is usually accompanied by cervicitis, may be purulent or non-purulent in character. In the former there is often a purulent discharge in the vagina, large quantities of which are retained in the uterus so that it is displaced over the brim of the pelvis. The cervix, if palpable, is usually enlarged and feels indurated. Chronic purulent metritis is caused mainly by *Corynebacterium pyogenes* or *Trichomonas foetus* infection. Other specific infections of the uterus in cattle include brucellosis and vibriosis. The former, which is caused by *Brucella abortus*, is manifested clinically by abortion, while the latter, caused by *Vibrio fetus*, gives rise to infertility, with an abortion incidence of between 5 and 30%. Other specific causes of abortion in cattle include *Trichomonas foetus, Leptospira pomona, Listeria monocytogenes, Salmonella* spp., *Aspergillus* spp., *Absidia* spp. and a virus of the psittacosis–lymphogranuloma group. The severity of the metritis caused by these agents is related to the age of the fetus when death occurs, and whether or not the placenta is retained. Specific diagnosis is based upon macroscopic and microscopic examination of aborted fetuses and/or placentae, coupled with cultural investigations or retrospective serological examinations.

In the smaller species of domestic animals, including the sheep and bitch, pregnancy may be recognized by means of abdominal palpation. Otherwise, in the sow and sheep, failure to show oestrum following mating and, in the later stages of gestation, obvious mammary gland development occurring in association with an increase in the size of the abdomen, are some of the criteria commonly relied upon. Inflammation of the uterus (metritis) in the sow often occurs following abortion, dystocia or farrowing. Affected sows are febrile and inappetant with some of the mammary glands hot, swollen and oedematous. The associated vulval discharge varies in character from whitish-yellow to watery, serohaemorrhagic and foul-smelling. Metritis results from retained fetuses, or laceration or pressure necrosis caused during assisted parturition. The well-known puerperal fever syndrome occurring in sows will be discussed at a later stage in this section. Abortion and stillbirth in sows are recognized to be important causes of economic loss in pigs of preweaning age. The causes remain largely undetermined, surveys revealing specific infectious agents in less than 30% of abortions.

In sheep infection of the uterus is more easily established in association with pregnancy, so that abortion is one of the most obvious clinical indicators. The specific micro-organisms involved include *Brucella melitensis, Br. abortus,*

Br. ovis, Vibrio fetus, Salmonella abortus ovis, S. typhimurium, Listeria monocytogenes, virus of psittacosis–lymphogranuloma group and *Toxoplasma gondii*. In those conditions, including vibriosis, enzootic virus abortion, listeriosis and salmonellosis, in which retention of the placenta is a not unusual sequel to abortion, the incidence of metritis is considerable. Specific diagnosis depends upon the results of microscopic and/or cultural examination of aborted fetuses or placentae, or retrospective serological examinations.

In bitches, provided there is no undue resentment to abdominal palpation, pregnancy can be diagnosed between the fourth and fifth weeks after conception by identifying the spherical enlargements spaced along the uterine horns, and which are about 2–4 cm in diameter. Later, the uterus is difficult or impossible to identify because, although the organ increases in size, the fetal enlargements become confluent and as the fetal fluids increase in volume there is less resistance to pressure. In advanced pregnancy, abdominal palpation of the fetus is possible in many instances. From the end of the seventh week after conception, until the termination of pregnancy, radiographic examination will reveal pregnancy, because at this stage sufficient mineralization of the skeletal structure has taken place to produce a diagnostic radiograph. Pseudocyesis (phantom pregnancy), which is considered to result from the action of excess luteinizing hormone arising from delayed regression of the corpora lutea during metoestrus, is frequently confused with pregnancy. In many cases, differentiation is only readily made by radiographic examination, which is undertaken when the clinical signs become obvious 60–70 days following oestrus. At this time bitches so affected exhibit all the signs of approaching parturition.

Acute metritis in the bitch is a sequel to abortion or some abnormal event in relation to whelping, such as retained fetus or placenta, injudicious instrumentation or malpractice by lay persons during whelping. Affected bitches are severely toxaemic, and a dark, foetid, mucopurulent discharge can be observed escaping from the vagina. The history of the recent events, and the clinical condition of the animal, coupled with inspection of the cervix by means of an illuminated vaginal speculum, will indicate the site and nature of the trouble.

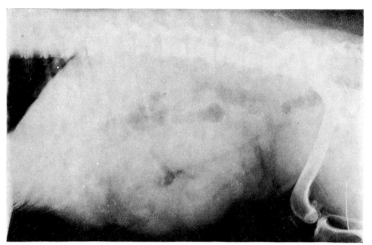

Fig. 177. *A radiograph showing marked distension of the uterus in a bitch affected with cystic endometrial hyperplasia (pyometra).*

Hyperplastic endometritis (pyometra) causes a variable degree of uterine enlargement which may be saccular in character. It is most prevalent in older bitches, usually occurring 1–2 months following oestrus, and is often associated with pseudocyesis. The abdomen increases in size, proportionately to the distension of the uterus, and may become pendulous. In the advanced stages toxaemia may develop, the indications consisting of depression and vomiting. The enlarged uterine horns, which are visualized radiographically (Fig. 177), can often be palpated posterior to the costal arch and towards the ventral part of the abdomen, and the vulva is usually swollen, although vaginal discharge or vaginitis is not a constant feature. Although not constantly present, bacteria such as *Escherichia coli* and *Staphylococcus aureus* may invade the damaged uterus and produce metritis. Cystic endometrial hyperplasia . is thought to result from the sequential changes in ovarian activity leading to endocrine imbalance, with overactivity by progesterone being a major factor. The use of progestational compounds to suppress oestrus in bitches, has, in recent years, caused cystic endometrial hyperplasia to occur in young bitches.

Mammary Glands and Teats

Anatomical Considerations

The mammary glands in the mare are two in number and are situated in the prepubic region.

Each gland forms a short cone which is transversely flattened. The teat, which constitutes the apex of each gland, has a transversely flattened pyramidal shape. There are usually two small lactiferous duct orifices on the extremity of each teat. The superficial inguinal lymph nodes are situated between the base of each gland and the abdominal wall.

The mammary glands of the cow, normally four in number, are generally known as the udder. They are considerably larger than the mammary glands of the mare, and are somewhat ellipsoidal in shape. Each gland is attached to the abdominal wall by a suspensory ligament which extends backwards to become attached to the pelvic symphysis. The base of each of the two posterior glands is related to the supramammary lymph nodes. Each gland (quarter) has a single teat which is about 8 cm long and has a single lactiferous duct which opens at the apex of the teat through a narrow orifice (streak canal) surrounded by a sphincter. Towards the base of the teat, the lactiferous duct widens considerably to join the lactiferous sinus.

The mammary glands of the sheep, two in number, are roughly globular in shape; they are relatively large. In the sow the mammary glands, ten to fourteen in number, are arranged in two rows extending from the posterior part of the pectoral region to the prepubic region. Each teat —one to each gland—has two lactiferous ducts. The mammary glands of the bitch have a similar anatomical location to those of the sow. The teats are comparatively short, each having between six and twelve small duct orifices on their apex.

Clinical Examination of the Mammary Glands and Teats

Examination of individual mammary glands in the mare, sow, sheep and bitch, of each division of the udder (quarter) in cows and of each teat must be performed at separate stages. The supramammary (inguinal) lymph nodes, which are situated in the inguinal region or perineum, should be subjected to examination by palpation whenever possible if mammary disease is suspected. Inspection of the glands reveals the presence of swelling in mammary oedema and in mastitis (Fig. 178), and of reduction in size when lactation is in physiological abeyance or is reduced because of pathological change (chronic mastitis in cattle), as well as eruptions (see Fig. 48, p. 53), ulceration (see Fig. 52, p. 54) and superficial injuries, all of which are more common and obvious on the teats. Rupture of the suspensory ligament, a condition which occurs in older cows, is readily recognized by the dropped position of the udder as well as by the marked increase in size of all quarters. By means of palpation (Figs 179, 180) increased temperature, changes in consistency

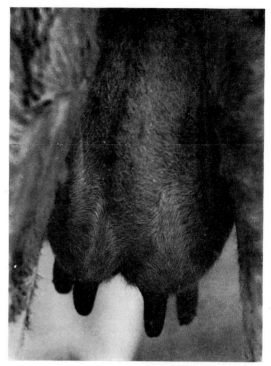

Fig. 178. *Chronic mastitis in a dairy cow, with enlargement of the right hindquarter of the mammary gland, which is nearly twice as large as the opposite quarter. Note the difference in level of the teats and the displacement of the midline of the udder towards the left.*

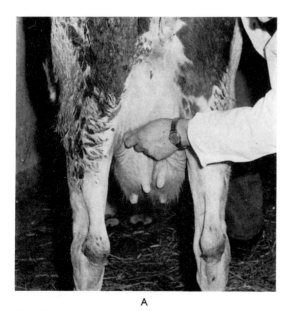

A

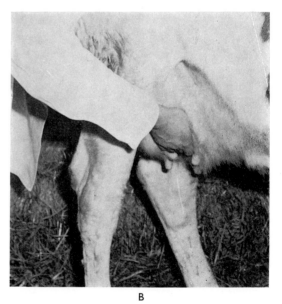

B

Fig. 179. *Examination of the udder in a cow. Note that the examination commences with inspection and palpation of the two hindquarters and is then continued in the same manner from the right side.*

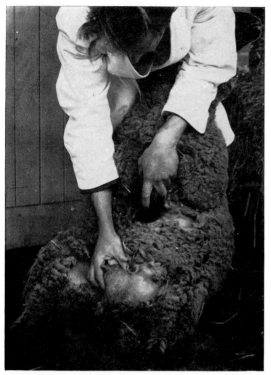

Fig. 180. *Examination of the udder of a ewe. Note that the animal's neck is held between the operator's left elbow and thigh and both forelegs in the left hand, thus leaving the right hand free.*

and texture of the gland and pain, which together suggest acute or subacute mastitis, and the deep nodular lesions associated with tuberculosis, chronic abscessation or neoplasia, can be recognized.

Mammary disease is relatively infrequent in mares. Pregnant mares, more particularly primipara, may develop extensive oedema of the udder and/or ventral abdominal wall 2–3 weeks before gestation terminates. The udder increases in size and becomes firm and painful. Later obvious oedema develops and extends along the ventral aspect of the abdomen, involving the subcutaneous tissues. Slight digital pressure causes pitting in the oedema areas. It is thought that hypoproteinaemia, by reducing the colloid osmotic property of the blood, thereby disturbing tissue fluid homeostasis, is an important causal factor for the condition.

Mastitis is of occasional occurrence and assumes acute or milder intensity. Its development may be associated with preceding oedema —in which instance, because of pain, the mare

discourages sucking by the foal—or with weaning. In both circumstances the presence of excessive amounts of mammary secretion provides a ready-made medium for bacterial growth. The bacterial flora associated with equine mastitis include *Streptococcus equi, Str. genitalium, Staphylococcus aureus, Escherichia coli*, etc. Mares with acute mastitis manifest systemic signs consisting of elevated temperature, increased pulse and respiratory rates, with anorexia, depression and stiffness of gait. Occasional cases of equine mastitis arise as a complication of strangles in the foal, the infection being transferred to the mammary gland in the nasal discharge. Cultural examination of mammary secretion from cases of mastitis will yield a specific diagnosis. Specimen samples should be collected in the manner described for the procedure in cows.

Through the medium of selective breeding for high milk yield, the udder of the present-day dairy cow, in comparison with that of other animals, is very large. Because of this factor, and also because its position exposes it to traumatic influences, it is frequently the site of disease. In this context also, the process of milking, more particularly mechanical milking, is of considerable significance. As a consequence of these factors the incidence of mastitis in cows in dairy herds is quite high. Milk of bovine origin is an important article of human food, consequently early clinical recognition of mastitis is of economic significance.

Examination of the udder consists of detailed inspection and systematic palpation followed by macroscopic, and when considered necessary, chemical and cultural examination of milk samples. Inspection of the udder should include viewing the hindquarters from behind the animal (Fig. 178) by grasping and pulling the tail to one side with the right hand. When the two hindquarters are revealed in this way they should be compared in respect of size and symmetry, and the direction and level of the teats observed. Observation is aided by grasping the skin over the posterior aspect of the glands with the left hand and lifting in an upward direction (Fig. 179A). The two forequarters may be brought into view by this means, provided the udder is not too pendulous. The two quarters on the same side of the body should be examined and compared in this manner. It is necessary, when making a closer examination of the teats—this part of the examination should never be omitted —to bend down on the milking side and, by grasping each teat individually, carry out careful palpation of the whole structure, paying particular attention to the lactiferous duct and sinus. Then the teat should be pulled laterally so that the condition of the surface skin can be ascertained, including that of the tip in the vicinity of the sphincter. Palpation of each mammary gland involves consideration of the more superficial, as well as of the deeper parts. For this purpose both hands (Fig. 179B) should be employed. In high-yielding cows, and heifers and cows with mammary oedema, which is noted to occur in late pregnancy and persists for a few weeks following calving, the groove between the lateral aspect of the udder and the medial aspect of the thigh should be examined for evidence of frictional dermatitis. Other conditions affecting the skin of the udder that would be revealed in this way include udder impetigo and cutaneous gangrene. The lesions in both of these diseases develop on the skin of the udder at the base of the teats, and show a tendency to spread to the teats and, less frequently, to other parts of the udder.

Inspection of the udder in the manner described reveals any disproportion in the size of the diametrically opposed quarters, which is generally taken to be an indication of mastitis. Enlargement or swelling occurs in acute and subacute mastitis, and in tuberculous mastitis. Reduction in the size of any gland is an indication of atrophy which is the result of induration and fibrosis; it is a characteristic feature of advanced chronic mastitis. The incidence of mastitis increases with age in dairy cows; this is probably an expression of increased patency of the teat sphincter and/or injury to the streak canal (teat orifice). Inspection of the apex of the teat in machine-milked cattle is a useful aid in determining the functional efficiency of the mechanical equipment. When the teats are exposed to excessive vacuum (more than 40 cmHg), or extreme fluctuations in vacuum pressure, the terminal portion of the streak canal becomes everted; this is recognized in the form of a circular, blanched area, about 0·5 cm in diameter, with shallow radiating fissures.

In all acute and subacute forms of mastitis, palpation will reveal the presence of heat, swelling and pain, which vary in degree according to the intensity of the inflammatory reaction.

The degree of systemic involvement is also related to the severity of the mammary disease, and is indicated by elevated temperature, increased respiratory and pulse rates, and loss of appetite. In the advanced stages of so-called 'summer mastitis' and of acute gangrenous mastitis, toxaemia causes profound depression with apathy, recumbency and subnormal temperature. In acute gangrenous mastitis the affected quarter and teat are initially swollen and hot. Within a matter of hours the teat becomes cold, and a sharply demarcated blue discoloration develops in the skin of the teat, and over a variable portion of that covering the gland. The associated changes in the character of the gland secretion are readily appreciated.

Chronic bovine mastitis is not responsible for a systemic reaction; acute or more usually, subacute mastitis, may, however, develop as the result of a flare-up of a chronic infection. Otherwise chronic mastitis is characterized by extending induration which usually commences in the vicinity of the lactiferous sinus. Changes in the physical character of the foremilk, which are continuous or intermittent, in the form of clots, flakes, pus or watery appearance, are the most typical features of chronic mastitis.

Acute and subacute mastitis may be caused by *Staphylococcus aureus*, *Escherichia coli*, *Streptococcus agalactiae*, *Str. dysgalactiae*, *Str. uberis* and *Aerobacter aerogenes*. Rare outbreaks have been attributed to *Klebsiella pneumoniae*, *Nocardia asteroides*, *Mycoplasma* spp. and fungi including *Cryptococcus neoformans*, *Candida* spp., etc. Fungal mastitis has been noted to occur following intramammary antibiotic therapy for bacterial mastitis in a number of instances.

Chronic mastitis not infrequently develops as a sequel to an acute attack and may therefore be caused by any of the specific agents enumerated above. In many cases, however, the affection is clinically mild from the outset; a large proportion of such cases may in fact have resulted from an infected condition of the udder established some considerable time before clinical signs are noted. These 'latent' infections are of considerable importance in relation to the spread of infection in the herd. Although chronic mastitis caused by *Mycobacterium tuberculosis* is rarely seen nowadays because of the success of bovine tuberculosis eradication programmes, its detection and diagnosis still requires consideration. In the early stages of the disease the lesions are frequently impossible to recognize by means of mammary palpation. If infection has gained entry via the teat duct, nodular thickening may develop in the tissues surrounding the lactiferous sinus at the apex of the gland. Later, when the disease has progressed, the affected gland becomes enlarged and indurated. In advanced cases, the enlargement assumes considerable proportions, obviously destroying the normal symmetry of the udder, and on palpation the normal rather regular lobulation is replaced by irregular nodulation. Certain other acid-fast bacteria, including *Mycobacterium lacticola*, have on rare occasions been found to produce similar effects which, however, are not usually permanent. Occasional cases of tuberculous mastitis assume rather acute proportions, more often during the later stages when rapid spread is occurring.

The organic status of the mammary tissues in milking cows can be most thoroughly investigated by examination of the secretion. In all instances the initial procedure is to employ the strip cup for the detection of visible particles and other physical changes in the foremilk. This procedure provides the opportunity to assess the patency of the streak canal. The regular use of the strip cup should be recognized as an important procedure in the early identification of clinical cases of mastitis. When normal milking procedures cause pain because of the existence of teat lesions, or there is traumatic injury involving the apex of the teat, milk samples can be obtained with the aid of a sterilized teat syphon. Abnormality of the milk may be detectable with the naked eye, or a special examination may be required. The colour, smell and consistency should be noted. In a proportion of cows and goats, early in the lactation period, varying amounts of blood may occur in the milk, in the absence of any readily recognizable lesions of disease. It is probable that many such cases are the result of trauma to which the udder is more freely exposed, because of its greater size, at a time when it is highly vascularized. Blood will appear in the milk in poisoning by coumarin derivatives and by dicoumarol, and in *Leptospira pomona* infection; in these instances the milk from all four quarters is affected.

In acute mastitis the secretion of the affected gland is scanty and, when it has been drawn, assumes a straw-coloured appearance like serum, with a clot. Large numbers of erythrocytes give the secretion a reddish tinge. Gangrenous mastitis, usually caused by *Staph. aureus* infection, is associated with suppression of secretion and a small amount of blood-stained fluid which later becomes darker in colour.

The changes in the character of the mammary secretion in chronic mastitis vary from the obvious to those which can only be detected by means of the strip cup or a chemical test. The most characteristic feature is the presence of flakes and clots in the foremilk, which may occur intermittently or in a persistent pattern. When clots are present, the foremilk often has a thin, watery appearance. The macroscopic appearance of the secretion in tuberculous mastitis varies according to the extent of mammary involvement. In the early stages it appears normal, no recognizable change occurring until the disease process is well established throughout the quarter, at which time the secretion becomes thin and watery in appearance. When the disease process is more active, the secretion, at least in the later stages, assumes a greyish-yellow colour with a heavy, flocculent deposit which settles out on standing; otherwise, at this stage, it consists of a small volume of honey-coloured secretion.

The odour of the mammary secretion is characteristically foetid in dry cows and pregnant heifers affected with 'summer mastitis'. A number of bacteria including *Str. dysgalactiae*, *C. pyogenes* and *Micrococcus indolicus* have been incriminated in the aetiology. It is contended that *M. indolicus* is responsible for the unpleasant odour. Cases of 'summer mastitis' occur in which the abnormal secretion does not have the foetid odour, and *C. pyogenes* is also capable of causing mastitis in lactating cows.

When a milk sample is required for laboratory examination, particularly in relation to the recognition of mastitis, it should be collected with due regard to the necessity to avoid all extraneous contamination. After washing and drying the udder, the foremilk from the affected quarter is discarded into the strip cup, and then the tip of the teat is wiped clean with a swab of cotton wool moistened with 70% alcohol and allowed to dry. The milk sample is then drawn into a suitable wide-mouthed screw-capped bottle which is held in an almost horizontal position (Fig. 181). Care should be taken to prevent any part of the animal from coming into contact with the sample bottle or tube, and the cap should be replaced while the container is in the horizontal position. If samples are required from all four quarters in

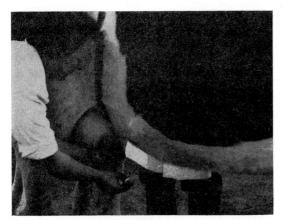

Fig. 181. *Collection of a milk sample required for bacteriological investigation. Note that the sample bottle is held in an almost horizontal position to avoid contamination with extraneous particles. An udder kinch is in use to prevent kicking; this is rarely necessary in a healthy dairy cow, but may be required when the udder is inflamed and painful.*

any individual animal, they should be taken from the two nearest quarters first, in order to avoid contaminating the ends of the teats by reaching across to the quarters on the far side. Samples of milk for examination from cases of suspected tuberculous mastitis should consist of about 200 ml of strippings.

Laboratory Examination of Milk Samples

The examination of milk samples in the laboratory consists of the application of physical and chemical tests (indirect) and, to make these procedures most effective, microscopic and cultural examination (direct test) (whenever advisable the latter should be followed by an *in-vitro* antibiotic sensitivity determination for any specific pathogen that may be isolated). Some of the chemical tests have been modified to make them suitable for field use. Changes in the physical quality of milk may be sufficiently gross as to be recognized by means of the strip cup. Chemical tests are adopted in order to determine the pH, and changes in chloride concentration and in the number of inflammatory cells in the milk. The pH of normal milk varies between 6·4 and 6·8; in mastitis, because the concentrations of lactose and casein are reduced, and sodium chloride and sodium bicarbonate are increased, the milk is more alkaline. Similar changes occur towards the termination of lactation. The pH of milk can be determined by means of a series of

chemical indicators including bromcresol purple, bromthymol blue, etc. The indicators are available in liquid form or as impregnated paper strips. A rapid field test for determination of milk chlorides is available, but results are difficult to interpret because colostrum and late lactation milk have elevated chloride levels as well as mastitic and physiologically suppressed milk.

An inflammatory reaction occurring in the mammary gland, irrespective of whether its cause is specific or traumatic in character, is associated with a cellular reaction which varies in intensity and character. Consequently an increased number of neutrophil leucocytes, as well as other cells, will be present in milk under such circumstances. It is possible to determine the number of leucocytes per millilitre of milk by microscopic examination of a suitably prepared and stained smear. The technique demands high standards of exactitude and is laborious. Milk from healthy udders rarely contains more than 500 000 cells/ml; samples from diseased quarters may have cell counts of the order of several millions.

Although a catalase determination will indicate roughly the number of tissue cells present in a milk sample, the test is of no practical value because mastitis milk cannot be differentiated from colostrum or late lactation milk by this means. In order to overcome the technical disadvantages of the cell counting method, chemical tests have been evolved which, although less accurate, lend themselves to field application. Of these, the modified Whiteside test, one of the first to be developed, is claimed to give a reaction —the milk separating into flakes and shreds or a viscous gel with a watery background in positive cases on the addition of normal (4%) sodium hydroxide—which is closely correlated to the total leucocyte count. The reaction varies in degree according to the amount of desoxyribonucleic acid (DNA) released from the cells. The presence of milk fat appears to be an essential factor in the test which can, therefore, be performed on a sample from the bulk milk of individual cows. A modification of the Whiteside test (Negretti) has been developed for field use.

The so-called California mastitis test (CMT) employs a reagent consisting of an anionic detergent which, when diluted to a standard concentration, reacts with DNA liberated from cells in milk. The inclusion of bromcresol purple in the reagent is helpful in recognizing pH changes in the milk. A variety of anionic detergents have been found to be satisfactory provided the method is standardized. The results of the test, which can be applied to foremilk, strippings, or mixed bucket or bulk samples, are calibrated as follows:

Trace	Slight precipitate forms which dissolves with mixing
1+	Slimy gel forms
2+	Gel becomes thick and flocculent
3+	Gel becomes viscous and tacky

With foremilk from individual cows a 1+ reaction should be classified as suspicious and 2+ and 3+ reactions as indicating mastitis. A 1+ reaction with herd bulk milk suggest that at least 20% of the lactating cows have mastitis or that a large percentage of them are nearing the end of their lactations. Recent observations suggest that the most reliable results are obtained when the test is performed with milk drawn 3–5 hours after normal milking. The reactions occurring in the CMT have been correlated with cell counts as follows:

1+	400 000–1500 000 cells/ml
2+	800 000–5000 000 cells/ml
3+	> 5000 000 cells/ml

In performing the test about 3 ml of **milk** from each quarter are drawn into one of the four shallow cups of the paddle (Fig. 182), and then an equal volume of the test reagent is squirted from a squeeze bottle into each pool of milk. More certain results are obtained with an

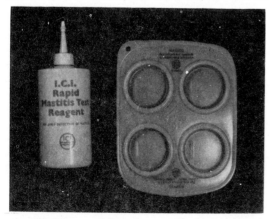

Fig. 182. *Plastic paddle and squeeze bottle of reagent for the California mastitis test. Note that the paddle has four shallow cups which can be marked to correspond to the four quarters of the udder, all of which can be examined simultaneously.*

excess of the reagent. The milk and reagent are mixed by gentle circular rotation of the paddle held horizontally. Milk more than 36 hours old, or which has undergone souring, is likely to give false negative reactions. The various modifications of the CMT include the Brabant test, the Michigan mastitis test and the Wisconsin test. Although the various types of CMT are subject to considerable personal error in performance and interpretation they are capable of detecting up to 90% of positive cases. It must also be appreciated that this type of test does not indicate the nature or degree of the infection, and also that the degree of reaction obtained in the test is not directly related to the numbers of bacteria. When, however, they are employed by experienced operatives these tests are the most efficient of the indirect tests for mastitis, and they are excellent screens for detecting problem herds and assessing the extent of the disease in an individual herd. The development of electronic cell counting equipment has enabled rapid and repeated screening of bulk milk to be undertaken in the laboratory; many such monitoring programmes are operated as part of a control scheme which includes economic penalties for high cell counts.

When the application of an indirect test reveals the presence of a significant proportion of disease in a herd, direct tests can then be employed to further elucidate the nature of the affection. Of the direct tests that can be applied, the incubated smear technique is the simplest and can be readily undertaken without the need for expensive equipment. If milk samples, collected in the recommended manner, are kept in a reasonably warm place for 24 hours most bacteria, with the exception of the tubercle bacillus, will multiply to a sufficient degree to be recognizable on a stained smear. The presence of inflammatory cells, especially neutrophil leucocytes, is of considerable assistance in interpreting the significance of organisms found under these circumstances. Newman's stain, which defats, fixes and stains bacteria and tissue cells, is recommended for use with this method. It is important to appreciate that reasonably satisfactory results (about 65% positive infections are identified) can only be expected when pretreatment milk samples are examined. The presence in the milk sample of any antibiotic, or other antibacterial chemotherapeutic residue, may retard or even completely inhibit bacterial growth unless drug resistance has been acquired.

Newman's stain consists of:

Methylene blue	1 g
Glacial acetic acid	6 ml
Tetrachlorethane	40 ml
Ethyl alcohol (95%)	54 ml

The staining procedure is simple and direct. After thoroughly mixing the milk sample a smear is made which is then dried slowly and flooded with the stain. The stain is allowed to act for 15 seconds and is then poured away and the slide is air dried before washing away the excess stain. The smear is then dried and prepared for microscopic examination in the usual way. This method is also satisfactory for staining smears for milk cell counts. In this case 0·01 ml of milk is spread over an area of 1 cm² on a microscope slide, which is then processed as described.

Isolation of bacteria from milk samples by cultural methods involves specialized laboratory procedures which, on economic grounds, are generally considered to be outside the scope of routine veterinary practice. The general availability of dried media, which are readily reconstituted and prepared for use, and packs of sterile disposable Petri dishes has made it possible for well-run practices to adopt such procedures. In addition prepared materials which are commercially available make it a relatively simple matter to undertake *in vitro* antibiotic sensitivity determinations.

The diagnosis of tuberculous mastitis is dependent upon recognizing *Mycobacterium tuberculosis*, by reason of its morphological features and staining characteristics, in suitably stained smears prepared from sediment obtained by centrifuging at least 50 ml of strippings from the suspect quarter. The search for tubercle bacilli is sometimes shortened if the microscopic examination is initially directed to finding epithelioid cell groups, and then concentrating on these areas in the smear. If confirmation is not obtained by this means then repeated examinations are necessary at short intervals, or a biological test should be considered. This is a laboratory procedure for which the guinea-pig is generally employed. For the test at least 120 ml of milk in the form of strippings are required in order to provide a reasonable quantity of deposit to inject into the animals. Although very efficient in detecting tubercle bacilli, the biological test does not provide an early answer. A tuberculin test is of little assistance in the differential diagnosis of tuberculous mastitis.

In sheep both acute and chronic forms of mastitis occur. As a rule the shorter the interval between lambing and the appearance of the disease the more likely it is to be severe in character. Acute mastitis is associated with signs indicating septicaemia or toxaemia. The degree of systemic involvement is probably greatest in acute gangrenous mastitis. The disease may occur in a sporadic or an enzootic pattern. In many cases its development is related to injury to the teat caused by the lamb, some mechanical injury or a lesion of a specific exanthematous disease, e.g. contagious pustular dermatitis (contagious ecthyma). Otherwise, towards the end of the normal rearing period, weaning the lambs or any other event, such as removing the fleece, which causes self-weaning and leads to retention of milk will predispose to chronic mastitis.

The bacteria associated with enzootic mastitis in sheep include *Pasteurella haemolytica, P. multocida, Staphylococcus aureus* (acute gangrenous mastitis), *Streptococcus uberis, Str. agalactiae, Escherichia coli* and *Corynebacterium pyogenes*. Sporadic mastitis is usually caused by streptococci, staphylococci, *E. coli* or *C. pyogenes*. The clinical signs and diagnostic methods are similar to those in cattle.

Mastitis in the goat is usually mild or chronic in intensity. The more important bacterial causes include *Str. agalactiae, Str. dysgalactiae, Str. pyogenes* and *Staph. aureus*.

Mastitis in sows occurs sporadically and is acute or, more rarely, chronic in intensity. Udder and teat injuries caused by the sharp canine teeth of nursing piglets is considered to provide a portal of entry for many of the bacteria which cause mastitis. Acute gangrenous mastitis caused by coliform infection usually develops rapidly and occurs within a few days after farrowing. Affected sows are severely toxaemic; temperature varies between subnormal and hyperthermic, appetite is absent, and there is great depression. A varying number of the inguinal and abdominal mammary glands are involved, being enlarged with blood-stained serous secretion, and the overlying skin is cyanosed. The extent of the skin discoloration depends on the degree of gangrene and is invariably followed by sloughing of the affected tissues. The specific bacterial causes include *Escherichia coli* and *Aerobacter aerogenes*. Other causes of mastitis in sows are *Streptococcus agalactiae*, *Str. dysgalactiae*, *Str. uberis*, *Sphaerophorus necrophorus*, *C. pyogenes* and *Staphylococcus aureus*; the last named is invariably associated with chronic mastitis, which in most cases involves one or a few only of the mammary glands, with no obvious indications of systemic involvement. In nursing sows chronically affected glands show reduced or complete absence of secretion, with permanent damage as a legacy. Infection with *Staph. aureus*, *Actinobacillus lignieresi*, *Actinomyces bovis* or *M. tuberculosis* often results in the development of granulomatous areas which progressively enlarge and involve the skin, so that the affected gland presents an appearance like a tumour, and becomes pendulous.

A puerperal syndrome consisting of fever, partial or complete anorexia and agalactia, the mammary glands being firm and congested, occurs occasionally as a herd problem in sows with, in some cases, a copious mucoid discharge from the vulva. The aetiology of the syndrome is not clear and although *Escherichia coli* and *Mycoplasma* spp. have been isolated from the uterine discharges and also from the mammary secretion, it is not certain that a primary metritis or mastitis occurs. Other causes of agalactia or hypogalactia in sows include absence of milk secretion, painful conditions of the teats, sharp teeth in the piglets, inverted nipples, which may have an hereditary origin, failure of milk let-down (noted especially in gilts) and excessive engorgement and oedema of the mammary glands. Partial or complete absence of milk flow in sows is important because young piglets are very susceptible to hypoglycaemia.

In the bitch mastitis occurs most frequently soon after whelping, at which time it is usually acute, although a chronic form of the disease is recognized. Traumatic damage, in the form of injury and bruising, may also act as a predisposing influence apart from whelping. One or more glands may be affected. In the acute form, and more particularly when it develops soon after parturition, it is usual for several glands to be involved. The systemic signs include elevated temperature, increased pulse and respiratory rates, and loss of appetite. Affected glands are hot, swollen and painful with hyperaemic dis-coloration. The gland secretion is abnormal in colour and consistency. In chronic mastitis the local changes mainly involve the secretion, although local abscesses may develop. The bacterial causes of mastitis in the bitch are variable and include staphylococci, streptococci and coliforms among others.

Functional disturbances of the mammary gland in the bitch are by no means uncommon and include galactostasis and agalactia. The former occurs in bitches when productive capacity exceeds the food demands of the puppies. The resulting back pressure leads to suppression of milk secretion. Agalactia occurs when there is inadequate mammary development or as the result of the suppressive action of a general anaesthetic in caesarean section.

Mammary Neoplasms

Tumours of the mammary gland are most frequently seen in the bitch, the incidence being highest in animals over 5 years of age. Occasionally gross enlargement of the supramammary lymph nodes occurs in cows affected with leucosis (lymphomatosis), giving an impression that there is a primary tumour of the udder. In the sow, chronic mastitis caused by *Actinomyces bovis*, *Staphylococcus aureus* or the tubercle bacillus may result in an enlarged pendulous gland which presents a tumour-like appearance. In the bitch, fibrocystic disease may be confused with mammary neoplasia, more especially because the former is a precancerous state so that both conditions may occur simultaneously. Fibrocystic disease affects mainly the inguinal and abdominal glands in the form of single or multiple thin-walled cysts which are small or large, and arise from the alveoli and ducts. The condition is most prevalent in bitches over 5 years of age.

Canine mammary tumours are benign or malignant and occur in many structural types. Benign neoplasms manifest mixed characteristics and are often composed of bone, cartilage, adenomatous gland tissue and fibrous tissue. Malignant tumours, which are relatively rare, may be recognized by their irregular contours and their tendency to metastasize and involve local nymph nodes and lungs. Because mammary neoplasms infrequently develop in ovariectomized bitches it is suggested that they are a product of endocrine fluctuation.

13

The Blood and Blood-forming Organs

The blood consists of a fluid medium with suspended cellular constituents, the latter being the product of the haematopoietic tissues, which is circulated round the body by the heart while being retained in the arteries and veins. The static blood cell forming organs comprise the bone marrow, liver, spleen, lymph nodes and the reticulo-endothelial tissues. The cellular elements are largely produced in these tissues, and the circulating blood comes directly or indirectly into intimate association with the vast majority of the functioning cells of the body. Its main functions are to supply oxygen, essential nutrients, enzymes, hormones, water and electrolytes and buffering systems to the tissue cells, and to remove the metabolic waste products as the first stage of their elimination from the body. In addition certain of the blood cells provide a defence mechanism against invasion of the body by living pathogenic agents. Even more significant protection against such agencies is provided by the immune globulins (Ig) of the circulating blood.

In spite of the relatively rapid changeover in the population of blood cells, due to a short life span, and the constant demands made for water, electrolytes and other constituents, the composition of the blood in normal animals is reasonably constant and falls within the fairly narrow limits, or normal range, that can be prescribed for any one particular species. This balancing mechanism is, however, very delicate and when disease exists in the body it is likely to produce changes in the composition of the blood of sufficient magnitude to cause the development of clinical signs or, alternately, to be recognized by means of appropriate laboratory techniques. Dysfunction of the blood is associated with circumstances such as a decrease in circulating blood volume, abnormalities of the cellular constituents, and abnormal variation in the non-cellular components including protein, electrolytes and buffering systems.

The study of the peripheral blood can provide significant information, additional to that resulting from the general clinical examination of the patient. Various techniques embodying many recent advances, including microanalysis, spectrophotometry, electrophoresis, enzyme determinations and the employment of radio-isotopes, are applicable to the study of the blood and blood-forming organs. Intelligent and informative evaluation of the results of such studies necessitates a knowledge of the normal range of the various cellular and non-cellular constituents in the blood of the various species of animals.

Blood Sampling

When a disease involving the blood is suspected to exist, or it is considered necessary to investigate the possibility that a significant change in blood composition exists in an animal, the blood can be subjected to examination. The methods of examination are of three main types, viz. haematological, biochemical and serological. The character of the examination considered necessary will dictate the type of sample required. The majority of haematological examinations are performed on unclotted samples, but in order to secure reasonable accuracy suitable anticoagulants must be used. When making blood smears for cell type differentiation, and where it is possible to perform dilution techniques in the presence of the animal, freshly withdrawn unclotted blood can be used. The biochemical group of examinations demand a

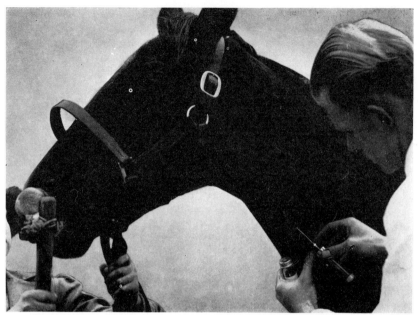

Fig. 183. *Collection of a blood sample of a horse. The jugular vein has been raised by a tourniquet round the neck and the operator is tensing the skin over the vein before inserting the needle. The barrel of a hypodermic syringe is being used as a handle. The animal is restrained by means of a twitch on the upper lip, held by a reliable assistant.*

variety of methods of treatment for blood, sampling depending upon the character of the test required. Laboratories which undertake to perform such tests will usually provide sample containers suitably prepared for particular biochemical determinations. Serological tests are, with few exceptions, usually undertaken with serum, so that clotted samples of blood are required in this case.

When collecting a blood sample from an animal it is essential to avoid exciting it, otherwise significant changes in composition may result, even in healthy animals. In addition, care is necessary in order to avoid too prolonged an application of pressure when raising a superficial vein, otherwise haemoconcentration may occur leading to an erroneous conclusion. The erythrocytes of the dog and ox are relatively fragile and prone to haemolysis unless a precise, expeditious technique is effected.

If only a small quantity of blood is required, as for blood smears, cell counts or haemoglobin determinations, it can be obtained by shaving an area on the outer surface of the pinna of the ear near the margin; then, after wiping the exposed skin with alcohol or ether and allowing it to dry, the marginal ear vein is visible and can be

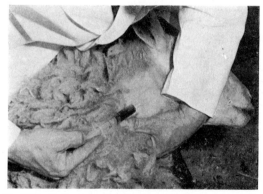

Fig. 184. *Collection of a blood sample from a sheep. The animal is placed with the hindquarters between the operator's feet and its withers are held tightly between the knees. The animal's head is restrained between the left arm and the body as shown. Pressure is applied with the left hand to distend the jugular vein.* (R. P. Lee (1956) Irish vet. J., *19*, 84)

punctured with a sharp-pointed surgical blade or needle. This method is suitable for all small animals including rabbits, mink, guinea pigs and chinchilla, and can be repeated as required. Shaving an area of interdigital skin, followed by incising a vein, made visible by spreading the foot over a suitable source of illumination, is a

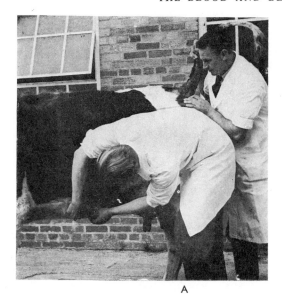

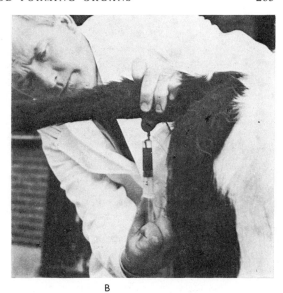

A   B

Fig. 185. *Collection of a blood sample from a cow.* A, *Mammary vein. Note that the operator keeps his back to the animal's hindquarters to avoid the risk of injury to the face or abdominal region should the cow kick forwards in spite of the holding up of the tail by an assistant.* B, *Middle coccygeal vein. Note that the needle is at a right angle to the tail.*

satisfactory method of obtaining blood in the ferret and mink.

When a larger quantity of blood is required venepuncture with a hypodermic needle and syringe is performed on any one of the superficial veins. The jugular vein is conveniently available in the horse, ox, sheep, goat and dog (Figs 183, 184); the subcutaneous abdominal (anterior mammary) vein is satisfactory in lactating cattle (Fig. 185A) provided a relatively small diameter needle (size 18 BWG) is used, otherwise there is a risk of haematoma formation. The middle coccygeal vein is also conveniently available in cattle. This method has a number of advantages in that very little restraint is required beyond elevating the tail as far as possible, the animal rarely becomes excited and it can be performed in most types of cow-bails and shutes. The site for insertion of the needle (size 18 BWG, 20 mm) is on the ventral aspect of either the second or third coccygeal intervertebral space posterior to the point where the tail joins the body (Fig. 185B). The needle is inserted at right angles to the tail to a depth of about 1 cm between the vertebrae and then withdrawn until a flow of blood is obtained. Lowering the tail slightly at this point may increase the flow of blood. The cephalic (radial) or recurrent tarsal (saphenous) vein is used in the cat and dog (Figs 186, 187), although for the dog experienced clinicians

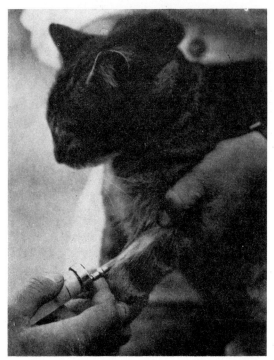

Fig. 186. *Collection of a blood sample from a cat. The cephalic vein is used. (This vein may also be used in the dog.) An assistant grasps the animal by the nape of the neck with the right hand, and holds the foreleg at the elbow with the left hand, raising the vein by pressure with the thumb. A 22 BWG needle and a syringe with an excentric nozzle are used.*

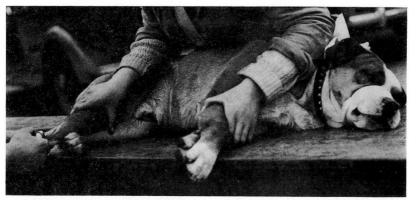

Fig. 187. *Collection of a blood sample from a dog (recurrent tarsal vein) (see also Fig. 186). The vein is raised by the assistant's grasp on the upper part of the hindleg. A tape muzzle has been applied. For all but very quiet dogs it is advisable to have two assistants —one to hold the hindlegs and the other the head and forelegs.*

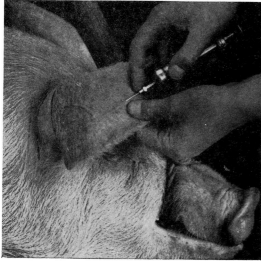

Fig. 188. *Collection of a blood sample from a pig. A twitch has been applied to the upper jaw. The ear veins have been raised by a rubber band around the base of the ear (the band is hidden by a fold of skin in this illustration). A 22 BWG needle and a syringe with an excentric nozzle are used.*

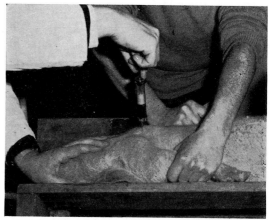

Fig. 189. *Collection of a blood sample from a pig using the anterior vena cava. The pig is restrained in dorsal recumbency with the head extended in a V-shaped trough. Note the direction of the needle, and that it is inserted in the right side.*

claim that the jugular vein is more readily entered. Pigs, which are usually difficult to restrain, are bled from an ear vein (Fig. 188), by amputation of the tip of the tail or by puncturing the middle coccygeal vein a little below the level of the anus.

More certain and uniform results are obtained when pigs are bled from the anterior vena cava. For this purpose small pigs are restrained by placing them in dorsal recumbency in a V-shaped trough (Fig. 189). Larger pigs are restrained in the standing position by means of a loop noose around the snout with the animal drawn up to a stout post or stanchion. An 18 or 20 BWG needle 6–8 cm long is attached to a hypodermic syringe and the point of the needle is inserted through the skin at a point varying from 1 to 5 cm, according to the size of the animal, from the apex of the cariniform cartilage, on a line extending from the extremity of the cartilage to the base of the ear. When the pig is in dorsal recumbency the point of the needle is directed medially downwards and backwards in the direction of the area between the first pair of ribs. If it is in the correct position the needle enters the anterior vena cava near the junction of the jugular veins and brachial veins.

Samples of blood can be obtained from rabbits, guinea pigs, mink, chinchilla, rats, etc. by means of cardiac puncture.

Whenever possible needles and hypodermic syringes used for blood sampling should be perfectly dry, otherwise haemolysis will occur. This stipulation is particularly important when the blood is to be collected directly into a hypodermic syringe. (Sterile disposable packs are ideal for the purpose; self-filling tubes (vacuumized) have the disadvantage that they cause haemolysis especially in canine and feline blood.) In an emergency a hypodermic syringe may be prepared by washing it out with 70% ethanol and then with ether. In all circumstances a separate needle and syringe should be used for each individual animal.

In undertaking puncture of a superficial vein, it is worth while to confirm that it is functional and patent by applying digital pressure for a few seconds until distension is detected. This marks the position of the vein so that the skin in the area can be prepared by clipping or shaving if necessary. It is impossible to sterilize the skin, but it is advisable to clean the area with surgical spirit or other suitable antiseptic in order to remove excess bacteria and debris. The antiseptic should be allowed to evaporate before proceeding to introduce the needle into the vein.

Except when the subcutaneous abdominal vein or the anterior vena cava is selected, it is generally necessary to distend the vein with blood by occluding it by the application of pressure with the fingers, or a suitable tourniquet (see Figs 183, 184, p. 262). Care should be taken that the tourniquet is not too tight, and that local venous stasis is not maintained for longer than 2 minutes before the sample is withdrawn, otherwise changes in the fluid and cellular proportions of the blood might occur. The skin is then gently tightened so that the vein is immobilized, and the hypodermic needle is inserted through the skin at an angle of $30°$ with the bevel at the point facing towards the skin. In all instances a sharp-edged needle is essential in order to minimize damage to the wall of the vein, and just sufficient pressure should be applied to ensure that the point of the needle enters the lumen of the vein in one smooth movement.

Gentle traction on the plunger of the syringe will quickly determine whether the vein has been entered. If it has, the traction is maintained until the required amount of blood has been obtained. Too strong traction will rapidly empty the vein so that it will collapse around the point of the needle, obstructing it (the likelihood of haemolysis is increased with strong traction). The needle is withdrawn, after allowing the vein to empty by releasing the pressure, by pressing on the skin at the point of insertion. Remove the needle from the syringe and gently discharge the contents of the latter into the collecting bottle or tube (Fig. 190). If an unclotted sample is required the blood is discharged into a container with a selected anticoagulant. Adequate mixing is ensured by inverting the tube or bottle several times, or by rolling it between the palms of the hands. Needles and syringes should be washed out with cold water immediately after the sample of blood has been obtained.

The choice of anticoagulant depends upon the type of examination to be carried out. For general haematological examination, commercially prepared bottles containing 5 mg disodium EDTA (Sequestrene) are satisfactory. In order to avoid errors arising from failure to prevent partial clotting, and disproportion between anticoagulant and blood, thorough mixing should be performed after introducing a measured 2·5 ml of blood. Otherwise reasonably satisfactory results, at little cost, can be obtained by placing 0·1 ml for each 5 ml of blood required of a solution containing 6% ammonium oxalate and 4% potassium oxalate in suitable screw-capped bottles and slowly evaporating to dryness. More uniform dispersal of the anticoagulant in the blood is achieved if the solution is distributed over the entire inner surface of the glass container by rotating it in an almost horizontal position prior to evaporation in a bacteriological incubator. Sodium oxalate or sodium citrate alone, at the rate of 2·4 mg/ml of blood, may be used in the same manner. Oxalates and sodium citrate prevent clotting by combining with calcium ions. When organic acid salt anticoagulants are in use, haematological examinations should be undertaken within an hour of taking the blood sample. In all cases it is preferable that blood smears are made within a few minutes (the freshly prepared smears should be fixed in absolute methyl alcohol for 2 minutes and then air-dried; this will minimize cellular degeneration), and if other procedures have to be delayed, the blood sample should be placed in a

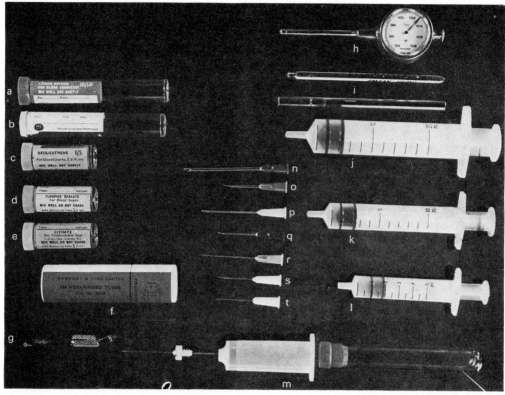

Fig. 190. A, *A vial containing lithium heparin (biochemical estimations).* B, *A vial containing no anticoagulant (serological examination).* C, *A vial containing sequestrene (haematology).* D, *A vial containing fluoride oxalate (inorganic phosphate and glucose estimation).* E, *A vial containing sodium citrate (prothrombin time, estimation).* F, *Heparinized capillary tubes.* G, *Needle director.* H, *Aneroid clinical thermometer.* I, *Clinical thermometer with case, blunt end.* J–L, *Disposable syringes, 20 ml, 10 ml and 5 ml.* M, *Heparinized glass container with tube-holder and two-way needle for blood collection (Vacutainer).* N–T, *A variety of disposable needles for collecting blood samples from animals.*

refrigerator as soon as possible, and discarded after 24 hours. It follows from this that many of the haematological determinations such as total erythrocyte and leucocyte counts, differential leucocyte counts, packed cell volume, etc. are considerably affected by delay and, more especially, by transmission of the blood sample through the post. The delay and, in the latter case, the shaking cause haemolysis (the erythrocyte count may be reduced by 10% or more), and the differential leucocyte count may be considerably modified by the fact that lymphocyte and monocyte cells disintegrate more readily than the neutrophils.

When biochemical examination of blood is required, heparin is probably the most useful anticoagulant; it is effective at the rate of 1 mg/5 ml of blood. Heparin is a natural anticoagulant which exists most abundantly in the liver, its action is achieved by preventing the conversion of prothrombin to thrombin. If samples have to be transmitted to a laboratory for phosphate determinations, sodium fluoride (10 mg/ml of blood) should be included. Ammonium oxalate should not be used as an anticoagulant when blood non-protein nitrogen or urea determinations are required. Although all biochemical tests give more satisfactory results if carried out on freshly obtained blood samples, the results of the tests likely to be used for routine diagnostic purposes are not seriously affected by suitable storage for 24 hours, except in the case of blood sugar, the test for which must be initiated within 1 hour of sampling.

Haematological Methods

With even relatively limited experience and simple equipment, the clinician is able to perform a number of haematological examinations. These include: (a) microscopic examination of an unstained preparation; (b) preparation and examination of a stained smear; (c) haemoglobin estimation; (d) packed cell volume determination; (e) erythrocyte count; and (f) total and differential leucocyte counts. Additional determinations which can be undertaken in selected instances include platelet count, sedimentation rate, clotting time and colour of the plasma.

Unstained preparation. This is made by placing a very small drop of blood on the surface of a perfectly clean cover-slip and inverting it onto the surface of an equally clean microscope slide. If the glass slide and cover-slip are clean, and the drop of blood is not too large, the blood spreads out into a thin film. If the cytological variations from normal are marked, it is sometimes possible, with experience, to recognize whether the changes indicative of anaemia, including increased transparency of the erythrocytes (hypochromia), variation in shape (poikilocytosis) and unequal size (anisocytosis), are present, and whether the leucocyte numbers are markedly increased or decreased. In addition, certain blood parasites can be recognized by this method, particularly microfilariae and trypanosomes (both by means of a low power objective), in exceptional circumstances even piroplasms (with an oil-immersion objective).

Stained preparation. For determining the species of blood parasites and the recognition of the different types of leucocyte cells, a stained preparation must be made. To prepare the film, select several good quality, clean, grease-free slides, and cut off a corner of one slide, shortening its width by one-third, to form a 'spreader'. Then place a small drop of well-mixed blood near the right-hand end of a glass slide placed horizontally on the bench and, while holding this slide with the thumb and forefinger of the left hand, place the cut-off end of the 'spreader' in the centre of the slide so that it forms an angle of 45°. Draw the 'spreader' slide towards the right until it comes into contact with the drop of blood, and then pause until the blood spreads along the area of contact between the two slides. At this point push the 'spreader' to the left, gradually decreasing the angle to less than 30°, thereby thinning off the film. When the film is spread, dry it quickly by waving it in the air in order to avoid crenation and fragmentation of erythrocytes. Drying can be hastened by holding the freshly

made blood film in the current of warm air produced by a spirit lamp or low-burning Bunsen (avoid overheating). Uniformly better quality blood films can be produced with limited experience by using a 2 cm² No. 1 coverslip as a 'spreader'. The prepared slide can be made readily identifiable by writing in the date and client's name, or a reference number, along the middle part of the smear with a pencil. Whenever possible stain blood films immediately they are prepared, otherwise fix them in absolute methanol and then store in a clean box until they can be stained.

Staining methods. The method selected to stain a blood film depends on the purpose for which it is made. For the diagnosis of anthrax in the septicaemic form, which is characteristic in ruminant species but more unusual in other species, fairly thick blood smears are made by means of a bacteriological swab. The smear is fixed by holding the glass slide above a small flame until the back of the slide becomes almost too hot to hold against the back of the hand (take care not to transfer any contamination to the exposed hand). Then place the film on the staining rack and flood it with 1% aqueous solution of methylene blue; allow the stain to act for 2 minutes and then wash off with water and dry in the flame. If blotting or filter paper is used for drying purposes, make certain it is disposed of by burning. During the septicaemic phase of infection the anthrax bacilli are usually fairly numerous in the blood of cattle and can be recognized microscopically (see Fig. 149A, p. 175) in the form of large blue rods with truncated extremities, sometimes in short chains, and associated with a characteristically purplish-coloured background. The purple-stained asymmetrical capsules are usually clearly visible. Excessive heating of the film during fixing, or carcase decomposition, may disperse the purple staining material, giving the capsules a halo-like appearance. Post mortem invaders, including *Clostridium* spp. and many others, which may be extremely numerous when putrefaction is advanced, are darker in colour, have rounded extremities, may have sporulated and in most instances lack a capsule (*Clostridium welchii* may occasionally possess a capsule which, however, shows no staining reaction) and the purple background. In the case of pigs and carnivorous species similar smears should be prepared from the oedematous swelling of the pharynx, the submaxillary lymph node and the fluid in the peritoneal cavity. Final confirmation of the diagnosis necessitates cultural identification of *Bacillus anthracis*.

Staining methods commonly employed for cellular characterization in haematology, and for the identification of protozoan and other parasites in blood, include the use of Leishman or Giemsa's stain. Both these stains are prepared from interaction between eosin and methylene blue. In the Leishman method the dried film is placed on the rack and sufficient of the stain, which is dissolved in absolute methyl alcohol, is applied until the whole area of the blood smear is flooded. The stain is allowed to act for 1 minute and then twice the volume of neutral distilled water is added, thorough mixing being performed by means of a Pasteur pipette. The addition of water precipitates the dyes out of solution, thereby aiding differential staining (the acid eosin is attracted to the alkaline cytoplasm, and the basic azures derived from the methylene blue are attracted to the acid nuclei of the cells). The diluted stain is allowed to remain on the slide for a period of time (2–10 minutes) sufficient to ensure a reasonable degree of differential staining. The requisite time may vary with different batches of stain and this has to be ascertained by experience. Then flush off the stain by flooding the slide with neutral distilled water or phosphate buffer (pH 6·6) solution. Further differentiation is achieved by repeatedly washing the film for a few seconds. Then dry the film with filter paper and allow a period for complete evaporation to occur before proceeding with the examination.

In Giemsa's method, the air-dried film is fixed with methyl alcohol for 3 minutes, followed by the application of freshly prepared staining solution consisting of one part Giemsa's stain to 10 parts of neutral distilled water, for at least 15 minutes. Better results are obtained if the slide or cover-slip smear is inverted onto the surface of the stain, as in this way deposits from the stain fall away from the blood film. The final procedure follows that for the Leishman method. Even better results are obtained by the use of a coplin jar. In this case the fixed blood film is placed in a jar containing one drop of Giemsa's stain for each millilitre of neutral distilled water. The slide should be left in the jar for 30 minutes and then washed for 30 seconds with the distilled water and allowed to dry.

Examination procedure. The initial step in the examination of a blood film is to place the dried slide on the microscope stage and observe it with the low-power objective in order to ascertain whether the leucocytes are regularly distributed, and whether the staining is adequate and uniform, with a good degree of cellular differentiation. If the film is not of reasonable quality in these respects, it should be discarded and another film prepared. With a satisfactorily prepared and stained film, immersion oil is applied over the whole surface and the examination is continued with the oil-immersion objective. If a more permanent preparation is required, and for the examination of cover glass films, a drop of Canada balsam or other suitable mounting fluid is applied to the surface and a cover-slip or microscope slide placed on top as required. A standard procedure such as the battlement or meander method (Fig. 191), the straight edge or

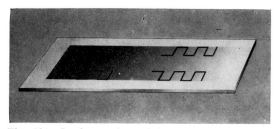

Fig. 191. *Battlement (meander) method of examining blood smears for cellular differentiation. It is particularly suitable for differentiating leucocytes. Note that four areas towards the ends and the periphery of the smear are selected for examination.*

the cross-sectional method should be employed in examining blood smears for the purpose of cellular differentiation. The same methods are applicable to examination of the erythrocytes when an inherent abnormality, or a protozoan or other prasitic disease is suspected. The value of examining blood films increases with greater experience and knowledge, and a basic requirement is appreciation of the normal picture presented by stained blood cells of animals.

Cellular Components of the Blood

Erythrocytes

The red blood cells of mammals, which are normally produced only in the bone marrow through the medium of a humoral factor, erythropoietin, are non-nucleated, circular biconcave discs. Certain pathological states may bring about erythrogenesis in the liver, spleen and lymph nodes. The erythrocytes of many species apart from mammals are elliptical in shape and nucleated. In some anaemic states circulating nucleated erythrocytes may occur in mammals.

The life span of the normal erythrocyte varies in the different species of domestic animals, averages being as follows: horse 140–150 days; ox 80 days; sheep 52 days; pig 62–70 days; dog 110–120 days; cat 68–77 days. Erythrogenesis is a constant process, its rate being influenced by variations in demand for blood-cell repopulation. On average in healthy animals, according to the species, 0·75–1·25% of the circulating erythrocytes are disposed of as being effete each day, i.e. about 35 million every second. Approximately 95–99% of the circulating cells are mature forms; the remainder are the less mature reticulocytes which are not ordinarily identifiable in smears stained by the modified Romanowsky methods. Reticulocytes are not seen in the blood of normal dogs, cats and pigs. The reticulocyte cell can be revealed by spreading a drop of blood on a slide previously prepared with a film of a suitable stain. The slide is prepared by making a film with one drop of a saturated solution of brilliant cresyl blue in alcohol, as for a blood smear. The film of stain is air-dried and the slide can be stored until required. Staining is achieved by placing a drop of capillary or venous blood on the central portion of the stained part of the slide; a cover-slip is applied and the preparation left standing for a minimum period of 15 minutes. The cover-slip may then be rimmed with lens immersion oil and the examination made, or it may be pulled off the slide in a parallel direction, thus drawing the blood out into a thin film. A permanent preparation can be obtained by counter-staining with Leishman's stain and mounting in the usual way. Supravital staining of reticulocytes can also be performed with brilliant cresyl blue 1% in 0·85% saline. Blood and stain in equal amounts are mixed in a small tube or on the surface of a clean slide. After an interval of 5 minutes a film is prepared as for blood and when dry it is counter-stained by the Leishman or Giemsa method. New methylene blue (0·5% in 0·85% saline with 1% formalin as a preservative) may offer some advantages as a supra-vital stain. The stain may be applied to a clean glass slide or cover-slip which is then placed on the surface of the blood

film on a cover-slip or slide respectively, the preparation being suitable for immediate examination. Under the microscope, supravitally stained reticulocytes are orange-coloured with a purple network.

Erythrocyte count. Red cell counts can be made on either capillary or venous blood. With the former the necessary precounting dilution must be performed immediately the blood is collected in the pipette, while with the latter the use of a suitable anticoagulant enables the requisite quantity of blood to be transported to the laboratory. Because of the large population of erythrocytes in the blood of all normal animals, enumeration is only possible when a reasonable degree of dilution is effected. For this purpose suitable diluting fluids and pipettes are required. Recommended diluting fluids include Hayem's (sodium chloride 1 g; sodium sulphate 5 g; mercuric chloride 0·5 g; distilled water 200 ml; filter occasionally), and Dacies' (99 ml of 3% aqueous solution sodium citrate; 1 ml of 40% formaldehyde) which, in addition to keeping well, preserves the shape of the erythrocytes. Because of inter-reaction with blood proteins both the foregoing dilutants occasionally cause clumping of the erythrocytes. If agglutination does occur it can be overcome by the use of physiological saline as a diluent.

Both macro- and micro-pipettes marked to give dilutions of 1 in 100 or 1 in 200 are available. Except in cases of obvious, or severe anaemia the 1 in 200 dilution is reasonably satisfactory for erythrocyte counts in all species of animals. Some authorities suggest that higher dilutions give more accurate counts. In the recommended method, the tip of a Thoma red cell diluting pipette (Fig. 192) is applied to a free-flowing source of capillary blood, or inserted beneath the surface of an unclotted blood sample which has been well mixed by rotation, and gentle suction applied to the glass mouthpiece of the attached rubber tube.

During this procedure the pipette should be held in an almost horizontal position so that when the column of blood reaches the 0·5 mark on the stem, further filling is terminated. If the column of blood extends beyond the selected mark, it can be drawn back by holding the open end of the pipette in contact with a piece of clean filter paper which can also be used to wipe the film of blood off the outside of the tip. Then insert the pipette, held in the vertical position,

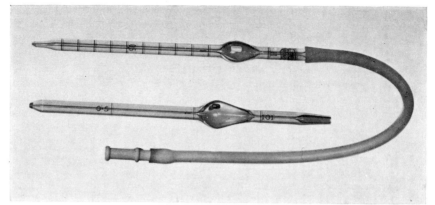

Fig. 192. *Thoma blood cell diluting pipettes. Note that the red cell pipette is marked 0·5, 1·0 and 101 in order to give blood dilutions of 1 in 200 and 1 in 100 respectively. The white cell pipette is marked 0·5, 1·0 and 11 respectively, blood dilutions of 1 in 20 and 1 in 10 respectively.*

into the diluting fluid, at the same time applying suction and gently rotating it as the bulb is filling. When the fluid level nears the 101 mark on the stem beyond the bulb, gently compress the rubber tubing in order to slow down the filling process, stop suction when the mark is reached and withdraw the pipette, placing the index finger over the tip. The diluting fluid should be wiped away from the outer surface of the pipette. Mixing is performed by holding the pipette horizontally with the thumb at one end and the second finger on the other end and shaking for about 2 minutes. The bulb of the pipette contains blood at a dilution of 1 in 200, and the stem portion diluting fluid only which is disposed of by discharging at least 25% of the bulb contents.

A macro-method of dilution can be undertaken with a Sahli haemoglobinometer pipette marked at 20 mm³ (see Fig. 200, p. 281). In this case the contents of the pipette are discharged into a small tube containing 4 ml of diluting fluid. The

small error (0·5%) introduced by the 1 in 201 dilution can be disregarded.

A variety of haemocytometers are available, the most suitable being those with two chambers separated by a central moat and the improved Neubauer ruling in which the central square millimeter in each chamber is divided into 400 small squares arranged in 25 groups of 16 squares each. This is achieved by making each fifth vertical and horizontal line a thick one (Fig. 193). It is important to ensure that the haemocytometer, including its cover-glass, is clean and free from grease. Prior to loading it is placed on a level surface and any dust removed with a camel-hair brush. The cover-glass is placed in position by holding the ends between the thumb and index finger, and then gently lowering it onto the counting chambers, with the long axes of both parallel, so that it rests on the raised bars on each side of the moats surrounding the ruled areas. Filling the counting chambers is achieved by placing the tip of the

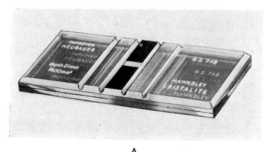

A

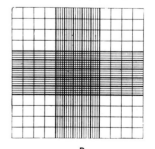

B

Fig. 193. A, *A double cell counting chamber with Neubauer ruling and a metallized central platform. An enlarged view* B, *of the Neubauer ruling.*

pipette containing freshly diluted blood, prepared as described to ensure thorough mixing, against the edge of the cover-glass at an angle of 45° immediately opposite one of the cells which is allowed to fill, at the same time taking care to prevent any of the fluid from spilling over into the moat area, or bubbles to form beneath the cover-glass. The second cell of the counting chamber is filled in the same way from the opposite side of the cover-glass. With the macro-dilution method, filling of the haemocytometer is effected by means of a capillary pipette after thorough mixing of the diluted blood.

In commencing the actual enumeration of the erythrocytes the haemocytometer is placed on the microscope stage and the counting areas examined through the low-power objective. If fluid has overflowed into the moat, or if the cells are unevenly distributed, counting is not proceeded with, the haemocytometer should be cleaned and reloaded in the prescribed manner until satisfactory cell distribution is apparent. At this stage the counting chamber should be allowed to rest on the microscope stage for a few minutes to allow the blood cells to come to rest and settle.

The erythrocytes are enumerated with the 0·4 cm objective, and in order to ensure that a reasonably representative distribution of cells is taken, it is recommended to select the four corner groups, and the central group of 16 smallest squares, giving a total of 80 out of the total of 400. In order to avoid counting the same cell twice a uniform method is adopted which involves counting only those erythrocytes which touch the left-hand and upper lines of any square, disregarding those touching the right-hand and bottom lines. Leucocyte cells are not differentiated and should routinely appear in the count. They can be discounted later if the total leucocyte count is found to be high. The cells in the second ruled area are counted in the same way and, provided the numbers obtained for each side do not differ by more than 5%, an average of the two counts is taken. The use of a mechanical tally is recommended in order to avoid mistakes in counting. In order to minimize the degree of error inherent in the technique, it is advisable to continue counting until at least 500 cells have been enumerated on each side of the chamber. If it is necessary to count considerably more than the eighty small squares recommended, it might be wise to repeat the whole

procedure with the particular blood sample diluted at 1 in 100.

The calculation of the erythrocyte population per mm^3 is made by multiplying the number of cells counted (R) (average of two fields) by both the dilution factor and the volume factor. Each smallest square has an area of 1/400 mm^2, and a depth of 1/10 mm giving a volume of 1/4000 mm^3. A total of 80 squares were included in the count, i.e. 1/50 mm^3. The dilution factor was 200 so that the total erythrocyte count per mm^3 is obtained as follows:

$$200 \times 50 \times R \text{ cells} = 10\,000 \times R$$

Example:

$$10\,000 \times \left(\frac{661 + 685}{2} \right) = 6730\,000/\text{mm}^3$$

Even with experience, and a standard technique, the margin of error is at least 5%, i.e. 250 000 in a count of 5000 000. In laboratories specializing in haematological work large numbers of blood cell counts can be performed in a standardized manner by means of electronic counting equipment. The normal erythrocyte populations per mm^3 of blood for the various species of animals are given in Table 13.

TABLE 13. NORMAL ERYTHROCYTE VALUES

Species	Normal Value
Horse	5·4–13·5 (8·5)
Ox	5·0– 9·0 (7·3)
Sheep	8·0–13·5 (10·5)
Goat	10·5–20·0 (14·3)
Pig	5·0– 8·5 (6·8)
Dog	5·0– 8·5 (6·5)
Cat	6·0– 9·5 (7·5)

Erythrocytes in disease. A significant increase in erythrocyte numbers occurs in polycythaemia vera and in disturbed tissue fluid balance such as occurs in dehydration and certain other states. In polycythaemia vera, a rare condition in animals but which has been recognized in dogs and cattle, there is a primary absolute elevation in the circulating erythrocyte population. Dehydration and other similar derangements of tissue fluid balance give rise to elevated erythrocyte counts because of a decrease in circulating plasma volume. In either case, erythrocyte counts and a packed-cell volume (PCV) (see below) determination would reveal the abnormal situation, the nature of which might be recognized by correlation with the clinical findings. Secondary polycythaemia may also occur in diseases in which there is impairment of respiratory efficiency, e.g.

congestive heart failure, chronic respiratory diseases and pulmonary and mediastinal neoplasia. In these situations tissue hypoxia causes increased production of erythropoietin, which leads to an increase in the circulating erythrocyte numbers.

Reduction below the normal range of the erythrocyte numbers, which if persistent is often associated with a reduced haemoglobin value per cell, is termed anaemia. This state, the degree of which is revealed by haematological investigations, is an important clinical sign of disease, the nature and cause of which may be revealed by evaluation of the history and clinical signs or by demonstration of specific parasites in the blood. On an aetiological basis anaemia may be classified into:

1. Blood loss anaemia.
2. Haemolytic anaemia.
3. Dyshaemopoietic anaemia.
4. Hypoplastic or aplastic anaemia.

In blood loss anaemia the extent of erythrocyte reduction and regeneration are related to the rate and amount of blood lost. The manner of blood loss includes chronic bleeding from gastrointestinal ulcers, enteritis, coccidiosis, neoplasms, haemophilia in dogs and foals, vitamin C and K deficiencies; blood-sucking parasites including *Haemonchus* spp., hookworms and ectoparasites, e.g. ticks, blood-sucking lice; and acute bleeding in warfarin poisoning, sweet clover poisoning in cattle, bracken fern poisoning in cattle, traumatic injuries and surgical operations, hypersplenism, idiopathic thrombocytopenic purpura.

The haemolytic anaemias are infectious or toxic in origin or caused by antigen-antibody reactions. The infectious causes include piroplasmosis caused by *Babesia* spp., anaplasmosis (*Anaplasma* spp.) in cattle, sheep and goats; feline infectious anaemia (haemobartonellosis), the causal organism of which is *Eperythrozoon felis*, eperythrozoonosis in dogs and cattle, bacillary haemoglobinuria (*Clostridium haemolyticum*) in cattle and equine infectious anaemia. Haemolytic anaemia due to toxic factors occurs in cumulative copper poisoning (observed most frequently in sheep, less so in calves and pigs), lead poisoning, rape or kale poisoning in cattle, phenothiazine poisoning in horses and mercury poisoning in sheep. Other diseases in which a haemolytic crisis may occur include leukaemia

and gangrenous mastitis caused by alpha-toxin producing *Staphylococcus aureus*. Antigen–antibody haemolytic reactions occur in isoimmunization of newborn foals, piglets and puppies, as well as in acquired autoimmune haemolytic anaemia in dogs and in incompatible blood transfusion reactions.

In dyshaemopoietic anaemia there is selective depression of erythrogenesis. This type of anaemia may be caused by nutritional deficiency, parasitic disease, infectious disease or organic or glandular disorders. Nutritional deficiencies which depress bone marrow function include iron, copper, cobalt, protein and vitamins including folic acid, thiamin, riboflavin and cyanocobalamin (B12). Bone marrow activity is reduced in trichostrongylidosis (non-blood-sucking gastrointestinal worms) in cattle and sheep. In all chronic infectious diseases depression of erythrogenesis occurs in 4–6 weeks and gradually intensifies. Selective depression of bone marrow function is an important aspect of hypothyroidism, extensive or diffuse neoplasia and of the advanced stages of chronic interstitial nephritis, more especially in the dog.

In hypoplastic or aplastic anaemia the circulating granulocytes and thrombocytes are also reduced. The recognized causes of this type of anaemia include bracken fern in cattle, trichloroethylene-extracted soyabean meal in calves, irradiation sickness, and sulphonamide poisoning.

Abnormal types of erythrocytes result from either increased erythrogenesis or from irregularities in the maturation of the red cells causing the appearance of circulating nucleated erythrocytes (erythroblasts). The blood of newborn animals contains a variable number of nucleated erythrocytes which usually disappear within 3 weeks of birth. Bone marrow stress may also result in the release of red cells which are stained uniformly blue (polychromasia). or which contain bluish granules (punctate basophilia, basophilic stippling) (basophilic stippling occurs in the cow and sheep when as the result of severe anaemia the erythrogenic stimulus is intense) and in some instances a single, eccentrically placed magenta-staining Howell–Jolly body. Such bodies occur in up to 1% of the erythrocytes from normal cats and horses. Heinz bodies are refractile structures which are not revealed in blood films stained by standard Romanowsky methods; for their detection smears should be stained with new methylene blue. Heinz bodies develop as a manifestation of toxicity by certain chemicals and drugs, e.g. phenothiazine toxicity in the horse. Less intensely stained (hypochromatic) and very faintly stained (oligochromatic) erythrocytes are a feature in certain forms of anaemia.

Variation in erythrocyte size (anisocytosis) is a not uncommon feature in animals, in fact as far as cattle are concerned it may be regarded as a normal feature. Variation in shape (poikilocytosis) with many aberrant forms may be regarded as an indication of degeneration.

Certain blood parasites associated with the erythrocytes can be detected only by means of the oil-immersion lens, e.g. *Anaplasma marginale, Babesia divergens* (Fig. 194), *Eperythrozoon felis*

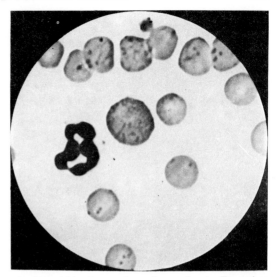

Fig. 195. *A blood smear from the cat showing* Eperythrozoon felis. *Note the characteristic position of the parasite at the circumference of the erythrocytes.*

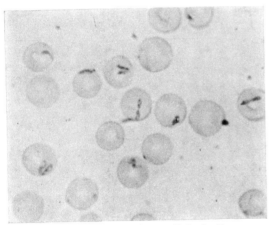

Fig. 194. *A blood smear showing* Babesia divergens.

(Fig. 195), *Theileria parva*, etc. Other, larger blood parasites, including trypanosomes and microfilariae, may be more readily observed in wet preparations, particularly when relatively large numbers occur; specific identification will necessitate examination of a stained blood film. Microfilariasis occurs in the blood of the dog; concentration methods may be required to reveal their presence (Fig. 196). When microfilariae are detected it is necessary to distinguish between *Dirofilaria immitis* and *Depetalonema* spp. because the latter are not regarded as being pathogenic.

Leucocytes

The white blood cells (leucocytes) (Fig. 197) consist of two main types: polymorphonuclear leucocytes (granulocytes) and mononuclear leucocytes (agranulocytes). The leucocytes use

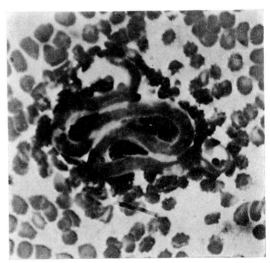

Fig. 196. *A blood smear from the dog showing microfilaria of* Dirofilaria immitis.

the blood as a transport medium between their source of origin and the various tissues of the body—liver, spleen, kidney, bone marrow—where, after performing specific functions, they are destroyed. Considerable numbers escape from the body into the saliva, the milk and the respiratory and alimentary tracts. It is suggested that elimination of leucocytes by these various routes is a mechanism for protection against disease. The leucocytes have a comparatively short life, a matter of a few hours in the case of

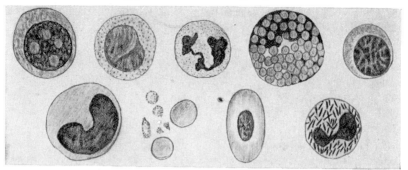

Fig. 197. *Blood cells.* Top (left to right), *Myeloblast, myelocyte, neutrophil, eosinophil* (*horse*), *lymphocyte.* Bottom (left to right), *Monocyte, two erythrocytes and several platelets* (*mammalian blood*), *erythrocyte, pseudo-eosinophil* (*fowl*).

lymphocytes, and not more than 14 days for the granulocyte cells.

The polymorphonuclear leucocytes include the neutrophils, eosinophils and basophils, all of which are produced extravascularly in the bone marrow from a stem cell, the myeloblast (Fig. 197). In the process of proliferation the myeloblast develops to a progranulocyte which produces the next generation, the myelocyte. At this stage the specific granules characteristic of the mature leucocyte appear, so that it is possible to identify neutrophilic, eosinophilic and basophilic myelocytes. Further successive stages of maturation of the neutrophilic myelocyte are metamyelocyte, band cell and segmented cell. Normally the proportion of immature cells of the granulocyte series present in the blood of animals is quite small. The bone marrow can, however, evince a rapid response to infection or stress, the end effect of which, as far as the blood is concerned, being the appearance of an increased proportion of circulating immature granulocytes. In this context it is useful to identify and classify the various types of leucocyte cells on a selected smear as a means of assessing the response of the myeloid tissues to disease.

The mature neutrophil leucocyte has either a monolobular nucleus, or its nucleus may have up to five lobes which are joined by thin strands giving it a segmented appearance. In both types the rather ragged appearance of the nuclear membrane is an indication that the cell is mature. In properly stained blood films, neutrophil leucocytes have faintly acidophilic cytoplasm with a deeply basophilic staining nucleus. The cytoplasm of the band neutrophil is less granular than that in the mature form, and the nucleus is

sausage-shaped or coiled, and the nuclear membrane is smooth. The metamyelocyte is morphologically similar to the band cell except that the nucleus is kidney-bean shaped. The myelocyte is a comparatively large cell with bluish staining granular cytoplasm and an oval or elliptical nucleus.

Neutrophils perform an important function as a cellular defence mechanism protecting the body tissues when they are threatened by inflammation or by bacterial invasion, especially by staphylococci and streptococci.

Eosinophil leucocytes are readily recognized in stained blood smears by the presence in the cytoplasm of numerous small, regularly circular orange-red granules (Fig. 197) which may cause the cell to bulge. The nucleus of the eosinophil is frequently non-segmented and the cytoplasm, when visible, is pale grey. In some breeds of dogs, particularly the greyhound, eosinophilic granules are lacking and non-staining vacuole-like inclusions are observed.

Eosinophils appear to have an important function in detoxification with particular reference to the inactivation of histamine. Being chemotactically influenced by histamine, eosinophils accumulate at the site of antigen-antibody reactions.

Basophil leucocytes characteristically have purplish staining granules scattered throughout the cytoplasm and over the surface of the nucleus which is less intensely stained. Basophils occur only rarely in the blood of the dog and cat.

There appears to be a close relationship between the basophil leucocyte and the tissue mast cell and as the granules of both contain histamine and heparin the cells probably perform a similar function. Following tissue injury,

TABLE 14. NORMAL TOTAL AND DIFFERENTIAL LEUCOCYTE COUNTS

Leucocyte count	Horse	Dog	Cat	Ox	Sheep	Pig
Total count (per mm³)	6000–13 000	9000–13 000	8800–20 000	6000–10 000	4000–13 000	10 000–20 000
Differential count (%)						
Segmented neutrophils	50–64	60–75	35–72	15–40	15–30	40–60
Band neutrophils	0–4	3–6	0–3	0–5	0–4	0–2
Lymphocytes	20–40	15–30	20–56	40–70	55–75	30–50
Eosinophils	4–10	2–8	1–12	2–20	0–10	1–5
Basophils	0–2	0–1	0–1	0–1	0–1	0
Monocytes	3–10	1–8	0·5–4	3–10	0–6	2–8

basophil and mast cells release heparin and histamine at the site so that an inflammatory reaction follows as the result of the ensuing increased capillary permeability and dilatation. The later arriving eosinophils help to curtail the spread of the inflammation.

In the horse, dog, pig and cat the granulocytes consist predominantly of neutrophils, but in ruminant species they may comprise a considerable proportion of eosinophils (Table 14). This is probably attributable not to an absolutely greater number of eosinophil cells in the blood of cattle and sheep, but to the smaller absolute number of granulocytes. In the various species of domestic mammals the absolute number of eosinophils varies considerably, but in health it rarely exceeds 15%. Basophils are very rare in all species, comprising about 0·2% of the total leucocyte population. As a general rule the total leucocyte count is higher in young than in adult animals of the various species. This is probably most marked in dairy cows. Thoroughbred horses give white cell counts which are slightly higher than those for standardbred and other types. Dogs and cats which struggle during the blood sampling procedure frequently evince physiological leucocytosis.

The mononuclear leucocytes comprise the lymphocytes and monocytes. The lymphocytes, which are formed in the lymphatic follicles of the lymph nodes, in the tonsils, spleen, thymus and lymphoreticular tissues (Peyer's patches) in the intestine, are of two varieties. The commonest form is of small size (less than 10 μm in diameter) with a large, almost circular or slightly indented nucleus and a narrow peripheral zone of blue-stained cytoplasm. The cytoplasm may contain a group of comparatively large, dark blue or red (azurophilic) granules. The larger lymphocytes have proportionately more cytoplasm, which stains pale blue and may contain small vacuoles, thus causing some confusion with monocytes.

The lymphocyte has been assigned many functions including that of transformation to many other types of nucleated blood and tissue cells. There is a close relationship between the lymphocyte and the plasma cell. Lymphocytes are an important source of gammaglobulin, which is released when these cells shed their cytoplasm into the lymph. Dissolution of lymphocytes is brought about by the action of adrenocorticosteroids. The life span of the lymphocyte is said to vary from a few hours to a month or longer; a variable proportion of the time is spent in the tissues.

The monocyte is the largest cell in the leucocyte series; it originates in any part of the reticulo-endothelial system. In stained smears monocytes are not unlike large lymphocytes, but their nuclei are more varied morphologically, being oval, elliptical or horse-shoe shaped and, in some instances, even segmented. The nuclear chromatin is stranded in a net-like pattern. In addition the cytoplasm is faintly granular, stains distinctly basophilic and may have a vacuolated or foamy appearance; this latter feature is most apparent in the monocytes of cattle. Monocytes appear to be capable of performing a variety of diverse functions, the chief of which is, in their capacity as macrophages, to deal with the specific causal agents of chronic infective processes including fungi, *Brucella* spp., *Mycobacterium tuberculosis* and protozoa. In many chronic infective processes the circulating monocyte population is increased; a similar response can be induced by corticosteroid compounds administered parenterally.

In the horse, dog and cat, differential white cell counts indicate that the granulocyte/lymphocyte ratio is about 60 : 30. In the pig, the granular leucocytes are slightly in excess of the lymphocytes. Generally the proportion of lymphocyte cells varies inversely with the granular leucocytes from species to species, being highest in cattle and sheep, and lowest in the dog (Table 14). Monocytes comprise less than 10% of the total white cell population in normal domestic animals of any species.

Thrombocytes or blood platelets are additional formed elements in the blood which originate from a detached portion or fragment of the cytoplasm of the megakaryocyte, or giant cell of the bone marrow, possibly also of the spleen or lung. The functions of the platelets, which are non-nucleated, is concerned with the process of blood clotting and clot retraction. In stained blood films they appear in groups of varying numbers, and may be round, oval or rod-shaped, staining light blue with red or purple granules (azurophilic). Accurate platelet counts necessitate the use of silicon-coated hypodermic needles, syringes, and diluting tubes, otherwise clumping will make counting difficult or impossible. Their number in the blood of normal animals varies from 250 000 to 600 000/mm³. Lambs and calves have more and puppies have fewer than adult animals of their species. Platelets survive in the circulating blood for 8–11 days at most. Significant reduction in the number of platelets occurs in thrombocytopenic purpura in dogs, in thrombocytopenia in young pigs, and as the result of depressed bone marrow function in poisoning by bracken fern and trichloroethylene-extracted soyabean meal in ruminants, and in radiation sickness.

Total and differential leucocyte counts. Total leucocyte counts are of reduced value when performed on blood samples more than 24 hours after collection. To ensure the greatest possible degree of accuracy the sample container is inverted or rolled between the hands to ensure thorough mixing. Suitable diluting fluids include 1% glacial acetic acid or 1/10 normal hydrochloric acid, to which 1% aqueous solution of gentian violet may be added at the rate of 1%. By means of a suitable pipette (see Fig. 192, p. 270) the blood is diluted 1 in 20. For this procedure a technique similar to that described for erythrocyte counting is employed. The diluting pipette is filled with an unbroken column of blood to the 0·5 mark and, after wiping off the blood from the outer surface, is then filled with diluting fluid to the 11 mark on the stem distal to the bulb. The bulb of the pipette now contains blood at a dilution of 1 in 20, and the stem portion diluting fluid. This latter is disposed of by discharging at least 25%

of the bulb contents. A variety of haemocytometer slides are available for counting leucocytes, the most suitable being those with two chambers and Neubauer type ruling as recommended for erythrocyte counts. In preparing the haemocytometer the same procedure is adopted as for a red cell count, and loading the two counting areas is achieved in a similar manner also.

For the actual count the haemocytometer is placed on the stage of the microscope, allowed to stand for 3 minutes, giving the leucocytes time to settle, and the 0·8 cm objective focused until the ruled lines of one counting area are clearly observed. The large square (1 mm²) in the upper left-hand corner, consisting of 16 smaller squares, is brought into view and the nucleated cells in the first small square are counted and then those in the small square on the immediate right, progressing across the top row from left to right. The second row of squares is counted from right to left and the procedure is continued for the 16 small squares. In order to avoid confusion and error from overcounting it is customary to count those cells which are in contact with any part of the upper or left-hand lines, and to disregard those touching the right-hand and bottom lines of each individual square. The leucocyte cells in the 3 remaining large squares at the corners of the ruled area should then be enumerated in a similar manner. The same procedure is applied to the second counting area when either the total number of leucocytes for the first four squares is less than 120, or there is considerable disparity between the numbers for different squares. A written record of the total for each square is made in order to obtain the final result.

The calculation of the total count is made by multiplying the number of cells (L) in 1 mm³ of the diluted sample obtained proportionally, by the dilution factor. Each large corner square has an average area of 1 mm² and a depth of 0·1 mm giving a volume of 0·1 mm³. The dilution factor is 20, and if four squares have been counted the total count per mm³ is obtained as follows:

$$20 \times \frac{1}{0·4} \times L \text{ cells} = 50 \times L \text{ cells}$$

Example:

68 + 70 + 65 + 67 = 270 × 50 = 13 500 leucocytes/mm³

The differential leucocyte count is frequently more revealing than the total count and should also be undertaken whenever the latter is performed. In the majority of even well prepared blood films the leucocytes will be marginated near the lateral edges of the smear. The examination is made with the 0·2 cm oil-immersion objective, and to allow for uneven distribution the battlement or meander method, counting and differentiating 50 cells at each of the four corners of the film will suffice for most purposes, (Fig. 191). The cells are classified into lobulated and non-lobulated neutrophil leucocytes, eosinophils, basophils, lymphocytes and monocytes according to their staining reactions, general and nuclear morphology and the characterization of any cytoplasmic granules that may occur. The individual cells can be tabulated in columns on a prepared sheet of paper, or a series of tallies can be used. In the event that gross discrepancy occurs in the proportion of any one series of fifty cells compared with the numbers in the other groups, either 400–500 cells should be differentiated, or a further blood film should be examined.

Because of the important relationship existing between adrenocortical activity and the number of circulating eosinophils methods have been developed for the direct counting of this particular leucocyte. An increase in the functional activity of the adrenal cortex, brought about by endogenously derived or parenterally administered adrenocorticotrophic hormone (ACTH), will decrease the number of circulating eosinophils. Direct eosinophil counts are possible with a diluting fluid containing propylene glycol and sodium carbonate; the former lyses the erythrocytes and the latter all the leucocytes except the eosinophils. Phloxine is included as a staining reagent at a final concentration of 0·1%. The count is made by the same method as that described for the total leucocyte count. Electronic systems for counting leucocytes employ the same type of equipment as for erythrocyte counts.

Leucocyte reactions in disease. Alterations in the leucocyte picture may not only involve changes in the total number of circulating leucocytes, or of one particular cell type, but also include the appearance of toxic changes affecting the cytoplasm and/or nucleus of a proportion of the cells, and the presence of immature forms.

Alterations in total number consist of an increase (leucocytosis) or a decrease (leucopenia). Leucocytosis may be the result of a general increase in the number of all the white blood cells, but is more usually attributable to a disproportionate increase in one of the main groups—neutrophils (neutrophilia) or lymphocytes (lymphocytosis). In order to identify and assess the significance of such alterations it is necessary to perform both total and differential leucocyte counts; the validity of the findings will be enhanced if a sequence of counts is made. Neutrophilia is caused by many factors, probably the most important of which is infection by pyogenic bacteria, but many so-called stress influences, including muscular exercise, pain, fear, exposure to cold and consumption of food, are regarded as physiological causes.

The total leucocyte count provides a basis for assessing the reactivity of the bone marrow to bacterial infection, while the proportion of immature neutrophils is related to the severity of the infection. In general the neutrophil shows the most significant alterations in numbers and in morphological characteristics in response to infective or inflammatory processes. The range and type of such responses, however, show some variation according to the species of animal.

In the dog, the myeloid tissues are capable of considerable response, so that total leucocyte counts of 30 000–50 000 occur during infective processes and stress syndromes. The bone marrow of the cat shows a lesser response to bacterial infection than does that of the dog, so total counts rarely reach the maximum figures for the dog. It is important to bear in mind that the normal cat can evince a remarkable degree of physiological lymphocytosis from fear, in which lymphocytes may equal or even exceed the neutrophil numbers. In the horse infective processes engender a leucocyte response which ranges on average from 15 000 to 25 000. As a rule the bone marrow in cattle is only mildly responsive to infective processes, so that total leucocyte counts range from 4000 to 12 000. Neutrophilia is an associated feature and is often pronounced.

An important aspect of neutrophilia is the appearance of immature neutrophils in the circulating blood. This gives rise to the so-called 'left shift' which varies from mild (band neutrophils) to moderate (both band and metamyelocyte neutrophils) or marked (myelocytes and progranulocytes) when regeneration is occurring.

In 'degenerative left shift' considerable numbers of immature neutrophils occur in the blood while the total leucocyte count is normal or only slightly elevated.

The abnormal features occurring in the neutrophils which are regarded as manifestations of toxicity include diffuse basophilia of the cytoplasm, blue-black or reddish granules in varying number in the cytoplasm (toxic granulation), giant neutrophils showing diffuse basophilia (seen in toxaemic states in the cat), and peripherally located vacuoles (common in the dog).

Lymphocytosis is of rarer occurrence than neutrophilia in animals. In relative form it is a feature of conditions associated with neutropenia and of the recovery phase of acute infections, and as a transient reaction to the injection of tuberculin, or the induction of various emotional states (fear, anger). Absolute lymphocytosis may occur at some time during the course of the 'leukaemia complex' (lymphosarcoma), more usually in the later stages, in cattle, dogs and cats. Lymph node enlargement and occasionally absolute lymphocytosis may be associated with certain protozoan infections including *Babesia*, *Trypanosoma* and *Theileria* spp.

Monocytosis is an increase in the number of monocytes. It may occur in relative form, as a transient feature, heralding the beginning of recovery from acute infections. It occurs also in certain protozoal infections, in chronic infections such as pyometra and brucellosis and in infection with *Listeria monocytogenes*. In the dog it may occur as a response to an increased output of corticosteroids under conditions of stress. Eosinophilia, an increase in the number of circulating eosinophils, occurs as a transient feature and to a variable degree in antigen–antibody reactions, and in allergic conditions including those forms of parasitism in which the parasite invades the tissues of its animal host (*Toxocara canis*, *Ancylostoma caninum*, *Fasciola hepatica*). A pronounced eosinophilia may occur in eosinophilic myositis and chronic allergic dermatitis. Eosinophilia not infrequently occurs in chronic suppurative conditions; when there is an accompanying lymphopenia the situation of the animal is grave.

Leucopenia may arise from a general decrease in the number of all types of circulating leucocyte cells (panleucopenia) or it may be, as is more likely, attributable to a disproportionate decrease in any one of the main types of leucocytes. Neutropenia occurs during the earlier phases of many virus infections, e.g. equine viral arteritis, mucosal disease in cattle, rinderpest, swine fever, canine distemper and canine infectious hepatitis. Because the neutropenia may be of short duration it is often not detected in routine haematological investigations. Panleucopenia is a feature of infectious feline enteritis. The majority of bacterial infections are usually accompanied by leucocytosis but leptospirosis in cattle is often associated with leucopenia. Reduction in all the cellular elements of the blood (pancytopenia), including the leucocytes, is observed in bracken fern and trichloroethylene-extracted soyabean meal poisoning and in irradiation sickness. In these conditions the activity of the bone marrow, spleen and lymph nodes is depressed. In some species, especially dogs, the repeated administration of antihistamine drugs can produce a severe degree of neutropenia. Lymphopenia occurs, to a variable degree, during many acute infections, more especially those caused by virus agents, and also as an early feature in stress syndromes and irradiation sickness. Persistent lymphopenia accompanied by a 'degenerative left shift' in the neutrophil picture is a bad prognostic sign.

Other causes of leucopenia include acute local inflammations, more especially when a septic focus is established; drugs such as sulphonamides and other chemicals that competitively utilize folic acid which is required for blood cell propagation; and deficiency of protein, nicotinic acid or folic acid.

In a proportion of infectious and other inflammatory diseases, the course is accompanied by a more or less regular pattern of changes in the leucocyte picture. In the early stages there may be a transient neutropenia (most marked in virus diseases), followed by a period of absolute neutrophilia with an increase in the proportion of immature neutrophils, the lymphocyte numbers are (quite often only relatively) reduced, and eosinophils may be absent. When the intensity of the disease subsides the neutrophils decrease in numbers, the lymphocytes and monocytes increase. The phase of recovery is marked by an increase in lymphocytes and eosinophils, followed by a gradual return of the leucocyte picture to normal. It must be realized that the foregoing is a general oversimplification of the potentiality for change that exists as far as the leucocyte cells are concerned, and that the value

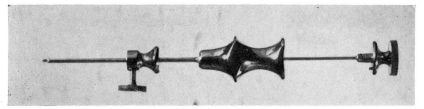

Fig. 198. *A Salah needle with a stilette and adjustable stop for bone marrow aspiration. The needle is inserted through the bone cortex with the stilette in position.*

of a single white cell count for diagnostic, and even more important, for prognostic purposes, is limited.

The leukaemia complex. Malignant tumours not infrequently develop areas of focal necrosis which causes an increase in the number of circulating neutrophils. In leukaemia, which is a neoplastic disease involving one or more of the blood cell types produced by the haematopoietic tissues, immature cells do not uniformly occur in the blood (aleukaemia) so that the circulating leucocyte count is not always elevated. Whenever possible it is advisable to identify the neoplastic cell type, e.g. lymphocytic, granulocytic, etc.; at the aleukaemia stage this will necessitate bone marrow examination or lymph node biopsy.

In domestic animals the commonest form of leucocytic neoplasic disease is the lymphosarcoma. Occasional cases of granulocytic leukaemia have been observed in most species, and rare cases of plasma cell myelomatosis in the cat and horse. In lymphosarcoma the distribution of neoplastic proliferations enables the disease to be classified into: (*a*) multicentric (all body lymph nodes with spleen, liver and kidneys), (*b*) thymic (thymus and most body lymph nodes) and (*c*) alimentary types (gastrointestinal tract, associated lymph nodes, liver frequently, body lymph nodes rarely). The majority of cases occur in animals more than five years of age. The main clinical signs consist of gross enlargement of the lymph nodes, wasting and anaemia. The greater proportion of the proliferating lymphocytes is immature. The initial haematological changes result from necrosis in the lymphoid masses and consist of neutrophilia and anaemia; in some cases these variations persist throughout the course of the disease with a tendency to become more marked, while in other instances a terminal spillover of lymphocytes into the blood occurs so that there may be a considerable numerical increase (counts of over 200 000/mm³ are not uncommon). The immature lymphocytes, many

of which present bizarre morphological characters, may account for over 90 % of the circulating leucocytes.

Bone Marrow Examination

The granular leucocytes, including the neutrophil, eosinophil and basophil cells, along with the erythrocytes and thrombocytes, are produced in the bone marrow. The production of polymorphonuclear leucocytes (granular leucopoiesis) is reduced when bone marrow function is depressed, giving rise to a variable degree of agranulocytosis. A study of the bone marrow cellular picture, through the medium of smears, will reveal whether the formation and maturation of the granulocytes, erythrocytes and thrombocytes are progressing normally. Cellular variation exists in the bone marrow from different parts of the skeleton. Bone marrow which is active haematopoietically is red in colour, and in adult animals is confined to the flat bones such as the ribs, pelvis, vertebrae, cranial bones and epiphyseal portions of the long bones. The nonproductive (yellow) marrow, which consists of endothelial, reticular and fat cells, occupies the shafts of the long bones. When in adult life there is an increased haematopoietic demand, red marrow expansion can replace the inactive yellow marrow. The varying activity of the bone marrow reflects, in some degree, the wide interspecies and individual animal differences in the erythrocyte population of the blood.

Aspiration of bone marrow is readily achieved using the iliac crest in horses and cattle. Local analgesia is induced and after the skin has been incised a Salah needle (Fig. 198) is forced through the cortex of the bone by means of a rotating movement. The cortex has been penetrated when there is a sudden reduction in resistance to penetration of the needle. At this point, the stilette is withdrawn from the needle and suction applied by attaching a 20 ml syringe containing an appropriate anticoagulant. In old animals the haematopoietically active marrow recedes so that the iliac crest does not provide a satisfactory sample. An alternative site is the second or third sternal segment on its lateral aspect; the animal should be cast when this site is chosen. The trochanteric fossa of the femur is the most convenient site in the dog and cat (the iliac crest is a suitable alternative), in which species a similar technique is employed as for other animals. Aspiration is commenced by pulling out the plunger of the syringe until fluid appears, when the suction process should be terminated in order to avoid excessive dilution with blood, which makes interpretation of the resulting smears more difficult. The contents of the syringe can be discharged into a prepared bottle or used immediately to prepare smears in the same manner as for blood films. The marrow smears should then be processed by a similar method.

The number of nucleated cells per unit volume of bone marrow can be determined with the haemocytometer, using a dilution technique. Counts of 100 000/mm³, or slightly over, indicate that relatively little dilution with blood has

occurred; it is generally agreed, however, that total nucleated cell counts are an unreliable indicator of the haematopoietic activity of the bone marrow. In examining bone marrow smears a differential count is made of 500 nucleated cells. Valid interpretation of pathological bone marrow smears requires considerable experience with cellular ratios in normal marrow, so that veterinary clinicians are unlikely to be directly concerned in the use of the technique. There are occasions, however, when it may be desirable to assess the degree of hyperplasia or hypoplasia in the bone marrow, for which purpose appropriate specimens may be submitted to a haematology laboratory.

Haemoglobin Determinations

Two types of colorimetric procedures are available for clinical haemoglobin determinations. In the direct procedures, such as the Tallquist method, which is very insensitive (margin of error up to 40%) and capable of indicating only wide variations from normal haemoglobin values, the colour of whole blood is compared with a colour standard which is

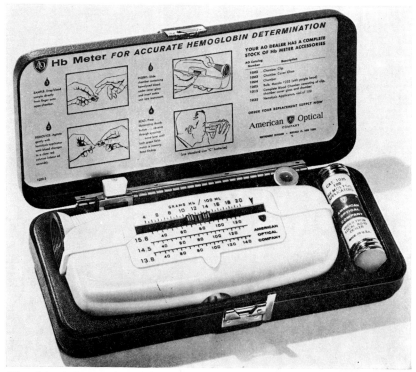

Fig. 199. *A Spencer haemoglobinometer including a read-out scale, a glass laking chamber and haemolysis applicator sticks.* (American Optical Company)

sometimes impossible to match with blood from animals. The indirect methods consist of converting haemoglobin to a more stable colour compound, and then measuring its density by direct comparison methods, or by means of a suitable photoelectric colorimeter or spectrophotometer.

Tallquist method. A drop of blood obtained by needle prick, or directly from a vein or from an unclotted sample of blood, is placed on a piece of white blotting paper and when dry compared with a colour scale the intensity of which corresponds to various percentages of haemoglobin (100% is equivalent to 13·8 g/100 ml). The method is very insensitive and at best should only be used for screening purposes.

Oxyhaemaglobin method. This is a direct method employing the Spencer haemoglobinometer (Fig. 199) which measures oxyhaemoglobin by light absorption using a green filter. A drop of blood is placed in the well of the small glass chamber after removing the glass cover and haemolysed by means of a prepared applicator stick. When the laked blood changes to a clear red solution the cover is applied and the mounted unit pressed into the holding clip and the whole inserted into the haemoglobinometer. The illuminating button is then pressed and, while maintaining observation through the eyepiece, the lever on the right side is moved horizontally until both green fields match in intensity. The haemoglobin value can be read off the scale on the side of the instrument.

Haematin methods. Of the indirect methods the acid haematin or Sahli is probably one of the most practical for routine clinical use. A special haemoglobinometer and pipette (Fig. 200) are required, and the method depends on the formation of acid haematin which is compared with a standard in the form of a tinted glass rod which does not fade. Add $N/10$ hydrochloric acid to the 20 mark on the graduated tube. Then fill the capillary pipette to the 20 mm³ mark from a freely flowing source of blood, or from a well-mixed unclotted sample, by gentle suction. Wipe off all the blood adhering to the outer surface of the pipette with cotton-wool, and expel the blood into the acid solution in the graduated tube; rinse out the pipette with the solution and thoroughly mix the tube contents. Remove from bright light and allow to stand for the recommended period of time. Maximum colour intensity develops in 40

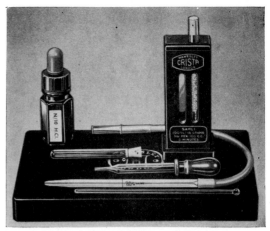

Fig. 200. *A haemoglobinometer, consisting of tinted glass standard a graduated tube and a pipette.*

minutes but the various haemoglobinometers are adjusted for colour matching at a stated period of time varying from 1 to 30 minutes. Then dilute with $N/10$ hydrochloric acid or distilled water, mixing thoroughly at each addition, until the colour matches that of the standard. Read off the figure which corresponds to the level of fluid in the graduated tube, and from this determine the haemoglobin content of the blood by means of the correction factor for the instrument which is usually given in grams/100 ml. If a standardized technique is employed the error in the acid haematin method is less than 10%.

In the alkaline haematin method adding dilute alkali to blood converts haemoglobin to alkaline haematin. With a micro-pipette 0·05 ml of freshly drawn, or well-mixed unclotted blood is added to 4·95 ml of $N/10$ sodium hydroxide solution in a selected glass tube. Mix thoroughly, and heat the tube and contents in a boiling water bath for 4 minutes. Cool the mixture and compare it with a known haemoglobin standard, similarly treated, in a photoelectric colorimeter.

Cyanmethaemoglobin method. When carefully performed this is a reasonably accurate method of haemoglobin measurement. Because of the risks associated with the use of the potassium cyanide reagent, and also to ensure greater accuracy, an automatic pipette calibrated to deliver 5 ml should be used (Fig. 201). The procedure consists of adding 0·02 ml of well-mixed blood to 4 ml of modified Drabkin's solution (potassium cyanide 0·05 g, potassium ferrocyanide 0·20 g, distilled water to 1 litre). The tube is stoppered with a rubber bung,

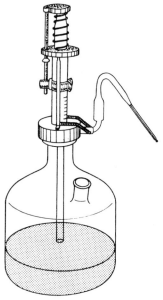

Fig. 201. *An automatic pipette which can be calibrated to deliver a predetermined volume up to 10 ml.*

inverted several times and then allowed to stand for 10 minutes. The solution of cyanmethaemoglobin is then ready for comparison with a standard in a photoelectric colorimeter with a suitable yellow-green filter. A cyanmethaemoglobin standard is available from commercial sources (C. Davis Keeler Ltd).

Carboxyhaemoglobin method. This method which compares in accuracy with the preceding one requires a source of carbon monoxide; it is now rarely employed.

The normal ranges of haemoglobin in the blood of the various species of domestic animals is given in Table 15. As a general rule very

TABLE 15. NORMAL HAEMOGLOBIN AND HAEMATOCRIT VALUES (RANGE AND MEAN)

	Haemoglobin (g/100 ml)	Haematocrit (PCV %)
Horse	8·5–13·0 (11·0)	28·0–45·2 (36·0)
Ox	8·5–13·5 (11·2)	28·3–42·3 (35·0)
Sheep	9·3–14·8 (11·5)	27·3–43·0 (35·0)
Goat	8·8–13·8 (11·3)	25·0–40·0 (34·0)
Pig	8·3–12·7 (10·4)	32·2–46·3 (39·6)
Dog	11·7–16·9 (14·3)	36·6–51·6 (43·6)
Cat	8·1–13·5 (11·2)	30·6–46·0 (38·6)

young animals have lower values than adolescent and young adult animals of the same species. Also animals that have been accustomed to being handled for blood sampling have proportionately lower erythrocyte counts, packed cell

volumes and haemoglobin values than animals not so handled.

A reduction in the amount of haemoglobin per unit volume of blood (usually expressed as grams/100 ml) gives rise to the state of anaemia. This state may or may not be due to a reduction in the erythrocyte population and/or in the packed cell volume (volume of erythrocytes in proportion to that of the plasma). Haematologists usually classify anaemia on such criteria as the morphology of the erythrocytes, the activity of the bone marrow or the aetiology involved (for a discussion on the last see p. 272). Morphological differentiation involves consideration of the cell size, e.g. macrocytic, normocytic or microcytic, and variations in staining intensity which are taken to reflect differences in haemoglobin content, e.g. normochromic, hypochromic. Some of the techniques employed to make these assessments have already been described, others will be referred to later.

For the clinician, classification on the basis of aetiology is probably most revealing because it is based on disease entities. Broadly speaking, on this basis, anaemia may be associated with four main groups of aetiological factors (see p. 272). It is necessary to point out that not infrequently a combination of factors may operate, more or less simultaneously, to produce anaemia.

Packed Cell Volume (Haematocrit) Determination

This procedure enables the volume of the erythrocytes to be measured and compared with the proportions of the other blood constituents. The volume of the erythrocytes in normal blood is directly proportional to their number and to the haemoglobin value. The results of the determination are informative, it is readily performed, and the margin of error is small. The measurement of the various cellular and fluid proportions of the blood, which comprises the principle of the test, is achieved by centrifuging unclotted blood in a special tube. Distortion of the erythrocytes is minimised when EDTA is used as the anticoagulant. Two main methods are suitable for routine use.

Wintrobe method. Wintrobe haematocrit tubes (Fig. 202), approximately 1 ml volume, closed at one end and calibrated by a 100 mm scale, are filled to the 10 cm mark with well-mixed blood by means of a pipette with a long slender tip. Air bubbles are avoided by inserting the tip of the pipette to the bottom of the tube and gently

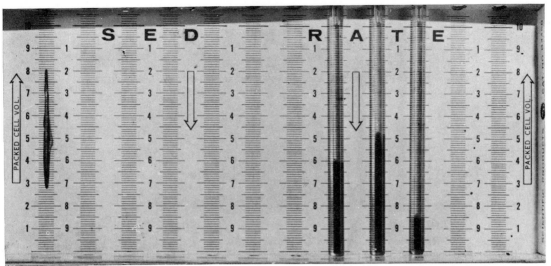

Fig. 202. *Haematocrit tubes (Wintrobe) used for determining the sedimentation rate and packed cell volume of a blood sample. Note the wide variation in packed cell volumes between the different tubes.*

withdrawing it as the blood level in the tube rises. The filled tubes are placed in a suitable holder in the bucket of a centrifuge with a head radius of not less than 22·5 cm and capable of 3000 rpm. These conditions will give the minimum required *g* force of 2260. The time required for satisfactory packing of the cells varies according to the speed and radius of the centrifuge arm, and the species of animal. A standard time of 60 minutes is recommended although prolonging centrifugation does not compensate for inadequate speed, i.e. below 3000 rpm. Because of greater variation in size and less tendency to rouleaux formation, erythrocytes of cattle, and more so those of sheep and goats, do not pack as readily as those of horses, dogs and cats. The method is tedious, time-consuming and expensive because of the high breakage rate of tubes and excessive wear of centrifuges.

The volume of red cells, as a percentage, when packed, is obtained by reading the graduation on the Wintrobe tube corresponding to the upper level of the erythrocytes. Immediately above the packed erythrocytes is a narrow band of leucocytes and thrombocytes (buffy coat) on which the plasma is superimposed. If erythrogenesis has been profound a narrow band of reticulocytes and nucleated red cells may be superimposed on the column of normal erythrocytes. The normal ranges of PCV values for the different species of animals are included in Table 15.

Microhaematocrit method (capillary tube method). This method gives better packing than the Wintrobe method with PCV values which are 2–3% lower. It requires the use of a special microhaematocrit centrifuge (Fig. 203) which is fiitted with a head for carrying up to 24 capillary tubes and capable of 12 000 rpm. An automatic switch set to a time of 5 minutes, which has been ascertained to give reasonably consistent results, can be incorporated into the centrifuge to ensure uniform treatment for all samples.

The tube, in the form of a short, slender cylinder, fills readily by capillarity from any source of unclotted blood, and when filled one end is sealed off by heating in a flame. The filled tube is placed in a slot in the centrifuge head with the sealed end outwards. Plain tubes are available for use with blood containing an anticoagulant, and heparinized tubes for blood directly available from capillary or venepuncture. The tubes are discarded after use.

A special scale, the microhaematocrit reader, is necessary to obtain the packed cell volume percentage, the depth of the buffy coat and the plasma layer, in the same terms.

By comparing the packed cell volume determination for a blood sample with the figure for normal animals, it is possible to appreciate the presence of anaemia, normal erythrocyte mass or the existence of haemoconcentration. Standardization of technique is necessary to ensure reproducible results. Potassium oxalate by causing shrinkage of the red cells will give low

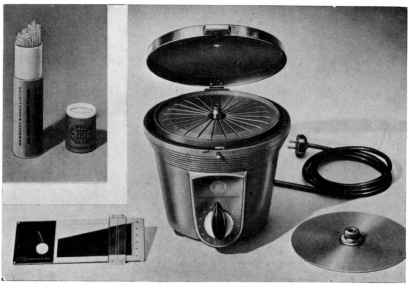

Fig. 203. *A microhaematocrit centrifuge, scale reader and capillary tubes for determining packed cell volume.*

PCV readings and should not be used on its own as an anticoagulant; EDTA or heparin is more satisfactory. False haemoconcentration can result if prolonged venous stasis occurs at the time the blood is withdrawn.

The cubical volume (mean corpuscular volume or MCV) of the erythrocytes can be determined by multiplying the PCV by 10 and then dividing the result by the erythrocyte count in millions/mm^3. The amount of haemoglobin expressed in picograms (pg) in each erythrocyte (mean corpuscular haemoglobin or MCH) is obtained by multiplying the haemoglobin value in g/100 ml by 10 and then dividing the result by the erythrocyte count in millions/mm^3. The average concentration of haemoglobin in each erythrocyte (mean corpuscular haemoglobin concentration or MCHC) is determined by multiplying the haemoglobin value in g/100 ml by 100 and then dividing the result by the PCV value. Values for these various parameters, which are of value in classifying anaemia, are available for the various species of domestic animals. For details textbooks on veterinary haematology should be consulted.

Sedimentation Rate

When it is considered necessary to determine the sedimentation rate of the blood cells, care must be taken to ensure that a standard amount of anticoagulant is present in each unit volume of blood. If possible make this measurement within 30 minutes after the blood has been collected if an oxalate anticoagulant has been used; a delay of up to 6 hours is acceptable when the anticoagulant is EDTA. For the test well-mixed venous blood is filled into a Wintrobe (Fig. 202) or other graduated haematocrit tube which is then placed in a perfectly vertical position; a well-made sedimentation rack will ensure that this is achieved. For optimal reproducibility and comparison, the room temperature should be near 20°C at all times, and the result should be read in exactly 1 hour. The rate of fall of the erythrocytes varies in the different species of animals and for all practical purposes ESR determinations are only of value in the dog. The rate at which erythrocytes sediment is inversely related to the number of red cells so that when interpreting the results of the test a correction factor based on the PCV value has to be introduced.

Bleeding Time and Coagulation Time

The bleeding time is determined by making a deep puncture with a sharp-pointed scalpel blade in the skin or the mucous membrane of the lower lip. At intervals of 30 seconds the blood should be removed by absorbing with a piece of filter paper. Note the interval which elapses before bleeding ceases. In normal animals it varies between 1 and 5 minutes.

Differences between the bleeding time and clotting time in an individual animal are largely attributable to variations in temperature and the inherent errors in the techniques employed. Coagulation time determinations should include the blood of normal controls in every instance. Techniques using venous or capillary blood may be used. Venous blood is allowed to flow freely from a hypodermic needle inserted into a superficial vein and a number of capillary tubes about 15 cm long and 1 mm diameter are filled by holding one end in contact with the blood emerging from the needle. Without delay one end of the filled tubes is plugged with plasticine and they are placed upright in a thermos jar containing water at a temperature between 37° and 40°C. The procedure is timed and, commencing after an interval of 30 seconds, portions of the tubes containing blood are broken off every 30 seconds. The coagulation time is the interval which elapses between filling the capillary tubes and the first appearance of fibrin thread on breaking a tube. The capillary tubes may be filled with blood obtained by the method employed for determining the bleeding time.

The Lee and White method, which is relatively efficient, consists of placing 4 chemically clean 2 ml testtubes in a suitable rack. With a sterile dry 10 ml syringe at least 5 ml of blood are withdrawn from a vein without any delay in entering the chosen vessel. Gentle suction only must be applied otherwise the vein may collapse and/or air bubbles may be produced. Withdraw the syringe and, after removing the needle, expel 1 ml of blood into each of 3 tubes and at least 2 ml into a fourth. Place the first three tubes in a waterbath heated to 37°C. After 2 minutes from when the blood first enters the syringe remove the first tube and tilt it gently to determine if the blood is still fluid. Continue to examine the first tube at 30 second intervals until coagulation is sufficiently advanced to permit the tube to be inverted without spilling blood. The second tube is then examined every 30 seconds in the same manner, and so on for the third tube until coagulation has occurred.

The coagulation time for normal animals varies and the times obtained with the capillary method are shorter than for the tube method. Generally clotting times are longest in the horse and ox, but the within-species variation is considerable. The normal range for the horse and ox extends from 4 to 15 minutes, and in the dog from 2·5 to 13 minutes.

Defects in blood clotting are relatively uncommon in animals, the incidence being highest in the dog. Poisoning by dicoumarol derivatives (sweet clover, warfarin) occurring in cattle, dogs and pigs, bracken fern in cattle and trichloroethylene-extracted soyabean meal in calves, and some diseases involving the liver, e.g. canine infectious hepatitis, are some of the recognized causes. The primary defects in these conditions are vitamin K antagonism leading to hypoprothrombinaemia, failure of vitamin K absorption with a similar effect or thrombocytopenia. Thrombocytopenic purpura has been observed in dogs. A bleeding defect genetically and pathologically similar to haemophilia B (Christmas disease) in man has been described in male cairn terrier dogs. Lack of antihaemophilic globulin has been recognized in male dogs exhibiting all the clinical and pathological signs occurring in haemophilia A of man. A similar situation has been described in thoroughbred and standardbred male foals.

Blood Groups and Blood Compatibility

Most animal species inherit specific erythrocyte agglutinogens and lysins as simple Mendelian dominants, so that so-called blood groups occur as in man. In cattle there are ten systems of blood groups incorporating more than sixty red cell antigens. Blood group determination in cattle is a valuable aid in confirming parentage in pedigree lines. Sheep have seven recognized blood groups containing many antigenic factors. Pigs have at least sixteen individual red cell antigens which have been classified in three systems—A–O, E and K. The dog has been shown to have five red cell antigens, named A (a variant A^1), B, C, D and E. The blood groupings of the cat have not been fully investigated.

Blood incompatibility reactions are produced when erythrocytes with an associated agglutinogen are introduced into the vascular system of a recipient animal, the serum of which contains the specific antagonistic agglutinin. Cross-matching the erythrocytes and serum of donor and recipient would indicate when such a reaction is likely to occur. Usually in animals the agglutinins (iso-antibodies) are either present in very low titre or are entirely lacking, so that the first blood transfusion is unlikely, except in the horse, to produce a severe intravascular reaction. A second transfusion, particularly with blood from the same donor, is likely to cause an incompatibility reaction sufficiently severe to jeopardize the life of the recipient. Except sometimes in the horse, *in-vitro* testing of serum of recipient animals is not likely to reveal potential iso-antibody reactions. Adequate cross-matching of blood in animals is possible only by the use of specific typing sera, as in the direct or indirect Coombs test.

In cross-matching bloods the selected method should be capable of detecting erythrocyte agglutination and haemolysis. In cattle and sheep haemolysins are of primary importance, while in dogs and cats agglutinins are dominant, and in horses both factors need to be considered. Blood is collected from both donor and recipient, one clotted and one unclotted sample in each case. The red cells from both unclotted samples are centrifuged and washed three times in 0·9% saline solution and a final 10% suspension prepared in each case. Two drops of the recipient's serum and a similar amount of the donor's red cell suspension are placed in a small testtube and mixed. Similarly for the recipient's red cells and the donor's serum. Controls consisting of the donor's cells and serum and the recipient's cells and serum should be included. The tubes are allowed to stand for 30 minutes at room temperature and then centrifuged for 1 minute at 5000–100 000 rpm. The supernatant is examined for evidence of haemolysis. Agglutination is detected by tapping each tube with the finger.

The Spleen and Lymphoid Tissues

The major portion of the lymphoid tissues of the body is contained in the spleen and lymph nodes; other important lymphocyte containing tissues include the thymus and the Peyer's patches in the small intestine and the similar nodules in the lungs and mucosa of the urogenital system. The main functions of lymphoreticular tissues include the production of lymphocytes and, in the case of the lymph nodes to filter the lymph by allowing the endothelial cells to phagocytose bacteria, senile cells and foreign matter; the spleen and haemolymph nodes perform a similar function in respect of the blood.

Spleen

The shape and size of the spleen show considerable variations as between normal animals of different species. In the monogastric species it is situated in close relationship to the greater curvature of the stomach on the left of the median plane, but it does not normally extend beyond the costal arch to a sufficient extent to be recognizable by means of palpation. In cattle and sheep the spleen is related intimately on its medial surface to the dorsal curvature of the rumen just below the left pillar of the diaphragm. Although the dorsal border extends just beyond the last rib, the normal spleen is not palpable in these species. The position of the spleen is influenced in monogastric animals by the degree of fullness of the stomach. In the dog, when the stomach is full of food, the spleen is situated medially to the last rib on the left side. Recognition of the organ by palpation, even under these circumstances, is doubtful.

The spleen, which is the largest organized mass of lymphoid tissue in the body, performs a variety of functions, the chief of which are destruction of effete or abnormal erythrocytes (during this procedure haemoglobin is degraded to bilirubin and haemosiderin, the latter being stored in the spleen), a reservoir for blood and haematopoiesis during fetal development, with continuation of this function in respect of the mononuclear cells of the blood during postnatal existence (lymphocyte production is important in relation to potential protection by antibodies). None of these functions is vital as, following splenectomy, animals exhibit no disturbance of health apart from an increased propensity, in the case of cattle, to succumb to repeated attacks of certain protozoan diseases, e.g. babesiasis.

Clinical examination of the spleen is limited mainly to palpation and percussion, which may reveal the presence of pain or gross enlargement. Palpation of the spleen in the horse is only likely to be achieved during rectal exploration when the organ is grossly enlarged or when its position is so modified, because of overfilling of the stomach, that its posterior border is within reach. Careful percussion may suggest when splenomegaly exists in cattle, although this technique is more likely to reveal a pain reaction in splenitis which, in this species, may develop as a further complication of traumatic reticulo-peritonitis. Otherwise splenitis may be due to splenic abscesses which result from lodgement of septic emboli. External palpation of the left anterior abdomen in the dog will, in the majority of instances, suggest when significant enlargement of the spleen exists by reason of detecting a vague indeterminate mass in this position. The enlargement is frequently the result of neoplastic involvement, in which case other, more general, clinical signs are likely to be exhibited.

Enlargement of the spleen may be of temporary or permanent duration. A degree of splenomegaly occurs during the course of septicaemic diseases, as well as in those conditions characterized by intravascular haemolytic reactions. In those circumstances the splenic enlargement is usually diffusely uniform. Nodular splenic enlargement may be the result of neoplasia, haematoma, hydatidosis or hyperplasia, although the latter, occurring particularly in old dogs, is not usually sufficient in degree to be appreciated by means of palpation. In malignant lymphomatosis (lymphosarcoma, leucosis) the spleen may in some instances be diffusely enlarged in addition to a variable number of the lymph nodes.

Lymph Nodes

The size of the lymph nodes varies greatly in normal animals; even in individual members of the same species the lymph nodes are by no means equal in size. They are usually larger in young animals than in adults and are comparatively large in the dog. Normal lymph nodes are firm in consistency; the smaller nodes appear to have a smooth structure on palpation, but lobulation is distinctly palpable in the larger nodes, e.g. the submaxillary lymph node in the horse. The skin is always freely movable over a superficially situated lymph node, and the node itself is somewhat mobile in relation to the neighbouring tissues.

The following lymph nodes are of importance in a clinical examination. Reference should be made to a textbook of veterinary anatomy for the exact size, shape, position and area drained by individual nodes in each species.

1. *Submaxillary lymph nodes.* In the horse these nodes are situated beneath the skin towards the posterior part of the intermaxillary space; they are as thick as a finger and converge anteriorly. In the ox and dog the corresponding lymph nodes lie behind the intermaxillary space near the angle of the mandible. There are at least two, more often even four or five, nodes in this group in the dog.

2. *Pharyngeal lymph nodes.* These consist of two groups. (*a*) The *subparotid* (*parapharyngeal* in the horse) lymph nodes are situated on the posterior part of the masseter muscle beneath the parotid salivary gland. In the horse the nodes lie on the upper part of the lateral surface of the pharynx, just below the guttural pouch, where they are not directly palpable. They are readily palpable in the ox and dog. (*b*) The *retropharyngeal* (or *suprapharyngeal*) lymph nodes in the horse and ox are situated on the posterior part of the pharynx; in the dog the relationship is dorsal to the pharynx. The nodes are comparatively small in the horse and because of their situation they are sometimes known as the guttural pouch lymph nodes.

3. *Anterior, middle and posterior cervical* (*prepectoral*) *lymph nodes*, which are situated respectively in the vicinity of the thyroid gland (under cover of the posterior part of the parotid salivary gland in the horse), in the middle of the neck on the trachea and near the entrance to the thorax, ventral to the trachea. These lymph nodes are not present as definitely recognizable masses in the dog.

4. *Prescapular lymph nodes*, which are situated in front and slightly dorsal to the point of the shoulder. In the horse they lie on the anterior border of the anterior deep pectoral muscle; in the ox and dog, at the anterior border of the supraspinatus muscle.

5. *Cubital lymph nodes* (regularly present only in the horse), which are situated on the medial aspect of the humerus between the elbow and the wall of the thorax; they are covered by muscle and are palpable only in a lean animal.

6. *Axillary lymph nodes* are situated deeply in the axilla beneath muscle masses which prohibit effective palpation in the horse and ox. In the dog, abduction of the limb enables these nodes to be recognized by palpation, more readily in lean animals.

7. *Precrural* (*prefemoral*) *lymph nodes*, which are situated above the fold of the flank on the anterior border of the tensor fasciae latae, dorsal to the stifle. They are absent in the dog.

8. *Popliteal lymph nodes*, which are situated between the biceps femoris and semitendinosus muscles posterior to the gastrocnemius muscle. In the dog, these nodes are relatively superficially situated on the gastrocnemius muscle, at the level of the stifle joint, where they can be palpated.

9. (*a*) *Supramammary lymph nodes* are situated in the perineum above the mammary gland. In the cow there are usually two, sometimes more, nodes on each side; the larger nodes of the

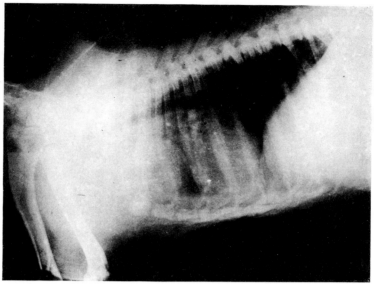

Fig. 204. *A radiograph showing a mass in the anterior mediastinum (lymph node or thymic in origin) in the dog.*

group, which are posterior, resemble sheep kidneys set on edge, flattened from side to side and approximately 4 cm in height. They are often fused posteriorly, giving the impression of a single mass when they are palpated. Palpation of these nodes in the cow is performed from behind the animal, using both hands and commencing in the upper third of the hindquarters and working towards the perineum. If the posterior nodes are situated near the skin, or the udder is to any degree pendulous they are usually palpable, but when the mammary gland is closely attached to the abdominal wall, or the lymph nodes are deeply situated, palpation is not possible. In female animals of other species the nodes are palpated in front of the hindlimb, and in the bitch they are readily recognized dorsal to the inguinal mammary gland. (*b*) *Superficial inguinal lymph nodes* in the stallion form an elongated group on either side of the penis. In the bull and ram they are situated in fatty tissue posterior to the spermatic cord at the neck of the scrotum. These nodes in the dog are related medially to the penis, below the external inguinal ring.

10. *External iliac lymph nodes* which are situated in the posterior part of the flank medial to the ilium, are not palpable from the exterior.

11. *Bronchial and mediastinal lymph nodes.* The lymph nodes of the thoracic cavity are sometimes visualized in a radiograph of the dog and cat, especially when they are enlarged (Fig. 204).

In the sheep, with the exceptions mentioned, the lymph nodes occupy the same positions as in the ox. None of the lymph nodes in the pig is ordinarily palpable.

12. Certain other lymph nodes are of clinical importance, but as a rule they can only be identified when they are enlarged and are palpable per rectum in large animals, or through the abdominal wall in the dog. In cattle enlargement of the *posterior mediastinal* lymph nodes (lymphosarcoma, actinobacillosis, tuberculosis), which may cause compression stenosis of the oesophagus and so reduce its lumen, can sometimes be recognized by passing a stomach tube. The condition is suggested by encountering a sudden increase in resistance well before the instrument enters the cardia. During withdrawal the sequence of events is reversed. Occasionally, swollen lymph nodes can be palpated at other sites, such as the subcutaneous tissues at the base of the ear or on the wall of the thorax and abdomen.

Clinical Examination of the Lymph Nodes and Vessels

Clinical examination of the palpable lymph nodes involves inspection and palpation. Biopsy specimens can be obtained for histopathological examination in selected cases; by this means the nature of primary or other neoplasms may be ascertained. Inspection reveals changes in normal contours caused by enlargement of a lymph node. Palpation provides more critical evaluation of the changes that may exist. The following points are noted: sizes; pain reaction; lobulation; consistency; temperature of the overlying skin; abscess formation, maturation and discharge; adhesions between the lymph node and the skin or surrounding tissues; and the number of the palpable lymph nodes involved and whether the involvement is unilateral or bilateral.

In all pathological processes of any significance there is a reaction in the associated lymph nodes, that is, those draining the affected area, although any increase in size is not always great enough to be recognizable clinically. When assessing the significance of an increase in the size of a lymph node it should be remembered that the enlargement may represent (a) an acute local inflammatory reaction which may either resolve completely (non-specific wound infection, sporadic lymphangitis in the horse, ephemeral fever) or lead to suppuration (strangles, epizoötic lymphangitis); (b) part of a systemic reaction to a major specific disease (anthrax, pasteurella septicaemia, malignant catarrhal fever, East Coast fever, swine fever); (c) a chronic inflammatory reaction (chronic suppuration of the sinuses or guttural pouch, early stages of glanders or tuberculosis, caseous lymphadenitis of sheep, some cases of actinobacillosis and actinomycosis (Fig. 205);

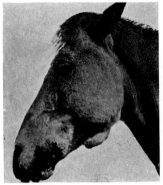

Fig. 205. *Severe swelling of the submaxillary lymph nodes and ulceration at the angle of the mouth. Actinomycosis.*

(d) neoplasia, which may be primary (lymphosarcoma) or secondary (metastasis) as the result of spread from the neighbouring tissues (carci-

noma); or (e) part of a generalized neoplasia of lymphatic tissue (lymphomatosis, myeloid leukaemia). In acute inflammatory conditions the swollen lymph node is hot and painful and the lobulation is indistinct. In chronic diseases, on the other hand, the lymph node when enlarged is painless, firm, normal in temperature and sometimes adherent to the skin, or the contiguous tissues; lobulation may still be perceptible. In pyogenic involvement of lymph nodes fluctuation may be demonstrated and the overlying skin may be hot, and the surrounding tissues painful and swollen (collateral inflammatory oedema and lymph stasis).

Unilateral enlargement of the pharyngeal lymph nodes indicates that there is a unilateral affection of the head, such as suppuration in a sinus or guttural pouch, whereas bilateral enlargement of the lymph nodes indicates that the disease involves both sides of the head. The submaxillary lymph nodes are bilaterally involved in strangles, bilateral nasal glanders and actinobacillosis of the tongue. As already indicated, generalized enlargement of the lymph nodes is usually associated with acute systemic infectious diseases or with certain neoplastic conditions. Differentiation between lymphadenitis and lymph node neoplasia can be established by histological examination of a biopsy specimen.

When grossly enlarged, lymph nodes may exert pressure on important structures in their vicinity and so produce secondary clinical signs, e.g. dysphagia or recurrent ruminal tympany as a result of enlargement of the posterior mediastinal lymph nodes; dyspnoea from swellings of the retropharyngeal or bronchial lymph nodes; obstructive oedema of the head and neck (see Fig. 82, p. 77) through pressure on the jugular vein by enlarged posterior cervical lymph nodes; and retention of urine in the horse through pressure on the urethra by enlarged superficial inguinal lymph nodes.

The peripheral lymphatic vessels may be grossly distended as a result of inflammation (lymphangitis), forming tortuous branching cords as in sporadic lymphangitis, cutaneous glanders, epizoötic lymphangitis, streptococcal lymphangitis in foals and ulcerative lymphangitis. If suppuration develops the abscesses and resultant nodular swellings occur at approximately equal distances apart, owing to the presence of valves in the vessels, at which invading bacteria tend to be arrested. This produces the 'pearl necklace'

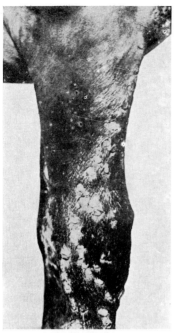

Fig. 206. *Swelling of the lymphatic vessels with 'pearl necklace' distribution of ulcers on the forelegs of a horse. Epizoötic lymphangitis.*

arrangement of nodular swellings (Fig. 206), noted in glanders, epizoötic lymphangitis, sporotrichosis, so-called 'skin tuberculosis', etc. When mature the pyogenic foci discharge onto the skin surface and are converted into ulcers. In chronic lymphangitis, fibrous tissue proliferation occurs in the subcutis along with thickening of the skin.

Clinical Blood Chemistry

Chemical analysis of the blood is of considerable value in confirming the diagnosis (in some diseases retrospectively) prognosis and response to treatment in a variety of diseases. The majority of the techniques involved require specialized facilities and experience, so are beyond the scope of most veterinary practices. It is necessary, however, in order to be able to interpret the results of such analyses accurately, to possess a sound knowledge of the normal range of some of the more important chemical constituents of the blood, and to appreciate the importance of any significant variation. When a decision is made to submit a blood sample to a laboratory for determination of some particular constituent, it is necessary to appreciate the need to ensure that the specimen is obtained in the proper manner, depending upon whether clotted or unclotted blood is necessary, and that it is accompanied by a clear request indicating the nature of the analysis required, based upon sufficient information about the patient to assist the analyst. The value of biochemical tests carried out on blood is related to the care taken when deciding which tests are to be requested, and in the actual collection of the specimen. Employing such procedures on a spot-check basis will lead to frustration for the clinical chemist and clinician alike.

For clinical purposes, biochemical analysis of blood is limited to determinations of glucose, non-protein nitrogen, ketones, calcium, inorganic phosphorus, magnesium, bilirubin and transaminases. Blood values can also be obtained for sodium, potassium, chloride, plasma proteins, alkaline phosphatase and tocopherals, as well as for 'trace elements' such as copper and cobalt and toxic elements including fluorine, lead and molybdenum. The majority of the determinations can be made on serum, so that clotted blood is suitable. All equipment used, including the needle and syringe, must be dry and chemically clean, otherwise haemolysis or contamination will cause errors in the result. If sterilization can only be performed by boiling, distilled or deionized water should be used, and the equipment removed from the boiling water and air-dried. When glucose or nitrogenous substances are to be determined, blood is collected in containers with potassium oxalate or EDTA. For accurate determination of chloride and other electrolytes, the blood must be collected under mineral oil in order to protect it from exposure to air. In all instances blood stasis must be avoided during collection of the sample by slightly loosening the tourniquet when the needle has entered the vein and then slowly aspirating the required amount of blood.

Delay in carrying out the analytical procedure will reduce the accuracy of the results. This is more marked with some constituents, including glucose, inorganic phosphate and non-protein nitrogen. The addition of 10 mg sodium fluoride and 1 mg thymol per millilitre of blood will preserve it for 2–3 days, provided the blood is sterile, so that reasonably satisfactory results are obtained. Laboratories which are prepared to undertake blood chemical determinations will usually provide sample bottles prepared for use.

TABLE 16. NORMAL VALUES (MG/100 ML) OF SOME CLINICALLY IMPORTANT CHEMICAL CONSTITUENTS

Species	Whole Blood Preformed Creatinine	Whole Blood Urea	Serum Calcium	Serum Inorganic Phosphate	Serum Magnesium	Serum Total Bilirubin
Horse	1·2–1·9	5–20	10·0–14·0	2·4–4·5	2·2–4·5	0·8–3·0
Ox	1·0–2·0	5–20	10·0–12·25	3·2–8·4	2·0–3·0	0–0·5
Sheep	1·2–1·8	5–20	9·0–12·25	2·9–7·4	2·6–3·5	0–0·4
Goat	0·9–1·8	5–20	9·25–11·5	4·0–9·7	2·7–3·5	0–0·1
Pig	1·0–2·7	5–20	9·0–12·5	4·6–10·2	2·4–3·6	0–0·4
Dog	1·0–1·7	5–40	8·5–11·5	2·4–4·2	1·8–2·8	0–0·3
Cat	0·9–1·7	5–40	8·0–9·5	2·5–4·3	2·0–2·8	0–0·2

The normal range of a number of chemical constituents in the blood of domestic animals and which are of possible clinical significance are given in Table 16.

Blood glucose. A minimum of 2 ml of unclotted blood is required for quantitative glucose determination. If there is likely to be any delay in making the measurement, sodium fluoride should be included in the sample bottle as recommended. The commonly used methods for measuring blood glucose are based on reduction of an alkaline copper solution. With the possible exception of the Nelson/Somogyi method they all overestimate glucose by up to 30%. The glucose oxidase method is more accurate.

Isolated blood glucose determinations have limited value in animals unless the results are carefully correlated with the clinical findings, and the results of other tests of metabolic function are also available. Even more meaningful is a metabolic profile compiled from periodic chemical determinations of all the animals in the herd or group. In normal cattle and sheep the blood sugar level ranges from 38 to 60 mg/100 ml. Dairy cattle with ketosis and sheep with pregnancy toxaemia invariably have blood glucose values below 35 mg/100 ml. The severity of the ketonaemia in both conditions, however, is such that the results of chemical tests for ketones, in association with the clinical findings, make a blood sugar determination unnecessary.

During the neonatal period the carbohydrate metabolism of the young pig is unstable and almost entirely dependent upon a regular milk intake, although energy requirements from carbohydrate sources are increased by low environmental temperatures. The circumstances which contribute to primary and secondary hypoglycaemia in the piglet are readily recognized so that blood sugar determination is not usually necessary in establishing the diagnosis. Blood glucose values in normal pigs range from 65 to 100 mg/100 ml.

The fasting blood glucose level in normal dogs ranges from 60 to 100 mg/100 ml and in cats from 70 to 100 mg/100 ml. If the renal threshold for glucose (between 160 and 190 mg/100 ml) is exceeded the glucose spills over into the urine (glucosuria). An important, infrequent, cause of hyperglycaemia and glucosuria in the dog and cat is diabetes mellitus which develops because of hypoinsulinism. The impaired carbohydrate metabolism is, however, accompanied by keto-naemia and ketonuria, so that chemical detection of glucose and ketones in the urine obviates the need for blood glucose determinations, at least as far as the diagnosis is concerned. A more exact prognosis in such a case demands a determination of the blood glucose level after the animal has been fasted for 24 hours. Replacement therapy with insulin, and dietary control measures can be more accurately assessed on the basis of the information obtained from regular blood glucose determinations.

Non-protein nitrogen. In normal animals of all species at least 90% of the nitrogen derived from protein of dietary origin is removed from the blood by the kidneys and excreted in the urine as non-protein nitrogenous compounds of which urea comprises from 70 to 95%, the remainder consisting mainly of ammonia (1–10%), and creatinine (1–10%). The excretion of urea is regarded as being one of the most important functions of the kidney, therefore the blood urea level may be considered to be an index of renal efficiency. It must be appreciated, however, that the blood non-protein nitrogen level is influenced by the proportion of protein in the diet, the volume of urine, and the occurrence and rate of endogenous protein catabolism.

For the measurement of urea 1 ml of well-mixed unclotted blood (avoid ammonium oxalate as an anticoagulant) is required. The normal blood urea values differ only slightly among the different species of domestic animals and, excluding the dog, range from 5 to 20 mg/100 ml. The within-species variation is greatest in the dog; urea nitrogen values of up to 40 mg/100 ml may be found in healthy animals on a meat diet, urea being an end-product of protein deaminization. In renal insufficiency associated with nephritis in dogs, the blood urea level may range from 80 to 400 mg/100 ml, the amount not necessarily being proportional to the severity of the kidney disease. In this context it is necessary to appreciate that urea at these levels is in itself relatively non-toxic, and that the so-called uraemic signs are probably produced by other unidentified substances. Generally, in a confirmed case of renal insufficiency arising from nephritis, the blood urea value is of some assistance in formulating a prognosis. Other clinical features reflecting kidney function, such as anuria or persistent oliguria in acute nephritis, or polyuria and polydipsia with urine of low specific gravity should, however, also be taken into account when blood urea nitrogen levels are elevated to over 100 mg/100 ml. It goes without saying that it is necessary to differentiate between prerenal and renal diseases when considering the significance of raised blood-urea values. Prerenal conditions causing so-called pseudouraemia (extrarenal azotaemia) include severe haemorrhage, shock, severe dehydration, prolonged vomiting, intestinal obstruction, protracted constipation, etc. Provided the patient survives long enough many of these states can be alleviated, thereby reversing the blood urea elevation.

Creatinine. Creatinine is the end product of protein catabolism and its concentration in the blood and urine of animals is not significantly influenced by the diet. Creatinine values for normal animals are given in Table 16. Because it is a non-threshold substance as far as the kidney is concerned, i.e. it is filtered by the glomerulus (more readily in fact than urea) and not reabsorbed by the tubules, when there is severe renal damage a rise in blood creatinine occurs. The degree of this rise can be more accurately correlated to the extent of the kidney damage in chronic nephritis than in acute renal impairment, in which excessive protein catabolism will artificially elevate the blood creatinine value.

Calcium. Blood calcium determination is performed on serum. The range for the different species of animals is given in Table 16. Age appears to have no significant influence on serum calcium values although young calves have been shown to have rather high levels for the first 8 weeks of life. The usual methods used to determine serum calcium measure the total calcium, which exists in three forms; a protein-bound fraction, an ionized portion and a third fraction which is combined with organic substances such as citrate.

Calcium, in association with phosphorus, is necessary to ensure normal bone growth in animals. A sudden increase in calcium mobilization from the skeletal reserves is desirable in parturient animals, more especially, perhaps, in the cow, ewe and bitch, to avoid the possibility of acute hypocalcaemia, leading to tetany. Total serum calcium levels are likely to be depressed by deficient calcium absorption from the intestine (this has been shown to be of considerable significance in relation to milk fever), by reduction in plasma protein, by decrease in the amount of parathyroid hormone, by increased secretion of thyrocalcitonin and by increase in the serum content of inorganic phosphorus. Reduction in the plasma protein value affects the physiologically inactive portion of the blood calcium which, however, appears to be readily unbound, at least by simple physicochemical procedures. The blood inorganic phosphorus level is increased in advanced renal insufficiency in the dog, leading to increased intestinal excretion of phosphate which brings about precipitation of dietary calcium in the form of insoluble tertiary calcium phosphate and hypocalcaemia. Active bone resorption is initiated in an attempt to supply ionized calcium and leads to demineralization of the bones, particularly those of the face, mandibles and extremities.

Calcium is stored in the body in the bones where, in association with phosphorus and magnesium, it forms complexes which are responsible for skeletal rigidity. In young animals, dietary deficiency of calcium or phosphorus, or too wide a calcium/phosphorus ratio or inadequacy of vitamin D is followed by the development of rickets, which is usually most obvious in the long bones of the limbs. The factors responsible vary according to the species, as a general rule calcium and vitamin D deficiency together is responsible in young carnivores, although in cats excess of phosphorus, producing imbalance in the ratio between this element and calcium, is likely when they are confined indoors and fed diets consisting almost entirely of fish and meat.

In adult animals, similar circumstances lead to the appearance of osteomalacia. Deficiency of vitamin D is, however, of relatively minor importance in the development of osteomalacia in domestic animals. Lack of vitamin D may, however, contribute to the development of the disease in certain species of monkeys. The bone lesion in osteomalacia results from demineralization, particularly of the diaphyses where metabolic activity is greatest during adult life.

The clinical syndromes resulting from disturbance of calcium metabolism are readily recognized in most cases, confirmation is usually provided by blood calcium determination and/or radiological examination. A satisfactory response to replacement therapy may be regarded as being confirmatory in parturient paresis (milk fever). In the absence of suggestive clinical evidence, too much significance should not be attached to the results of sporadic calcium or inorganic phosphate determinations on blood samples from an ailing animal. A more accurate picture of the status of animals in respect of calcium is obtained by examining samples from a proportion of the group, or in an individual animal, by retesting at stated intervals after dietary adjustments have been made.

Elevation of the serum calcium value (hypercalcaemia) above the normal range for animals of any species occurs with hyperparathyroidism or is induced following the administration of vitamin D and certain other steroid substances. Prolonged hypercalcaemia may cause calcium to be precipitated in the intima of arteries, particularly those directly connected to the heart.

Inorganic phosphate. Over 80% of the total body phosphorus is contained in the skeleton and teeth. The remainder is present in the body fluids in variable concentrations, those for the blood of normal animals being given in Table 16. The functions of phosphorus, outside the skeleton, are concerned with carbohydrate metabolism and the acid–base balance of the body. During periods of high carbohydrate utilization the blood levels of inorganic phosphate fall, and during fasting they usually rise.

There is also, but invariably, an inverse relationship between the inorganic phosphate and calcium levels in the tissue fluids. Phosphorus is present in the blood in at least three forms; inorganic phosphorus (this is the fraction that is usually determined and referred to in clinical discussion, organic or esterified phosphorus and lipid phosphorus which comprises 50% or more of the whole. The esterified phosphorus is contained in the erythrocytes, so that if a blood sample is, even partially, haemolysed the inorganic phosphate value will be increased because of the ease with which phosphate esters undergo hydrolysis. Young animals have somewhat higher levels of serum inorganic phosphate than adults, and with advancing years cattle show a marked fall in organic phosphate. No correlation has been established between variations in esterified phosphorus and disease in animals.

The inter-relationships between calcium, phosphorus and vitamin D have already been referred to in discussing calcium. The ratio between the calcium and phosphorus present in the diet will influence the absorption of both elements. When the ratio departs further from the optimum $2:1$, $1:2$, the vitamin D requirement increases and may become of primary significance. Reference has already been made to the possible significance of dietary phosphorus in the development of rickets, particularly in the ruminant species. Osteomalacia in adult animals of the ruminant species occurs as an expression of chronic aphosphorosis. During periods of inadequate dietary phosphorus intake, the serum inorganic phosphate levels will invariably fall. However, because of the inter-relationship between this element and both calcium and vitamin D, and the influence of factors such as phytates on intestinal absorption of phosphorus, and others, including alkaline phosphatase, parathyroid hormone and thyrocalcitonin on mobilization, utilization and excretion, too much significance should not be attached to variations from normal serum values. Generally, in aphosphorosis, it is found that affected animals have below normal serum inorganic phosphate levels and normal calcium and magnesium values. Diets, such as green growing cereals (oats, barley, etc.), containing high levels of carotene which has an anti-vitamin D effect have been recognized to cause osteomalacia and hypophosphataemia in grazing sheep. A similar situation involving lush pasture has been recognized to cause rickets in foals. Aphosphorosis causing severe hypophosphataemia manifest by hindleg lameness, occurs in high-yielding dairy cows ('milk-lameness'). Hypophosphataemia is considered to be an important factor in the development of post-parturient haemoglobinuria in dairy cattle and, in conjunction with a haemolysin, is responsible for intravascular haemolysis and the other clinical signs. Feeding on cruciferous crops (kale, rape, etc.) is a recognized precipitating factor for the condition.

Hyperphosphataemia occurs in advanced chronic renal insufficiency, and during the repair period of fracture healing. Osteodystrophia fibrosa, occurring in horses, goats and pigs fed on diets containing excessive amounts of phosphorus or inadequate calcium, and manifested clinically by lameness with softening, swelling and even fracture of bones, is associated with an early rise in serum inorganic phosphate and a later fall in serum calcium. These various conditions are connected with secondary hyperparathyroidism which is a compensatory reaction to hypocalcaemia. In young carnivorous animals feeding an unsupplemented meat diet, which has a calcium to phosphorus ratio of about 1 : 12, causes osteogenesis imperfecta characterized by extreme fragility of the skeleton. There is secondary hyperparathyroidism. Blood analyses reveal hyperphosphataemia and mild hypocalcaemia. Radiographic examination is likely to prove most revealing.

Alkaline phosphatase. Phosphatases are enzyme catalysts which split off inorganic phosphate from certain esterified forms of phosphorus by a process of hydrolysis. Alkaline phosphatases possess maximum activity at pH 8·5–9·5 (they are fairly active at the pH of blood), and they are activated by magnesium ions. There appears to be a wide range of serum phosphatase levels within each animal species, although in each individual animal the values tend to be rather restricted. In ruminant species serum phosphatase values progressively decline during adolescence, becoming, more or less stabilized during adult life. Pregnancy is associated with a slight increase which becomes quite marked as parturition becomes imminent (see Table 17).

In bone disease, serum alkaline phosphatase levels are increased when bone regeneration is being attempted or is actually taking place. When bone destruction is occurring in the absence of

regeneration, the serum enzyme value is normal. Young calves made hypophosphataemic by dietary means usually have increased serum phosphatase activity. The estimation of serum alkaline phosphatase activity is infrequently undertaken as a diagnostic procedure in domestic animals. Alkaline phosphatase is excreted in the bile so that when bile production or excretion is impaired serum values will increase (this is particularly so in extra- and intrahepatic biliary obstruction). Because the cat excretes alkaline phosphatase via the kidneys this situation does not arise

Magnesium. Reductions in blood magnesium levels are responsible for clinical disorders in cattle and sheep only among the domestic animals. In the rapidly developing form of hypomagnesaemic tetany the clinical course is short, so that the animal is not often observed until it is either in convulsive seizures or dead. During the convulsive episodes, magnesium is translocated into the blood from the soft tissues, and determining the serum magnesium content at this time is usually misleading. Assessment of the bone-ash magnesium, using rib or coccygeal vertebrae, is a post mortem means of identifying the hypomagnesaemic tetany syndrome in milk-fed calves.

A sample of clotted blood is required for magnesium estimation. The serum magnesium levels for normal animals of the domestic species are given in Table 16. In cattle, in contradistinction to other species of animals, the magnesium level is higher in the serum than in the erythrocytes. About one-third of the 70% of the total body magnesium which is present in the skeleton is a mobilizable source of the element, called upon when the dietary intake is inadequate. The rate of mobilization is, however, much slower in adult cattle compared with calves, so that the former often die from hypomagnesaemic tetany with no significant reduction in bone magnesium content.

Functionally, magnesium is an activator of a number of intracellular enzymes including phosphatases, and those catalysing reactions involving adenosine triphosphate (ATP). Because of the many diverse functions in which ATP is required it would appear that magnesium is involved in all the important anabolic and catabolic processes of the body. Extracellularly, magnesium exerts an important function in the production and the destruction of acetylcholine.

It appears that it is the depletion of the magnesium ion in the extracellular fluid surrounding the neuromuscular junctions and synapses which appears to be responsible for the tetanic muscular contractions observed in clinical hypomagnesaemia. The role of calcium in relation to hypomagnesaemia is not clear, although during the course of the disease, in a large proportion of adult cattle, a variable degree of hypocalcaemia exists.

Hypomagnesaemia in calves, manifested by typical tetanic seizures, is an expression of dietary deficiency of magnesium which occurs particularly in those animals which are growing fastest, when their food consists almost entirely of whole milk for considerable periods of time. Under these circumstances serum magnesium levels will fall gradually to about 0·7 mg/100 ml, at which point clinical signs are likely to develop. There is usually no significant change in serum calcium or inorganic phosphate values. During the period preceding the appearance of clinical disease, the bone magnesium stores are mobilized with a corresponding reduction in their magnesium status. The magnesium content of the bone ash from normal calves is around 0·8%, and in calves with serum magnesium values of 0·7 mg/100 ml, or less, the bone ash contains 0·4–0·5% of magnesium.

Clinical hypomagnesaemia in adult cattle has a complex aetiological pattern of inter-related factors which bring about a gradual or rapid fall in serum magnesium levels, thereby producing the clinical signs of the disease. In seasonal hypomagnesaemia there is a gradual fall in serum magnesium during the late autumn and winter (this is particularly marked in animals at pasture during periods of wet, cold and windy weather without supplementary feeding or shelter). So-called 'winter tetany', which occurs in beef cattle while being stall-fed or grazing during the winter when pasture growth has ceased, often develops when rather poor quality rations are being fed. Under these circumstances certain cows which appear to be clinically normal may be hypomagnesaemic, and an occasional animal may suddenly develop clinical signs within a few weeks after calving. Clinical cases of hypomagnesaemic tetany usually occur when the serum magnesium values are lowest and a variable degree of hypocalcaemia (around 8 mg/100 ml) exists. In so-called grass tetany, clinical hypomagnesaemia develops in cattle within a few weeks after they are turned out to graze in the spring. Young spring grass is high in water (85%), phosphorus, soluble carbohydrate and crude protein content, and low in crude fibre and calcium, while the magnesium content is theoretically adequate. In tetany-inducing situations it is usually found that the magnesium content of the herbage is below 0·2% (dry matter). As a rule a considerable proportion of the associated apparently normal grazing cattle will be found to have serum magnesium values near 1 mg/100 ml.

Ketone bodies. The ketone bodies which are important in cattle and sheep include acetoacetate, beta-hydroxybutyrate, acetone and isopropanol. Only the first three occur in other species. Total blood ketone values in normal cattle and sheep are less than 10 mg/100 ml. In non-ruminant species the liver is probably the only site of ketogenesis, while in ruminant species, although the liver is the main source, supplementary production of ketone bodies takes place in the rumen and mammary gland. Ketone bodies diffuse into all the body fluids so that in hyperketonaemia there are appreciable amounts in the urine and milk. Abnormally high blood ketone levels are a feature of bovine ketosis, pregnancy toxaemia, starvation (particularly in ruminants) and diabetes mellitus, which last occurs most frequently in dogs.

Total blood ketones can be determined quantitatively as acetone by the salicylaldehyde method, or one of its modifications, but the simple, rapid qualitative methods of detection, applied to urine or milk, are sufficiently accurate for diagnostic purposes. Renal concentration of ketones gives rise to many false positive results with urine of normal cows. Diluting one part of urine with ten parts of water may increase the diagnostic value of tests for urinary ketones. In lactating cows, the milk ketone levels approximate those of the blood, so that the results of a qualitative test on the milk may be a fair indication of the degree of hyperketonaemia, if it exists. The rapid qualitative tests can be applied to blood serum when it is diluted 1 : 1 with water, and are particularly valuable as an aid in the diagnosis of pregnancy toxaemia in sheep because of the difficulty of obtaining samples of other body fluids. In these various diseases, it is important to realize that the degree of ketonaemia does not directly reflect the severity of the clinical signs.

The qualitative tests consisting of various modifications of Rothera's test, and recent developments of them, which are employed for the detection of ketones in the various body fluids are described on p. 231.

Bilirubin. Because of the general use of the van den Bergh reaction, variations in serum bilirubin values in animals were a source of confusion and almost impossible to interpret. The application of chromatographic techniques revealed that the 'direct reacting' fraction in the van den Bergh test is a glucuronide conjugate of bilirubin, and the 'indirect reaction' fraction is free and unconjugated. Conversion of free to conjugated bilirubin is activated by glucuronyl transferase, a non-specific enzyme, in the liver. Deficiency of this enzyme, a condition which is genetically derived, gives rise to a number of syndromes in man, and appears as a mutant condition in Southdown sheep.

The van den Bergh test can be performed in a qualitative or quantitative manner. As a practical diagnostic procedure the qualitative test is of little value. Serum bilirubin values for normal animals of the various domestic species are included in Table 16. The interpretation of quantitative bilirubin values varies according to the species and, on the whole, is disappointing as an aid to classifying icterus. In the dog, bile metabolism in disease follows more closely the pattern in man, when compared with that of the other domestic animals. Increased serum levels of conjugated bilirubin in the dog indicate intra- or extrahepatic biliary obstruction. When the total bilirubin value is elevated, and more than 50% is of the conjugated variety, liver cell damage has probably occurred. A corresponding situation with a preponderance of free bilirubin suggests a prehepatic haemolytic disease. Because the renal threshold for conjugated bilirubin is low, moderate or even slight increases in serum levels may indicate the existence of hepatocellular disease. The significance of such determinations must be interpreted on a basis of correlation with the clinical condition of the animal.

In the horse the significance of elevated serum bilirubin values is frequently difficult to interpret, not least because hyperbilirubinaemia and icterus do not always coincide. The major part of the bilirubin in the serum of horses with either haemolytic or hepatic jaundice is of the free or indirect reacting variety. Confusion is added to the situation by reason of the rapid rise (up to 8-fold in 2–4 days) in blood bilirubin values which occur as the result of fasting. Consequently other more organ-specific function tests are likely to prove of greater efficiency in detecting liver disease in this species.

In cattle severe and extensive hepatopathy causes only a slight elevation in serum bilirubin value. Haemolytic jaundice causes a significant hyperbilirubinaemia. In ragwort poisoning in cattle it appears that disturbance of bilirubin excretion is a terminal event. Changes in conjugated and free serum bilirubin values in sheep, goats and pigs follow the same pattern as in cattle. In all these species fasting induces a rise in bilirubin values.

Serum enzyme activity. Serum normally contains a number of enzymes which can be measured by means of their biochemical activity. The factors which bring about variations in the serum concentration of the enzymes and their possible sources are discussed on p. 212. The enzymes include glutamic pyruvic transaminase (SGPT) and glutamic oxalacetic transaminase (SGOT), as well as arginase, isocitric dehydrogenase (SICD), sorbitol dehydrogenase (SD), glutamic dehydrogenase (GD), ornithine carbamyl transferase (OCT) and lactic dehydrogenase (LDH), which are present in many tissue cells, more particularly those of the liver, heart and skeletal musculature, so that necrosis or altered membrane permeability of these cells is associated with elevated serum values. In addition there are alkaline phosphatase (SAP), the serum concentration of which rises in obstructive jaundice, and choline esterase, the concentration of which falls when liver synthesis is impaired. The hepatic tissues of the dog, cat and primates contain high concentrations of SGPT, and in all ureotelic animals, including man, dog, sheep, ox and rat, the levels of arginase are high at this site. Following hepatic necrosis it would be logical to expect an increase in the blood concentration of these enzymes. Other tissues besides the liver possess high levels of SGOT and SICD, so that only when all tissues, apart from the liver, are normal, would it be possible to interpret the significance of elevated blood values. As a means of measuring the degree of hepatic necrosis, from mild to severe, the so-called 'liver-specific' enzyme tests (SGPT and arginase) are most satisfactory.

Normal serum values for the various enzymes

TABLE 17. SERUM ENZYME VALUES IN NORMAL ANIMALS

Species	Glutamic Oxalacetic Transaminase (Sigma–Frankel units/ml)	Glutamic Pyruvic Transaminase (Sigma–Frankel units/ml)	Arginase (units/ml)	Isocitric Dehydrogenase (W-Wa units/ml)	Alkaline Phosphatase	Creatinine Phosphokinase (IU/litre)
Horse	110–200	5–15	0–4·5	250–1000	5·1–14·8 King-Armstrong units/ml	0–3·5
Ox	38–60	7–35	0–1·8	500–1250	0·04–0·60 King-Armstrong units/ml	—
Sheep	90–130	15–30	0–2·5	25–600	0·25–0·35	0–3·0
Pig	15–45	20–35	—	—	—	—
Dog	13–55	5–40	0–0·30	25–400	0·4–4·0 Bodansky units/ml	0–7·5
Cat	12–30	6–25	—	100–650	—	0–3·0

(Table 17) vary for each species and also according to the age of the animal, being lower in young than in adult animals of each species. A variety of methods, including rapid kit techniques which are available from commercial sources (Boehringer, Dade, Roche, Sigma and many others) can be used to measure these enzymes.

Interpreting the significance of elevated serum levels often presents difficulties and should never be attempted, except in the context of the clinical condition of the animal. As a means of identifying liver damage it must be realized that so-called liver specific enzymes only occur in the dog, cat and primates, and also that significant increases are most likely when the assault is recent and severe. Hepatic necrosis in adult horses, cattle, sheep and pigs produces insignificant increases in SGPT blood levels so that when elevated values are observed in these species, other sites of tissue damage must be looked for. Diseases such as muscular dystrophy, azoturia and myocardial ischaemia will, in addition to liver disease, give rise to increased SGOT values in the horse, cow, pig, dog and cat. Clinical cases of muscular dystrophy in calves have been observed with serum values of 300–900 units/ml, and in lambs 2000–3000 units/ml.

The presence of relatively large amounts of the mitochondrial enzyme arginase in the liver of the dog, sheep and cattle, suggests a means of identifying hepatic necrosis. Because of its source, the blood level of this enzyme returns more rapidly to normal in comparison with SGOT and SGPT, when the progress of liver necrosis is halted. A combination of arginase and transaminase determinations can be used for prognostic as well as diagnostic purposes.

Copper. This element is required in trace amounts for the utilization of iron in haemoglobin synthesis and as a stimulus to haematopoiesis. It also plays an important part in cellular respiration through the medium of cytochrome oxidase systems, or at least by supplementing them. The other enzymes which contain copper include tyrosinase, ascorbic acid oxidase, plasma monoamine oxidase, ceruloplasmin and uricase; their functional activity is dependent on this element.

Dietary supplies of copper (minimum 1–2 ppm for cattle and sheep and 4–6 ppm for pigs) are required almost constantly because the element is continuously being excreted in the faeces. Ordinarily, it appears that sheep and cattle are most prone to be affected with copper deficiency syndromes, although young pigs have also been recognized to be at risk in this respect. In grazing animals copper deficiency may be primary when there is an inadequate amount in the soil and, therefore, in the herbage, or secondary when the soil and herbage content of molybdenum and inorganic sulphate is high. Cattle appear to be much more susceptible to the interfering effects of molybdenum than sheep.

Apart from anaemia, other clinical syndromes associated with copper deficiency include bone disorders (spontaneous fractures, osteoporosis), neonatal ataxia (swayback in lambs), depigmentation and abnormal growth of hair or wool, reduced growth rate and fertility, and intestinal hypermotility (molybdenosis in cattle).

When it appears desirable to determine the copper status of a group of animals, because of wide individual variations in blood copper levels, samples should be obtained from a proportionate number of the group, and only if there is a uniform reduction compared with normal values can a diagnosis of copper deficiency be justified. Samples of blood for copper determination must be collected in special polythene bottles which are obtainable from laboratories prepared to perform this analysis. Blood copper values in normal sheep range from 0·07 to 0·13 mg/100 ml. In primary copper deficiency the levels fall to between 0·01 and 0·02 mg/100 ml, and in secondary copper deficiency the figures range from 0·04 to 0·07 mg/100 ml. For cattle the corresponding values are 0·07–0·17 mg/100 ml, 0·01–0·02 mg/100 ml and 0·03–0·05 mg/100 ml.

Liver copper values are a more reliable indicator of the copper status of a group of animals. When considering liver biopsy specimens as a source of material for copper estimations, it is necessary to sample a number of animals in the group and also to consider the range of values obtained in defining their significance, as with blood values. The technique for liver biopsy sampling has been described earlier. Levels of copper in the liver of normal adult sheep range from above 200 ppm DM and for cattle more than 100 ppm DM. Sheep affected with primary copper deficiency have liver copper levels of 20 ppm DM or less; in secondary copper deficiency the figure is usually around 15 ppm DM. The corresponding values for cattle are 2–5 ppm DM and 12 ppm DM. Soil and herbage copper, molybdenum and inorganic sulphate determinations are often revealing when investigating copper deficiency states in grazing animals.

An excess of copper in the diet has been recognized to give rise to so-called chronic copper poisoning which is usually manifested as an acute haemolytic crisis. In some countries certain plants (heliotrope, *Heliotropium europaeum*, subterranean clover, *Trifolium subterraneum*) growing in pastures are capable of accumulating copper (in some cases even when soil copper values are relatively low) and,

therefore, of inducing excessive retention of copper in the grazing animal, so that the presence of liver damage or exposing the animal to severe stress triggers off a 'haemolytic jaundice' crisis which proves fatal in the majority of cases. In some instances, copper sulphate included as a growth promotant at high levels (250 ppm) in diets will cause chronic poisoning in pigs with liver dystrophy, or when they are exposed to stress, as well as in sheep and cattle.

In chronic copper poisoning blood levels do not rise significantly until the haemolytic crisis has occurred; but liver copper values of above 1000 ppm DM in sheep, 2000 ppm in calves and 5000 ppm in pigs are not unusual shortly before clinical signs appear. It is also usual to find SGPT levels markedly increased beforehand.

Cobalt. Estimations of cobalt values in the blood of ruminant animals are usually valueless in relation to the recognition of deficiency syndromes. Estimation of vitamin B12 is usually more rewarding and for this purpose rumen contents, faeces and blood plasma are suitable. In ruminant species cobalt is required for vitamin B12 synthesis by the rumen microflora. In these species deficiency of the vitamin results in anorexia, wasting of skeletal muscle, fatty liver and anaemia. The high demand for vitamin B12 arises from its function as a coenzyme in energy (propionate) metabolism; it also fulfils an important role in the synthesis of deoxyribonucleic acid (DNA) which regulates cell division and growth.

In normal animals plasma vitamin B12 values range from 4 to 6 μg/ml; after a prolonged period on a cobalt deficient diet the values fall to less than 0·2 μg/ml. Liver cobalt and vitamin B12 values may also prove of diagnostic value. In normal sheep the liver cobalt levels are usually above 0·2 ppm DM, those for vitamin B12 are around 0·3 ppm, while the figures for normal cattle are 0·15 ppm DM and 0·3 ppm respectively. Signs of cobalt deficiency in sheep are associated with liver cobalt values of less than 0·07 ppm DM and liver vitamin B12 values of around 0·1 ppm. In cattle clinical signs are associated with liver vitamin B12 values of less than 0·1 ppm DM.

Because cobalt deficiency is primary in origin, resulting from an insufficient amount of the element in the soil, analysis of pasture and/or soil often proves helpful in diagnosis. Soil containing less than 2 ppm of cobalt is likely to produce pasture supplying inadequate cobalt to maintain health in grazing ruminant animals. Clinical signs may develop in sheep grazing pasture containing below 0·07 ppm DM and in cattle below 0·04 ppm of cobalt.

Blood electrolytes. Some of the clinically important blood electrolytes including calcium, inorganic phosphate and magnesium have already been considered. Others of significance are sodium, potassium, chloride and bicarbonate. A range of values for these electrolytes in the blood of normal animals is given in Table 18.

TABLE 18. BLOOD ELECTROLYTES IN ANIMALS

Electrolyte	Normal Range (mEq/l)
Sodium	135·0–160·0
Potassium	2·7– 9·0
Chloride	97·0–125·0
Bicarbonate	17·0– 29·0

The main functions of the electrolytes consist of maintaining the pH and osmotic balance of the body fluids and blood pressure, as well as ensuring their electroneutrality, and in addition securing polarization of cellular membranes and acting as structural components of many tissues. Normal tissue function is vitally dependent on the maintenance of a stable pH.

The cation sodium balanced by the anions chloride and bicarbonate are mainly distributed in the extracellular fluids including the blood in which the plasma proteins are an additional component. The major cations of the cellular fluid are potassium and magnesium which are balanced by organic phosphate, proteinate and sulphate. The erythrocytes, however, have chlorides as a major anion. As a consequence of the manner in which the various electrolytes are distributed in the fluid containing compartments of the body, in dehydration, especially when it is the result of alimentary tract dysfunction, or renal disease, large amounts of sodium and chloride are lost. Replacement requirements necessitate measurement of the haematocrit, urine specific gravity and blood electrolytes. Reduction in serum potassium values (hypokalaemia) only occurs when large amounts (up to 50%) of intracellular potassium are lost from the body. As a consequence replacement requirements are difficult to estimate.

Lead. Following ingestion lead can be detected in the faeces, blood, urine and milk of living animals. The interpretation of the results of lead analysis is assisted when a number of specimens are examined. Urinary lead values are not always a reliable indicator of the lead status of the animal, and faecal lead may represent harmless, insoluble and, therefore, unabsorbed lead, as well as lead being excreted from the body tissues, so that the results of faecal analyses should be considered in conjunction with blood lead values. Ingestion of lead over a short period (a few days) is associated with high faecal values which persist for 2–3 weeks, and high blood levels which are usually maintained for several months

In normal cattle and sheep the faeces contain from 1 to 35 ppm DM and the whole blood 0·05–0·25 ppm lead. Animals with lead intoxication of clinical severity may excrete faeces with lead values between 100 and 1000 ppm, depending upon the interval which has elapsed since lead was last ingested, and have blood levels ranging from 0·25 to 2·5 ppm. When submitting samples from a living animal to a laboratory for lead analysis, send at least 30 ml of blood containing a suitable anticoagulant, and about 56 g of faeces. Post mortem confirmation of lead poisoning in ruminant species can be achieved by analysis of kidney cortex, which tissue is more reliable than liver as an index of the lead status of an animal. Kidney cortex values above 25 ppm can be considered significant, with a similar interpretation when the liver contains 10–20 ppm. The livers of horses dying of chronic lead poisoning have been assayed and found to contain between 4 and 7 ppm of lead.

The need to institute an analysis for lead in living animals is usually indicated by the circumstances. Poisoning by this element is most frequently observed in housed, young calves. Affected animals exhibit a staggering gait with muscle tremor, champing the jaws, nystagmus and bellowing, with apparent blindness, terminal convulsions, coma and death. Less severely affected animals may exhibit hyperaesthesia, incoordination of gait, signs of abdominal pain and constipation followed by foetid diarrhoea.

Fluorine. The continued ingestion of small amounts of fluorine in the food or drinking water may produce fluorosis which is characterized by osteoporosis and excessive wear of the teeth with mottling of those which developed during the relevant period. The toxic level of fluorine in the diet varies according to the type of fluorine compound present. Contamination of pasture by certain industrial processes (electrolytic production of aluminium, brickmaking, glass and enamel works, steel manufacture, etc.) is a considerable hazard when the fluorine intake by grazing animals is in excess of 15 ppm of either hydrofluoric acid or silicontetrafluoride. Sodium fluoride, which is twice as toxic as fluorine in rock phosphate, produces disease when, on a dry matter basis, the diet contains more than 50 ppm. In drinking water, levels as low as between 5 and 10 ppm may produce mild dental changes, higher values being proportionately more toxic.

When the fluorine intake is small it is deposited in the permanent teeth during the pre-eruption phase in young animals, and in the bones where the greatest concentration is on the periosteal surface, where exostoses may be a feature. With larger intakes the fluorine levels in the blood and urine rise significantly. In assessing the fluorine status of animals a reasonable proportion of the group should be sampled. In normal cattle and sheep blood levels of fluorine do not exceed 0·2 mg/100 ml and urine values range from 2 to 6 ppm. Cases of fluorotoxicosis in cattle may have blood fluorine values of 0–6 mg/100 ml and urine levels of at least 16 ppm. Urine values should always be corrected to a specific gravity of 1·040.

Unclotted blood in amounts of 20–50 ml is required, in addition to a specimen of urine, for fluorine analysis in living animals. Confirmation of chronic fluorosis can be obtained from bone analysis after death has occurred. In this case the abnormal bone may contain levels of fluorine in excess of 100 ppm. During life affected animals usually have normal serum calcium and inorganic phosphate levels, but the serum alkaline phosphatase level is increased. It is likely that there is a relationship between the increased phosphatase activity and the abnormal bone structure. Herbage and dietary analyses can prove extremely helpful in recognizing the source of excess fluorine.

14

The Nervous System

The nervous system comprises the most extensive and complex control and coordinating mechanism in existence; its controlling influence affects those functions which are concerned with the relationship of the animal organism to its environment and with endogenous homeostasis. All the component divisions of the nervous system are involved in ensuring that the relationship is maintained at the highest level of harmony. Thus the sensory together with the motor system is responsible for maintenance of normal posture and gait; the autonomic nervous system controls the activity of smooth muscle and also that of the endocrine glands (the latter is important in relation to the internal environment of the body; some of the hormones of the endocrine system have feedback effects); the system of special senses, in part, assists in maintaining normal posture and gait; and the psychic system controls the mental state of the animal. The overall function of the nervous system is based on reaction, in the form of instructions to effectors (muscles, glands), and on information from sensors (sensory receptors). The integrity of both afferent and efferent nerve pathways is essential to the reception of exogenous and endogenous stimuli and their transduction into activity.

Anatomical Considerations

The nervous system, comprising all of the nervous tissues of the body, consists of two major divisions, the central nervous system and the peripheral nervous system. The former, which includes the brain and spinal cord, is enclosed, for reasons of protection, within the bony casing of the cranium and vertebral column and so is not readily accessible for clinical examination. The latter comprises the cranial and spinal nerves, their ganglia and end-organs, and the autonomic nervous system. For proper appreciation of the situation, type and degree of nervous dysfunction, a reasonable knowledge of the anatomical ramifications and physiological functions of the component parts of the nervous system is necessary, in addition to an appreciation of the modes by which nervous dysfunction can be expressed.

The brain and spinal cord are further protected from injurious influences by being enclosed in the meningeal membranes, the dura mater and the pia mater. The dura mater is quite substantial, being composed of dense fibrous tissue, the cerebral portion of which is adherent to the internal surface of the cranium. Two projecting septa from the dura extend into the cranial cavity and occupy the major fissures which subdivide the brain. The falx cerebri is situated in the dorsal longitudinal fissure between the cerebral hemispheres, while the tentorium cerebelli projects into the transverse fissure between the cerebellum and cerebral hemispheres. The spinal portion of the dura mater forms a cylindrical tube around the spinal cord throughout its length, and is separated from the periosteum of the neural canal by the epidural space, which is filled with fat, supporting tissue and blood vessels.

The arachnoid membrane, which is situated between the dura mater and pia mater, is a very delicate structure, its outer surface forming the inner wall of the subdural space which contains a small quantity of lymph-like fluid. The deeper surface of the arachnoid membrane has an intimate attachment to the pia mater through the medium of a network of fibres. The subarachnoid space so formed contains cerebrospinal fluid. At various points the arachnoid and pia mater are more widely and extensively separated from each other. These enlarged cavities are termed cisterns, the most important of which is the cisterna magna, or cerebellar–medullary cistern, situated at the angle formed by the posterior aspect of the cerebellum and the dorsal surface of the medulla oblongata. Medially it connects with the fourth ventricle of the brain through small openings in the lateral wall of the latter, and behind there is free communication with the subarachnoid space of the spinal cord.

The pia mater forms a somewhat delicate vascular membrane which is closely applied to the brain and spinal cord. The cerebral portion follows closely all the fissures and sulci of the cerebrum and cerebellum. Its external surface forms the deep boundary of the subarachnoid space.

That portion of the central nervous system situated within the cranial cavity comprising the brain, includes the cerebrum, cerebellum and brain stem which merges imperceptibly at its posterior part with the spinal cord. The cerebrum consists of the cerebral hemispheres and the olfactory bulbs. The cerebral hemispheres form two large ovoid masses filling the greater part of the cranial cavity and are separated by a median fissure, the floor of which consists of a band of white matter, the corpus callosum, connecting the hemispheres and forming the roof of the lateral ventricles. The convex upper and lateral surfaces of the cerebral hemispheres are indented by shallow fissures and grooves giving rise to the readily recognized convolutions. The base of each cerebral hemisphere is irregular. At its anterior part it is in contact with the ventral portion of the olfactory bulb and the olfactory tract. Behind the olfactory tract, the relationship is with the optic nerve which runs backwards and medially to converge at the optic chiasma and continues as the optic tract, which extends laterally and backwards, crossing the anterior part of the cerebral peduncle connecting the mid-brain to the cerebral hemisphere on each side. Immediately posterior to the optic chiasma is a small prominence from which a thin stalk-like structure, the infundibulum, emerges to connect the base of the cerebrum with the pituitary gland which is closely invested by the dura mater. The remainder of the base of each cerebral hemisphere is related to the anterior part of the cerebellum from which it is separated

by a deep transverse fissure which is occupied by a projection of dura mater.

The olfactory bulb forms a ribbon-like enlargement extending upwards over the anterior pole of each cerebral hemisphere. The convex anterior surface is accommodated in the fossa of the ethmoid bone where it is penetrated by numerous olfactory nerve fibres. Arising from the olfactory bulb as a short, wide band of white matter, the olfactory tract extends back to enter the base of each cerebral hemisphere at two points.

The interior of each cerebral hemisphere is occupied by an irregular cavity called the lateral ventricle, which communicates anteriorly, by means of a narrow canal with the cavity of the olfactory bulb, and medially with the third ventricle through the interventricular foramen. The roof of the lateral ventricles is formed by the corpus callosum, a downward projection of which goes to form the medial division between them. The floor of each ventricle is formed, anteriorly, by a pear-shaped projection, the caudate nucleus, and posteriorly by a convex body, the hippocampus.

The cerebellum, which is situated in the posterior area of the cranium, dorsal to the medulla oblongata and pons, is composed of a median portion which is curved in a sagittal direction, and two lateral hemispheres. The anterior surface of the cerebellum is separated from the occipital pole of the cerebral hemispheres by a projection of dura mater. The posterior aspect is irregularly vertical, while the base, which is superimposed on the fourth ventricle, is related by three pairs of peduncles, to the medulla, pons and mid-brain. The surface of the cerebellum is intersected by numerous furrows, the paramedian fissure on each side separating the lateral hemispheres from the central vermis, being especially deep. The three pairs of peduncles unite the base of the cerebellum to the upper surface of the medulla and mid-brain on each side.

The brain stem consists of the medulla oblongata behind, the central pons and the corpora quadrigemina and cerebral peduncles in front. The medullary portion, which is situated on the base of the occipital bone, is shaped like a flattened wedge with the widest part in front. The ventral surface is convex with a median fissure, on each side of which is a longitudinal elevation, the pyramid, which extends forward to cross over the corpus trapezoideum, a transverse band, to join the pons. The dorsal surface of the medulla is almost entirely hidden by the cerebellum where the former provides the greater part of the floor of the fourth ventricle.

The medulla connects in front with the pons, a ventrally placed elongated transverse projection which is convex in both directions. Laterally, it has a connection with the base of the cerebellum through the middle cerebellar peduncle, while dorsally, at the anterior part, union is effected through the anterior cerebellar peduncles.

The two cerebral peduncles, the ventral visible part of the mid-brain, originate from the anterior aspect of the pons at the base of the brain in the form of thick columns which diverge as they pass upwards and forwards to penetrate the ventral aspect of the cerebral hemispheres. The depression formed by the diverging peduncles is largely covered by the pituitary gland. At this point each cerebral peduncle is crossed obliquely by the optic tract. The dorsal part of the mid-brain, the corpora quadrigemina, consisting of four rounded projections, is concealed by the posterior part of the cerebral hemispheres. Lying obliquely across the dorsal part of each cerebral peduncle is a large egg-shaped mass, the thalamus, which connects with the two larger anterior eminences of the corpora quadrigemina.

The third ventricle of the brain consists of a narrow, ring-like cavity situated between the thalami. Anteriorly it connects directly with the lateral ventricle on each side by means of the interventricular foramen, and behind it communicates with the fourth ventricle via the cerebral aqueduct which is situated beneath the posterior pair of corpora quadrigemina. The fourth ventricle is elongated in a saggital direction. The floor is formed by the medulla oblongata and pons, the lateral walls by the restiform body and the anterior cerebellar peduncles, and the roof by part of the vermis of the cerebellum. It is connected in front with the third ventricle as as described, and posteriorly with the central canal of the spinal cord. It communicates with the subarachnoid space at the cisterna magna through the apertures situated in the lateral recesses of the ventricle.

The Cranial Nerves

These comprise twelve paired nerves, the identity, origin and main functional properties of which are given below.

The *olfactory nerve* consists of small bundles of non-medullated (non-myelinated) fibres which are the central processes of sensory cells in the nasal mucous membrane. The fibres terminate in the olfactory bulb from where secondary fibres transmit impulses to the cortical olfactory areas in the hippocampus.

The *optic nerve* consists of a relatively thick trunk derived from the grouping of the central processes of visual cells in the retina at the optic papilla, where the nerve so formed pierces the choroid and sclera at the posterior part of the eyeball. Passing backwards, the nerve enters the optic foramen and forms the optic decussation when it converges and meets its fellow nerve, and is then continued as the optic tract on each side, containing nerve fibres from the lateral part of the retina on the same side and the medial part of the retina on the opposite side. The fibres terminate in the thalamus from where visual impulses are relayed to the cortical areas of vision.

The *oculomotor nerve* emerges from the ventral aspect of the cerebral peduncle. This nerve, through its two branches, provides motor function to the extrinsic muscles of the eyeball with the exception of the superior oblique, retractor and external rectus and, via the medium of the ciliary ganglion, to the sphincter pupillae muscle of the iris. The function of the nerve is concerned with elevating the upper eyelid, positioning the eyeball, and modifying the amount of light entering the eye through alteration of the size of the pupil (pupillary reflex). The fibres of the oculomotor nerve originate from cells located in the oculomotor nucleus in the mid-brain.

The *trochlear nerve* emerges from the anterior peduncle of the cerebellum immediately behind the corpora quadrigemina. At its termination it passes along the medial wall of the orbit to penetrate the superior oblique muscle of the eyeball, to which it supplies motor power. The cells of origin of the trochlear nerve fibres are located in the mid-brain.

The *trigeminal nerve*, the largest of the cranial group, consists of a large sensory root and a smaller motor root both of which originate from the lateral aspect of the pons. The nerve trunk divides into three major branches the ophthalmic, maxillary and mandibular nerves. The ophthalmic segment, which is entirely sensory, divides into three branches. The lacrimal nerve innervates the lacrimal gland and skin of the upper eyelid. The frontal nerve is distributed to the skin of the poll and upper eyelid. The nasociliary nerve innervates the mucous membrane of the nasal cavity and the dorsal turbinate bone, as well as the skin of the medial canthus and the conjunctiva, including the membrana nictitans.

The maxillary nerve is also purely sensory; it also divides into three main branches, the zygomatic, sphenopalatine and infra-orbital nerves. The zygomatic nerve is distributed to the skin of the lower eyelid and surrounding areas. The sphenopalatine nerve innervates the mucous membrane of the lower part of the nasal septum, the hard and soft palate and the gums. The infra-orbital nerve is distributed to the teeth, alveoli and gums of the maxilla.

The mandibular nerve is composed of a large sensory root and a small motor root, and is distributed through the medium of seven branches. The masseteric, deep temporal, buccinator and pterygoid nerves supply motor innervation to the corresponding muscles. In addition, the buccinator nerve supplies sensory fibres to the mucous membrane of the lips in the vicinity of the commissures, and the pterygoid nerve supplies motor fibres to the tensor palati and tensor tympani muscles, and the Eustachian tube. The superficial temporal nerve supplies sensory innervation to the skin of the cheek, the guttural pouch, the external ear, the tympanic membrane and the skin of the external auditory meatus. The mandibular alveolar nerve provides sensory fibres to the skin of the anterior part of the intermandibular space, the lower lip, chin, teeth and gums, as well as motor fibres to the mylohyoid and anterior portion of the digastricus muscles. The lingual nerve ensures sensory innervation to the mucous membrane of the tongue and the floor of the mouth.

The sensory root of the trigeminal nerve has several ramifications, the most important of which are the cerebral cortex via the thalamus, the cerebellar cortex through the posterior peduncle, and with the origins of the hypoglossal and facial nerves, and of the motor part of the trigeminal nerve itself. The motor root arises mainly from the deeper parts of the pons.

The *abducent nerve* makes its exit from the brain posterior to the pons, immediately lateral to the pyramid. In the retrobulbar part of the orbital cavity it is distributed to the lateral rectus and retractor muscles of the eyeball, which it innervates. The fibres of the nerve originate as axons from large cells situated beneath the floor of the fourth ventricle.

The *facial nerve* emerges from the brain on the lateral aspect of the corpus trapezoideum, immediately behind the pons. The nerve consists mainly of motor fibres along with a small contingent of sensory fibres. Through the medium of its many branches it innervates the stapedius muscle, the muscles of the ear, base of the tongue, upper and lower lips and nostril, as well as the orbicularis oculi and corrugator supercilii muscles. It also supplies sensory function to the skin of the inner and outer surfaces of the conchal cartilage, and to the end-organs of taste in the mucous membrane of the anterior two-thirds of the tongue, via the chorda tympani nerve, which also supplies secretory fibres to the submaxillary and sublingual salivary glands. The motor fibres of the facial nerve originate from cells in the medulla; the sensory fibres terminate in the same part of the medulla as the glossopharyngeal and vagus nerves.

The *auditory* (*acoustic*) *nerve* consisting of two roots, vestibular and cochlear, emerges from the lateral aspect of the medulla. The vestibular nerve is concerned with spatial orientation and balance, for which purpose its peripheral fibres originate in the semicircular canals, and the saccule and utricle of the internal ear. The cochlear nerve of hearing has its peripheral origin in relation to the hair cells of the organ of Corti in the cochlea of the internal ear. The nerve fibres terminate through numerous ramifications beneath the floor of the fourth ventricle.

The *glossopharyngeal nerve* is comprised of the combination of several filaments which emerge from the lateral aspect of the medulla. The peripheral branches of the nerve provide sensory perception to the pharynx and posterior third of the tongue, as well as taste sensation to this part of the tongue. In addition, the nerve supplies secretory fibres to the parotid salivary gland and motor fibres to the muscles of the pharynx. The central connection of the major sensory portion of the nerve is the floor of the fourth ventricle, while the motor fibres originate in the medulla.

The *vagus nerve* is characterized by its considerable length, wide distribution and extensive ramifications with contiguous nerves and with the cervical sympathetic. The major branches of the vagus nerve and their terminations are as follows: the pharyngeal nerve which ensures motor function in the muscles of the pharynx, those of the soft palate except the tensor palati (supplied by the mandibular branch of the trigeminal nerve) and the commencement of the oesophagus; the anterior laryngeal nerve, which supplies sensation to the mucous membrane of the floor of the pharynx, the larynx and the entrance to the oesophagus. The motor segment of this nerve supplies the cricothyroid and crico-pharyngeus muscles of the larynx. The recurrent laryngeal nerve has a different point of origin and initial course on the two sides. The right nerve leaves the main trunk opposite the second rib where it turns medially round the costo-cervical artery, and is continued forwards on the ventral aspect of the carotid artery, beneath the trachea. The left nerve originates at the point where the vagus crosses the aortic arch, passing backwards it turns medially round the aortic arch, and is continued forward ventral to the carotid artery. At its termination the nerve is distributed to the lateral and dorsal crico-arytenoid, ventricular and vocal muscles of the larynx. The nerve also supplies branches to the anterior laryngeal nerve, the trachea, oesophagus, and posterior cervical ganglion of the sympa-thetic. The cardiac nerves, in conjunction with filaments from the recurrent laryngeal nerves and the sympathetic, form the cardiac pexus, which is distributed to the heart and great vessels. The small tracheal and oesophageal nerves, which originate from the vagus in the thorax, combine with fibres from the laryngeal nerve, and from the sympathetic ganglia, to form plexuses from which the trachea, oesophagus, heart and large vessels are innervated. The bronchial nerves arise beyond the division of the trachea and after combining with sympathetic fibres, travel along the bronchi and blood vessels to supply the substance of the lungs.

The dorsal and ventral oesophageal trunks are formed by the division of each vagus nerve into two branches in the vicinity of the bronchi. The trunks run backward in the posterior mediasti-num and enter the abdominal cavity with the oesophagus. In the abdomen branches are supplied to the stomach, duodenum, liver and pancreas; other parts of the gastrointestinal tract are innervated through the medium of plexuses and ganglia.

The vagus nerve emerges from the brain at the lateral aspect of the medulla behind the glosso-pharyngeal nerve and in front of the spinal accessory nerve. As the vagus emerges from the cranium it communicates with the glossopharyn-geal, the spinal accessory, and the hypoglossal nerves. In its passage along the neck, dorsal to the carotid artery, it is accompanied by the cervical sympathetic trunk.

The sensory fibres of the vagus nerve terminate centrally in the posterior part of the floor of the fourth ventricle, and in the vicinity of the decussation of the pyramidal tracts. The motor components originate from cells in the depth of the medulla at the level of the posterior part of the floor of the fourth ventricle.

The *spinal accessory nerve*, which is entirely motor, consists of two parts each differing in origin and function. The medullary segment emerges from the lateral aspect of the medulla posterior to the origin of the vagus nerve, the several roots uniting together and with the spinal part, which originates from the spinal cord at the level of the fifth cervical vertebra and extends forwards to enter the cranial cavity through the foramen magnum. The medullary portion of the nerve is almost immediately distributed to the vagus and glossopharyngeal nerves, while the remainder of the trunk passes backward down the neck to innervate the trape-zius and sternocephalicus muscles. The spinal segment of the nerve originates from cells in the lateral part of the ventral grey column of the spinal cord as far back as the fifth cervical vertebra.

The *hypoglossal nerve* originates by the combination of a series of roots which emerge from the ventral aspect of the medulla, lateral to the posterior part of the pyramid. It extends anteriorly across the wall of the pharynx and ramifies in the muscles which attach the tongue to the hyoid bone, and in the tongue itself. The fibres of the nerve originate from cells which are medially situated beneath the floor of the posterior part of the fourth ventricle.

Spinal Cord and Spinal Nerves

The spinal cord is continuous with the medulla oblongata and extends from the foramen magnum to the mid-point of the sacrum. It is situated in the vertebral canal and is somewhat cylindrical in transverse section, being flattened dorsoventrally. In general the spinal cord tapers gradually in a posterior direction but those parts from which the nerves of the limbs originate show obvious enlargements. These comprise the cervical enlargement in the vicinity of the fifth cervical to the second thoracic vertebrae, and the lumbar enlargement contiguous to the fourth and fifth lumbar vertebrae.

The spinal nerves are paired and emerge from the lateral aspect of the cord after the conjunction of a number of dorsal and ventral roots. They vary from 36 to 42 pairs according to the species, the largest number occurring in the horse. At its termination the spinal cord, enclosed in the meninges, tapers to a point where it is surrounded by the roots of the sacral and coccygeal nerves, which extend backwards in the neural canal, so forming the cauda equina. The division of the spinal cord into cervical, thoracic, lumbar and sacral parts reflects its relationship to the appropriate vertebrae.

The surface of the spinal cord is composed of white matter (myelin), the depth of which varies because of the uneven distribution of the underlying grey matter, so that it is divided into three columns on each side of the dorsal septum and ventral median fissure. The columns are classified according to their position as dorsal, lateral, and ventral. The grey material is deeply situated and, on transverse section of the spinal cord, is seen to be aggregated roughly in the form of an H with, on each side, the projecting dorsal and ventral columns, or horns. The distribution of the white and grey material in the cerebrum is the reverse of that for the spinal cord, so that the major portion of the brain surface is grey.

The autonomic nervous system, consisting of the cranial and sacral divisions comprising the parasympathetic, and the thoracolumbar or sympathetic division, innervates the glands and visceral musculature of the body. The overall function of the autonomic nervous system is to maintain internal homeokinesis. Reference has previously been made to the cranial portion of the system. Many of the structures concerned are supplied by both sympathetic and parasympathetic components which are frequently mutually antagonistic.

General Considerations

Diseases of the nervous system may be primary or secondary in origin. The former arise as the result of the actions of infective agents such as bacteria, viruses, helminth parasites and protozoa. Specific examples caused by these several agencies are listeriosis, tetanus, louping-ill, rabies, pseudorabies, coenurosis, toxoplasmosis,

etc. Primary disease of the nervous system is also a possible result of nutritional deficiency, e.g. Chastek paralysis in the dog caused by thiamine deficiency and pantothenic acid deficiency in the pig, or of intoxication as in lead or strychnine poisoning. Developmental defects of the central nervous system may have a genetic basis (inherited cerebellar hypoplasia of calves, inherited congenital hydrocephalus, inherited congenital chondrodystrophy, etc.), a nutritional basis (brain compression caused by vitamin A deficiency, swayback and enzootic ataxia in lambs), an infective basis as in virus infection in early pregnancy (following vaccination with modified swine fever virus, following vaccination with attenuated bluetongue virus) and infection of the brain (toxoplasmosis) or an obscure origin (myoclonia congenita of pigs, 'barkers' and 'wanderers' in foals, arthrogryposis and hydranencephaly of calves, etc.). Degenerative changes, affecting the cerebral and/or spinal white matter causing demyelination, give rise in lambs to enzootic ataxia and swayback, of which the former is a primary and the latter a primary or secondary copper deficiency.

In secondary disease of the nervous system, infective processes elsewhere in the body, through the medium of general debilitation and injury to vascular and other tissues, invade the nervous system, thereby causing the development of further clinical signs. It appears that the protection normally given to the central nervous system by the so-called blood–brain barrier is most readily overcome by a prolonged febrile reaction, such as is associated with tick-borne fever infection in sheep, and which is of significance in the development of clinical louping-ill and toxaemia. Certain of the infective agents, more particularly some members of the virus group, appear to invade the nervous system rather easily. This may be a matter of particle size or is a reflection of biological adaptation to which the term neurotropic is applicable.

The component structures of the nervous system, including the meninges, brain, spinal cord and cranial and spinal nerves, can be involved in disease processes to a variable degree. Although specific agents manifest a tendency to invade particular areas of the nervous system, because of the limited range of reactivity of nervous tissue it is not possible in all cases, by consideration of the clinical signs alone, to identify the nature of the affection.

Diseases which are responsible for signs indicating derangement of nervous function, and in which no observable lesion can be found, are termed functional. In parturient paresis and hypomagnesaemic tetany, the disturbance of nervous function is due to biochemical abnormality, and in either instance the clinical signs usually follow a rather constant pattern. In these conditions effective treatment usually results in complete recovery with no evidence of residual damage to the nervous system as a legacy. When the metabolic change develops more slowly, or persists for a longer time, as in ketosis in sheep (pregnancy toxaemia), irreversible encephalopathic damage is likely owing to the marked hypoglycaemia which is a feature of the disease. Epileptiform-like convulsions of varying severity in dogs may result from organic lesions such as the encephalitides, or in some cases from mimicry when the hysteria threshold is low, in the absence of detectable brain damage. Similarly, the convulsions which sometimes occur in severe vitamin E deficiency in calves are most likely an indication of cerebral hypoxia because of cardiac insufficiency, rather than actual brain injury.

In addition to those diseases occurring elsewhere in the body, and which because of the toxaemia they induce influence the functional status of the nervous system, there are a variety of others which have a reflex effect. In this category can be included the convulsive syndrome occasionally observed in calves because of an abnormal mass, which may consist of hair, baling twine or inspissated curd clot, in the pyloric portion of the abomasum. Painful conditions, whether local or general, have a variable reflex effect on the nervous system through mediating elevation of temperature, increase in the pulse and respiratory rates with, in addition, a degree of excitement and restlessness. The significance of intestinal infestation with ascarid parasites in relation to convulsive syndromes in puppies appears indisputable, but the mechanism involved has not been clarified, although hypocalcaemia has been determined to be present in many puppies so affected.

Clinical Examination

Neurological examination is most rewarding in the dog and cat, in which species techniques can be employed which are not applicable to farm animals because of their size. Size alone,

however, is not the only limiting factor because, although young lambs and piglets are satisfactory in this respect, it is unlikely that the responses to many of the neurological tests will prove valuable.

In general, a routine clinical examination should be performed and if it becomes apparent during this procedure that clinical signs of neurological malfunction exist then certain aspects will require detailed consideration. Of these, the history is especially important in order that all the relevant information appertaining to the duration of the signs, the manner of onset, whether sudden or gradual, acute or mild, the mode of expression and the pattern of the clinical signs, e.g. periodic or continuous, should be considered. Modes of nervous dysfunction are broadly divisible into two forms, depressed activity and exaggerated activity.

Depressed activity may be attributable to depression of metabolism of the nerve cells as the result of inadequate supply of oxygen and other essential nutrients; the terminal stage of complete paralysis occurs when nervous tissue is destroyed. Depression of function with final complete paralysis may follow an initial period of exaggerated activity which is a not unusual occurrence when the nerve cell becomes infected. Paralysis may arise from involvement of the motor and/or the sensory nervous system. The main manifestation in the former consists of muscular paresis or paralysis and in the latter hypoaesthesia or anaesthesia. Nervous shock caused by an acute lesion is associated with loss of function in the damaged nerve cells with, in addition, a variable degree of loss of function in other parts of the nervous system not directly affected.

Exaggerated activity on the part of nerve cells can be caused by many factors including inflammation, early or mild hypoxia, hypoglycaemia (factors which when present in severe degree cause depression of nerve cell function) and stimulant drugs. The greater excitability of the nerve cells is evidenced by increased activity of the reactor organ. Increased activity may also take the form of irritation phenomena such as convulsions and muscle tremor, and hyperaesthesia and paraesthesia in the motor and sensory systems respectively. Irritation signs may result from causes such as inflammation caused by viruses, bacteria, certain poisons, severe hypoxia and increased intracranial pressure when there is sufficient interference with local circulation to cause local anaemic hypoxia. Exaggeration of nervous system activity also occurs when spinal centres are released from the inhibitory control of brain centres. The lack of cerebellar control in cerebellar ataxia causes limb movements to be exaggerated in rate, range, force and direction.

With regard to investigating neurological dysfunction in a group of animals, the number affected, the rate of spread and the mortality rate are other significant features. In some cases the significant clinical features are only available through elucidation of the history, as for instance in canine epilepsy or convulsive seizures, in which the clinical episodes can be of short duration. An appreciation of the duration, frequency and pattern of convulsive seizures will often be found helpful in achieving a diagnosis, e.g. sodium poisoning in the pig is associated with convulsive episodes which recur at fairly regular intervals, whereas in strychnine poisoning the clonic convulsions reappear after ever-shortening intervals unless recovery is occurring. Other aspects of convulsive episodes which require consideration include whether the movements were general or local in extent, tonic or clonic in character, and whether consciousness was affected. Some of these points could only be decided if the patient is in a convulsive state at the time of examination.

The history is also important in those cases in which neurological signs develop following trauma and in which external injury is not evident. Further useful evidence is whether or not the clinical signs are associated with fever or pain. In this context it is necessary to appreciate that convulsive episodes will invariably cause body temperature to rise, so that in such circumstances this finding should not be given too much significance, otherwise the possibility of an infective or toxaemic process should be considered as a possible cause.

Clinical examination of the nervous system largely consists of observations based on the animal's behaviour in response to various stimuli and other interferences, designed to reveal changes in functional control. The normal functions are concerned with the maintenance of the body's relationship with the environment through the medium of the sensorimotor system, which is concerned with posture and gait, the autonomic nervous system controlling the activity of plain muscle and endocrine glands, the segments of the sensory system comprising the special senses, and the psychic element which controls the animal's mental state. Direct examination of the central nervous system is prohibited by the bony structures surrounding it, except for the optic papilla, which can be observed with the ophthalmoscope, and the cerebrospinal fluid. The latter is withdrawn from the subarachnoid space by means of lumbosacral or cisternal puncture, if required for examination.

Diseases of the nervous system, in the majority of cases, are suspected because of abnormal behaviour on the part of the animal, the significance of which is interpreted by consideration of the clinical evidence in conjunction with, where practicable and desirable, the results of other methods of examination such as various radiological techniques, and examination of the cerebrospinal fluid. The preliminary inspection of the animal, performed whenever possible without its being aware of the clinician's presence, or at least in an undisturbed state, may have already suggested that the nervous system is the site of disease. It should be borne in mind, however, that mere inspection is not a sufficient degree of examination on which to base a diagnosis of a nervous disorder. Unwillingness to use a limb on account of a painful lesion may be mistaken for paralysis, muscular weakness for ataxia, the depression of malnutrition for disease of the brain or the frenzy caused by a bone impacted between the arcades of the upper molar teeth in a dog for rabies.

The systematic examination of the nervous system should commence with inspection and palpation of the cranial area, noting whether there are any changes in shape and contour (Fig. 207), the presence of pain and areas of

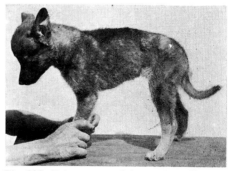

Fig. 207. *Enlargement of the cranium. Congenital hydrocephalus.*

softening. The vertebral column should be included in the examination, in which case departures from normal, including upward curvature (kyphosis), downward curvature (lordosis) and lateral curvature (scoliosis), may be sufficiently obvious to be recognized. It should be noted that slight deformity of the vertebral column is not necessarily associated with clinical disease of the nervous system (see Figs 14, 15, p. 17), and may be an expression of senility or a mild developmental defect. In small animals, the vertebral column can be examined by manual manipulation (Fig. 208).

Localization of clinical signs will necessitate their consideration in relation to a detailed

in function of a motor nerve causes partial paralysis or paresis. If there is total loss of function, the result is paralysis. Increased activity in a sensory nerve produces a condition of hyperaesthesia or hypersensitivity; loss of function in a sensory nerve causes anaesthesia or loss of sensitivity; reduction in functional activity causes hypoaesthesia or reduced sensitivity.

Qualitative disturbances of the motor nerves are known as parakineses or motor aberrations, and of the sensory nerves as paraesthesiae or sensory aberrations.

The voluntary movements and postural relationships in normal animals are initiated and

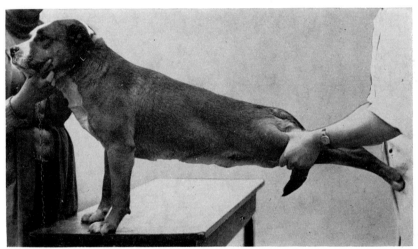

Fig. 208. *Physical examination of the vertebral column, pelvis and associated structures by means of palpation, in association with extension of the hindlegs.*

investigation into the state of locomotion, perception, consciousness and mental state exhibited by the animal. A nervous disorder is described as central, peripheral or autonomic according to whether it originates in the brain or spinal cord, in the peripheral nerves or in the sympathetic or parasympathetic nervous system. Depending upon which nerve component is affected, the disturbance may be motor, sensory or both. Where a motor nerve is affected, there may be a change in the amount of movement (quantitative disturbance) or in the way in which movement is performed (qualitative disturbance).

Quantitative disturbances vary in degree from gross exaggeration to complete suppression. If a motor nerve increases in activity a condition of continuous spasm may be produced; reduction

governed by certain areas in the cerebral cortex in conjunction with the pyramidal and the extrapyramidal motor system (the latter is of much greater importance in animals than is the case in man), with the support of muscle tone, skin sensations, sense of sight, and joint, tendon, muscle and various other reflexes. The clinical signs associated with cerebral affections include those of increased motor nerve activity in the form of muscular spasms, convulsions, paresis or paralysis, alteration in cutaneous perceptivity, disturbances of vision, hearing or consciousness.

The cerebellum is largely concerned with the coordination of those voluntary movements which ensure equilibrium, so that diseases of the cerebellum cause the appearance of clinical signs such as incoordination of the limbs with varying degrees of spasticity, falling, and nystagamus. The main function of the spinal cord and peripheral nerves is the transmission of sensory and motor impulses. Diseases of this segment of the nervous system are usually expressed by regional spasticity, paresis or paralysis according to the nature and situation of the injury.

Motor Disturbances

Paralysis. This may be subdivided, according to the anatomical position of the lesion, into peripheral and central paralysis. Central paralysis includes spinal and cerebral paralysis. Peripheral paralysis affects only the region supplied by one or a few nerves (monoplegia). The paralysis is of the flaccid type, i.e. muscle tone is absent and passive movement of the affected part is not actively resisted. Reflex responses, pain induced or otherwise, are lost, and visible wasting of the muscles soon occurs (degenerative atrophy). Spinal paralysis is usually bilateral (paraplegia) (Figs 209–212), its extent

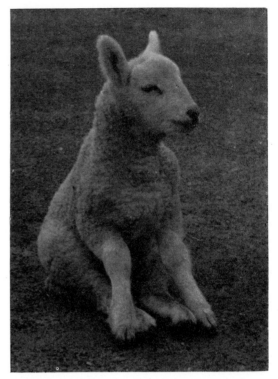

Fig. 210. *Hindlegs, lacking tone, are extended between the forelegs. There was complete motor and sensory paralysis of the hindquarters in the lamb, which had an abscess in the spinal canal at the level of the fifth lumbar vertebra (compare with Figs 209 and 211).*

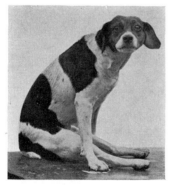

Fig. 209. *Hindlegs extended stiffly between the forelegs of a dog. Spastic paralysis of the hindquarters (compare with Fig. 212).*

depending upon the location and degree of the damage in the spinal cord. Initially, in many cases, the paralysis is of the spastic type, i.e. muscle tone is increased so that the hindlimbs are extended stiffly, and passive movements are resisted. The reflex responses may be reduced or exaggerated. No obvious degenerative change takes place in the muscles unless the disease process is progressive and flaccid paralysis supervenes. Severe damage to the spinal cord will cause flaccid paralysis from the onset. Cerebral paralysis is frequently accompanied by loss of consciousness. The loss of function is often

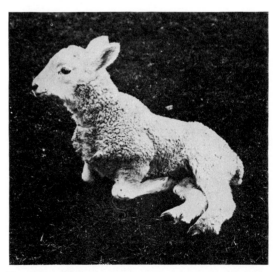

Fig. 211. *Hindlegs, lacking tone, lying in extension. Flaccid paralysis of the hindquarters in a lamb suffering from tick pyaemia.*

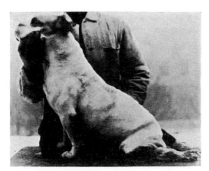

Fig. 212. *Hindlegs trailing behind the animal, producing a seal-like posture. Placcid paralysis of the hindquarters (compare with Fig. 209).*

unilateral (hemiplegia). The function of some of the cranial nerves is altered. The paralysis is spastic in character. The reflex responses may be reduced or exaggerated. No obvious wasting of muscles occurs.

An alternative method of classification of paralyses is to group them according to the position of the injury in relation to the nuclei of the affected nerves (Fig. 213). As indicated,

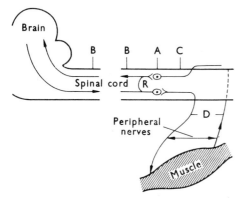

Fig. 213. *Diagram of the types of paralysis.* A, *Site of injury causing nuclear paralysis.* B, *Site of injury causing supranuclear paralysis.* C, D, *Sites of injury causing infranuclear paralysis.* R, *reflex arc.*

nuclear paralysis includes all those forms that arise through injury to the nuclei of the cranial nerves, or to those of the equivalent ventral horn cells of the spinal cord. Infranuclear paralysis is caused by injury to the lower part of a nervous pathway (the axons of the cranial nerve cells, or those of the ventral horn cells of the spinal cord). Supranuclear paralysis, in contradistinction, originates in injury to the upper part of a motor pathway (upper motor

neurone lesion). In nuclear and infranuclear paralysis, reflexes and muscle tone are absent, and severe atrophy of the muscles soon becomes apparent (degenerative atrophy). In supranuclear paralysis the reflexes are exaggerated on account of the removal of the inhibitory control of the cerebrum and muscular atrophy is slight (atrophy of inactivity).

Muscular atrophy. With the passage of time a muscle which is partially or completely deprived of motor innervation becomes weaker and begins to waste (Fig. 214). Muscular atrophy, to which

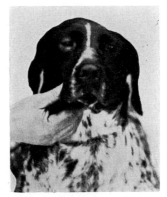

Fig. 214. *Atrophy of the left temporal muscle.*

in long-standing affections is added contracture (permanent shortening of muscle fibres), occurs in two forms: (*a*) simple atrophy or atrophy of inactivity, which is caused by disease of the muscle, develops very slowly and occurs, for example, in supranuclear paralysis, as well as from local diseases of joints and other structures; and (*b*) degenerative atrophy, which develops rapidly and soon reaches an advanced state, it occurs in nuclear and infranuclear paralysis. The great rapidity with which advanced atrophy develops in these cases is because no nervous impulses are able to reach the muscle, so that it is deprived of reflex stimulation, whereas in supranuclear paralysis, the muscle still receives reflex stimuli.

Spasm. This is a pathologically exaggerated contraction of muscle associated with greatly increased tone which may be clinically recognizable. Continuous spasm is described as being tonic, e.g. in trismus (spasm of the jaw muscles) or tetanus (Figs 215–217). In clonic spasm, which is a feature of strychnine poisoning, there is alternation between muscular contraction and

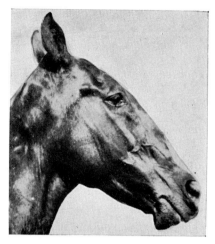

Fig. 215. *Fixed expression; muscles of upper and lower lips and cheeks clearly defined; chin prominent; angle in palpebrral margin of upper eyelid. Tetanus.*

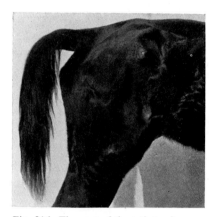

Fig. 216. *The root of the tail standing out from the perianal region. Tetanus.*

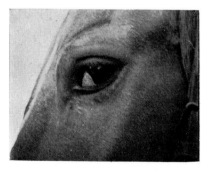

Fig. 217. *Formation of an angle in the palpebral margin of the upper eyelid and protrusion of the membrana nictitans. Tetanus.*

relaxation. If clonic spasms are so violent that the whole body is shaken, they are described as convulsions or 'fits'. Attacks comprising first tonic and then clonic spasms of all the body muscles, with loss of consciousness, are described as being 'epileptiform'. Reflex spasms are those evoked by stimulation of another organ, e.g. by a painful operative procedure, by strong light falling on the eye, etc.

Tetany. This is a generalized condition in which there is tonic muscular spasm, excitement and panting, which should not be confused with tetanus. It is usually associated with metabolic disturbances such as hypomagnesaemic tetany of cattle and sheep, and transit tetany of horses and cattle.

Tremor. This is a rapid sequence of limited clonic muscular contractions which produces quivering of the muscles but little or no movement of any part of the body, except in severe cases. Tremors are described as being coarse or fine according to the degree of muscle contraction. (Note the difference between tremors and rigors.) Contraction of individual bundles of muscle fibres is known as fibrillary twitching. Serious chloride loss from the body in association with dehydration is a cause of tremor. When physical exertion causes tremor to intensify, the possibility of cerebellar dysfunction should be considered.

The clonic muscular contractions which produce jerking (spastic) movements of single muscles or muscle groups, often occurring in dogs as a sequel to distemper, may be so slight as to be detected only on palpation, but usually they cause visible movements of a limb or a larger part of the body. The choreiform movements seen in man, consisting of irregularly repeated, purposeless movements of a limb or the face, do not occur in animals.

Nystagmus. This consists of jerking movements of the eyeball from left to right (horizontal nystagmus), from above to below (vertical nystagmus) or in a circular direction (rotatory nystagmus). It occurs in spasm of the eye muscles innervated by the oculomotor, trochlear and abducent nerves, and is also frequently seen in cerebral meningitis and in diseases of the cerebellum and membranous labyrinth. The importance of cerebral hypoxia as a cause of nystagmus should not be overlooked.

Ataxia. This type of locomotor disturbance exists when the power of individual muscles is

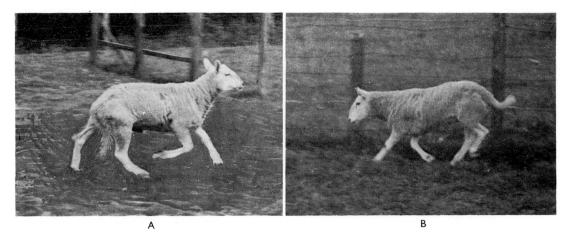

Fig. 218. A, *The peculiar gait ('cuddie trot') of a sheep affected with scrapie; the animal trots unsteadily, with the ears moving loosely up and down.* B, *The fast gait of a normal sheep; the animal canters with the ears pricked. The normal sheep rarely trots.*

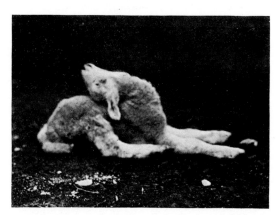

Fig. 219. *Abnormal position of the head. A 'daft' lamb. Corticocerebellar atrophy.*

unaffected (thus there is no paralysis) but there is lack of functional coordination between the several members of a group of muscles (Figs 218, 219). As a result of this situation, movements become uncertain, groping and exaggerated. Ataxia is caused by disturbances of the coordinating activity of the central nervous system involving the cerebellum, cerebrum and spinal cord. It is particularly severe in diseases of the cerebellum, e.g. cerebellar hypoplasia. If there is doubt as to the presence of ataxia, the animal should be blindfolded. In ataxia the locomotor disturbance is thereby increased, whereas in lameness or muscular weakness it is not.

Forced movements. These are fully coordinated muscular movements that are caused by stimulation of the motor centres and are repeated again and again, always following the same pattern. They usually indicate the presence of a circumscribed lesion of the brain, e.g. focal encephalitis, haemorrhage, parasites or neoplasm, but may occur also in generalized disease of the brain as the result of the almost inevitable rise in intracranial pressure. They may take the form of rotatory movements in which the animal moves its hindquarters in a circle round the stationary forequarters, or vice versa. In circular, or circus, movements the animal walks in small or large circles (observed in listeriosis and coenurosis in ruminants); sometimes it presses forward or backward against a wall. Some animals, particularly rabid dogs, may stray for long distances, even as much as 130 km, as if in response to some inward compulsion. In unilateral disease of the middle ear, vestibular nerve or vestibular nucleus in the medulla, and in diseases of the cerebellum and the external auditory meatus, not only is the head carried obliquely (Fig. 220), but the animal may stagger from side to side, fall to the ground and even roll over on the ground until it meets an obstruction. When the head is rotated the animal invariably falls to that side, otherwise if the head is deviated only, as may occur when the vestibular nucleus is affected in listeriosis or in coenurosis, the animal falls in the opposite direction towards the normal side. In such cases varying degrees of

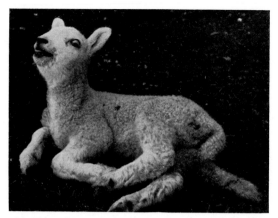

Fig. 220. *Abnormal position of the head, with staring eyes. Staphylococcal encephalitis.*

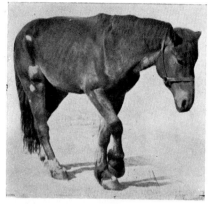

Fig. 221. *Abnormal attitude in disturbance of consciousness: forelegs crossed, hindlegs adducted, head low. Chronic acquired hydrocephalus.*

squinting often occur also; in rotation of the head, one eye is directed downwards and inwards and the other upwards and outwards.

Abnormal movements or attitudes may be caused not only by paralysis or spasm of individual muscles or of a muscle group, but also by injury to muscles, tendons or bones, or by unilateral disturbances.

The maintenance of normal posture is assisted through the medium of statokinetic and statotonic reflexes involving muscles, ligaments and joints, vision and the thalamic and cortical areas of the brain. It has been shown that, without awareness, man receives precise information as to the state and position of his muscles, ligaments, etc., from the proprioreceptors in these structures. The same situation is presumed to exist in animals. If these reflexes are disturbed, unnatural movements and attitudes are seen, e.g. crossing (Fig. 221) or excessive lifting of the feet, stumbling or resting the foot on the dorsal surface. Such behaviour indicates space-occupying lesions of the brain, e.g. hydrocephalus, neoplasia, etc.

Sensory Disturbances

General. Disturbances of perception may affect all five senses (touch, sight, smell, taste and hearing). Loss of any one is very difficult to demonstrate in animals because of the absence of subjective signs. It is permissible to speak of a disturbance in perception only when repeated examinations unquestionably yield the same results. Otherwise any opinion must be guarded and the suspected disturbance is best described as being 'apparently' present. A disturbance of perception may be described as of nervous origin only if the peripheral sense organs themselves (eye, nasal mucosa, ear, tongue, skin) are normal. Nervous animals, because of fear, may give no outward sign of having perceived a sensory stimulus, although perception has actually taken place (false insensibility), or in spite of absence of perception the animal may behave as if perception had occurred (false sensibility). Individual gradation of sensory perception also occurs.

Absence of sensitivity (anaesthesia). Diminished sensitivity of the skin is shown by a reduction in the reaction to palpation and the application of a pain-inducing stimulus. Complete insensibility to pain is termed analgesia. It is assessed by pricking the skin at various points with a needle. The most sensitive skin areas include the lips, around the eyes, the withers and the perineum. Elsewhere the skin is normally less sensitive. In considering the significance of the response to the infliction of painful stimuli, due regard should be paid to species and individual animal variation. Cattle, especially bulls, react slowly, horses are more sensitive and dogs are most sensitive of all the domestic species. Individual variations in skin sensitivity are related to sex, age, physical condition and previous experience of exposure to pain-inducing stimuli. Generally, aged male animals in poor physical condition react more slowly, and to a less marked degree, than young female animals in good condition. If the retina becomes insensitive to variations in light intensity, a type of blindness develops in which there is no obvious structural damage, but the pupillary reflex is absent. This is known as amaurosis and in animals usually results from poisoning by santonin and male fern. In domestic animals more than half the fibres of each optic nerve decussate in the optic chiasma, so that a lesion situated between the chiasma and the brain causes partial bilateral blindness and not complete unilateral loss of sight.

Lack of auditory preception is known as deafness. It is sometimes hereditary in certain breeds of dog and cat, particularly those with a white coat in which it is the result of defective development of the organ of Corti, and has been described as a sequel to carbon monoxide poisoning in both these species. Deafness is not necessarily absolute; it may apply only to sounds within a certain frequency range.

Absence of the sense of smell is known as anosmia. Its existence may be difficult to detect except in those species in which sniffing at objects is a characteristic behaviour pattern. In the dog it may result from severe rhinitis as in distemper.

Hypersensitivity (*hyperaesthesia*). This develops in cases of inflammatory injury or compression of the peripheral nerves and dorsal spinal roots, the latter frequently being involved in spinal meningitis. Hypersensitivity to light is shown by photophobia; it is only rarely nervous in origin. Hypersensitivity to sound, odour and flavour cannot satisfactorily be demonstrated in animals. In the horse, hypersensitivity of particular areas of skin may cause restiveness during grooming and harnessing or unwillingness to work (pressure of harness, particularly the collar). Persistent head-shaking in the horse, in the absence of demonstrable lesions of disease, may be the result of hypersensitivity of some part of the external ear or adjacent skin—the lightest touch causes the animal to cringe and cry out. A similarly exaggerated response to pressure, particularly in the region of the loins, may occur in cattle in certain metabolic disorders associated with hypophosphataemia.

Sensory aberration (*paraesthesia*) may be expressed in a limited number of ways. Severe cutaneous pruritus of nervous origin causes violent rubbing, scratching and even biting, which may be induced by the lightest touch. The abnormal behaviour may be carried as far as self-mutilation, in which loss of sensitivity to pain may also play its part. These signs, in varying degrees, are a feature of rabies, pseudo-rabies (Aujeszky's disease) and scrapie. Paraes-

thesia of the eyes is exhibited by 'fly-catching'; the animal snaps as if at flies which do not in fact exist (rabies, encephalitis, early stages of ophthalmia). Paraesthesia of the other senses cannot be demonstrated in animals and, at most, is only occasionally suspected.

Disturbances of the Autonomic Nervous System

The action of this division of the nervous system is involuntary, being mainly motivated by reflex mechanisms comprising afferent sensory neurones and efferent visceral motor neurones. By this means the equilibrium of many dynamic processes is so effectively controlled that they may appear to be static. Some of the nerve fibres comprising the autonomic nerves are associated with those from other sources in the cranial and spinal nerves, with the result that disease of the latter may be accompanied not only by motor and sensory, but also by autonomic disturbances. The most important functions mediated by this division of the nervous system are respiration, cardiac activity, vasomotor tone, visual accommodation, secretion of sweat, deglutition, emesis, secretion of digestive juices, gastric motility, intestinal peristalsis, defaecation, urination, uterine contraction, erection of the penis and milk letdown.

The heart rate is decreased by paralysis of the sympathetic (cardiac accelerator) or by stimulation of the vagus (cardiac inhibitor), and is increased by opposite conditions. The cardiovascular reflex centres are situated in the medulla along with those controlling respiration; the heat regulatory centre is located in the hypothalamus. The spinal centres for defaecation and urination lie in the posterior portion of the lumbar section of the spinal cord. The clinical signs produced by dysfunction of the various components of the craniosacral (parasympathetic) and thoracolumbar (sympathetic) divisions of the autonomic nervous system will be discussed in more detail in relation to the particular nerves concerned.

Reflexes

The functional status of the nervous system is largely assessed by determining the integrity of reflex arcs. A reflex is the involuntary activity induced in a muscle or gland in response to a stimulus. Activity may be absent, diminished or exaggerated. A reflex is diminished or absent when the effector organ is diseased, when the reflex arc is interrupted at any point (e.g. in nuclear and infranuclear paralysis) or when reflex excitability as a whole is reduced without organic change in the reflex arc as in loss of consciousness, narcosis and collapse. Reflexes are exaggerated when the inhibitory action of the cerebrum or hypothalamus is removed or when there is irritation of the reflex arc or its centre. The value in diagnosis of the examination of the different reflex arcs varies; the most important are the corneal, pupillary, cutaneous and tendon reflexes. In addition for the dog and cat, postural and righting reflexes are important; these reflexes cannot be satisfactorily examined in farm animal species.

Corneal reflex. Touching the cornea, preferably the peripheral part, with the moistened fingertip, or with a clean feather, causes the animal to blink. Touching the palpebral conjunctiva, e.g. at the medial canthus, produces the same effect and serves the same diagnostic purpose since the innervation of the two structures is the same. The reflex arc is activated through the sensory fibres in the ophthalmic and maxillary branches of the trigeminal nerve, and the motor fibres in the facial nerve.

Pupillary reflex. The reflex pathway concerned is located in the optic nerve (sensory), in the oculomotor nerve (constrictor) and in the cervical sympathetic nerve (dilator). The reflex is examined by first shading both eyes and then directing a pencil beam of light on to one of the eyes. Normally the pupil dilates in the dark and rapidly becomes constricted on exposure to light. In mammals, on account of the decussation of the optic nerves at the chiasma, variations in light intensity which alter the size of the pupil of one eye will have a somewhat similar influence on the pupil of the other eye. This is termed the consensual reaction of the pupil and it does not occur in avian species. In severe pain, fright or excitement there is a transitory dilatation of the pupil. The pupil is constricted (miosis) and the pupillary reflex is absent in poisoning with eserine, pilocarpine, nicotine or morphine (stimulation of the oculomotor centre), and when there is increased intracranial tension, disease of the cervical section of the spinal cord and of the cervical sympathetic nerve or ganglia, injury to the cranial bones, etc. The pupillary reflex is absent, with the pupil in the dilated state (mydriasis), in loss of consciousness as in epileptiform convulsions, in disease of the optic tract

and retina, e.g. retinal detachment or atrophy, in poisoning with atropine or botulinus toxin, and in injury to the oculomotor nerve or its centre. When the pupil is completely immobile, in the absence of adhesions of the iris to the cornea or lens (anterior or posterior synechia), disease of the retina or optic disc or recognizable poisoning, it may be taken as an indication of serious disease of the brain.

When there is a neoplasm or parasitic cyst involving the brain in the region of the optic radiation, the animal behaves as if blind, although the optic nerves are intact and the pupillary reflex, in consequence, is retained. The animal can see, but what is seen conveys no meaning, because the power of recollecting images has been lost. An equivalent condition may affect auditory perception. Such syndromes are known as mental or cortical blindness (or deafness) or optic (acoustic) amnesia.

Cutaneous reflexes. These are tested by touching or lightly pricking the skin with a pin or hypodermic needle in certain parts of the body. The pedal reflex is examined by pinching an interdigital fold of skin (dog and cat) between forefinger and thumbnail, or pricking the skin of the coronet (horse and cow). In the normal animal the leg is promptly withdrawn. The test is performed with the animal in the recumbent position and, ordinarily, it would not be applied unless it cannot rise or stand unless supported. The anal or perineal reflex is tested by touching the anus or the contiguous skin. In the normal animal this results in a short series of jerky contractions of the anal sphincter, with tensing of the surrounding skin. Determining the state of this reflex is particularly important in the recumbent cow or horse as the absence of a response indicates serious nerve dysfunction. The cutaneous muscle reflex is tested by touching the animal's body with the finger—the area behind the shoulder is most responsive—whereupon the cutaneous muscle twitches and the animal usually turns its head towards the examiner. In the dog exaggeration of cutaneous sensitivity is a feature of spinal cord compression. Identifying the distribution of the hypersensitive areas is an important guide in locating the site of injury. The examination is made by lightly pricking the skin, starting at the tail, and proceeding anteriorly on each side of the vertebral column. The normal dog is relatively insensitive to pin-prick in the lumbar area and only slightly reactive in the vicinity of the thoracolumbar area.

Tendon reflexes. This group of reflexes, along with others, is concerned with posture and gait. The most important one is the patellar reflex. The need to apply the test occurs only with the recumbent animal which is apparently unable to rise. In addition, since the patient must be in a position of lateral recumbency, with the limbs relaxed and in the partially flexed position, it is obvious that the test can conveniently be applied only to small animals. The patellar ligament is tapped smartly by flicking the index finger, or with the handle of a percussion hammer or other suitable instrument. Where it is possible to apply the test to a large animal, the middle patellar ligament is struck with the head of the hammer or the back edge of the hand. When the reflex arc is intact there is immediate contraction of the quadriceps femoris muscle with forward extension of the leg. If the animal, although recumbent, resists the positioning of the limb for the test it may be taken that some degree of neuromuscular function exists. The hock reflex can be tested similarly by striking the tendon of the gastrocnemius muscle, with the limb partially flexed.

Postural reflexes. A number of additional reflexes, which are of considerable value in assessing neuromuscular function for the purpose of locating lesions in nerve tissue, can be examined in the dog and cat. These include placing and righting reflexes which can be tested with or without blindfolding the animal. The placing reflex is applicable to either the fore- or hindlimbs and, when the test is performed with the animal in the blindfolded state, requires for its execution normal cutaneous sensitivity and functional peripheral nerves, spinal cord tracts and motor responses. The animal is held off the floor in the normal standing position and slowly advanced until the distal radial or tibial region of the limbs touches the edge of a table or chair. The normal dog or cat will immediately lift both fore- or hindlegs and place them on the table or chair. With unobstructed vision, when the animal is advanced towards the table or chair, if vision and neuromuscular control are satisfactory, it will raise the feet before any contact is made and place them on the surface of the obstacle.

For the righting reflex, the dog or cat is held in the inverted position at twice its height over a deep bed of straw or a large soft cushion. When released the normal dog or cat, during its fall, will attempt to right itself and so land on its feet or sternum. In the blindfolded animal this reflex tests the function of the utricle, vestibular branch of the auditory nerve, cerebellum, and portions of the spinal cord. In the non-blindfolded animal the optical apparatus is also subjected to examination.

Disturbances of Consciousness

It is not known whether animals, like man, possess a consciousness of the ego, but if an animal behaves appropriately in relation to its environment it is said, by analogy with man, to be conscious. Behaviour, intellect or personality traits in man are governed by areas of the cerebral cortex, particularly the frontal lobes and temporal cortex, both of which are relatively poorly developed in animals, so that significant areas regulating consciousness are unknown. The state of consciousness is tested by applying stimuli of various kinds and observing whether, and how, the animal reacts to them. Disturbances in consciousness may take the form of a decrease (dullness, depression) or an increase (excitation states including mania and frenzy). When dull or depressed, the animal reacts to external stimuli such as a shout, skin prick, touching of the skin or cornea or light directed into the eye, either tardily and slowly or not at all; the reflexes are reduced or absent. The animal has a vacant expression and reacts as if partially asleep. The mildest state is a dazed condition (Fig. 222); somnolence is a more advanced stage (Fig. 223). The final stage is complete loss of consciousness (coma), which is demonstrated by absence of blinking when the cornea is touched

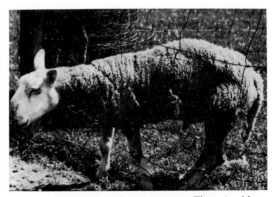

Fig. 222. *Disturbance of consciousness. The animal has a dazed expression and is unable to extricate itself from the fence. Scrapie.*

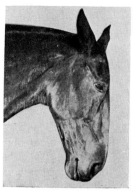

Fig. 223. *Sleepy indifferent expression. Chronic acquired hydrocephalus.*

and of pupillary response (constriction) when a light is shone into the eye. In total loss of consciousness all the non-visceral reflexes are abolished and only the autonomic system continues to function, ensuring the operation of the vegetative reflexes controlling respiration, cardiac activity, maintenance of body temperature, etc.

Sudden loss of consciousness, known as syncope (fainting), occurs in acute cerebral hypoxia due to acute heart failure, anaemia, cerebral haemorrhage, thrombosis or embolism, concussion and contusion, electrocution and lightning strike. The development of unconsciousness is more gradual in coma, which is the more usual mode, and occurs at the termination of clinical uraemia, heat stroke and many infections and poisonings in which the brain becomes involved. A dazed condition is present in hyperpyrexial states, in severe inflammatory processes and in severe fatigue, as the result of the action of toxic waste products causing depression of cerebral function. Mental confusion of varying degree is caused also by haemorrhage, by increased intracranial tension produced by space-occupying lesions and by certain poisons, e.g. alcohol by ingestion, carbon tetrachloride by inhalation. Slight signs of disturbed consciousness can sometimes be exaggerated by causing the animal to exert itself.

When an animal suffering from a disorder of consciousness fails to respond to a needle prick or some other stimulus, it does not invariably mean that the skin of the area is insensitive or that the corresponding muscle is paralysed, but only that the stimulus has failed to reach the level of conscious appreciation in spite of the nervous mechanism for the reception and conduction of the sensation being unimpaired.

Excitation is shown by exaggerated responses to stimuli. The sound of the voice or the clapping of the hands may cause the animal to cringe. In extreme cases it may become frenzied, may injure itself or cause damage by shying, bolting while at work or throwing itself against the walls if indoors. In rabies a biting mania commonly occurs, being most marked in dogs, with repeated compulsive biting even at solid objects. Cattle affected with the nervous form of ketosis manifest depraved appetite, compulsive licking and incoordinated movements. The syndrome, which is suggestive of delirium rather than frenzy, is probably the result of persisting hypoglycaemia. Frenzied behaviour, manifested by violent, uncontrolled movements with a tendency to attack, is exhibited during the early stages of furious rabies and some other forms of encephalomyelitis, and in acute lead poisoning.

Psychical Disturbances

Although it is generally accepted that certain of the domestic animals are capable of such simple mental activities as memory, expressing pleasure or displeasure and so on, it is very doubtful whether the higher mental faculties of imagination, reasoning ability etc., are present in even the slightest degree. When what appear to be psychical manifestations are exhibited, therefore, it is important always to look for evidence of organic disease. For example, the change in temperament occurring in rabies in the dog is not a true mental disorder or psychosis, because it arises from an organic lesion in the cerebral cortex and not primarily from a derangement of the functions of that part of the brain. It must be appreciated, however, that a number of diseases of animals do occur in which manifestations of disturbed nervous function are a feature without any histological evidence of disease. In some such conditions it is possible that the derangement is the result of biochemical abnormality. Such psychotic diseases (neuroses) are regarded as being of rare occurrence in domestic animals. The vices of crib-biting (cribbing) and weaving in the horse have been placed within this category, along with farrowing hysteria in sows, and a number of inherited functional diseases occurring in cattle, including inherited idiopathic epilepsy in the Brown Swiss breed, inherited spastic paresis and inherited periodic spasticity. It is probable that epilepsy affecting young dogs, more particularly those of the brachycephalic breeds, is of the same nature.

Determination of the Site of the Lesion in the Central Nervous System

Diseases of the Brain

In general the character of the clinical signs arising from disease of the central nervous system depends on the localization, rather than on the nature of the lesion. Generalized diseases, such as severe diffuse encephalitis and meningitis, or increased intracranial pressure are usually accompanied by disturbances in consciousness —excitement may have occurred transiently during the early stages—epileptiform seizures and sometimes compulsive movements. The function of some of the cranial nerves is abnormal and appreciation of the nerves involved is of assistance in assessing the severity and extent of the brain injury. The existence of compulsive movements usually, but not invariably, indicates disease of a circumscribed area of the frontal or prefrontal lobe of the cerebral cortex.

In meningitis, since the adjacent brain substance is always involved, the signs are similar to those occurring in generalized disease of the brain, particularly disturbances of consciousness.

In attempting to elucidate the site of disease in the brain, attention should be paid to recognizing the existence of overactivity or paralysis of the cranial nerves. If the base of the brain is affected, the clinical signs depend on which nerve origins are involved, so that there may occur, for example, loss of the sense of smell (olfactory lobe or tract), unilateral or bilateral blindness (optic or oculomotor nerve, or corpora quadrigemina), paralysis of extrinsic muscles of the eye (oculomotor, trochlear or abducent nerve). Indications of cerebral involvement may also have some significance; for example, depressed consciousness (frontal lobe), apparent deafness (temporal lobe) and changes in mentality (temporal and frontal lobes). Compulsive circling movements suggest unilateral disease of the middle ear, membranous labyrinth, basal ganglia or brain stem. Circling is towards the side of the lesion (ipsilateral) if the lesion is posterior to the mid-brain stem region, and away from the lesion

(contralateral) if it is situated forward of the anterior brain stem. Involvement of the cerebellum, vestibular apparatus, basal ganglia or anterior brain stem is indicated if there is falling or rolling to one side; this occurs in the ipsilateral direction when the major damage occurs behind the anterior brain stem, otherwise it is contralateral. Abnormal muscle movements such as twitching or trembling are most likely caused by fear, although the former is a feature of hypomagnesaemic tetany in cattle, and the latter may indicate an anterior cerebellar lesion. Extensor rigidity is a feature of tetanus and strychnine poisoning, otherwise it results from brainstem lesions, trauma to the cerebellum or a pressure lesion of the spinal cord. Tonic/clonic spasms of muscles indicate the existence of a chronic basal ganglion lesion; they occur characteristically in some cases following an attack of canine distemper. Epileptiform convulsions and psychotic behaviour indicate that the cerebral cortex (temporal area) is affected.

In animals it is often extremely difficult to establish the site of major brain damage, not only because of the lack of cooperation from the patient, but also because exact knowledge of the course of some nerve tracts is lacking.

Diseases of the Spinal Cord

Injuries transecting the spinal cord cause bilateral motor paralysis and loss of sensation below the site of injury. Complete section of the anterior part of the cervical spinal cord results in immediate death from respiratory paralysis. Complete division of the cord at the cervical enlargement produces flaccid paralysis of all four limbs and loss of cutaneous sensitivity below the site of the lesion. Because of spinal shock, all the spinal reflexes, including those controlling urination and defaecation, are in abeyance, at least in the early stages. Respiration depends upon diaphragm activity through the medium of the phrenic nerve, the thorax and abdomen both being immobile. There is bilateral dilatation of the pupils and the eye reflexes are functional. In complete section of the spinal cord in the thoracic or lumbar regions the flaccid paralysis and loss of sensation affect only the posterior parts of the abdomen and hindlimbs. Urination and defaecation are suppressed but the reflexes, excepting the patella and extensor thrust, are maintained.

Compression injury to the lumbar section of

the spinal cord, which may be caused by vertebral fracture, dislocation, abscessation, haematoma, degenerative changes in the vertebrae, intervertebral disc protrusion or neoplasia, initially results in spastic paralysis with the hindlegs extended stiffly between the forelegs (see Fig. 209, p. 310); this is a usual feature in the dog affected with intervertebral disc protrusion. At a later stage, because of spinal cord degeneration, other signs, varying somewhat according to the precise site of the injury, make their appearance. When the anterior part of the lumbar division is so affected there is flaccid paralysis of the hindlimbs (see Figs 210–212, p. 310) with preservation of reflexes elsewhere and suppression of urination and defaecation, which is due either to inability by the animal to assume the usual posture for these acts, or to deranged nervous function. The urine is retained, but when the bladder becomes very full, or if pressure is applied, complete evacuation occurs which is not dependent on the continuance of pressure (supranuclear paralysis of the bladder; overflow incontinence). If, however, the lesion is in the posterior part of the lumbar spinal cord, there is, in addition to flaccid paralysis of the hindquarters, almost complete loss of reflexes and incontinence of urine and faeces (nuclear and infranuclear paralysis of the bladder) (see Fig. 213, p. 311). Loss of trophic reflexes leads to severe muscle atrophy and the early appearance of pressure ulcers. Severe disease of the cauda equina leads to retention of urine and faeces, paralysis of the tail, relaxation of the anal sphincter and loss of sensory perception in the perineal region. Priapism (frequent erection of the penis) or self-mutilation are not uncommon signs of spinal cord disease.

Assessment of the state of the spinal reflexes will assist in evaluating spinal cord injuries caused by compression, and in differentiating them from inflammatory and degenerative conditions and those caused by poisoning with insecticides and other toxic substances such as strychnine, lead and arsenic. The patellar tendon reflex is absent when the femoral nerve is paralysed, the spinal cord is extensively damaged, or the portion of the cord extending from the fourth to the sixth lumbar vertebrae is affected (nuclear or infranuclear paralysis). This reflex is exaggerated when pressure injury involves the thoracolumbar area of the spinal cord (supranuclear paralysis).

The pedal reflex is assessed by observing the degree of limb flexion and central pain response to pinching or pin-pricking. Limb flexion is absent in the forelimb when the cervicothoracic section of the spinal cord is damaged; in the hindlimb when the cord area posterior to the fourth thoracic vertebra is affected, or in diffuse myelitis. Pain appreciation, central or local, is absent whenever severe or extensive spinal cord damage exists. A retarded, somewhat limited degree of limb flexion indicates injury to the cord in the cervical, thoracic or anterior lumbar region. An exaggerated superficial pain reaction, revealed by the animal attempting to kick or bite when the skin is touched or pricked, is a useful guide in determining the location of the lesion.

When multiple lesions of the spinal cord and brain are present, the clinical picture varies according to the site and extent of the damage, e.g. the neurological sequelae to canine distemper include continuous spastic twitching of individual muscles or groups of muscles, transient recurrent epileptiform seizures, flaccid paralysis of muscles, sensory disturbances and even psychotic signs.

Clinical Signs Caused by Dysfunction of the Principal Nerves

In order to recognize defects of the more important nerves a knowledge of their individual functions is necessary. A fair measure of assessment is possible through the medium of tests of sensory perceptivity and measurement of muscle tone and function.

Cranial nerves. In animals the cranial nerves, especially near their origin, are fairly well protected from traumatic injury. Apart, however, from inflammatory and degenerative diseases of the brain, which may be associated with dysfunction of one or more of the cranial nerves in addition to other more common clinical signs, such as cranial fracture, haemorrhage or concussion in the vicinity of the origin of one of these nerves may cause dysfunction.

Olfactory nerve. The function of the olfactory nerve may be impaired, temporarily, in rhinitis if the inflammatory reaction involves the olfactory area of the nasal mucosa. More permanent dysfunction may result from a tumour involving the bones comprising the nasal cavities and face. Tests of the sense of smell in animals usually fail to give an unequivocal result because they are conditioned to the sounds and movements associated with food preparation and presentation.

Optic nerve. Abnormalities of vision (partial or complete, unilateral or bilateral blindness) are caused by a defect at any one of several sites including the lens, retina and optic disc, nerve, tract and centres. In the case of disease of the lens, vision is only appreciably impaired when opacity (cataract) is advanced to the stage at which it is readily recognized by direct examination. The deeper structures of the eye, including the retina and optic disc, can only be examined satisfactorily by means of the ophthalmoscope. The more important diseases affecting the ocular fundus which cause blindness are retinal degeneration, retinal detachment and retinitis. Progressive retinal degeneration (atrophy) is recognized to have an hereditary basis in certain breeds of dogs including the Irish setter, Gordon setter, miniature poodle and certain other breeds. Diseases of the optic nerve are relatively rare in animals, and only when they produce a change in the condition of the optic disc will they be recognized during ophthalmoscopic examination.

Tests of visual acuity, which involve the functional activity of a number of eye structures, often produce results which are difficult to interpret because of the virtual impossibility of excluding other senses from reacting to the applied stimuli. Tests which are applicable include the corneal and conjunctival reflexes (eye preservation), and the retinal reflex. The eye preservation reflexes are readily tested by gently moving the index finger, or a swab-stick, towards each eye in turn and noting if, and at what point, closure of the eyelids occurs. Otherwise visual efficiency may be tested by throwing a small ball of cottonwool at a plastic sheet held in front of the eyes and noting whether any head movement occurs. In both these tests it is important to avoid producing air currents which may give rise to a confusing response. The retinal reflex can also be examined by walking the animal over ground on which have been placed a number of small obstacles of varying height up to 22 cm or so, and spaced at irregular distances. This method is particularly suitable for the horse, provided the groom walks along with the animal at a regular pace, taking uniform steps and does not adjust his stride to step over an obstacle. By increased movement of the ears (which can be observed) the horse may attempt to overcome a defect of vision through greater application of the sense of hearing. For dogs, a useful test of visual perceptivity is to make the animal walk up a stairway to which it is not accustomed, or to bring it into a room with a number of free-standing pieces of furniture. It may be noted that when afflicted with a visual defect, the dog will attempt to orientate itself through its sense of smell by slightly raising the head and sniffing. The history regarding the behaviour of the animal, as related by the owner, often contains information that is grounds for suspecting impaired vision. In mammals, owing to the decussation of the fibres of the optic nerve at the optic chiasma, a lesion of the nerve anterior to the chiasma will affect the vision of only one eye, whereas a lesion posterior to the chiasma will affect the vision of both eyes.

Ophthalmoscopic examination. Two main types of ophthalmoscope are available for use in the examination of the ocular fundus: the simple ophthalmoscope and the electric ophthalmoscope (see Fig, 85B, p. 82). Because the former requires a fixed light source behind the animal which can be reflected into the eye, satisfactory conditions are not readily achieved. The latter instrument provides its own illumination which is projected into the eye through the medium of a prism, the position of which can be varied in relation to the light source, thereby regulating the divergence of the light beam to suit the method of ophthalmoscopy in use. The electric ophthalmoscope provides only limited illumination, so that the examination must be undertaken in a partially darkened place.

Ophthalmoscopic examination can be performed by either the direct or indirect method. Direct ophthalmoscopy, which is undertaken without the need to interpose a condensing convex lens between the instrument and the patient's eye, provides an upright image of the ocular fundus. It is the only practical method of this type of examination in animals, and for all general purposes the electric ophthalmoscope is the most suitable instrument. The structures of the ocular fundus which can be observed include the optic disc, tapetum lucidum, tapetum nigrum, and the retinal vessels. If the patient is examined in an environment from which light is excluded, chemical dilatation of the pupil is not likely to be necessary. Otherwise mydriatic agents such as homatropine hydrobromide (2% solution) should be instilled into the conjunctival sac 15 minutes, or more, before the examination is made. On completion of the examination the induced mydriasis is counteracted almost immediately by instillation of a few drops of physostigmine salicylate solution (0·5%), otherwise pupillary dilatation, which persists for about 12 hours, will interfere with accommodation.

Electric ophthalmoscopes are fitted with a series of convex and concave lenses around the periphery of a circular disc, so that any individual lens can be rotated into position during the examination procedure. In use, the ophthalmoscope is held so that the observer obtains the widest possible field of vision through the viewing aperture, with the back of the instrument about 2–5 cm away from the patient's eye (see Fig. 89, p. 85). Difficulty in observer accommodation is overcome by rotating a suitable concave lens (usually about −2D or −3D) into position until the clearest view of the fundus structure is obtained. Then by rotation of lenses back through the concave to the convex series, the refracting structures anterior to the fundus, including the vitreous humour, lens, anterior chamber and cornea are brought into focus. It is necessary during ophthalmoscopic examination to identify the location of any lesion which affects the refracting media. With some experience it is possible to achieve this by noting the particular lens giving the clearest image of the lesion. Opacities in the vitreous humour are best seen with lenses in the series 0 to +8D, lens cataracts in the range +8D to +12D and corneal changes at up to +20D; the visual efficiency of the clinician will affect the lens selection.

Recognition of abnormalities of the ocular fundus necessitates an appreciation of normal structure and arrangement in the different species of animals. The tapetum lucidum, which extends over the greater part of the fundus and occupies the dorsal sector, is variously coloured in the different species and breeds of animals. The colours commonly observed are blues, yellows and greens, or varying shades or combinations of these colours, produced by reflection of light from the iridescent, pigmented epithelium of the choroid which overlies the retina. The lower sector of the fundus, the tapetum nigrum, is usually brown, chocolate or black in colour because of the presence of melanin which is, however, absent in albinos. The boundary between the tapetal zones is usually quite distinct because of the difference in pigmentation.

The optic disc (papilla) is the portion of the fundus at which the retinal fibres of the optic nerve are aggregated together and penetrate the overlying choroid. It forms a disc-like elevation, situated slightly towards the temporal canthus, from the periphery or centre of which relatively large blood vessels radiate. In the horse the optic disc, which is elliptical, is surrounded by the tapetum nigrum with blood vessels appearing at the periphery and running radially for a short distance before disappearing. The optic papilla in cattle is relatively small and rather poorly defined; it is surrounded by the tapetum lucidum, with blood vessels arising from the periphery which sometimes run across one another. Other ruminant species possess optic discs showing somewhat similar characteristics to those of cattle. In the dog, the optic disc, which shows a variable relation with the tapetal areas is also variable in shape with centrally originating blood vessels which extend almost to the periphery of the tapetum lucidum. The cat has a circular optic disc with the blood vessels showing the same general characteristics as in the dog.

In general the blood vessels have a more or less straight, branching course and the arteries can be distinguished from the veins by being narrower and not so dark in colour.

Some of the more important diseases of the retina and optic nerve that may be recognized by means of ophthalmoscopy include anatomical defects, retinal detachment, retinal degeneration or atrophy, retinitis and diseases of the optic nerve.

Slight anatomical defects such as partial absence of tapetal structure require careful examination, otherwise they may be overlooked. Detachment of the retina, which in most cases is secondary to some other disease of the eye, is usually associated with a history of sudden blindness. Ophthalmoscopic examination during the early stages of detachment reveals folds in the retina around the optic disc; at a later stage there may be larger undulating folds. Complete detachment exists when the retina presents the form of a funnel, the narrow end of which is related to the optic papilla where it is still attached. Following the course of the blood vessels is a useful means of recognizing when retinal detachment exists.

Secondary retinal degeneration arising as a sequel to systemic viral diseases, e.g. canine distemper, equine viral arteritis, may be readily confused with progressive retinal atrophy. The history of a dog with the latter condition is highly relevant for differential diagnosis; points of particular significance are visual defects in dim-light vision, indicated by bumping into objects, and cautious movements, in an animal of certain breeds, with no history of an antecedent illness likely to be of significance. In the later stages, as the retinal atrophy progresses, the owner may have noted increasing visual impairment with more obvious tapetal reflectivity. In the early phases there is a degree of increased pupillary dilatation which becomes more marked as the retinal degeneration progresses. At this time the pigmentation of the choroid appears more intense, and the blood vessels are reduced in number and diameter, and become threadlike. The optic disc becomes almost white in colour and loses its regular outline.

Retinitis is, in the majority of cases, associated with and probably arises as an extension of choroiditis. Its presence is indicated by observing white to grey patches on the fundus, or a uniform greyish exudate which gives the tapetum lucidum a somewhat dull appearance and obscures the blood vessels.

Haemorrhages into the retina are relatively rarely seen in animals. Vascular hypertension has been stated to be a cause, but conclusive proof is lacking; otherwise it may occur in septicaemic diseases, acute leptospiral infection and certain forms of poisoning, e.g. warfarin, and in purpura haemorrhagica. Retinal haemorrhages usually surround a blood vessel in the form of small discrete spots or large blotches.

The optic disc shows changes when there is atrophy of the optic nerve, and when intracranial or intraocular pressure is increased. Atrophy of the optic nerve may be caused by a variety of factors including retinal degeneration and retinitis, as well as elevated intraocular pressure, or a severe blow on the occipital region of the head. In addition a form of optic atrophy has been recognized in Jersey and Guernsey cattle which is attributed to the influence of an autosomal recessive factor. Deficiency of vitamin A in the diet during adolescence is another established cause. Whatever the cause, atrophy arises in association with failure of the optic foramen to enlarge, so that the nerve is constricted. Optic atrophy is indicated by finding that the disc is reduced in size and is pallid, with reduction in the number of blood vessels. Elevated intra-

cranial pressure, which may result from cerebral coenurosis, chronic acquired hydrocephalus or meningitis, may give rise to a variable degree of oedema of the optic disc, recognizable by its mushroom-like appearance, in conjunction with arterial constriction and venous dilatation. Increased intraocular pressure is indicated by 'cupping' of the optic papilla, the periphery of the disc being raised with reduction in the size and length of the blood vessels.

Oculomotor nerve. Loss of function of this nerve influences the condition of the eye and some associated structures. When the parasympathetic filaments are involved the pupillary reflex does not operate so that the pupil is dilated (mydriasis). Drooping of the upper eyelid (ptosis) occurs when the motor supply to the levator palpebrae superioris muscle is lacking, with restriction of movement of the eyeball, which is deviated laterally and downwards, when the inferior oblique and rectus muscles, excluding the external, are deprived of their motor innervation. The degree of pupillary response to variations in light intensity is best tested by directing the light beam from a pencil torch into the eye with the animal in a darkened place. When the reflex is normal the pupil constricts in response to increased light. The range of movement of the eyeball can be tested by moving one hand in front of the animal's face.

Trochlear nerve. Loss of function of this nerve deprives the superior oblique muscle of motor function so that the eyeball is turned inward and slightly upward.

Trigeminal nerve. When the motor component (mandibular branch) of this nerve is paralysed—this might result from trauma or fracture of the cranial bones, or tumours involving the nerve or contiguous structures—there is some difficulty in closing the mouth, and when the animal is relaxed the lower jaw is dropped (Fig. 224). Unilateral paralysis causes slight deviation of the lower jaw towards the normal side. The masseter and temporalis muscles will atrophy if the paralysis persists for some weeks. Paralysis of the mandibular branch is also associated with loss of sensory appreciation in the lower part of the face, lower lip, tongue, teeth and associated structures. The tongue may show evidence of injury. Loss of function of the ophthalmic and maxillary branches, which are purely sensory, will deprive the temporal region, eye, poll, ear, eyelids, nasal mucous membrane, teeth of the

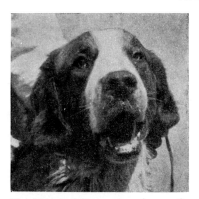

Fig. 224. *Inability to close the mouth; the lower jaw hangs loosely. Paralysis of the masticatory muscles caused by injury to the mandibular branch of the trigeminal nerve.*

upper jaw and the hard and soft palate of sensory perceptivity. This state can be recognized quite readily by means of the application of a pain inducing stimulus. The most sensitive test, however, for paralysis of the ophthalmic branch is that involving the corneal or conjunctival reflex. The absence of these may be indicated by the development of secondary keratitis.

Abducent nerve. Loss of function in this nerve is indicated by medial rotation of the eyeball with inability to direct the axis of vision in a lateral direction due to lack of motor action by the external rectus muscle.

Facial nerve. Paralysis of this nerve may arise centrally or peripherally, the latter usually being unilateral. Central paralysis affects the lower part of the face and is characterized by narrowing of the nostril on the affected side (horse), drooping of the lower lip, with the upper lip drawn towards the unaffected side, and increased salivation. The tongue may protrude slightly from the mouth in the early stages. With peripheral paralysis, which is more common, as well as the foregoing signs, there is drooping of the ear (the upper eyelid is not involved), and inability to close the eye (lagophthalmos) because motor function is absent in the orbicularis oculi muscle. Inability to close the eyelids will lead to excessive tear production and conjunctivitis, if the conjunctival sac is irritated.

Auditory nerve. Defective function of the cochlear branch of the acoustic nerve will interfere with hearing. In suspected cases of deafness in animals, before concluding that there is a defect of auditory perception, it is necessary to exclude other abnormalities of the external ear as a cause. Accurate interpretation of the results of tests of hearing in animals is frequently difficult to achieve. The need to apply such tests is greatest in the dog, less so in the horse. Normally both these species possess very acute auditory perceptivity; this is very readily demonstrated in highly trained sheep dogs. In such dogs the history, as related by the owner, may provide highly relevant information regarding the animal's ability to hear, based on observation of failure to respond to customary sound signals. Noting the reaction of the animal to noises of increasing tone pitch, made out of sight, or getting the owner to call the dog by name, first at low volume and gradually louder, are useful tests.

Defective function of the vestibular segment of the auditory nerve interferes with the maintenance of equilibrium through the normal proprioceptive mechanisms associated with vision, the skeletal muscles, tendons, and joints. Signs of paralysis include nystagmus, strabismus, rotation of the head with the affected side downwards

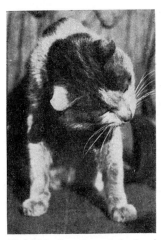

Fig. 225. *Rotation of the head and neck (torticollis). Injury to the vestibular segment of the auditory nerve.*

(Fig. 225), rolling movements and circling. If the paralysis is bilateral, coordinated movement is lacking. Defective function of this nerve occurs in middle-ear infection, in certain congenital defects of middle ear development and in dogs and cats from streptomycin intoxication.

Glossopharyngeal nerve. Because of its association with the vagus nerve in the pharyngeal region, loss of function in the glossopharyngeal nerve alone cannot readily be distinguished, unless there is no evidence of vagal dysfunction in other areas supplied by the latter nerve. Through the medium of its sensory and motor branches, the glossopharyngeal nerve is concerned in the pharyngeal reflex, the functional status of which can be readily assessed, at least in dogs and cats, by touching the posterior wall of the pharynx with a tongue depressor. Absence of the reflex is indicated by failure to stimulate a swallowing movement by the affected side of the pharynx. In large animals, the most obvious clinical sign is difficulty in swallowing (dysphagia), which becomes virtually impossible when the paralysis is bilateral.

Vagus nerve. A lesion situated near the origin of the vagus nerve, as well as involving the glossopharyngeal nerve, and possibly the spinal accessory, produces dysfunction over a considerable area. Peripheral lesions will have a limited, less serious effect. Loss of motor innervation to the pharynx will cause changes in, or complete loss of, voice and varying degrees of dyspnoea because of flaccidity of the vocal cords. This situation is most prevalent in the horse, in which paralysis of the recurrent laryngeal nerve (more usually the left) gives rise to 'roaring'. Difficulty in swallowing, with, in addition, regurgitation of fluid and food particles through the nostrils because of the flaccid state of the soft palate, occurs when there is loss of vagal motor innervation to these parts. Vagal paralysis involving particular nerve branches may result in dilatation of the stomach and increased pulse frequency. Increased vagal activity is a likely event because of failure of the sympathetic component of the autonomic nerve balance. Its existence is indicated by increased salivation, bradycardia, and intestinal hypermotility expressed by diarrhoea.

Spinal accessory nerve. Peripheral paralysis of the nerve causes slight dropping of the scapula on the affected side, with the head turning towards the normal side, because of flaccidity in the trapezius and sternocephalicus muscles, both of which will eventually undergo atrophy.

Hypoglossal nerve. In unilateral paralysis, when the tongue protrudes, it deviates towards the affected side; in established cases the tongue shows evidence of atrophy. Bilateral paralysis causes the tongue continuously to protrude from the mouth.

Spinal nerves. As lesions of the spinal nerves will affect the lower motor neurone components, the resultant paralysis will be accompanied by muscle atrophy, which will become apparent rather soon, and by the early development of bed sores, particularly in large animals, because of the lack of important trophic reflexes. Loss of function of individual spinal nerves is, in most instances, caused by injuries of various types. Identification of the particular nerve involved necessitates a sound knowledge of the anatomical distribution and function of those peripheral nerves likely to be affected. The clinical features resulting from loss of function of only the more important of these will be discussed.

Suprascapular nerve. Paralysis of this nerve is associated with adduction of the forelimb so that the point of the shoulder tends to roll outwards during progression. Voluntary abduction of the limb cannot be achieved. Atrophy of the supraspinatus and infraspinatus muscles is an early feature, so that the spine of the scapula becomes prominent.

Brachial plexus. Dysfunction of the group of nerves comprising the brachial plexus causes complete motor and sensory paralysis of the forelimb, which is dragged along hanging loosely from the shoulder. Excoriation of those parts of the limb which are in contact with the ground is a feature.

Radial nerve. The radial nerve trunk is liable to injury by fractures of the first rib, or by compression between the humerus and the first rib when horses or cattle are cast with hobbles. In paralysis of the nerve there is lack of motor function in the extensor muscles of the elbow, carpus and digits, as well as loss of sensation in the skin over the anterior and lateral aspects of the upper part of the forelimb, and the anterior aspect of the phalangeal region. The elbow is flexed (see Fig. 227, p. 331), even when the animal walks, and the foot is dragged along. If pressure is applied to the anterior aspect of the carpal region, so that it is maintained in the normal weightbearing position, the leg will support the animal's weight, but bends again as soon as the pressure on the carpus is removed. Absence of sensory perception in the upper part of the limb only, differentiates radial nerve from brachal plexus paralysis. When the radial nerve is injured distal to the origin of the branches supplying the triceps brachii muscle, the carpus shows a tendency to involuntary flexion so that the affected limb knuckles over onto the anterior aspect of the phalangeal region.

Lumbosacral plexus. This is derived from the last three lumbar and first two or three sacral nerves and supplies sensory and motor innervation to the croup and the whole of the hindlimb. Paralysis of the plexus is associated with atrophy and loss of sensation in all the muscles of the area. The hindleg can be lifted and brought forward but is lowered uncertainly, with the hock strongly flexed.

Sciatic nerve. Ensures motor innervation to the posterior thigh muscles as well as to the muscles which flex and extend both the hock and the digits, and sensory perceptivity to the skin, over the posterior and lateral aspects of the upper hindleg, and the whole of the lower limb. Loss of function of the nerve is associated with absence of sensation and paralysis of the muscles below the stifle. The dorsal aspect of the foot rests on the ground. Active support of the weight of the body is impossible, but the weight can be borne passively, i.e. when the hock is supported. The function of the hip-joint is maintained by the obturator and femoral nerves, the latter also ensuring extension of the stifle joint.

Tibial nerve. This nerve is one of the terminal branches of the sciatic nerve; it supplies sensory function to the skin over the plantar aspect of the phalangeal region, and motor innervation to the muscles which extend the hock and flex the digits. Loss of function causes the hock to remain flexed when the animal is walking, the flexion being accentuated if the limb bears weight. Voluntary extension of the hock and flexion of the phalangeal joints are impossible, but the limb can still be partially advanced and weight borne on it.

Peroneal nerve. This is the terminal branch of the sciatic nerve which ensures motor innervation to the muscles which flex the hock and extend the phalanges, and sensory perceptivity in the skin of the anterior aspect of the leg. When the function of the nerve is lost the leg is dragged along the ground with the dorsal aspect of the foot downwards, and the hock joint overextended (Fig. 226). If the phalangeal joints are supported, weight can be taken on the limb. There is muscular atrophy and loss of sensation in the anterior and lateral aspects of the limb below the stifle.

Femoral nerve. This nerve ensures motor

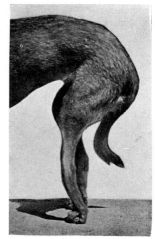

Fig. 226. *The hock can be pushed forward (overextended). Injury to the peroneal nerve.*

function in the quadriceps femoris muscle and sensory perception in the skin of the medial aspect of the limb. When the nerve is paralysed the stifle joint cannot be fixed and the limb can be advanced only incompletely. There is atrophy of the quadriceps femoris muscle and loss of sensation over the area supplied by the nerve.

Obturator nerve. Through the medium of its motor supply to the pectineus, adductor, external obturator and gracilis muscles this nerve enables the thigh to be adducted. If the nerve is paralysed the hindlimb is abducted during forward progression, producing a 'scything' action. When affected with bilateral obturator nerve paralysis (this is a not uncommon occurrence in cows at parturition, more particularly in heifers producing disproportionately large calves) an affected animal would 'do the splits' on a slippery surface.

Internal pudendal (pudic) nerve. This nerve ensures motor function in the external anal sphincter and the muscles of the penis, vulva and urethra, and sensory perceptivity in the skin of the associated areas. When the nerve is paralysed there is loss of sensation in the area, with relaxation of the external sphincter and absence of the perineal reflex. The penis protrudes from the prepuce and cannot be retracted. Secondary dependent oedema is a likely development.

Examination of the Cerebrospinal Fluid

The composition of the cerebrospinal fluid is maintained within rather narrow limits, so that disease of the central nervous system will give rise to detectable changes because of alteration in the rates of production and absorption and, in some instances, the existence of an inflammatory reaction. The major bulk of the cerebrospinal fluid is accommodated in the ventricles of the brain and in the subarachnoid space of the spinal cord where it provides an internal and external cushioning effect as well as a space compensating mechanism, and a transport medium between the blood and the nervous system and vice versa.

Cerebrospinal fluid can be collected from the cisterna magna or the spinal subarachnoid space in the lumbar region. Irrespective of the site used a suitable spinal needle, with its stilette in position, is required, otherwise the lumen becomes blocked with adipose or other tissue. General anaesthesia is recommended for cisternal puncture, whereas local anaesthesia may be found satisfactory for the lumbar site, although when further procedures, such as the introduction of contrast media, are envisaged, general anaesthesia is advisable. The technical aspects of the procedure require a precise knowledge of the anatomical relationships existing at the chosen sites. Because of this, the technique is not generally applied in veterinary clinical work where it is most extensively used in the dog; it is also applicable in the pig, sheep, calf and foal, for which species the basic technical procedure as recommended for the dog can be adopted.

The anaesthetized dog is placed in sternal recumbency with the head firmly held at an angle of 90° to, and in line with, the cervical vertebrae. Following preparation of the site a spinal needle (22 WG, 8 cm long) is inserted through the skin in the midline, at a point midway between the external occipital protuberance and a transverse line joining the most anterior point of the wings of the atlas. The needle, with its stilette in position, is directed through the muscular tissues towards the atlanto-occipital interspace, while being maintained perpendicular to the cervical vertebrae. The passage of the needle through the ligamentum nuchae, which immediately overlies the dura mater, requires slightly greater pressure. Immediately the dura mater is penetrated there is a slight contraction of the skeletal musculature, and resistance to the further passage of the needle disappears. When the stilette is withdrawn, welling of fluid from the needle hub confirms that it is in the correct position, and the requisite

sample can be collected by attaching a sterile hypodermic syringe and applying gentle suction.

Lumbar puncture is, technically, a more difficult procedure than that of the cisterna magna. The anaesthetized animal should be placed in sternal recumbency with the head at the higher end of a table tilted to an angle of 75°, with the object of providing the maximum quantity of spinal fluid in the lumbar area. The subarachnoid space can be punctured at any of the vertebral interspaces in the lumbar region. The recommended procedure is to insert a suitable spinal needle through the skin in the midline, almost immediately anterior to the dorsal spine of the vertebra, and continue the insertion until further progress is arrested by bone. At this stage the interarcual space between the contiguous vertebrae can be identified by altering the direction of the needle, which can then be pushed through the dura mater into the subarachnoid space.

Cerebrospinal fluid pressure. This can be determined during cisternal puncture by means of a suitable manometer containing Ringer's solution which should be connected to the spinal needle, with the animal in the lateral position, before any cerebrospinal fluid has been removed. Because the volume of the cranial cavity is relatively fixed any variation in the volume of one of the contained components (brain, blood and cerebrospinal fluid) will be compensated by changes in the other two. A small change in the volume of the cerebrospinal fluid results in a large change in pressure. Normal pressures for animals range between 75 and 140 mm Ringer's solution. For accurate interpretation a uniform technique must be employed, embodying the use of a standard needle, and the avoidance of pressure on any part of the body, more particularly over the jugular veins which causes a marked rise of fluid in the manometer (jugular compression in the dog can increase the pressure from 120 mm to as high as 310 mm). In general a significant rise in pressure readings occurs in meningitis, meningo-encephalitis, central nervous system haemorrhage, coenurosis, intracranial tumours, abscesses, hydrocephalus, etc. In calves and pigs low vitamin A status is associated with cerebrospinal fluid pressures above 200 mm.

Composition of cerebrospinal fluid. Normal cerebrospinal fluid is water clear, with a specific gravity only slightly above that of pure water, and contains no protein. The composition is different from that of blood plasma and is to some extent independent from it. The number of leucocytes (predominantly lymphocytes) present is usually less than 5/mm³. Other substances that may be significantly altered include glucose, chlorides, sodium, potassium, calcium, magnesium, phosphorus and urea. In bacterial infection of the meninges or brain, the presence of the causal organism in the cerebrospinal fluid will be revealed by the adoption of appropriate cultural techniques.

Radiological Examination

This method of examination of the central nervous system is not generally applicable to the larger farm animal species. Under general practice conditions, the quality of the radiographic equipment that is usually available is such that its relevant principal use is in the detection of fractures in bones associated with the central nervous system. In certain hereditary bone diseases, e.g. chondrodystrophic dwarfism in calves, the abnormal bone features are sufficiently gross to be recognized during the first 2 weeks of life in radiographs of the lumbar vertebrae. Prior to considering the use of radiographic methods for neurodiagnosis, it is imperative that a detailed clinical examination should be performed, and a careful analysis made of the neurological signs, in order that the possible nature and site of the pathological lesion can be indicated.

Radiological methods for examination of the central nervous system have been more thoroughly worked out in the dog than for any other species. Because of the small size of the lesions in many instances, and their relatively low resistance to the passage of the X-rays, in contrast to other structures such as the surrounding bone, which itself shows considerable variation in density, the quality of the radiographic equipment and of the technique, become of prime importance. Minimizing movement of the animal is a first essential; this can be achieved by the use of a sedative, tranquillizer or suitable general anaesthetic.

The technique of myelography is applicable in cases of spinal cord compression resulting from an intervertebral disc protrusion not revealed by direct radiography, or a meningeal tumour or haemorrhage, or a spinal abscess. For this purpose cisternal or lumbar subarachnoid puncture is performed and a small quantity of cerebrospinal fluid is removed and replaced by an equal volume of a suitable contrast medium. Posterior migration of the contrast medium is promoted by tilting the table on which the dog is placed, to an angle of about 60°. Rotating the animal while in this position will assist distribution of the medium throughout the spinal fluid. Exposure of films at intervals will reveal the point at which posterior migration of the contrast medium ceases.

Contrast procedures which have been developed to assist the radiographic examination of the brain include cerebral angiography, pneumoencephalography and ventriculography. Cerebral angiography, which is virtually an experimental technique, involves placing a needle or cannula in the common carotid artery, following which an injection of diatriazoate sodium, or some other suitable contrast medium, is made and films exposed in rapid sequence. Pneumoencephalography consists of introducing air, or oxygen into the subarachnoid space by means of cisternal or lumbar puncture. With appropriate head positioning, the air or oxygen rises and the subarachnoid space and cerebral ventricles are outlined on exposed X-ray films. The method is not always reliable, this is particularly so when the lumbar site is employed. Cisternal pneumoencephalography may successfully reveal space-occupying lesions or obstructive hydrocephalus.

Ventriculography involves a more direct approach to replacing the ventricular fluid by air or a radiopaque medium. This is achieved by means of a spinal needle which is forced through a small trephine hole in the skull, sited midway between the lateral canthus of the eye and the external occipital protuberance. After insertion through the burr hole, the needle is pushed vertically downwards for a distance of about 1–2 cm. The stilette is withdrawn, and if the lateral ventricle has been punctured fluid will appear in the needle. When the correct position has been reached, as much as possible of the ventricular fluid is withdrawn and 5–15 ml of air or 1–3 ml of contrast medium are slowly injected. Movement of the head will assist distribution of the medium; air will disperse more readily.

Electroencephalography

Because of certain technical difficulties, and the rather high cost of essential equipment, electroencephalography has mainly been employed on an experimental basis in animals.

The variations in electric potential which occur in the cerebral cortex can be recorded by means of electrodes applied to certain areas of the scalp and connected to suitable amplifying and recording instruments. The degree of amplification required is of the order of one million times because of the low voltages (10–300 mV) emanating from the surface of the scalp. The type of electrode and the manner of their application are obviously of considerable importance in obtaining good quality electroencephalograms. The most suitable electrode for general use is a small cadmium-plated alligator clamp, which grasps a fold of skin firmly enough to ensure reasonable electrical contact and also resists movement. The skin at the point of electrode attachment should be defatted with acetone, and a long-acting analgesic drug injected, not only beneath the skin but also into the underlying muscle, in order to obviate contraction, prior to the application of the electrode paste and then the electrode itself.

The sites for electrode attachment are within the area of the cranium where the cerebral cortex is closest to the surface. Five areas, designated left frontal, right frontal, vertex, left occipital and right occipital, in association with an earth, the last being over the occipital protuberance, have been most extensively employed in the dog. Corresponding electrode attachment areas have been worked out for other species. When the thickness of the temporalis muscle interferes with the quality of the EEG, insulated needle electrodes, inserted through the muscle to the frontal bone, will overcome this handicap.

During the recording period the animal must be fully conscious but perfectly quiet, for which purpose physical restraint alone is practicable. There are many factors which influence the electrical activity of the cerebral cortex including species, breed, sex, and stimuli which reach the central nervous system through the medium of visual and auditory perception.

Electroencephalography has seldom been used as a method for assisting the evaluation of neurological function in clinical diagnosis in animals. In the dog, experimental studies have shown that the EEG is a valuable aid in confirming suspected cases of encephalitis. Otherwise, although changes in EEG patterns are a feature of brain damage, the variations cannot be related to specific pathological features.

15

The Musculoskeletal System

The primary function of the musculoskeletal system is to support the body in various ways in order to ensure normal locomotion and posture. In addition, particular skeletal structures are involved in such functions as respiration, mastication, urination and defaecation. Diseases of muscles, bones or joints give rise to abnormal locomotor action (lameness) and/or changes in posture as their major clinical features.

Disturbances of locomotion are revealed when the animal moves voluntarily, or is exercised at varying paces in the presence of the clinician. Some of the various types of disturbance have already been mentioned in connection with the preliminary general examination of the animal. Locomotor function is altered in many diseases of the nervous system (see Fig. 218, p. 313), and in other diseases in which the musculoskeletal system is not primarily involved. Severe systemic disease often results in muscular weakness and tremor, along with pain and incoordination, because of toxaemia. In such circumstances, it is unlikely that the primary affection will be overlooked if a methodical clinical examination is made. Likewise, alterations in posture may arise from abnormalities involving structures other than those of the musculoskeletal system (see Fig. 14, p. 17).

The component parts of the musculoskeletal system include the muscles and their attachments, the bones and the joints. Diseases that affect these structures can be classified on the basis of their clinical, aetiological or pathological features, but understanding of their nature is best realized by categorizing them as degenerative, inflammatory, proliferative and developmental types. The degenerative diseases of muscles, bones and joints are distinguished as myopathy, osteodystrophy and arthropathy respectively, and the corresponding inflammatory diseases as myositis, osteomyelitis and arthritis. Proliferative diseases (neoplasms) of these structures are relatively rare, but developmental defects, particularly of bone, are by no means uncommon.

The Muscles

The superficial muscles are examined by inspection and palpation. Function and tone can be assessed in a similar manner, although observed exercise should not be omitted as an examination procedure. Local changes are more readily detected when it is possible to compare corresponding muscles, or groups of muscles on both sides of the body. Reduction in the size or bulk of a muscle (atrophy), which is otherwise normal, occurs as the result of limited or curtailed use (see Fig. 214, p. 311). This is a feature in persistent radial nerve paralysis (most commonly seen in the horse and dog), and is also a development in painful conditions of bones and joints in which movement is limited voluntarily, and in ankylosis where there is mechanical interference with movement. In radial nerve paralysis the animal is unable to advance the limb, and the elbow is dropped owing to the absence of motor function in the triceps brachii muscle, and the carpus is flexed (Fig. 227). The extensor muscles show signs of atrophy within a few weeks.

Increased tone of the musculature may be continuous (tonic spasm) as in tetanus, or intermittent (clonic spasm) in strychnine intoxication in which the degree of spasm may be severe and generalized, so that the affected animal exhibits convulsive seizures during which

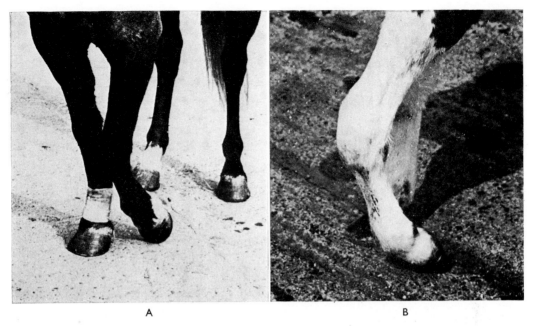

A B

Fig. 227. A, *Radial paralysis in a horse.* B, *Radial paralysis in a calf. Note the lowered position of the elbow, with flexion of all the joints except the shoulder, so that the toe and the anterior aspect of the foot rest on the ground.*

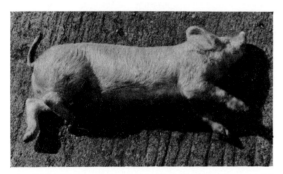

Fig. 228. *Abnormal elevation of the head and tail, with depression of the back and extension of the limbs (opisthotonus). Cerebrocortical necrosis.*

it assumes a laterally recumbent posture and manifests opisthotonus (Fig. 228). When muscular spasm is marked, the increased firmness and rigidity of the muscles are readily appreciated on palpation, and some of the individual superficial muscles are more clearly delineated. Tetany is a state of tonic muscular spasm in association with excitement and panting respirations. This syndrome is observed in hypomagnesaemic tetany of cattle and sheep, and in transport tetany of horses. Tremor, a repetitive twitching of the voluntary muscles, is readily observed and can be appreciated by palpation. It may have a biochemical or an organic basis. Dehydration and electrolyte imbalance, particularly chloride depletion, are important biochemical causes of muscle tremor. When deranged nervous function is responsible for muscle tremor it is usually intensified if the animal is forced to exert itself, more especially if the cerebellum is involved.

Myopathy

Clinically the non-inflammatory degenerative diseases of voluntary muscle (myopathies) are characterized by muscle weakness which gives rise to changes in posture or, in severe cases, to recumbency as well as significant alterations in cardiac function. In acute cases of myopathy of recent origin the affected muscles are swollen and hard, and at autopsy have an appearance like fish flesh because of hyaline degeneration.

One of the most important groups of myopathic conditions in animals is that classified as enzootic muscular dystrophy (white muscle disease), which is particularly prevalent in lambs and calves, but it has also been recognized to affect older members of these species as well as horses, pigs and dogs. The aetiology of muscular dystrophy is complex; it has been described as being due to primary or secondary vitamin E deficiency, inadequate dietary selenium or excess legumes or polyunsaturated fatty acids in the diet. Unaccustomed exercise is an important trigger mechanism for the condition. Affected animals are lethargic and unwilling to get up, with obvious stiffness of gait ('stiff-lamb disease'); there is, in many cases, respiratory and circulatory dysfunction. The muscular changes, which in the case of the skeletal system are invariably bilaterally symmetrical, can be detected by palpation, the involved muscles being hard and rubbery and, in the more acute phases, swollen. The distribution of the skeletal muscle

dullness and cardiac irregularity followed by sudden death.

Irrespective of the situation and extent of the muscle lesions, their character is uniformly similar, consisting of localized white or greyish areas of degeneration ('white muscle disease') in the form of streaks. Histologically, initial hyaline degeneration is followed by coagulation necrosis.

Confirmation of a clinical diagnosis of muscular dystrophy may be obtained by means of urinary creatine excretion studies and determination of the serum glutamic oxalacetic transaminase value; both the foregoing are increased in proportion to the severity of the

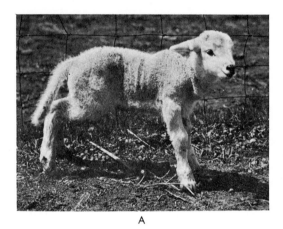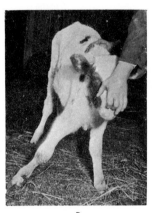

| A | B |

Fig. 229. A, *Abnormal posture with feet widespread and scapulae protruding above the line of the withers. Muscular dystrophy.* (Montana Veterinary Research Laboratories and H. Marsh (1965) Newson's Sheep Diseases, 3rd ed. London: Baillière, Tindall & Cassell). B, *Abnormal posture with marked abduction of the right forelimb. Muscular dystrophy in a calf.*

lesions varies in individual cases. In a proportion of the severe cases, the line of the back is lowered so that the upper borders of the scapulae, which are widely separated from the chest, extend above the normal height of the withers (Fig. 229). Involvement of the diaphragm and intercostal muscles is indicated by abnormal respiratory function including dyspnoea and abdominal type respiration.

Muscular dystrophy in pigs is predominantly associated with the myocardium (Herztod disease), although skeletal muscle lesions are also found at autopsy. The dystrophic changes have a somewhat similar distribution to this in some calves, but they occur less frequently in lambs. In cases of this type clinical signs are not always of great diagnostic value and consist of

muscle damage, and inversely to the interval which has elapsed since clinical signs developed. The urinary excretion rate of 200–300 mg creatine in normal calves may be increased to 1·3 g daily in animals with muscular dystrophy. In normal lambs, the creatine/creatinine ratio is less than 0·7 whereas in muscular dystrophy this figure is between 1 and 5. Blood and liver tocopherol levels will reflect the vitamin E status of the animal, although data on which to base an interpretation are not available. Because tocopherols are stored in the liver, values from this source are a more accurate index of vitamin E status.

Dystrophic muscular changes have been recognized in sheep showing clinical signs of scrapie. As similar lesions have been found in the musculature of apparently normal sheep, the significance of the muscle pathology in relation to scrapie has not been determined.

Characteristic degenerative changes in the gluteal and lumbar muscles in equine paralytic myoglobinuria (azoturia) give the affected tissues a hard board-like feel on palpation. The so-called 'tying-up' syndrome in saddle horses bears some similarity to azoturia but is usually associated with less severe myopathic lesions. In both conditions the muscular changes arise from coagulation necrosis of the fibres resulting in dysfunction and pain which cause stiffness, sweating and reluctance to continue work. In severe cases of azoturia the affected animal stumbles, sways from side to side and falls to the ground, with considerable struggling in spite of which it is unable to rise. The history of the development of such signs in a horse which has been rested for 2–7 days on full rations should suggest the diagnosis. The appearance of brownish-red discoloration of the urine from the presence of liberated myoglobin provides confirmatory evidence. Because of its relatively low molecular weight myoglobin is freely excreted by the kidneys and is not retained in the blood. Following recovery the affected muscles atrophy (Fig. 230).

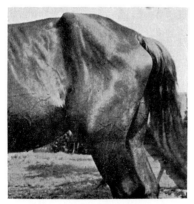

Fig. 230. *Atrophy of the tensor fasciae latae muscle after an attack of paralytic myoglobinuria.*

The 'tying-up' syndrome is seen most frequently in race horses and riding ponies, particularly mares, in good condition when working rigorously. The clinical signs consist of rigidity of the loin or croup muscles, lameness, accompanied by pain, unwillingness to move and myoglobinuria. In contradistinction to azoturia, kidney

damage is slight and recovery, which is usual, occurs fairly quickly.

In both the foregoing conditions, the degree of muscle damage at the acme of the disease can be assessed by determination of the urinary creatine value or the urine creatine/creatinine ratio, both of which are increased proportionately according to the severity and extent of the damage. In addition, the serum values for glutamic oxalacetic transaminase, lactic dehydrogenase and potassium (hyperkalaemia) are elevated. In the horse, muscle damage, in the absence of hepatic injury, is associated with SGOT values of over 1000 Sigma–Frankel units/ml. Horses which have been subjected to severe exercise may have serum levels slightly in excess of 1000 units.

A special form of myopathy occurs in spring and early summer in thoroughbred foals up to 5 months of age. Although the foals are usually running at grass with their dams, exercise has not been considered to be a causal factor. The condition, which develops suddenly, is characterized by deep depression, stiffness, disinclination to move, prostration and death in from 3 to 7 days. Less severe cases manifest lethargy and stiff gait. In addition there is pronounced swelling and firmness of the gluteal muscles and of the subcutaneous tissues at the base of the mane. The masseter muscles may also be involved causing dysphagia with apparent excessive salivation.

Secondary myopathy, occurring as the result of interruption of the nerve or blood supply, occurs in the hindlimbs of cattle which are recumbent for periods in excess of 48 hours.

Myositis

Inflammatory changes in muscle may arise from direct or indirect trauma during the course of such specific diseases as blackleg, actinobacillosis, bluetongue, foot-and-mouth disease and invasion by parasites in sarcosporidiosis and trichinosis. Myositis varies in clinical intensity being acute in blackleg and malignant oedema, and producing no obvious clinical signs in trichinosis and sarcosporidiosis.

In blackleg the muscle lesion, which is usually in the upper part of one leg but may occur in the psoas muscles, brisket, diaphragm or base of the tongue, is initially a hot, painful swelling, later becoming cold, painless and emphysematous. Systematic palpation of the musculature will reveal the situation of the lesion. The general signs are those of fever, which within a few hours become replaced by those of toxaemia. Diagnosis is based on the clinical features or on finding the characteristic muscle lesion on post mortem examination in cases of sudden death. Malignant oedema most often develops as the result of muscle wound contamination, so that almost any part of the body may be affected. The local lesion when near the body surface consists, initially, of a soft, doughy swelling which later becomes tense, with the previously erythematous skin now dark and tightly stretched.

Suppurative myositis develops in most cases, in dogs at least, as a complication of bacterial infection elsewhere in the body. Trauma and bruising are also likely to assist in the establishment of pyogenic infection. Severe local pain and swelling are usually fairly obvious features, which can assist in locating the site of the infection. The firm swellings later soften and fluctuate, but the pyogenic process does not always completely mature.

Actinobacillosis in cattle usually causes chronic myositis involving the tongue; more rarely the muscular tissues of the pharynx or larynx are affected, and very occasionally the superficial musculature of some other part of the body. The affected muscle, which is painless, becomes enlarged and firm; when the tongue is affected the mucous membrane frequently becomes ulcerated, more particularly along its lateral surfaces.

Eosinophilic myositis is an occasional disease of the dog and is manifested by intermittent attacks of muscular inflammation that persists for a few weeks, punctuated by periods of regression of variable length. The attacks are characterized by symmetrical swelling of the muscles of mastication including the masseter, temporalis and pterygoid groups. Pseudotrismus is usual, the mouth cannot be completely opened, or the incisor teeth brought into apposition (Fig. 231). Following repeated attacks, the masseter and temporalis muscles exhibit atrophy to a marked degree, and trismus is more severe and persistent and even permanent. In the early phases, the attacks of muscular inflammation coincide with a significant eosinophilia of 20–30% which is revealed when a differential leucocyte count is performed. The clinical features, as described, are sufficiently distinctive to enable acute attacks to be recognized readily.

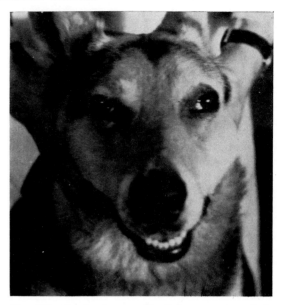

Fig. 231. *Pseudotrismus with slight narrowing of the eyelids in an Alsatian dog. Acute eosinophilic myositis.* (J. C. Whitney (1958) Vet. Rec., 70, 661)

The cause of the condition has not been identified. Histological examination of affected muscle tissue reveals infiltration with mature eosinophil leucocytes which later become replaced by mononuclear cells. An asymptomatic form of eosinophilic myositis occurs in beef cattle; its economic significance arises from carcass condemnation at slaughter.

Traumatic myositis, affecting some of the muscles of the limbs, and accompanied by severe lameness, swelling, heat and pain, occurs in horses, cattle and dogs. In horses the posterior thigh muscles are most commonly involved although, occasionally, the muscles of the forelimb are similarly affected. Subsidence of the acute inflammation may be followed by fibrous tissue proliferation with adhesions, and by subsequent calcification. The characteristically abnormal gait of affected horses consists of shortened stride, with sudden withdrawal of the extended foot when it almost reaches the ground.

Severe and/or extensive traumatic myositis may be accompanied by fever and toxaemia. Extreme exertion from running, or exhaustion during prolonged transport when they are unable to lie down, will cause myositis in cattle. Rupture of muscle tissue is invariably followed by an inflammatory reaction. The adductor muscles of the thigh in cattle are prone to rupture when the hindleg slips sideways on ice or on smooth concrete surfaces, causing excessive abduction of hindlimbs. Cows in the prerecumbent phase of parturient paresis occasionally rupture the gastrocnemius muscle. This is probably the result of sudden strain on the muscle at a time when functional tone is reduced, and the gait is unsteady with the animal reeling from side to side. In the majority of cases the condition is recognized when the animal attempts to stand up following effective treatment for milk fever. The muscle damage permits extension of the stifle and flexion of the hock joint, so that the tuber calcis is lowered and the weight is supported over the whole length of the metatarsal bone.

Muscular Hypertrophy

Selection for good beef characteristics has, in the case of certain breeds of cattle, led to the emergence of a genetic factor which is expressed by muscular hypertrophy (various colloquial names have been applied to the condition including, 'buffalo', doppelender, etc.). The condition has been described in the South Devon, Friesian, Charolais, Ayrshire, Piedmont and Hereford breeds of cattle. Muscular hypertrophy varies from slight to extensive and severe. The muscles of the hindquarters are most frequently affected, the hypertrophy together with the absence of fat accentuating the grooves between the muscles. The musculature of the forequarters, back and other parts of the body may be affected to a lesser degree. It is postulated that the genetic character concerned is an incomplete recessive which can be expressed in a variable manner. The significance of the condition is related to its importance as a cause of dystocia.

Developmental Defects

Developmental abnormality of muscles and tendons may be structural or functional, and genetically derived or acquired extrinsically. Inherited multiple tendon contracture, which occurs in calves and lambs, is associated with fixation of the limbs in flexion or extension, so that it is a cause of dystocia. Affected animals are unable to stand, and atrophy of the limb muscles is usual. Arthrogryposis is a non-inherited, congenital condition of calves which

is clinically similar to the foregoing; it is frequently accompanied by hydranencephaly as an additional feature. There is an absence of ventral horn cells in the spinal cord and myopathic degeneration. Inherited functional diseases involving the musculature include spastic paresis and periodic spasticity, both of which occur in cattle. In the former, the clinical signs, which appear during the first 6–9 months of life, consist of hypertonicity of the gastrocnemius muscle and overextension of the hock joint. Although the gastrocnemius and perforatus muscles are spastically contracted, the affected limb can be passively flexed. Inherited periodic spasticity usually makes its appearance in adult life. Initially the clinical signs only occur when the animal rises. The hindlegs are extended backwards, with marked tremor of the muscles of the hindquarters. In the early phases the attacks are transient in duration, but later they may persist for up to 30 minutes, during which time movement is virtually impossible.

Myofibrillar hypoplasia (splayleg) is a development defect of the skeletal musculature in newborn piglets. Although the condition has familial features it has not been conclusively demonstrated to be hereditary in origin. The clinical signs are apparent at birth and consist of inability to stand because of abduction (splaying) of the limbs. Recovery will occur over a period of a few weeks provided the piglets are protected from being trampled on or overlaid by the sow. Microscopic examination reveals immaturity of the muscle fibrils.

The Bones

Clinical examination of the bones consists primarily of inspection and palpation of those parts of the body where these skeletal structures are superficially situated and not overlaid by muscle masses. In addition, radiological examination is an extremely valuable adjunct in suitable cases, because it is capable of revealing the structure of bone. Some bone diseases may cause the animal to adopt rather characteristic aberrations of posture and gait.

By means of inspection and palpation of bones it is possible to recognize abnormalities in consistency, in addition to those of contour, shape and sensitivity. On these bases, it may be possible to decide whether any existing bone disease is localized to one part, or is generalized to a variable degree.

Developmental Defects

Abnormal bone formation resulting from developmental defects occurs in a variety of forms in animals. The defects vary in severity from those which are virtually incompatible with survival so that affected animals succumb in early life, to those that are clinically unrecognizable. Localized developmental defects are occasionally seen in the horse. Ankylosing lesions of the vertebral column, affecting both the coccygeal and sacral region and the lumbar vertebrae, are not likely to be a serious clinical problem. Enzootic incoordination ('wobbles'), which affects mainly young horses, arises from injury to the spinal cord as the result of intervertebral disc protrusion, or upward displacement of one cervical vertebra on another because of asymmetric articular facets (a form of cervical retrolisthesis). The existence of the defect only becomes apparent when incoordination develops. Local developmental defects of the appendicular skeleton are of minor clinical significance in the horse. Generalized developmental defects of bone are relatively rare; the most important, 'ankylosed foal', is not a primary bone disease, but results from severe shortening of the muscle tendons which causes the articular ends of the bones to be distorted. This is often expressed clinically by varying degrees of scoliosis.

Localized developmental defects of osseous structures in cattle include reduced phalanges and achondroplastic dwarfism. Both conditions have a genetic basis and are apparent at birth. In the former, the upper parts of the limbs are normal but the carpus and tarsus are abnormally short, and the first and second phalanges are missing, with the normal hooves and third phalanges attached by soft tissues. Calves affected with the latter exhibit short legs, with wide heads and protruding lower jaws. Some types of dwarfism in cattle are not readily recognized early in life because there is no obvious local anatomical disproportion (compact dwarfism in the Hereford and Shorthorn breeds). Abnormal mandibular development of varying severity (prognathism), with malocclusion of incisor teeth and dental pad, occurs as a rare event in all breeds of dairy cattle. Underdevelopment of the mandible, with shortening of the jaw has also been described, and may be so severe that the calf is unable to grasp the teat.

Generalized chondrodystrophy in cattle is demonstrated in the so-called 'bulldog' calf which occurs in the Dexter breed, and also in other breeds including Jersey, Guernsey and Friesian (Holstein). The condition is apparent at birth; some of the affected fetuses cause dystocia because of marked hydrocephalus. In addition, there is bulging of the frontal area of the head with shortening of the nose, which is dished. The neck is short and stout, and the limbs are thick. Chondrodystrophic changes also occur in 'acorn calves', which is a recognized congenital defect in cattle.

Developmental bone defects appear to be relatively uncommon in sheep and pigs. Mild degrees of mandibular prognathism (projecting jaw) have been described in Merino and Rambouillet sheep. In pigs, excessively thick forelegs, resulting from subcutaneous oedema, increased thickness of bone and irregularity of the periosteum, produce obvious signs at birth. Absence and deformity of the tail have also been described in Landrace and large white pigs.

Congenital deformities involving bone are relatively common in the dog. Hemivertebrae—a median cleft in the vertebral body which results from failure of the centres of ossification to unite—may cause scoliosis or kinking of the tail when only a few vertebrae are affected. When the condition is more extensive, because of vertebral compression, the spinal column will be obviously shortened. Although the clinical signs may suggest the existence of this bone defect, its exact nature is likely to be revealed only by radiography. Spina bifida, a more rare condition than the foregoing, arises from failure of union between the halves of the neural arches, resulting in a median cleft. When the cleft is sufficiently wide the meninges, spinal cord or both may prolapse, resulting in paralysis or limb contracture. Spina bifida is only likely to be identified accurately by radiological means.

Curvature of the radius in the dog has an uncertain and possibly multiple aetiology. Unequal growth rates at the medial and lateral aspects of the distal epiphysis, cause the shaft of the radius to become concave on its lateral aspect. The ulna is affected similarly, but usually to a lesser degree. The condition is most frequently bilateral. Affected dogs evince no sign of pain during manipulation of the carpus, or when the abnormal limb is subjected to the full weight of the animal. The foot is turned laterally distal to the carpus, which is usually in dorsiflexion.

Osteogenesis imperfecta is a generalized

developmental defect of bone occurring in new-born lambs, and in the dog and cat, which is considered to result from deficient periosteal and endosteal bone formation. Because enchondral osteogenesis proceeds normally, the bones are of normal length but lack thickness and strength. The condition is exposed clinically because of a predisposition to fracture when the bones are subjected to relatively minor stress. Recent fractures, lameness or malformation of the bones following repair of a previous fracture are the usual features. Specific diagnosis depends upon radiological examination revealing increased bone porosity and thinner than normal bone cortices. Thyroid hyperplasia is a feature of osteogenesis imperfecta in the cat in which species dietary deficiency of calcium appears to be of aetiological significance. It is suggested that the condition has a genetic basis in lambs.

Bone Degenerations

The degenerative diseases of bone occurring in animals, and grouped under the term osteodystrophy, arise from failure of normal bone development or from abnormal growth in mature bone. The dystrophic changes in the bones, which usually have a more or less generalized distribution, are attributable to nutritional deficiency, toxic factors and hereditary influences. The last have been considered in dealing with chondrodystrophy. Dietary deficiencies of calcium, phosphorus and vitamin D or imbalance of phosphorus and calcium cause rickets, osteomalacia or osteodystrophia fibrosa, according to the age or species of the animal concerned.

The most important nutritional bone disease in the horse is osteodystrophia fibrosa in which there is deposition of soft, cellular fibrous tissue as compared with the uncalcified osteoid tissue of osteomalacia. In advanced cases, the characteristic bone changes occur in the mandible, where swelling of the lower and alveolar margins is followed by bilateral enlargement of the facial bones. The earliest phase of the disease may be associated with shifting lameness with no readily discernible defects, and creaking sounds in the joints when walking. The condition is invariably caused by a primary, or by a secondary calcium deficiency arising from excessive dietary phosphorus because of feeding on cereals or bran. Affected horses may show no significant changes in blood chemistry. Radiological exami-

nation usually reveals reduced density of bone structure.

Calves develop rickets when grazing on phosphorus-deficient land or when fed cereals or hay grown in such areas. In calves housed for long periods, vitamin D deficiency may be responsible. The bones and teeth become abnormal because of inadequate mineralization of the cartilaginous matrix and excessive proliferation of epiphyseal cartilage. The clinical features, which eventually develop to the degree that they are readily recognized, include enlargement of the limb joints and of the costochondral junctions, with forward and outward curvature of the long bones of the forelimbs. In severely affected calves, involvement of the jaw bones prevents closure of the mouth. Blood chemical changes consist mainly of serum inorganic phosphate values below 3 mg/100 ml and elevation of plasma alkaline phosphatase. Radiographic examination provides valuable confirmatory evidence, even in the relatively early stages.

In adult cattle, osteomalacia develops in areas where there is significant deficiency of phosphorus in the soil. The initial bone lesion is demineralization, followed by deformity of the weakened bones, with production of large amounts of diaphyseal osteoid which remains uncalcified. Depraved appetite and reduced productivity, with painful stiff gait and crackling joint sounds while walking, are suggestive clinical signs. In very severe cases bone deformities are present, with persistent recumbency due to weakness as a culminating feature. The major changes in blood chemistry include decreased serum phosphorus and increased plasma alkaline phosphatase. The osteoporotic state of the limb bones is revealed by radiological examination. Lambs and sheep are less likely than calves and adult cattle to develop rickets or osteomalacia, and when the latter are clinically affected, the former only exhibit mild signs, although in lambs thickening and softening of the jaw bones, in conjunction with dental abnormalities, may prohibit closure of the mouth.

The clinical signs of rickets in young pigs simulate those occurring in other species of animals when so affected, and consist of increased thickness of bone at the region of the epiphyseal cartilage, with curvature of the long bones of the limbs. Lameness and failure to thrive are usual features. Under intensive conditions, feeding pigs on cereal diets containing excessive amounts of phosphate contributes to the development of rickets, more especially if dietary calcium and vitamin D, or its precursors, are inadequate. Young pigs fed on garbage are likely to receive a diet which is deficient in vitamin D and calcium. In adult pigs similar diets result in the development of osteodystrophia fibrosa, with clinical signs which resemble those described for the horse. Moderately severely affected pigs exhibit bending of the limb bones with lameness, the facial bones and joints remaining normal. In severely affected pigs there is, in addition, more marked distortion of limb bones with swelling of the facial bones and some of the joints. The changes in the nasal bones may cause narrowing of the nasal cavities to a degree sufficient to give rise to snuffling respirations.

Osteomalacia occurs most frequently in sows about 5–6 weeks after farrowing, in which case one of the main signs is inability to stand on the hindlegs. This is often due to fracture of the severely demineralized bones.

Curvature of the limbs and enlarged joints, which results from spreading of the metaphyses of the long bones (Fig. 232), is the usual clinical

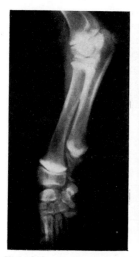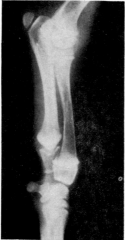

Fig. 232. *Radiographs showing the abnormal skeletal development in the radius and ulna, consisting of increased density of the metaphyses, which are mushroomed, with narrowing of the epiphyses. Rickets in a puppy.*

feature of rickets in the dog. In addition, enlargement of the ribs at the costochondral junctions is quite marked, producing the so-called 'ricketic rosary'. Lameness of varying severity is usual.

An abnormal calcium/phosphorus ratio and deficiency of vitamin D in the diet are the most important causal factors. The significance of vitamin D is greatest when there is a wide calcium/phosphorus ratio either way. Rickets is usually recognized on the basis of clinical observation, with confirmation by means of chemical determinations on blood, and from radiographic examination. Radiographically identifiable changes appear at the distal extremity of the radius and ulna (Fig. 232) prior to the development of clinical signs. Because of compaction of the soft uncalcified bone through weight-bearing, the ends of the diaphyses of the limb bones are dense and mushroomed in shape. The epiphyses appear narrow and the epiphyseal line is ragged. In osteomalacia, because of demineralization, the limb bones tend to fracture rather than bend, and because growth has ceased there is no disturbance of enchondral ossification.

The significance of vitamin C in relation to normal bone metabolism in animals is not clearly defined. In occasional instances in dogs, lameness, associated with local swelling of one or other of the long bones of a limb resulting from subperiosteal haemorrhage, has been considered to be related to a deficiency of or an inordinate demand for vitamin C. Calcification of the subperiosteal haemorrhages causes enlargement of the distal ends of the diaphyses which may be clinically apparent, or revealed by radiographic examination.

In young foals in areas of high soil molybdenum and/or low copper content enlargement of bones in the vicinity of joints, stiffness and failure to thrive have been observed. No direct evidence incriminating either molybdenum or copper as a causal factor has been obtained, and the character of the bone lesion has not been elucidated. Posterior paresis with impairment of gait caused by osteoporotic changes in the skeleton occur in young lambs exposed to high lead-containing diets during the first 3 months of life. In fluorosis, excessive mobilization of calcium and phosphorus causes osteomalacia, osteoporosis and exostoses. Palpable and visible enlargement is discernible in the mandible, sternum, metacarpal, metatarsal and phalangeal bones, with an appreciable pain reaction when pressure is applied to the lower limb bones.

Skeletal changes and metastatic calcification are features of secondary hyperparathyroidism, which in animals, especially the dog, results from renal insufficiency in chronic interstitial nephritis. In young dogs the bone defects are similar to those of rickets with, in addition, deposits of calcium in the kidneys, lungs and stomach. In similar circumstances, older dogs develop generalized osteodystrophia fibrosa which is characterized by demineralized softening of the mandible and maxilla, as well as of other bones of the head, giving rise to the state of 'rubber jaw'. The hyperfunction of the parathyroid gland in chronic renal insufficiency results from inability to excrete phosphates with a consequent hyperphosphataemia and hypocalcaemia. The elevated level of blood inorganic phosphate brought about by the inability of the damaged kidney to perform its normal excretory function, produces secondary hyperplasia of the parathyroid gland which then initiates excessive withdrawal of calcium from the bones.

Typical cases of renal rickets or osteodystrophy are easily recognized as the flexible state of the decalcified bones permits them to be bent readily. Less obvious cases can be identified by measuring the calcium and phosphorus blood levels, and by radiographic examination. In the late stages both the calcium and phosphorus values are usually elevated. The important radiographic change is one of general demineralization in which the phalanges are extensively involved (see p. 236).

Bilaterally symmetrical enlargement, affecting more especially the long bones, occurs in hypertrophic osteopathy (Marie's disease) which is more common in dogs than in other domestic animals, although it also affects horses, cattle and sheep. In established cases the enlargement is marked. Associated pain causes lameness, particularly during the early stages when there may be a variable degree of accompanying oedema. Clinical evidence of chronic pulmonary involvement in the form of coughing, or dyspnoea is a frequent accompaniment. The aetiology is obscure; one suggestion is that the skeletal changes result from a reflex vasomotor disturbance secondary to circulatory disturbance in the lungs. Diagnosis necessitates recognition of the clinical aspects, in conjunction with radiological examination of the abnormal bone and also of the chest area. Radiographically the disease is characterized by diffuse osteophytic apposition on the periosteal surfaces, particularly of the long bones of the limbs.

Similar changes occur in craniomandibular osteopathy ('lion jaw') of dogs affecting the mandibles, temporal and occipital bones. The condition occurs in Scottish terriers and West Highland White terriers, and because it is often seen in littermates a genetic origin has been suggested. It appears in puppies from four months of age upwards. The clinical signs include pain during eating and when the head is held, irregular enlargement of the mandibles and restricted jaw movement. The lesion is not uniformly and regularly progressive.

Inflammatory Diseases

Inflammation of bone (osteitis)—commonly referred to as osteomyelitis, which term should apply only to inflammation of the medullary cavity of bone—is somewhat uncommon in animals. The majority of cases arise as the result of infection consequent upon traumatic injury (exogenous). Specific infections (endogenous) in which osteomyelitis is a concomitant feature include joint-ill in foals, calves and lambs, actinomycosis in cattle, brucellosis and atrophic rhinitis of pigs and tuberculosis in the horse, cat, ox and pig. If a limb bone is affected by osteomyelitis then lameness, local swelling and pain are readily detected on examination. Inflammatory rarefaction and erosion of the bone cortex is succeeded by spread of the pyogenic infection to the surrounding tissues, and subsequent discharge of pus with the establishment of sinuses. Involvement of the bones of the jaw causes malalignment, and even shedding of teeth, so that pain and disability interfere with prehension and mastication.

Actinomycosis (caused by *Actinomyces bovis*) is a rarefying osteomyelitis with an associated granulomatous reaction. Initially it develops as a painless, bony swelling on the mandible or maxilla opposite the midpoint of the molar arcades. In many cases rapid enlargement takes place; in others development may be very slow. With rapid development there is usually considerable pain. The lesions invariably break through the skin and discharge small amounts of sticky, honey-like fluid containing minute, hard, yellow-white granules through several openings. Repair of some of the sinuses takes place in conjunction with the development of others. Spread of the infection to contiguous soft tissues occurs in severe cases.

The clinical signs of brucellosis in pigs occur in animals of breeding age and most obviously involve the genital tract. In addition, there is usually the gradual onset of lameness, incoordination and posterior paralysis caused by osteomyelitis of the bodies of the lumbar and sacral vertebrae; there is often an accompanying arthritis. In atrophic rhinitis the typical lesions are restricted to the nasal cavities. The early stages are characterized by inflammation, but later the mucous membrane becomes atrophic and there is decalcification and atrophy of the turbinate and ethmoid bones; the pathological process may spread to involve the facial sinuses. The clinical signs vary in intensity from mild sneezing with a slight impairment of food utilization to dyspnoea and cyanosis with deformity of the face due to arrested development of the bones, the nasal bones and premaxillae turning upwards. The aetiology of atrophic rhinitis is in doubt; the most acceptable view is that the disease is caused by an infectious agent (*Bordetella bronchiseptica* and *Pasteurella multocida* type B have some credibility in this respect), or by a dietary deficiency of calcium, or possibly by a combination of both these factors.

In tuberculous osteomyelitis in the horse, the cervical vertebrae are commonly affected and may undergo a considerable degree of rarefaction, which causes stiffness of the neck so that the animal is unable to eat off the ground. Specific recognition of the disease is assisted if other clinical indications, e.g. coughing due to pulmonary lesions, enlargement of palpable lymph nodes, fluctuating temperature, are present. The tuberculin test in the horse can only be reliably interpreted when it is negative. In the cat some of the vertebrae, or the bones of a limb when they become involved in tuberculous osteomyelitis undergo extensive rarefaction, resulting in the almost complete disappearance of the bone; in a proportion of cases, a discharging sinus is established which communicates between the lesions and the surface of the body. The presence of tubercle bacilli in the discharge is usual in many such cases, and may be revealed by means of prescribed bacteriological techniques. Tuberculous osteomyelitis in cattle and pigs most commonly affects the vertebrae with involvement of the meninges. The majority of cases of tuberculous osteomyelitis are specifically identified at post mortem examination.

Apart from the preceding specific infections, osteomyelitis can result from haematogenous infection in tick pyaemia of sheep, abscesses from tail-biting in pigs or infection of castration or docking wounds in lambs. In these circumstances the diagnosis necessitates consideration of the history and clinical signs including the local enlargement, deformity and tissue swelling with discharging sinuses. Again the nature and extent of the condition are often only recognized at autopsy. Haematological studies usually reveal marked leucocytosis, and on radiological examination the affected bones are increased in diameter with reduction in density of the cortex and, in severe cases, areas of cavitation.

Aseptic necrosis of bone and cartilage (osteochondritis) is a cause of lameness in young lightweight horses and in dogs. The areas of bone most commonly involved include some of the epiphyses or epiphyseal cartilages and contiguous bone. There is no general agreement regarding the aetiology of the condition, although it is accepted that trauma is a definite factor. The end result is avascular necrosis followed by hyperaemia of surrounding bone, with some degree of osteoporosis and resorption of the necrosed bone. Clinically, in addition to lameness, there is little of note to be seen apart from the possibility of a firm, local swelling on the medial aspect of the radius and metacarpal bone, at the level of the distal epiphyseal cartilage of the radius in 'epiphysitis' in young horses. Osteochondritis in the dog may involve the neck of the femur or the proximal tibial epiphysis and tuberosity. In the former, flattening (coxa plana) of the femoral head is almost inevitable, with unilateral or bilateral lameness which, in severe cases, is exhibited by the dog 'carrying' one hindleg. Lameness is also a feature of the latter condition, and may prevent the dog from getting up when lying down. When walking, dogs so affected exhibit a waddling gait. The only local feature during the early stages of the disease is pain on palpation of the anterior aspect of the femorotibial articulation.

The radiological features of 'epiphysitis' include compression and thinning of the cartilage, with evidence, at a later stage, of new bone formation. Aseptic necrosis of the head and neck of the femur is not detectable, on the basis of recognizable radiological change, in the early stages. Later, osteoporosis, at some points, gives rise to increased bone density in adjacent areas. At this stage, flattening of the head of the femur and variable degrees of damage to the acetabulum are usual.

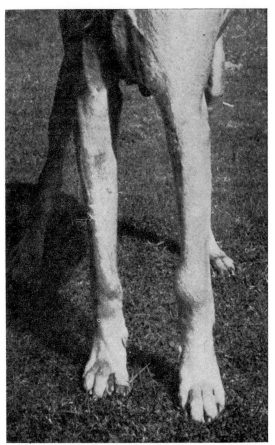

Fig. 233. *Swelling of the distal extremity of the radius in a dog. Osteosarcoma.*

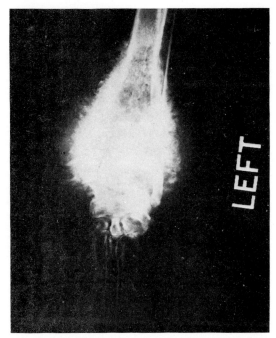

Fig. 234. *A radiograph of an osteosarcoma (telangiectic type) involving the distal part of matacarpal bone in a dog. Note the exploding nature of the lesion.*

Proliferative Diseases

Proliferative diseases of bone have a relatively low incidence in animals, with the possible exception of the dog. Hypertrophic osteopathy has already been considered in the context of degenerative diseases of bone. Osteopetrosis (marble bone disease) is a well-known proliferative bone disease of man which occurs in poultry but not in mammals.

The incidence of bone tumours in animals is, on the whole, relatively low, with the exception of the dog and to a lesser degree the cat. Primary bone neoplasms, including osteosarcoma and chondrosarcoma, usually evince a marked degree of malignancy. Metastatic tumours of bone occur infrequently; the most common type is the melanoma, the incidence of which is highest in the horse with, as a rule, involvement of the long bones or vertebrae.

Primary bone tumours are rare in horses, and when they occur show a predilection to involve the bones of the head. Mandibular tumours in young horses are either adamantinoma or osteosarcoma. The incidence of bone neoplasia in cattle and sheep is of the same order as that in the horse. The bone tumours seen most frequently in the dog are osteosarcoma and chondrosarcoma. The latter occurs most frequently in the nasal passages, although it may originate in any of the bones. In contrast, the osteosarcoma is usually confined to the extremities of the long bones (Fig. 233), and to the ribs above the costochondral junction. Two forms occur, which can be recognized by means of radiological examination. The sclerosing osteogenic sarcoma, although malignant, develops fairly slowly with increased density of the cortical bone, and deposition of similar bone, which has an irregular spicular surface, beneath the overlying periosteum. In the other type—telangiectic osteogenic sarcoma—malignancy is more marked. It appears to originate in the endosteal surface of the bone and erodes the cortex until it is displaced, causing a swelling to develop (Figs 233, 234). Both types of osteosarcoma are painful and give rise to obvious locomotor disability. In most cases the true nature of the affection, at least in the early phases, is revealed only by means of radiography.

Secondary neoplasia of bone in the dog occurs from metastasis of a squamous cell carcinoma of the nasal mucosa, which is one of the commonest tumours encountered in this species. Occasionally fibromas, originating from the periosteum, may cause erosion of cortical bone to a degree sufficient to cause clinical signs.

Bone tumours in cats, more especially those involving the long bones of the limbs, are usually of considerable size when the affected animal is presented for professional attention. This is an indication that, in general, neoplasms of bone cause only minor disability in this species until they reach large proportions. The commonest sites for primary osteosarcoma are the mandible and the humerus. Occasionally a squamous cell carcinoma, originating from the gum, may invade the underlying bone and, when the tumour is of fair size, give rise to obvious clinical signs.

The Joints

Clinical examination of the joints is performed in the same manner as for the rest of the skeleton. Inspection and palpation of the joints of the appendicular skeleton can be supplemented by observing the range of flexion and extension of the joints during exercise, or which is achievable by manual means. In the smaller animals indirect palpation of the vertebral column is worthwhile. Radiological examination is a valuable supplement in the same manner as for the bones. By means of inspection, performed with the animal at exercise and resting, and palpation, it is possible to recognize abnormalities of contour, shape and function of joints.

Congenital Defects

Inherited defects of joints are rare in large animals. In 'contracted foals' (congenital axial and appendicular contractures) there are multiple deformities including torticollis, scoliosis, asymmetry of the skull, flexion-contracture of the distal limb joints and thinning or absence of the ventral abdominal wall. A similar condition has been recorded in calves. Multiple ankylosis of all the limb joints occurs as an inherited, congenital defect in cattle. The flexion of limbs is such that the affected fetus is a cause of dystocia. A non-inherited, congenital form of severe joint contracture (arthrogryposis), which may

concern flexion or extension, occurs in calves. This state arises from tendon contraction. There is no joint abnormality and severe muscle wasting is a feature. Sporadic cases of joint deformity at birth are not unusual in foals and calves; the most common manifestation is excessive flexion of the metacarpophalangeal joints so that affected animals knuckle at the fetlock.

In the dog, congenital dislocation of joints is relatively common, particularly in the chondrodystrophic and dwarf breeds (poodle) as well as in the Labrador and Alsatian. The joints most frequently affected are the hip, elbow and stifle. Less severe degrees of acetabular dysplasia in the dog range from preluxation to subluxation of the hip joint. Clinical signs usually appear when the degenerative changes in the joint have caused considerable destruction and structural modification of the tissues. Affected dogs have difficulty in rising, are lame and walk with a swaying motion of the hindlegs. Pain is readily elicited by means of manipulation which may reveal looseness of the hip-joint. Radiological examination reveals that the acetabulum and femoral head and neck are abnormal to a varying degree. The acetabulum shows a reduction in depth which varies from very slight to very severe, in which case it becomes flattened, or even concave, while the head of the femur is flattened with a variable degree of expansion, giving it a mushroom-like shape, and the femoral neck is misaligned. Secondary joint dysfunction resulting from degeneration and vascular necrosis occurs in 'Legg–Perthes' disease which affects young dogs of the smaller breeds. It is said to be associated with blood vessel damage and sex and hormone imbalance.

Arthritis

Inflammation of the structures (synovial membrane and articular cartilages) comprising a joint is a relatively common event in animals during early life. Arthritis results from bacterial invasion which may take place following local trauma or, as is more likely, as an extension of specific bacterial infections in newborn animals (joint-ill, pyosepticaemia, omphalophlebitis). Extension of infection into a joint may occur from the surrounding tissues, as in pedal necrosis ('foot-rot', 'fouls') in cattle, or from pyogenic infections involving the endocardium, uterus or udder, and local abscesses. If neglected, cases of suppurative arthritis may become complicated by spread of infection locally (osteomyelitis) or generally (pyaemia, septicaemia).

The bacteria which invade joints vary somewhat in type according to the species of animal, although *Escherichia coli* and *Streptococcus* spp. cause arthritis in all species. In young foals *Shigella equirulis* and *Salmonella* spp. are important causes, the *Klebsiella genitalium* and *Corynebacterium pyogenes* are of somewhat lesser significance. Any one of the foregoing bacteria may be associated with the occasional cases of arthritis that occur in older horses. Individual cases and sporadic outbreaks of arthritis in calves arise from joint invasion by such species of bacteria as *C. pyogenes, Staphylococcus* spp. and *Sphaerophorus (Fusiformis) necrophorus,* and less frequently *Salmonella dublin* and *S. typhimurium,* and rarely *Erysipelothrix insidiosa.* The last named may also cause arthritis in young and recently docked lambs and also in occasional instances in sheep after they have been dipped; more commonly, however, it causes joint trouble in pigs at varying ages. Arthritis in newborn lambs is more commonly associated with invasion of the joints by *E. coli, Streptococcus* spp. (see Fig. 12, p. 16) or *Staphylococcus* spp., although the last named also cause general pyaemia with suppurative arthritis in tick pyaemia of older lambs. In addition rare cases in young lambs may be caused by *Pasteurella haemolytica* and *Haemophilus agni.* Polyarthritis of epidemic propensities has been shown to be caused by an organism of the psittacosis–lymphogranuloma group. The important bacteria associated with arthritis in young pigs include streptococci, which initially produce a septicaemic state terminating in death or with survival, polyarthritis and meningitis. *Salmonella* spp., *Brucella suis* (in older pigs) and *E. coli* have also been involved. Joint infection in the dog is associated with either staphylococcal or streptococcal invasion; in rare instances *Brucella abortus* may be responsible.

Specific diseases in which systemic involvement may precede or develop concomitantly with that of the joints occur in both young and other animals and include infectious polyarthritis of pigs (Glasser's disease), sheep and goats. Stiffness of gait, with disinclination to move, and evidence of pain on forcible flexion of the limbs are observed in many septicaemic and viraemic diseases. These features are usually somewhat less obvious in subacute bacterial endocarditis, and in certain toxaemic states such as occur in septic metritis and acute mastitis in cows in which conditions the joints of the tarsus are most frequently involved.

The clinical signs of arthritis consist of lameness with heat and pain on palpation, and resentment to passive movement of the affected joint. The pain, which varies in intensity, is caused by inflammation of the synovial membrane, and may be so severe that the animal 'carries' the limb if only one is involved. The degree of swelling of the joint is greatest when pyogenic bacteria are the responsible causal agents; otherwise, enlargement of the epiphyses, which is a usual feature in all forms of arthritis, is the main local change in non-pyogenic infections. Severe or extensive erosion of articular cartilage is indicated by crepitation when the joint is subjected to passive movement. In young and in recently born animals, several joints may be affected simultaneously, and in the neonatal cases there may be evidence of infection elsewhere, e.g. in the liver and the meninges. Following subsidence of the acute inflammation, when local damage is severe, and in chronic cases, fibrous thickening of the joint capsule, periarticular ossification, osteomyelitis and, in rare instances, ankylosis of the joint, are likely sequelae. The joints most commonly affected are the hock, stifle and carpus; less frequently the fetlock, interphalangeal and intervertebral joints are similarly involved.

Degenerative Diseases

It is extremely doubtful whether rheumatoid arthritis, as it affects man, occurs in animals. The suggestion that it occasionally occurs in the dog has not been authenticated. A non-septic form of arthropathy (osteoarthritis) is, however, of relatively common occurrence in animals. Accepted aetiological factors include bruises or strains arising from postural abnormalities and structural defects in such conditions as rickets, osteomalacia and osteodystrophia fibrosa. A proportion of the postural abnormalities which are associated with osteoarthritis, more particularly of the limb joints, are recognized to have an hereditary basis.

Because of the demand made upon its physical powers, the horse is a common subject of degenerative arthropathy. Important causes include poor conformation and various nutritional deficiencies including calcium, phosphorus, vitamin D and possibly copper. The significance of trauma as a cause is not clear, although in sporadic cases sufficient damage may be produced in the articular surfaces, menisci, synovial membrane and ligaments, including the cruciate ligament in the stifle joint, to give rise to progressive injury from inflammation.

Much the same factors are responsible for osteoarthritis in cattle, in which species the incidence is highest in beef bulls and aged dairy cows of the larger breeds. The hip or stifle joints are most commonly affected, and in a proportion of the cases due to nutritional causes, it is bilateral. Degenerative arthropathy occurs in young bulls between 6 and 18 months of age and is usually associated with rearing on nurse cows or with being fed on rations predominant in cereals or their byproducts, i.e. diets giving a high phosphorus : calcium ratio. In inherited osteoarthritis of cattle the stifle joint is most commonly affected. Manchester wasting disease is associated with calcification of many of the arterial and other tissues along with degenerative arthritis of many of the limb joints and calcification of tendons and ligaments. In pigs, chronic zinc poisoning results in degenerative lesions affecting the articular surface of the head of the humerus.

Arthrosis deformans (impotentia coeundi), a spastic condition involving the hindlimbs which develops after sexual maturity is reached, has been described in male pigs of the Landrace breed. The bone lesions take the form of degenerative changes in the femoral articular areas and are thought to have a genetic origin.

Clinically the most obvious and common manifestation of osteoarthritis of the limb joints is lameness, which varies in intensity according to the degree of joint damage. In severe cases crepitus may be detected owing to extreme joint mobility and looseness of the ligaments and joint capsule which last becomes distended with synovial fluid. Confusion with chronic arthritis is likely and differentiation may require recognition, from the herd and individual animal history, of preceding dietary deficiency or injury, and the revelation of an existing mineral deficiency or imbalance by means of calcium, phosphorus and alkaline phosphatase estimations on blood samples.

The pathological changes, which are localized to certain joints, consist in the early stages of patchy thinning of the joint cartilage. Later these areas are denuded and at some of them, where exposed bone is increased in density,

eburnation (polishing) is apparent. Rarefaction permits a degree of collapse of the articular surface, which then assumes an irregular or even a folded contour. Extensive erosion is usual in some of the exposed bone areas, and small osteophytes are present at the periphery of the articular surface which, as a rule, appears to encroach further onto the epiphysis. Other joint structures, including menisci, cartilages and ligaments, may persist as remnants or be entirely absent, and the excessive joint fluid is turbid or brown in colour. Occasionally a chip of bone may be found in the joint space. This is more likely to occur when the stifle joint is involved.

Osteoarthritis of the intervertebral articulations produces clinical signs when it causes pain, which is usually sudden in onset. In horses such changes involving the articular processes of the cervical and thoracic vertebrae appear to be an important feature of many cases of equine ataxia ('wobbles') which occurs sporadically in young animals. The development of pain is considered to result from compression of spinal nerve roots or the spinal cord itself, following protrusion of a vertebra or an intervertebral disc into the neural canal. In many cases the history suggests that the appearance of pain is a sudden event, but clinical examination, consisting of pressure over or sudden movement of the cervical vertebrae would elicit an obvious reaction indicating discomfort. Apart from restricted movements of the neck, there is clumsiness during turning, lurching and swaying when walking with dragging of the toes and knuckling over at the fetlocks. All these signs are increased in intensity when the horse is blindfolded. The history and clinical signs provide sufficient evidence on which to base a diagnosis. At post mortem the lesions of degenerative arthropathy are found, in most cases, to involve the third and fourth cervical vertebrae and are most marked over the opposing surfaces of the articular processes.

Degeneration of the intervertebral fibrocartilages (discs) is common in dogs, particularly in the chondrodystrophic breeds such as dachshunds. Each intervertebral disc occupies the space between the bodies of two adjacent vertebrae. The discs have a biconcave profile, being somewhat thinner at the centre; each consists of a soft jelly-like central nucleus pulposus and a peripheral fibrous ring (annulus fibrosus), which is thinner on its dorsal aspect, i.e. the surface nearest the neural canal. The functions of the intervertebral disc include maintaining the rigidity of the vertebral column and acting in the capacity of a shock absorber. The efficiency of the latter function is related, in some measure, to the water content of the disc which decreases when degenerative changes take place. In the chondrodystrophic breeds the changes, which develop when the animal is about one year of age, involve successively the nucleus pulposus and then the annulus fibrosus. Over a period of time the nucleus pulposus is converted into cartilaginous tissue which later undergoes degeneration and becomes calcified. Simultaneously

which is manifested by the animal keeping the vertebral column rigid and often arched upwards (kyphosis). There is often resentment to palpation. Motor disturbances, which are a later development, appear in both of the hindlimbs but not necessarily to an equal degree. The dysfunction varies from uncertain gait to paraplegia which latter may be of the spastic (see Fig. 209, p. 310) or flaccid type (see Fig. 210, p. 310). Diagnosis is assisted by means of radiography which will reveal calcification of the intervertebral discs or narrowing of the space (Fig. 235) between adjacent vertebrae when prolapse of the disc has occurred. In cases of doubt

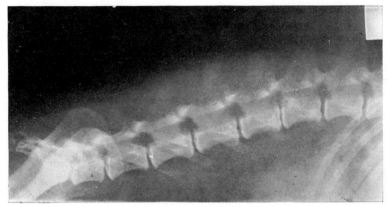

Fig. 235. *A radiograph of the lumbosacral portion of the vertebral column in a dog, showing narrowing of the interspace between the second and third lumbar vertebrae as a result of disc prolapse.*

the deeper parts of the annulus fibrosus degenerate. The changes which take place in the intervertebral discs of other breeds of dogs occur much later and are different in character. The earliest change, which involves the nucleus pulposus, appears at around 5 years and consists of deposition of collagen fibres. Degeneration occurs as the result of necrosis in the absence of calcification. The annulus fibrosus may then degenerate in the same manner.

The normal nucleus pulposus ensures that pressure changes are distributed evenly to the whole extent of the annulus fibrosus. When degenerate the pressure effects may impinge on the annulus fibrosus over a very limited area and thereby cause it to prolapse. This can occur in a ventral direction, giving rise to spondylitis, but more often it takes place dorsally into the neural canal where it exerts pressure on the spinal cord or spinal nerves. The earliest clinical sign is pain

spinal myelography may be availed of to reveal the site of disc protrusion.

Ankylosing spondylitis is a progressive form of inflammation of the vertebral bodies which usually affects older dogs of the chondrodystrophic breeds such as the dachshund, or large breeds including foxhounds, boxers and great Danes. Pain and disability when walking are the most constant clinical features, although the origin of the pain cannot easily be located. In many cases a history of recurrent pain and lameness leading to permanent stiffness is a feature.

The diagnosis of ankylosing spondylitis is usually based on a consideration of the history and clinical aspects in relation to the evidence obtained from a radiological examination. Radiographs of early cases reveal 'lipping' of the ventral part of the articular surfaces of the bodies of the vertebrae (more commonly the posterior

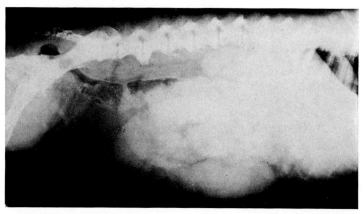

Fig. 236. *A radiograph of the abdomen showing ossifying spondylitis in a dog. Note the extensive bony bridging between the sixth and seventh lumbar vertebrae.*

thoracic and lumbar). When more advanced, the intervertebral spaces are bridged by an ossified mass which is convex on its ventral aspect (Fig. 236).

The Feet

A variety of diseases of the foot occurring in the horse may affect the animal's ability to work. Keratoma, sandcrack, false quarter, quittor and sidebone produce changes in the shape or size of the hoof which are fairly obvious and, therefore, readily recognized. Keratoma causes bulging of the hoof, more usually towards the toe. The growth of horn extends downwards from the coronary band and because of pressure on the sensitive laminae and os pedis is a cause of lameness. Sandcrack is a fissure in the wall of the hoof which commences at the coronary band and extends a variable distance downwards. It occurs at the quarters in the forefoot and at the toe of the hindfoot. Excessive dryness of the hoof is considered to be an important predisposing cause for the condition. 'False quarter' is usually the result of an injury to the coronary band which impairs horn growth. Residual evidence of the injury, in the form of scar tissue, may be evident. Less serious injury may result in one side of the hoof being flattened or even concave. In quittor, necrosis or suppuration of the lateral cartilage is associated with a sinus which connects with the coronet. With the disappearance of draught horses the condition is nowadays very rare. In sidebone a lateral cartilage has been partially or completely ossified.

Puncture wounds and corns may require thorough cleaning of the sole followed by careful examination, including paring away of the superficial layers before either can be identified. A corn is located at the angle of the sole between the wall of the foot and that portion of the wall forming the bar. It takes the form of a contusion from pressure by the heel of a shoe, more usually the inner branch. Radiological examination is essential in the diagnosis of navicular disease and may confirm the existence of sidebone, ringbone and pyramidal disease.

Defective epidermal horn formation, associated with vascular engorgement of the sensitive laminae, produces the syndrome of laminitis, the clinical signs of which are most marked in the horse although the condition also occurs in cattle and sheep. The basic causal factor is an allergy to protein in cereal diets, or protein breakdown products such as those derived from body tissue, bacterial infection, or fermentation of intestinal contents. The condition develops under various circumstances including sustained feeding on cereal concentrates, following retention of the placenta or metritis in mares which have recently foaled and after enforced standing for several days during transportation. The chronic form of the disease may follow a previously acute attack, or originate at this level of intensity in fat ponies at pasture which are given inadequate exercise. Important clinical signs consist of immobility with altered posture, whereby the hindfeet are drawn forward under the body, with the forefeet advanced, so that the centre of gravity is shifted posteriorly in order to reduce weight-bearing by the acutely painful

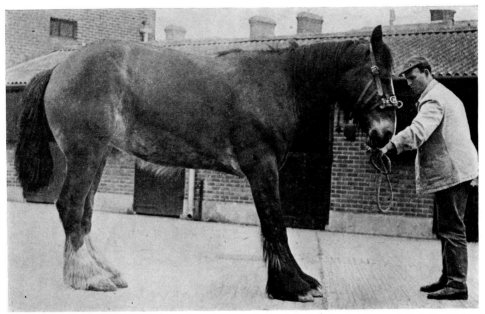

Fig. 237. *Acute laminitis in a horse. Note the extended position of the forefeet and that the hindfeet are drawn forward with the object of relieving pain.*

forefeet (Fig. 237). The abnormal warmth of the affected feet is readily detected by palpation which, when directed to the coronary band region, elicits a pain reaction. The intensity of the pain is indicated by the increased pulse (in acute laminitis there is usually marked pulsation in the digital arteries) and respiratory frequencies, with elevated temperature. In the chronic form of the disease, because of weakening of the attachment between the horny and sensitive laminae, the anterior border of the pedal bone drops until it may eventually penetrate through the sole. Prior to this stage the normally concave sole becomes convex and the slope of the anterior surface of the wall becomes concave, with marked horizontal ridges extending over its whole extent.

Laminitis in cattle usually occurs in animals that have been overfed, or have engorged on concentrate foods. Initially, because the affected animal lies down almost continuously, the condition of the feet is overlooked. Later the reluctant, stilted gait is readily appreciated and is followed by overgrowth of the hoofs, the walls of which become corrugated.

Overgrowth of the hoof wall and elongation of the toes (see Fig. 36, p. 44), associated with the lateral wall growing inwards beneath the sole is often seen in mature cattle. One or, more often, both of the lateral digits of the hindfeet are involved, although both toes on one or more feet may be affected. It is suggested that the lateral digit (fourth) is more often affected because it is occasionally slightly shorter and weaker than the medial digit. The condition is an important cause of lameness and, not infrequently, contributes to bruising of the sole of the foot with subsequent infection by acting as a receptacle for pieces of gravel and other foreign bodies.

Hyperplasia (interdigital fibroma) of the connective tissues of the anterior half of the interdigital space is not uncommon in overfat cows. The condition is readily recognized when the proliferating mass, which may be smooth or irregular on the surface, protrudes between the digits or causes them to be more widely separated than usual. Local irritation arising from infection with *Sphaerophorus necrophorus*, or pressure on surrounding tissues, may cause lameness.

Infectious footrot of cattle (infectious pododermatitis, foul in the foot) is one of the common causes of lameness in adult cattle. Because of severe pain and toxaemia, acutely affected cattle exhibit marked and rapid loss of body weight; the milk yield is also dramatically reduced. It is generally agreed that the disease develops following invasion of the tissues in the vicinity of the coronary band or interdigital cleft by *Sphaerophorus necrophorus*. Other bacteria including a

Gram-negative bacillus resembling *Sph. nodosus* and unidentified spirochaetes have been said to be aetiologically significant. Injury to the integument in the parts of the foot referred to by materials such as gravel, cinder, flints, etc., provide ready access for the causal bacteria.

Inspection of the appropriate parts of the foot, which is facilitated by washing and cleaning, will reveal the presence of necrosis over a variable extent of the interdigital space or coronary band. Pain with swelling are usually well marked. The lesion takes the form of a fissure, the swollen, protruding edges of which are covered with necrotic material. Extension of the infection, or secondary invasion by *Corynebacterium pyogenes*, may lead to suppurative arthritis of the coffin joint or suppurative tendosynovitis of the flexor tendon sheaths which, when affected, are usually distended.

Chronic ergotism in cattle, which is the most common form of the disease caused by *Claviceps purpurea*, is associated with a degree of lameness in the early stages so that affected animals may remain recumbent for long periods. The lower parts of the limbs, particularly of the hindlegs, are erythematous and somewhat swollen, later becoming cold and devoid of sensation, followed by the appearance of a blue-black colour with dryness of the skin, and after an interval of a few days separation occurs between the diseased and healthy tissues. The extremities of the ears and tail are also likely to be similarly affected. The disease known as 'fescue foot' which affects cattle 10–14 days after being introduced into pastures dominated by tall fescue grass (*Festuca arundinacea*) is clinically and pathologically similar to chronic ergot poisoning. The lesions are considered to arise following the action of a vasoconstrictive agent as in ergotism. Another condition (terminal dry gangrene) with similar features occurs in calves from three weeks to about six months of age. There is no association with ergot sclerotia and in most cases subacute salmonellosis precedes the development of gangrene of the extremities (Fig. 238). The initial vascular lesion is one of obliterating thrombosis brought about by the action of a toxic factor produced by certain serotypes of salmonellae.

Of the many foot affections causing lameness in sheep, infectious footrot is the most important from the economic aspect. In established cases (Fig. 239) the marked overgrowth and under-running of the horn, which can be lifted

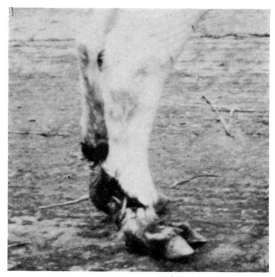

Fig. 238. *Terminal dry gangrene affecting the hindlegs of a calf following arthritis. Note the obvious line of demarcation between living and dead tissue.*

up and is associated with a small amount of foul-smelling discharge, is immediately apparent on inspection. In the early stages of the disease there is swelling and moistness of the skin of the interdigital cleft followed by necrosis which under-runs the horn in the region. When only one foot is affected it is carried, otherwise if two or more feet are involved the animal may walk and graze on its knees or remain recumbent. Rams appear to be more severely affected than other sheep. The presence of the specific causal organism *Sphaerophorus* (*Fusiformis*) *nodosus*, which possesses characteristic morphological features, is readily determined by means of smears prepared from the most active parts of the lesions. It is contended that the most severe and active form of the disease requires, in addition, invasion by *Spirochaeta penortha* which has been classed as an 'accessory' organism. The disease is most prevalent and serious in the spring season when the weather is warm and wet.

Other causes of lameness in sheep include foot scald and interdigital abscess. Foot scald, in the early stages, is rather similar to footrot. The skin in the interdigital region is hyperaemic and covered by a film of moist necrotic material and the horn becomes blanched and pitted. Separation of the horn occurs at the heel but under-running is limited to this part. Interdigital abscess usually affects adult sheep in a sporadic manner, more

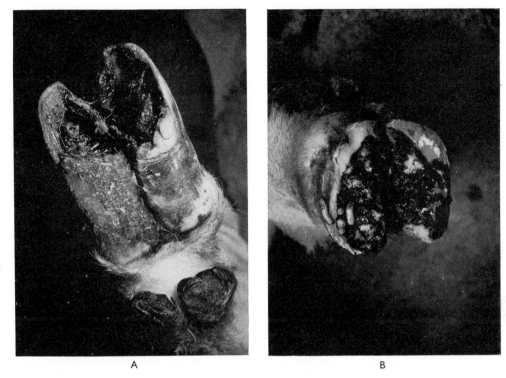

A   B

Fig. 239. A, *Gross overgrowth of the horn in footrot.* B, *Overgrown horn has been pared away to reveal under-running of the sole and wall of the hoof. Note the presence of blowfly larvae, a not infrequent complication during early summer.*

usually during wet weather, and takes the form of a localized abscess at the coronet or interdigital region. *C. pyogenes* is usually present in the lesion which shows a tendency to extend and is associated with swelling, heat and pain in the surrounding tissues. In laminitis, which occurs after cereal engorgement and may cause lameness and recumbency, the feet are hot and painful but no superficial lesions occur.

Acute lameness, often associated with recumbency, is a feature of foot-and-mouth disease in sheep, as well as in cattle and pigs. During the course of the disease, vesicles develop in the interdigital cleft and on the coronet, simultaneously with those in the mouth and elsewhere. Rupture of the vesicles causes great discomfort,

which is intensified by marked swelling of the coronary region. Severe involvement of the deeper structures of the foot may follow from secondary bacterial invasion. In pigs the severity of the reaction in the foot is indicated by a line of separation appearing in the horn of the wall below the coronet, or in some cases even complete ablation of the hoof may occur. This last more usually occurs in the accessory digits. Foot lesions consisting of laminitis and coronitis which cause lameness and recumbency occur in bluetongue. In addition, however, there is hyperaemia of the nasal and buccal mucosae with oedema of various mouth structures and the development of lenticular necrotic ulcers on the lateral aspect of the tongue.

16

Diagnostic Tests

Allergic Tests

An allergic test is one that elicits a sensitivity response in an animal following the injection into its tissues of a protein derivative of the specific organism with which the animal is, or has been, infected. Animals in the very early or the very late stages of the disease may fail to react to such a test, in the first instance because a state of hypersensitivity has not yet been developed at the time the test is applied, and in the second instance because the hypersensitivity has been lost following flooding of the tissues with antigen, a situation which is likely to occur in the advanced stages of some diseases. Certain other circumstances have been recognized to reduce the hypersensitiveness (or allergy) to a low level, the most important of which is parturition, when the reacting tissue antibody leaves the body in the colostrum. A positive response to an allergic test, on the other hand, does not mean that the animal is actively infected at the time of the test, but only that it may have been infected, perhaps subclinically, in the past.

In general terms, allergy is a state of tissue hypersensitivity made manifest as the result of an antigen–antibody reaction which varies in degree and extent. The signs, which are usually delayed in development, are localized, although in some instances more than one tissue may be involved. Severe allergic reactions may induce a delayed febrile response. In anaphylaxis, the clinical signs are severe, with signs of shock and are general in extent.

The two most important allergic tests used in veterinary practice are those employed in the control and eradication of tuberculosis and of glanders, using tuberculin and mallein respectively. Because there is lack of agreement regarding standardization of the antigens, an acceptable uniform international test for either of these diseases has not been evolved. The adoption of official control and eradication programmes in respect of glanders and bovine tuberculosis in so many countries has produced a situation in which a considerable variety of diagnostic tests are statutorily recognized and employed. Allergic tests have also been applied in the diagnosis of Johne's disease but, without exception, they have been shown to have a low level of specificity.

Tuberculin Tests

There are three major methods of applying the tuberculin test to animals; these are the intradermal, subcutaneous and ophthalmic. The ophthalmic test is rarely used nowadays because of its comparatively low degree of specificity, while the subcutaneous test has become unpopular because it is time-consuming and, being based on temperature response, is susceptible to interference by a number of extraneous factors. As a consequence, some form of the intradermal method is employed throughout the world.

Cattle. Since cattle may become sensitized not only to the bovine type of tubercle bacillus, but also to the human and avian types, and with immunogenically related organisms such as *Mycobacterium paratuberculosis*, and the acid-fast bacillus associated with so-called 'skin tuberculosis' (acid-fast lymphangitis), it has been considered advisable in national bovine tuberculosis eradication programmes in Britain, Ireland and the Netherlands to use a comparative tuberculin test. Two different types of tuberculin, mammalian and avian, are therefore injected into the skin simultaneously, fairly close together, so that any resulting reactions may be more readily compared for interpretation purposes.

The value of the comparative tuberculin test is associated with its considerable specificity in respect of the sensitizing antigen. For this test the intradermal route of injection is used, care being necessary to place the injections at the appropriate sites on the same side of the neck as skin sensitivity varies, being greater in sites nearer the head and in the vicinity of the jugular furrow, and reduced in sites near the shoulder and in those towards the nuchal crest. The middle portion of the neck should be selected as being preferable, and the sites prepared by clipping away the hair over each area; the upper site is placed at least 10 cm below the crest and the lower 12 cm away on a line roughly parallel with the slope of the shoulder. The avian tuberculin should be injected at the upper site and the mammalian tuberculin at the lower (Fig. 240).

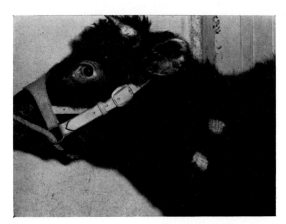

Fig. 240. *The clipped areas on the left side of the neck indicate sites for injection in the single intradermal comparative tuberculin test.*

Prior to injecting the tuberculins, the needles and syringes should be checked for efficiency; a useful way of doing this is to assemble the needle and syringe as if for use and then, after filling the syringe with water, insert the needle into a piece of good quality cork and proceed to inject 0·1 ml into it. If the equipment is working satisfactorily no water should escape when the injection is made into the cork. Needless to say, the needles and syringes should be sterilized before use in animals, and the needle wiped with a clean swab of cottonwool moistened with 70% methylated spirit between each injection. The injection site

should be cleaned with cottonwool soaked with methylated spirit. Prior to injecting the tuberculin, the thickness of the skin at each site is recorded by measuring with a caliper graduated in millimetres. The equipment required for the performance of the intradermal tuberculin test is illustrated in Fig. 241.

For making the injection a short dental type needle is used, which should be attached to the syringe so that the bevel edge at the tip is facing towards the user. When held at the correct angle, i.e. about 30° to the skin surface, and properly inserted, the point of the needle will penetrate to the deeper layers of the dermis. Some degree of pressure is necessary to deposit the required amount of tuberculin (0·1 ml) in the skin, and evidence that this has been achieved is usually apparent in the form of a small pea-sized swelling, which bulges outwards. The mechanism of the syringe should incorporate an automatic, or manual control for measuring the dose. The test is read by repeating the skin measurements 72 hours after the injection. A variable degree of desensitization will occur in the skin over the area of the injection site, so that when retesting is necessary, it is advisable to allow an interval of about 2 months to elapse, and the skin on the opposite side of the neck should be used.

In Britain and Ireland the mammalian tuberculin used is prepared from a human strain of the tubercle bacillus. The prepared product is standardized to contain 2 mg/ml purified tuberculoprotein and of which the recommended dose is 0·1 ml. The avian tuberculin used in the single intradermal comparative test contains 0·5 mg/ml purified protein derivative (PPD) tuberculin and the dose is again 0·1 ml. The value of avian tuberculin, when used simultaneously with mammalian, is that it aids in the classification of tuberculin sensitivity, an example of which is so-called non-specific infection, a category which should only be recognized in established herds of cattle under certain circumstances to be described later in this chapter.

Other European countries employ mammalian tuberculins prepared in a variety of ways from either the human or bovine types of the bacillus. In general, although there is little difference in specificity between these two types of tuberculin, that of bovine origin is less potent than that of human origin. Also, because of greater specificity and greater ease of standardization, PPD tuberculins are more generally used.

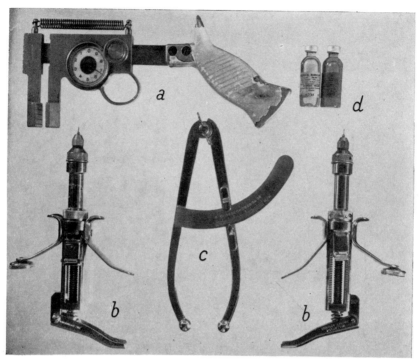

Fig. 241. *Equipment for performing tuberculin tests.* a, *Dial caliper for measuring skin fold thickness.* b, *Multidose resetting intradermal syringes.* c, *Hinged quadrant caliper.* d, left, *vial of mammalian tuberculin;* right, *vial of avian tuberculin.*

Various modifications of the intradermal tuberculin test are in use in different countries, although in Europe, generally, the neck site is employed. In the USA, Canada and Australia the caudal fold is the recommended injection site (in the USA the lip of the vulva at the muco-cutaneous junction is also included in routine tuberculin tests). Tuberculin prepared from cultures of *M. tuberculosis* or *M. bovis* is injected intradermally, the recommended amount being 0·05 ml. Intradermal deposition of the tuberculin is more certain at these sites than in the neck, although sensitivity is at a lower level. For these tests heat-concentrated tuberculin, prepared from a human strain of tubercle bacillus, is injected in the required amount of 0·1 ml for routine tests, and 0·2 ml when retesting a herd in which positive reactors have appeared. Doubtful reactors, or herds with a history of repeated breakdowns, are usually subjected to an intradermal tuberculin test using the neck site. In Australia a modified subcutaneous test ('short thermal test') is employed in similar circumstances.

Interpretation of results. It is necessary when reading the results of intradermal tuberculin tests to take note of the character of any swelling which appears at an injection site. In the first instance, even when a comparative test is being applied, the initial interpretation is made on an individual animal basis, hence underlying the need to apply the correct technique at all aspects. In Britain and Ireland it is officially recommended that the results of the single intradermal comparative tuberculin test should be interpreted on the following basis: Any swelling showing oedema should be regarded as a positive reaction. In the absence of oedema no skin swelling which shows an increase in skin thickness of more than 2 mm should be regarded as a negative reaction. Skin swellings giving an increase of 3 mm should be classified as doubtful and those of 4 mm or more as positive.

The importance of making a careful clinical examination at the time of the test is highly pertinent in the context of clinical tuberculosis, so-called 'skin tuberculosis' and Johne's disease, with particular emphasis in the case of reactor and inconclusively reacting animals.

It is necessary to clarify some of the terms used in connection with the interpretation of the test. Reaction means the changes which occur at the injection site in respect of skin thickness, or the development, or otherwise, of oedema, and is classified as negative, doubtful or positive as outlined above. A reactor, which is either positive or inconclusive, is the categorization of the animal as the result of interpreting not only its local reactions to the injections of mammalian and avian tuberculins, but also those of all the other animals in the herd in the light of whether, or not non-specific sensitization exists in the group. The term doubtful is applied to a reaction. when the increase in skin thickness is more than 2 mm and less than 4 mm, in the absence of local oedema. The use of the term inconclusive is restricted to those individual animals which, on the basis of a herd or group, single intradermal comparative tuberculin test, cannot be classified as being either positive or negative reactors.

The interpretation of the comparative test is influenced by the presence of non-specific infection in the herd. It is generally accepted that the existence of non-specific infection is established during the herd test by one or more animals giving a positive reaction to avian tuberculin, and a negative reaction to mammalian tuberculin; clinical evidence of Johne's disease or of so-called 'skin tuberculosis' are also considered to establish a similar situation.

With the information derived from the herd or group test, in conjunction with the results of a clinical examination and the previous tuberculin and health record, it is possible to classify the majority of animals in respect of the comparative tuberculin test as follows:

1. Animals showing a positive or doubtful reaction to avian tuberculin and a negative reaction to mammalian tuberculin are negative reactors and can be retained in the herd.

2. Animals giving a doubtful reaction to mammalian tuberculin and a negative reaction to avian tuberculin are inconclusive reactors and should be retested.

3. Animals showing a positive or doubtful reaction to avian tuberculin and a positive or doubtful reaction to mammalian tuberculin, provided the increase in skin measurement to mammalian tuberculin is not more than 4 mm greater than the increase to avian should be:
   a. Classified as negative reactors if non-specific infection is established.
   b. Classified as inconclusive reactors and subjected to a retest if non-specific infection is not established.

4. Animals giving a positive reaction to mammalian tuberculin and a negative reaction to avian tuberculin when the increase in skin measurement to mammalian tuberculin does not exceed the avian increase by more than 6 mm should be:
   a. Classified as inconclusive reactors and subjected to a retest if non-specific infection is established.
   b. Classified as reactors and removed from the herd if non-specific infection is not established.

5. Animals which give a positive reaction to mammalian tuberculin and a positive or doubtful reaction to avian tuberculin when the increase in skin measurement to mammalian tuberculin is 5 or 6 mm greater than the increase to avian tuberculin should be:
   a. Classified as inconclusive reactors and subjected to a retest if non-specific infection is established.
   b. Classified as reactors and removed from the herd if non-specific infection is not established.

6. In any test, animals showing a positive reaction to mammalian tuberculin and a positive, doubtful or negative reaction to avian tuberculin should be classified as reactors and removed from the herd when the increase in skin measurement to mammalian tuberculin is more than 6 mm greater than the increase to avian tuberculin.

The majority of herd or group tests can be satisfactorily interpreted on the foregoing bases but instances will occur in which some modification will be necessary. The tuberculin test record for the herd will be of value in deciding when a modified interpretation is desirable. The appearance of a number of reactors indicating bovine type infection, or a clinical case of tuberculosis, suggests the advisability of altogether ignoring evidence indicative of non-specific infection. It is also recommended that when there is a high incidence of non-specific sensitivity in the absence of so-called 'skin tuberculosis', and a few animals show increases in skin measurement to mammalian tuberculin of 7–8 mm greater than for avian tuberculin, they may be classified as inconclusive reactors and subjected to a retest rather than being removed from the

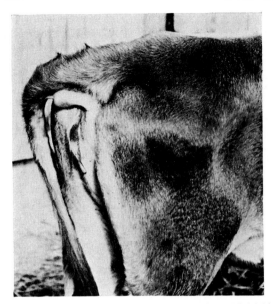

Fig. 242. *A positive tuberculin reaction at the caudal fold site.*

herd as reactors. Also animals with lesions of so-called 'skin tuberculosis' (acid-fast lymphangitis), which give reactions which would normally classify them as reactors and necessitate their removal from the herd, may be regarded as inconclusive reactors and retested. If a number of such instances occur in a herd test then other animals in the reactor category, not showing clinical evidence of so-called 'skin tuberculosis', may be dealt with on similar lines. Any animal showing large increases in skin measurements to both tuberculins, even though the mammalian increase is only equal to or slightly in excess of the avian increase, should be classified as an inconclusive reactor and subjected to a retest.

The reactions produced by the caudal fold test as employed in the USA, Canada and Australia are read between 72 and 96 hours after injection by comparison with the opposite fold. A positive reaction consists of a diffuse, oedematous, painful swelling at the injection site (Fig. 242). The same standards apply when the lip of the vulva is used as the injection site.

Although the traditional subcutaneous test has been generally discarded, modified tests of this type are in use in some countries, it being claimed that it provides useful clarification in cases of doubt, particularly those due to low sensitivity. In Australia the 'short thermal test' is employed involving the subcutaneous injection in the neck area of 4 ml of intradermal mammalian tuberculin. The rectal temperature is taken before the tuberculin is injected and the test is not proceeded with if it is higher than 39°C (102°F). If the temperature remains below this point for 2 hours after the injection and then rises and remains above 40°C (104°F) at 4 hours, 6 hours and 8 hours, the animal is classified as a positive reactor. It is claimed that the test possesses a high degree of efficiency in detecting infected cattle with low-level skin sensitivity to tuberculin. Occasionally an anaphylactic reaction occurs during the acme of the thermal response.

Horses. Tuberculin tests in the horse appear to possess a much lower degree of specificity compared with cattle. This is particularly the case in respect of the subcutaneous test which is virtually useless in this species. The horse is apparently highly sensitive to tuberculin, so that much smaller amounts of tuberculoprotein than those customarily employed might prove more satisfactory. There is lack of authoritative information on the subject and the consensus of opinion is that a negative reaction can be accepted as indicating the health status of the animal, but the significance of a positive reaction is not always clear, although it is contended that the occurrence of a systemic reaction in conjunction with a positive intradermal test can be accepted as indicating the presence of infection.

The technique of the single intradermal test is similar to that in cattle, due care being necessary because of the thin skin in the neck area to ensure that the tuberculin is deposited in the dermal tissues. It is advisable to measure the skin thickness at the injection site at 48 and 72 hours.

Sheep and goats. The single intradermal test has been recommended for use in these species. The test is not highly specific as reports indicate that loss of skin sensitivity occurs in a proportion of tuberculous animals. The caudal (anal) fold site is probably the most satisfactory for both species. The test is read 72 hours after injecting 0·1 ml of standard mammalian tuberculin; an increase of 5 mm in the thickness of the caudal fold constitutes a positive reaction. Many infected animals fail to react.

Pigs. In the majority of instances progressive tuberculosis in pigs is caused by either the avian or the bovine type of tubercle bacillus. The success of bovine tuberculosis eradication programmes in many countries has considerably reduced the proportion of bovine type infections in pigs. The simultaneous injection of avian and mammalian tuberculin, one in the right and the other in the left ear, may enable the type of infection present in the herd to be differentiated. The value of the test is highest in herds with a known history and in which repeated herd tests have been performed. It appears that many tuberculous pigs lose sensitivity to tuberculin in a rather short time. Two sites on the ear have been recommended. The most acceptable is the skin towards the base of the ear on its posterior or outer surface; otherwise the skin of the anterior border of the ear, towards its base, is selected. The dose of each tuberculin is 0·1 ml and the type used in cattle is satisfactory.

A positive reaction to either tuberculin consists of the development of a local inflammatory reaction at 24 hours, followed by haemorrhage, necrosis and ulceration at 48–72 hours. As a rule any reaction to avian tuberculin is delayed so that in this case the test should be read at 48–72 hours. In the case of either tuberculin an increase in skin thickness of 4 mm is classed as positive. It appears that in pigs maximum sensitivity to tuberculin occurs 3–9 weeks after infection; a retest in about 8 weeks will indicate whether the lesions of the disease are actively progressing.

Dogs and cats. Tuberculin tests in dogs and cats usually fail to give unequivocal reactions in naturally infected animals. For the intradermal test tuberculin may be injected into the skin of the flank in amounts of 0·1 ml and the site remeasured at 24 and 48 hours. A subcutaneous test may be performed by injecting 0·1 ml of a 1 in 10 dilution in normal saline of standard intradermal tuberculin. The test must not be undertaken if the animal's temperature is above 39·5°C (101·5°F). A positive reaction consists of a rise of temperature of 1·2–2·8°C (2–5°F) appearing between the 5th and 7th hour and persisting for 4–5 hours. In old-established, chronic infections a fall in temperature may result, often followed by collapse and death. A proportion of infected animals which fail to evince a thermal response may show a reaction in the form of swelling in some of the joints and lymph nodes.

Mallein Tests for Glanders

Mallein as employed in tests for the diagnosis of glanders is a bacteria-free filtrate from a fluid culture of *Actinobacillus* (*Malleomyces*) *mallei* which has been prepared by one of a variety of methods. Although mallein has a high degree of specificity, so that by its proper use a high proportion of infected animals can be identified, it must be appreciated that, as with other types of allergic sensitivity, false positive and false negative reactions can occur because of low-level sensitization, loss of sensitivity in the advanced stages of the disease and sensitization by other bacteria. Diagnostic antigens prepared from some strains of *Act. mallei* will cause reactions in horses sensitized to *Pseudomonas pseudomallei*. A number of mallein tests are in use including the intradermopalpebral, cutaneous, subcutaneous and ophthalmic. Of these the intradermopalpebral is most widely used.

Intradermopalpebral test. In this test, 0·1 ml of mallein is injected into the skin of the lower eyelid which is then re-examined in 48 hours. The intradermal tuberculin syringe and needle for cattle will be found suitable for this test but the animal will need to be effectively restrained to ensure that the injection is correctly made. Tensing the skin of the lower eyelid with the fingers of the free hand will assist needle penetration. When inserting the needle into the skin, the syringe should be held at an angle of 20° to the surface of the eyelid with the needle point about 1 cm away from the mid point of the palpebral margin. If correctly placed in the dermal tissues the deposited mallein produces a small, visible nodule. Alcohol swabbing of the site should not be employed in connection with this test. A positive reaction constitutes inflammatory oedema of the eyelid or even of the whole orbital area, and frequently severe purulent conjunctivitis (Fig. 243). The swelling, which is painful, develops

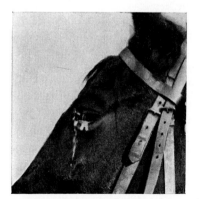

Fig. 243. *Positive reaction to the intradermopalpebral mallein test: purulent conjunctival discharge, swelling of the lower eyelid.*

slowly, is most intense between 24 and 48 hours and persists for at least another 48 hours.

Cutaneous tests. A variety of cutaneous tests, including superficial scarification of the skin following clipping and cleaning of the site and then the direct application of a few drops of mallein, and an intradermal test have been employed but because of comparatively low specificity they have been discarded.

The subcutaneous test and the ophthalmic test have fallen into disuse for a variety of reasons. The former is prohibited in countries such as Germany and Austria, where the control of glanders is based upon serological tests, e.g. complement-fixation, because there is a significant antibody response which may persist for several months following the subcutaneous injection of mallein. Otherwise this form of test is time-consuming and costly to perform. The ophthalmic test is of relatively low specificity.

Allergic Tests for Johne's Disease

Tests based on skin sensitivity are likely to be of value only during the later stages of the development of Johne's disease and, in the majority of cases, by the time clinical signs are fully established desensitization has occurred. In addition, the value of an allergic test is minimized by the likelihood that cattle infected with tubercle bacilli of any type, or those with acid-fast lymphangitis and those which have been vaccinated against Johne's disease, will give confusing reactions. For these reasons, tests to determine the sensitivity status of cattle are rarely used in the diagnosis of Johne's disease.

The single intradermal test has been the most extensively employed. It involves the injection of 0·2 ml PPD johnin into the skin of the neck. The test should be read at 48 hours, a positive reaction constituting an obviously oedematous swelling. In the USA an increase of skin thickness of 3 mm or more is regarded as a positive reaction. The comparatively low level of specificity of the test is indicated by it being possible to substitute avian PPD tuberculin for johnin without serious reduction in efficiency, although in this case the test is carried out in the same way as for a double intradermal tuberculin test. In any event there is local desensitization of skin for over three months following an injection of johnin. The test is of greatest value when employed on a herd basis although repeated testing

will help in the identification of early clinical cases.

The short thermal test for the detection of subclinical Johne's disease consists of injecting 10 ml of avian tuberculin intravenously. A positive reaction consists of a rise in temperature of 1°C (2°F) between 5 and 8 hours, in conjunction with a systemic reaction including anorexia, depression, dyspnoea and diarrhoea in some cases. A similar test has been devised using 2–4 ml of johnin, in which case a rise in temperature of over 0·75°C (1·5°F) within 3–7·5 hours is regarded as a positive reaction. Sensitization to group antigens associated with heterologous bacteria will give rise to a positive reaction in both these tests so that their specificity is rather low. The development of antibodies following the intravenous injection of either of these diagnostic antigens precludes the use of this type of test in countries where diagnosis is based on the complement fixation test.

Serological Tests

Although serological examination, which is based on the detection of specific antibodies in serum by employing selected specific antigenic systems, cannot, except in very few instances, be conveniently undertaken by the clinical veterinarian, it is essential to be aware of the various tests that are available and which are of value in assisting the diagnosis of certain infectious diseases. The majority of such tests are performed on serum. For this purpose 10 ml of blood are usually sufficient. Care should be exercised at all stages from obtaining the sample until clotting is complete in order to prevent haemolysis. Allowing it to stand undisturbed in an environmental temperature of 20°C (68°F) or higher will aid clot retraction and separation of the serum. If the serum can then be removed into a separate sterile container prior to dispatch to the laboratory, the risk of haemolysis is entirely eliminated. In all instances when dispatching blood samples for serological or other examination, or indeed any specimen to a laboratory, include a history and description of the case along with a precise request for the diagnostic service required. Each individual sample should be clearly labelled; and when a number are being submitted a separate list should be included.

Serological tests employed in this way may reveal evidence of recent or past infection, as the case may be, but in general the results obtained are often disappointing unless paired serum samples obtained at an interval of two to three weeks reveal a rising antibody titre. Such a situation provides retrospective confirmation of the diagnosis. Recognition of recent infection may also be established on a basis of clinical observation coupled with a high level of serological reaction in a single test. Certain types of serological tests are of considerable assistance in the establishment of a rapid diagnosis. These include immunofluorescent techniques and the complement fixation test in canine distemper. Conversely detection of the specific cause is possible by serological means in such conditions as contagious pustular dermatitis (orf), foot-and-mouth disease and rinderpest.

The principal serological tests employed in diagnosis include the following:

Agglutination Tests

Immunological tests of this type generally have a retrospective value in diagnosis because specific agglutinins only appear in the blood some time subsequent to the establishment of infection. In veterinary medicine the phenomenon of agglutination has had its greatest application in relation to detecting the presence of agglutinins to *Brucella abortus* in blood serum, milk, milk-whey, vaginal mucus and seminal plasma of cattle. For this purpose either a tube or plate agglutination test may be employed. In the absence of a generally accepted international standard *Brucella* antigen (some countries have adopted the WHO/ FAO Standard International Unit) it is difficult to interpret the significance of different concentrations (titres) of agglutinins. In the USA complete agglutination at a serum dilution of 1 in 50 in the tube test is regarded as a suspicious titre, and at 1:100 or above as indicating positive evidence of bovine brucellosis. In the case of animals known to have been vaccinated these criteria are applied at 1:10 and 1:200 respectively. In Britain and Ireland any titre above complete agglutination at 1:10 (30 I.U. *Brucella* antibody) is considered positive in unvaccinated animals, and at 1:200 (50 I.U.) in vaccinated animals. There is a tendency for vaccinated calves to retain agglutinin titres of 1 in 40 or above when they are reared in a *Brucella* contaminated environment. In the case of infected cows which have calved or aborted within the preceding three weeks, withdrawal of the agglutinins from the blood and their removal from the body in colostrum and uterine excretions is more than likely to give rise to false negative results if a serum agglutination test were undertaken.

The plate or rapid agglutination test has not been widely used except in the USA and although it is not as accurate as the tube agglutination test it has a place as an initial screening test when employed on a herd basis. The results are available within a few minutes so that it can be applied to cattle of unknown brucellosis status in sale-yards. A rapid whole blood plate test has also been devised but because the erythrocytes interfere somewhat with the agglutination reaction the test is not entirely dependable.

A modified rapid plate agglutination test for brucellosis, the Rose Bengal Plate Test (Card test), has been extensively used in the USA and more recently in Britain and Ireland. Serum samples are examined by placing one drop of each on a white enamel tile and then placing one drop of Rose Bengal stained *Brucella* antigen alongside the serum. Mixing is performed with an applicator stick and the tile rotated for 4 minutes, when the result is read as positive or negative. Comparative investigations have shown that this test is about as efficient as the complement-fixation test in identifying animals in the early stages of infection, surpassing the tube agglutination test in this respect. It also gives few false negative reactions and usefully excludes a significant proportion of post-vaccinal positive reactors to the tube agglutination test. The Rose Bengal test appears to meet many of the desirable requirements of a screening test in brucellosis eradication programmes.

The value of the agglutination tests on milk and milk-whey depends upon *Br. abortus* becoming localized in one or more quarters of the bovine udder, although transfer of blood agglutinins to milk occurs at certain times, more particularly in association with parturition and when clinical mastitis exists. The milk-whey tube and plate tests will give positive results in almost all cattle in which *Br. abortus* has invaded the supramammary lymph node or udder, but confusion will occur in the case of animals either recently calved or vaccinated because of false positive reactions which will persist for three months and two weeks respectively. The whey tube agglutination test has been found to be more reliable than the milk ring test in identifying adult *Brucella*-free vaccinated animals.

The milk ring test is claimed to be more efficient than the whey test in detecting cattle infected with *Br. abortus*, even although the organism has not localized in the udder. Its efficiency is said to be somewhat less than that of the tube serum agglutination test but it is claimed that the milk ring test is satisfactory for screening bulk herd samples. Milk from a cow which gives a positive ring-test reaction can be diluted with negatively reacting milk from 4 cows and still give a positive reaction; greater dilution would be likely to invalidate the result by causing a negative reaction. The milk ring test has been extensively employed in bovine brucellosis eradication programmes as a herd screening test, being of greatest value where only calfhood vaccination is permitted. On the basis of the disparity between the milk ring test reactions shown by milk samples from individual quarters infected cattle can, in many instances, be differentiated from those with vaccinal agglutinins in which case the quarter reaction is more or less uniform. The proportion of false positive milk ring test reactions is highest in recently calved and late lactation cows.

The test is simple to perform, requiring only limited materials. The procedure consists of adding two drops of tetrazolium-stained *Brucella abortus* antigen to 2 ml of well-mixed milk in a small tube. After thorough mixing of the contents the tube is incubated at 37°C for 1 hour. If *Brucella* agglutinins are present the stained antigen is agglutinated and carried to the surface with the rising fat globules to form a deep-blue creamline. In the absence of specific agglutinins the milk remains bluish with a normal cream layer. In doubtful reactions both cream layer and milk are uniformly stained.

The vaginal mucus agglutination test will, in general, give positive reactions only when the uterus is infected. The value of the test is largely offset by the technical complexities associated with acquiring and handling the mucus samples, and also the periodicity of agglutinin secretion. A pipette or tube technique should be used in preference to a tampon for collecting the mucus. In bulls *Br. abortus* may localize in the genital organs without the appearance of agglutinins in the blood. Testing the seminal plasma by means of a tube dilution technique similar to that of the serum agglutination test will invariably yield positive results in such cases.

Because brucellosis is a chronic disease the type of antibody present in the blood and elsewhere varies at different stages. During active infection and soon after vaccination with an agglutinogenic antigen, agglutinating (IgM) antibodies are detectable; at a later stage only non-agglutinating (IgG) antibodies exist. Treatment of serum samples with 2-mercaptoethanol destroys IgM type immunoglobulins thereby providing a means of differentiating between serum titres resulting from recent infection or vaccination and those associated with old-standing infection.

Some specific antibodies, even in high titre, are incapable of agglutinating *Br. abortus;* they have been classified as incomplete agglutinins. The presence of such immunoglobulins can be detected by means of a modified agglutination reaction. This is achieved by employing an anti-species (antiglobulin or Coombs') serum. When bacterial cells which have adsorbed non-agglutinating antibody are prepared by being washed twice in fresh saline solution after prior centrifugation and finally resuspended in saline containing the appropriate species antiglobulin they will be agglutinated by reason of the antiglobulin linking the *Brucella* antibodies together. The term antiglobulin and Coombs' test have been used for the procedure, but the latter has a special connotation in relation to blood grouping in human pathology and should not be employed in the context of bacterial agglutination phenomena.

The serum agglutination test also has a practical application in the diagnosis of brucellosis in other species of animals including goats, sheep, pigs, horses, camels, deer, etc. Because of the considerable variation in the serum agglutinin titre in individual animals, even when infected, it is recommended that for goats, sheep and pigs the test results should be interpreted on a herd basis, and that the presence of a single positive reactor in a herd or flock in which clinical brucellosis has been suspected justifies a positive diagnosis.

A serum agglutination test, although the simplest method, appears to have serious limitations in the diagnosis of brucellosis in pigs caused by *Brucella suis*. Following infection a positive titre is unlikely until about eight weeks have elapsed, and the majority of infected pigs evince only a low titre. The test should, therefore, be used to determine the herd status. As a guide to the interpretation of test results, herds with no history of infection and in which no individual pig has a titre greater than 1:100 are classified as negative; herds with a record of *Br. suis* infection in which any one pig has a titre greater than 1:25 are classified as positive.

Brucellosis in goats, cattle and sheep caused by *Brucella melitensis* may be diagnosed by means of a serum agglutination test. In assessing the status of individual animals the test has limitations because of the transient character of the infection in many cases. Interpreting the results on a herd basis gives more satisfactory results. Also, because of the prolonged persistence of mammary gland infection, at least in the goat, it is likely that a milk ring test would give a more accurate reflection of the disease status of individual animals.

Serum agglutination tests are of some value in detecting animals which have been infected by a particular *Salmonella* spp. As a general rule, agglutinins do not appear in the blood until about 2 weeks after the appearance of clinical signs of the disease. Also in young animals including foals and calves, infection tends to be eliminated and positive agglutinin titres usually disappear within 2–3 months. Conversely, infected adult animals, which may or may not evince overt signs of disease, tend to become 'carriers' and retain positive serum agglutinin titres. The application of agglutination tests in the diagnosis of salmonellosis in animals is precluded by the lack of knowledge regarding positive and negative criteria for the serum agglutinin titres in the different species. It appears that positive flagellar agglutinin titres are more likely to be significant than those obtained with somatic antigen. The efficiency of bacteriological methods in detecting the presence of salmonella infection in both clinically affected and carrier animals has reduced the significance of serological methods as diagnostic aids. Following isolation, specific identification and classification is achieved by means of somatic and flagellar agglutinin adsorption tests.

The presence of *Salmonella* infection in adult fowl can be determined by means of agglutination tests. The two most important serotypes *S. pullorum* and *S. gallinarum*, are antigenically identical so that a suspension of *S. pullorum* will detect infection with either of these bacteria. A tube dilution or a whole-blood plate test may be employed. In the tube test complete agglutination at 1:40 or a higher serum dilution is indicative of infection. The rapid whole-blood plate agglutination test has the advantage that it can be performed in the field, only a small quantity of blood is required, and reactor birds can be removed from the flock immediately on detection. For the test the wing vein is pierced and blood collected with a standard loop (0·02 ml), this is mixed with twice its volume of methyl violet stained antigen on a white porcelain tile. Agglutination within 2 minutes indicates a positive reaction. Some degree of agglutination will occur with *S. pullorum* antigen when it is admixed with serum from birds infected with other species of *Salmonellae* possessing some of the same somatic antigens. Under modern intensive systems of poultry production the incidence of pullorum disease and fowl typhoid is extremely low. Avian salmonellosis is nowadays more usually caused by individual members of a variety of serotypes which in many instances gain entrance to poultry units as contaminants of foodstuffs.

A serum agglutination test has been widely used in the detection of herds of cattle affected with vibriosis. Because of considerable variation in agglutinin titres and in their persistence in infected cattle, the test has been found to be of greatest value when applied on a herd basis. The local production of agglutinins by the female reproductive tract lends value to a modified form of agglutination test performed on vaginal mucus which can be collected by means of a pipette or by tampon. In the performance of the test the mucus is diluted with sodium chloride and formalin and then stored at 4°C for 24 hours before testing. Some possible anomalies, such as uncertainty in selecting infected cattle, variability in the time of appearance of the agglutinins, false positive reactions during oestrus and tendency for the titre to fall with time, all militate against the test being used on an individual animal basis. A similar situation prevails in respect of bovine trichomoniasis. The serum agglutination test may be of value in the diagnosis of vibrionic abortion in sheep; similar reservations apply as in the case of cattle.

Serum agglutination (tube or plate) or haemagglutination-lysis tests are the methods most commonly used to detect antibodies against *Leptospirae* spp. Recent infection may be confirmed when paired sera reveal a rising agglutinin titre. Otherwise positive titres at a serum dilution of 1:500 or over in cattle, 1:500 in pigs and

1:1000 in dogs may be taken to indicate recent or past infection. The specific serotype of *Leptospira* may be indicated by noting the antigen which gives a reaction at the highest dilution of serum; confirmation can be obtained by means of agglutinin-absorption tests. In leptospirosis, agglutinins are at a peak about 4 weeks after generalized infection has occurred and then begin to subside. They persist at significant levels for over three months in sheep, for over a year in cattle and pigs and even longer in horses.

The agglutination test employs an antigen composed of a formalized culture, whereas in the haemagglutination–lysis test the antigen consists of living organisms. The serum agglutinin titre is taken to be the dilution in which about 50% of the organism are agglutinated or lysed. Both tests necessitate the use of dark-ground microscopy for the final reading. Both tube and plate agglutination tests are available for the diagnosis of tularaemia. In pigs, because of unilateral cross-agglutination with *Brucella* spp. antigens, the tularaemia tube dilution test gives more satisfactory results when it is interpreted in conjunction with the herd history. A positive serum titre of 1:50 is regarded as being indicative of tularaemia in pigs while a titre of 1:200 is similarly interpreted in sheep in which species cross-agglutination between *Pasteurella tularensis* and *Brucella abortus* is much less common. Following infection agglutinin titres in sheep range from 1:640 to 1:1500; values around 1:320 7 months later are usual while in horses the titre reverts to normal values within 21 days.

Complement-fixation Test

The principle of the complement-fixation test is that complement, which is a normal constituent of serum, is taken up (fixed) on the formation of a specific antibody–antigen complex, and lysis of the antigenic component then occurs. In complement-fixation tests unknown sera are heated to 56°C for 30 minutes to destroy all the complement and then a known amount of complement in the form of guinea pig serum is added to each serum under test. Following the addition of known antigen the mixture is incubated at 37°C and if a specific complex is formed all the complement is used up, so that on the addition of the haemolytic system (sheep erythrocytes plus homologous red cell antiserum) no haemolysis will occur. The complement-fixation test can be adopted to detect either antibody, which

shows a rising titre during the course of certain diseases, or antigen. The latter form of the test yields rapid diagnostic results and is particularly useful in dealing with suspected cases of foot-and-mouth disease and rinderpest.

The complement-fixation test is regarded as being the most accurate of the serological tests for glanders in all species. Sufficient antibody develops to give a positive reaction within about seven days, following infection, and this situation exists for a prolonged period in chronically affected animals. A horse is considered to be infected with *Actinobacillus mallei* when 0·1 ml or less of its serum completely inhibits haemolysis. Similar values in relation to the quantities of serum required to produce positive and negative complement-fixation reactions are employed in the diagnosis of dourine and certain other types of trypanosomiasis.

The complement-fixation test is of value in detecting *Brucella* infected cattle; it is more efficient in the early stages of infection than any of the agglutination tests. Although the test is capable of distinguishing between post-vaccinal and post-infective antibodies this differentiation is only satisfactory when vaccination has antedated the test by a considerable period. Acceptable criteria for the complement-fixation test in bovine brucellosis are positive results at serum dilutions of 1:4 or less in animals with serum agglutination titres of 1:20 (50 I.U.).

The complement-fixation tests has been applied rather intermittently in the diagnosis of Johne's disease in both sheep and cattle. The virtual eradication of bovine tuberculosis has in recent years given a fresh impetus towards evaluating the efficiency of this test. At the present time its greatest usefulness is in confirming clinically suspect cases of Johne's disease (accuracy about 90%) which give positive reactions, even in the early phase. Under field conditions, however, some months may elapse between the establishment of infection and the appearance of detectable antibodies. The degree of specificity of the test in non-clinically affected animals and in animals with tuberculosis is rather low (25%) and it gives a considerable proportion of false positive results in normal animals. A number of countries throughout the world allow the importation of cattle only on the basis of a negative complement-fixation test in respect of Johne's disease.

Although the virus responsible for enzootic

abortion in ewes has common antigens with other viruses of the psittacosis–lymphogranuloma group, fixation of complement by the serum of an ewe which has aborted, in conjunction with a history of the disease in the flock, may be regarded as being diagnostically significant. Retrospective diagnosis of canine infectious hepatitis, or canine distemper, can be established by means of the complement fixation test.

Precipitin Test

The principle of this test is somewhat similar to that of the agglutination test except that the reaction occurs at the interface between soluble antibody, in the form of globulin and a prepared soluble extract of the antigen. The precipitation reaction may occur at room temperature but, in some cases, is hastened by exposure to temperatures from 37°C to 55°C (98·8–131°F). The test can be done as a gel diffusion test (immuno-diffusion) using small wells cut in an agar gel or in small tubes.

The tube precipitin test has had its greatest application in the classification of streptococci. More recently agar gel diffusion tests are extensively used in the study and diagnosis of many virus diseases, e.g. rinderpest, mucosal disease, swine fever. This type of test can be adopted to detect either antigen or antibody. A positive result takes the form of a white line of precipitation at the interface between antigen and antibody.

Haemagglutination Tests

These tests are not dependent on the formation of an antigen–antibody complex. Many viruses, when mixed with washed chicken erythrocytes, cause them to agglutinate. Homologous virus antibody will prevent the appearance of this phenomenon. In performing the test a standard suspension of erythrocytes is mixed with virus in a tube which is then allowed to stand for a few hours. If the red cells remain unagglutinated they sediment and collect as a mass in the bottom of the tube; when aggregated the cells form a thin film over the whole bottom of the tube. The method of the test can be adopted for the detection of either virus or antibody (haemagglutination inhibition test), the latter usually appears in the blood of affected animals and birds within a few days after the development of clinical signs of disease and has reached a high titre within a few weeks. Other factors apart from virus anti-body are known to inhibit haemagglutination; for myxoviruses these factors can be removed by treatment with trypsin and for arboviruses by extraction with acetone.

Virus neutralization Test

This type of serological test is only applicable in those instances in which homologous virus antibody is produced by the animal following infection. In this form the test is of retrospective value in diagnosis although it may be used for virus identification at an earlier stage. Because viruses will only grow in living cells the employment of this type of test depends upon the availability of suitable tissue cell cultures, chick embryos or a susceptible laboratory animal. A number of viruses are capable of causing microscopic cytopathogenic lesions in some of the cells in tissue cultures and/or in chick embryos. Adding homologous antibody to the virus in an appropriate amount by serially diluting the latter will prevent virus multiplication when it is introduced into susceptible cells. By this means the presence of homologous virus antibody is indicated when cytopathogenic lesions fail to develop.

Viruses which can be recognized by this means include those causing louping-ill, viral encephalomyelitis of pigs, pseudorabies (Aujeszky's disease), equine encephalomyelitis, infectious bovine rhinotracheitis, swine influenza, African horse sickness, etc.

Toxin Neutralization Test

The principle of this test is the detection of specific toxin in the tissues or intestinal contents of animals by means of injecting a filtrate of the unknown material together with one of a series of purified antitoxins into laboratory animals of a suitable species. Conversely antitoxin can be identified in the sera of recovered animals following initial titration with a range of known toxins. Diseases which can be recognized by this method include lamb dysentery, pulpy kidney, ovine enterotoxaemia, infectious necrotic hepatitis, tetanus, malignant oedema and ulcerative lymphangitis.

Immunofluorescence

The technique of labelling either antibodies or antigen with certain chemicals which possess the inherent property of fluorescing is of fairly recent development. That conjugation has occurred between specific labelled globulin and antigen can only be determined by means of special microscopes which have been developed for use with ultraviolet illumination. Because such microscopes are expensive to purchase the application of immunofluorescent methods in diagnosis is not in general use. It is, however, useful to have some knowledge of the capabilities of immunofluorescence in diagnosis, and of the type and nature of the materials that can be submitted to laboratories prepared to perform the examination.

In the labelling process fluorescein is generally used (it gives visible light of an apple-green colour) and because it is the antibodies which are most commonly labelled, the application of the method is described as the *fluorescent antibody* technique. The basic principle involved in the procedure is that microconjugation occurs on the microscope slide between the known labelled antibody and the specific pathogen, when the latter is present in even very small numbers, and either living or dead. Conversely by employing a known labelled antigen it is possible to determine whether an unknown serum contains any specific antibody. In addition to the direct methods as described in which one of the primary

reactants is labelled, a sandwich or indirect method may be employed, in which a labelled antiglobulin is used. This latter method is more versatile than the direct method.

Applications. By means of prepared smears the direct method can be employed for the rapid identification of specific pathogens while awaiting the results of traditional bacteriological techniques. By the use of specific labelled sera various species of clostridial organisms can be identified so that diseases such as lamb dysentery, pulpy kidney disease, enterotoxaemia, infectious necrotic hepatitis, tetanus, blackleg, etc. may be rapidly diagnosed. Other conditions which can be diagnosed in this way include listeriosis and rabies.

The indirect or sandwich technique can be used in the diagnosis of the same conditions as the direct test. Because of its greater range of application it is particularly valuable in detecting the presence of infectious canine hepatitis virus and *Toxoplasma gondii* in impression smears made from appropriate material. Only the indirect test is capable of detecting antibody instead of antigen. By this method the presence in sera of antibody to *Babesia bigemina* can be demonstrated.

Index